NURSING 3SS3

TABLE OF CONTENTS & ACKNOWLEDGEMENTS

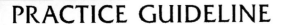

PRACTICE GUIDELINE

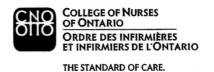

COLLEGE OF NURSES OF ONTARIO
ORDRE DES INFIRMIÈRES ET INFIRMIERS DE L'ONTARIO
THE STANDARD OF CARE.

RN and RPN Practice: The Client, the Nurse and the Environment

Table of Contents

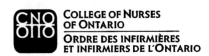

COLLEGE OF NURSES
OF ONTARIO
ORDRE DES INFIRMIÈRES
ET INFIRMIERS DE L'ONTARIO

THE STANDARD OF CARE.

VISION
Leading in regulatory excellence

MISSION
Regulating nursing in the public interest

RN and RPN practice: The Client, the Nurse and the Environment   Pub. No. 41062

ISBN 978-1-77116-100-8

Copyright © College of Nurses of Ontario, 2018.

First Published June 1996 as *A Guide to Health Care Consent and Substitute Decisions Legislation for RNs and RPNs*
Replaces Publication Published 1997, *Determining Appropriate Category of Care Provider*
First Published July 2002 as *Practice Expectations: A Guide for the Utilization of RNs and RPNs*, Reprinted December 2002,
Revised for Web June 2003, Reprinted January 2004, December 2005, May 2008. Updated June 2009.Revised Dec 2011 as *RN and RPN Practice: The Client, the Nurse and the Environment*, this document replaces *Utilization of RNs and RPNs*. Revised 2014 for Dispensing (ISBN 978-1-77116-013-1). *Revised January 2018 for Controlled Act of Psychotherapy.*

Additional copies of this booklet may be obtained by contacting CNO's Customer Service Centre at 416 928-0900 or toll-free in Canada at 1 800 387-5526.

College of Nurses of Ontario
101 Davenport Rd.
Toronto ON M5R 3P1

www.cno.org

Ce fascicule existe en français sous le titre : *L'exercice de l'IA et de l'IAA : l'infirmière, le client et l'environnement*, n° 51062

Practice guidelines are documents that help nurses understand their responsibilities and legal obligations to enable them to make safe and ethical decisions when practising. They provide an outline of professional accountabilities and relevant legislation.
— College of Nurses of Ontario

Introduction

Nursing is a profession that is focused on collaborative relationships that promote the best possible outcomes for **clients**. These relationships may be **interprofessional**, involving a variety of health care professionals working together to deliver quality care within and across settings; or it may be **intraprofessional**, with multiple members of the same profession working collaboratively to deliver quality care within and across settings.

This document focuses on three factors — the client, the nurse and the environment — to support nurses in making decisions that are specific to their intraprofessional responsibilities when providing client care.

These three factors have an impact on decision-making related to care-provider assignment (which nursing category (Registered Nurse [RN] or Registered Practical Nurse [RPN]) to match with client needs), as well as the need for consultation and collaboration among care providers.

Many of the concepts in this document apply to all nurses; however, references to nurses or intraprofessional care in this document refer only to RNs and RPNs — Nurse Practitioners are not included in this document because the complexity of client care does not define their involvement in care.

This document replaces the *Utilization of RNs and RPNs* practice guideline.

Purpose

The purpose of this document is to:
- help nurses, employers and others make effective

decisions about the utilization[1] of individual nurses in the provision of safe and ethical care
- outline expectations for nurses within the three-factor framework, highlighting the similarities and differences of foundational nursing knowledge and its impact on **autonomous practice**[2]
- highlight nurses' accountabilities when collaborating with one another
- identify attributes of practice environments that facilitate nursing assignments, enhance **collaboration** and lead to improved client outcomes and public protection.

Guiding Principles

The following principles guide nurses' practice expectations and are the basis for decision-making when working within the intraprofessional team:
- The goal of professional practice is to obtain the best possible outcome for clients.
- RNs and RPNs study from the same body of nursing knowledge. RNs study for a longer period of time, allowing for greater foundational knowledge in clinical practice, **decision-making**, critical thinking, **leadership**, research utilization and resource management. As a result of these differences, the level of autonomous practice of RNs differs from that of RPNs.
- The complexity of a client's condition influences the nursing knowledge required to provide the level of care the client needs. A more complex client situation and less stable environment create an increased need for consultation and/or the need for an RN to provide the full range of care requirements.
- Respecting and understanding the expectations and contributions of the **health care team** facilitates appropriate utilization of nurses, enhances collaboration and leads to improved client outcomes.

Legal Scope Of Practice

The *Regulated Health Professions Act, 1991* (RHPA) and the *Nursing Act, 1991* provide

---

[1] For the purpose of this document, utilization refers to determining the appropriateness of assigning client care to nurses, and of nurses accepting responsibility for client care.

[2] **Bolded** words are defined in the glossary on page 14.

the legislative framework for nursing practice. Components of the legislative framework are a scope of practice statement and a list of controlled acts authorized to nursing.

Controlled acts are activities that are considered to be potentially harmful if they are performed by unqualified persons. A profession's legal scope of practice is determined by its scope of practice statement and the controlled acts it has the authority to perform.

Members of regulated health professions are authorized to perform specific controlled acts appropriate to their profession's scope of practice. Having the authority to perform a procedure does not necessarily mean that the individual is competent or that it is appropriate for the individual to perform the procedure.

i. Nursing's Scope of Practice Statement

The scope of practice statement describes in a general way what the profession does and the methods that it uses; it refers to the profession as a whole, rather than what any individual can do.

The scope of practice statement for nursing states:

The practice of nursing is the promotion of health and the assessment of, the provision of, care for, and the treatment of, health conditions by supportive, preventive, therapeutic, palliative and rehabilitative means in order to attain or maintain optimal function.

Practice is so broad and varied that no one nurse is expected to be competent to carry out all the activities within the legal scope of practice; hence, the notion of "full scope of practice" is unlikely.

ii. Controlled Acts Authorized to Nurses

The *Nursing Act, 1991* authorizes nurses to perform the following controlled acts:
- performing a prescribed procedure below the dermis or mucous membrane
- administering a substance by injection or inhalation
- putting an instrument, hand or finger:
  - beyond the external ear canal

- beyond the point in the nasal passages where they normally narrow
- beyond the larynx
- beyond the opening of the urethra
- beyond the labia majora
- beyond the anal verge, or
- into an artificial opening in the body.
- dispensing a drug
- treating, by means of psychotherapy technique, delivered through a therapeutic relationship, an individual's serious disorder of thought, cognition, mood, emotional regulation, perception or memory that may seriously impair the individual's judgement, insight, behaviour, communication or social functioning.

There are differences between RNs and RPNs' authority to initiate controlled acts. Initiation refers to independently deciding that a specific procedure within a controlled act is required, and performing that procedure in the absence of an order. For more information, refer to the *Decisions About Procedures and Authority,* practice document at **www.cno.org/docs**.

Nurses' Accountability

Nurses show accountability by taking responsibility for their decisions and actions, taking appropriate action when needed and ensuring that practice is consistent with entry-to-practice **competencies**, standards of practice, guidelines and legislation.

Nurses are expected to consult with others when any situation is beyond their **competence**. A nurse is not accountable for the actions and decisions of other care providers when the nurse has no way of knowing of those actions.

The nurse is accountable for:
- her or his actions and decisions
- knowing and understanding the roles and responsibilities of other team members, and collaborating, consulting and taking action on client information when needed
- taking action to ensure client safety, including informing the employer of concerns related to the conduct and/or actions of other care providers, and

- collaborating with clients, with each other and with members of the interprofessional care team for the benefit of the client.

The designated nursing authority (which is the nurse with the highest level of authority for nursing in the practice environment) is accountable for ensuring there are mechanisms in place such as policies, procedures, guidelines and other resources to support the following:
- utilization decisions that take into account client, nurse and environment factors, and that are evidence-based
- nurse collaboration and consultation
- clear and well-understood role descriptions
- professional nursing practice, and
- continuity of client care.

The Three-Factor Framework

Making effective decisions about which nursing category (RN or RPN) to match with client needs involves considering three factors of equal importance: the client, the nurse and the environment, and deliberating on how they apply to the situation.

Client factors

Decisions about the utilization of an RN and an RPN are influenced by:

1. Complexity:
- the degree to which a client's condition and care requirements are identifiable and established
- the sum of the variables influencing a client's current health status, and
- the variability of a client's condition or care requirements.

2. Predictability:
- the extent to which a client's outcomes and future care requirements can be anticipated.

3. Risk of negative outcomes:
- the likelihood that a client will experience a negative outcome as a result of the client's health condition or as a response to treatment.

Client continuum

The three client factors described above combine to create a representation of the client that can be placed on a continuum. The continuum goes from less complex, more predictable and low risk for negative outcomes, to highly complex, unpredictable and high risk for negative outcomes. (See chart below.)

All nurses can autonomously care for clients who have been identified as less complex, more predictable and at low risk of negative outcomes. The more complex the care requirements, the greater the need for consultation and/or the need for an RN to provide the full spectrum of care.

Client Continuum

Less complex, more predictable, low risk for negative outcome(s)

Highly complex, unpredictable, high risk for negative outcome(s)

Autonomous RPN or RN practice

RN PRACTICE

Increasing need for RN consultation and collaboration

Client Factors	Autonomous RN or RPN Practice	RN Involved or Providing Care
Complexity (includes bio-psycho-social, cultural, emotional and health learning needs)	• care needs well defined and established • coping mechanisms and support systems in place and effective • health condition well controlled or managed • little fluctuation in health condition over time few factors influencing the client's health • client is an individual, family, group or community	• care needs not well defined/ established or changing • coping mechanisms and supports unknown, not functioning or not in place • health condition not well controlled or managed • requires close, frequent monitoring and reassessment • fluctuating health condition many factors influencing the client's health • client is an individual, family, group, community or population
Predictability	• predictable outcomes • predictable changes in health condition	• unpredictable outcomes • unpredictable changes in health condition
Risk of negative outcomes	• predictable, localized and manageable responses • signs and symptoms are obvious • low risk of negative outcomes	• unpredictable, systemic or wide-ranging responses • signs and symptoms subtle and difficult to detect • high risk of negative outcomes

Nurse factors

The factors that affect a nurse's ability to provide safe and ethical care to a given client include leadership, decision-making and critical-thinking skills. Other factors include the **application of knowledge**, knowing when and how to apply knowledge, and having the resources available to consult as needed.

It is important for nurses to be aware of the limits of their individual competence and their practice. Based on individual practice reflection and the current requirements of their practice environments, nurses must continually enhance their knowledge and competence through ongoing learning, education, experience and participation in quality assurance activities. Nurses can become experts in an area of practice within their own nursing category; however, enhanced competence through continuing education and experience does not mean that an RPN will acquire the same foundational competencies as an RN. This will only occur through the formal education and credentialing process.

Nurses consult with one another when a situation demands nursing expertise that is beyond their competence. Consultation involves seeking advice or information from a more experienced or knowledgeable nurse or other health care professional. The amount of consultation required is determined by the complexity of client care needs and the nurse's competence. The practice setting influences the availability and accessibility of these consultation resources.

An important aspect of efficient consultation is providing nurses with the time and resources needed to consult as often as is necessary to meet client needs.

Nurses also need to clarify their reasons for consulting and determine an appropriate course of action. Unless care is transferred, the nurse who sought consultation is still accountable for the client's care.

Consultation results in one of the following:
a) the nurse receiving advice and continuing to care for the client
b) the nurse transferring an aspect of care to the consultant
c) the nurse transferring all care to the consultant.

When any care is transferred from one nurse to another, the accountability for that care is also transferred.

When a care provider assignment involves the expectation of consultation, nurses must assess that the required consultative supports are available. When supports are inadequate to meet client needs and ensure quality care, nurses must take appropriate action.

Whenever the need for consultation exceeds the efficient delivery of care, it is most likely that the client requires an RN to provide all care.

Nurse Factors	RPN	RN
Client	• Individuals, families and groups and communities	• Individuals, families, groups, communities and populations
Direct practice assessment	• recognizes changes, probes further and manages or consults appropriately with RN or other health care team member	• anticipates and recognizes subtle changes, probes to assess further, identifies relevant factors, understands significance and manages appropriately
Direct practice decision-making	• transfers knowledge from similar situations through pattern recognition • makes decisions based on the analysis of available information • makes decisions by accessing a known range of options to solve problems	• analyzes and synthesizes a wide range of information using a variety of frameworks or theories • makes decisions after actively seeking information • makes decisions by drawing on a comprehensive range of options to interpret, analyze and solve problems • anticipates many possibilities and makes proactive decisions
Direct practice planning	• develops plans of care to achieve identified client goals when overall care needs are less complex, outcomes are predictable and risk of negative outcomes is low	• plans broadly and over a longer time period, incorporating a variety of options and resources
Direct practice care coordination	• coordinates care for less-complex clients	• coordinates care for complex clients

Nurse Factors	RPN	RN
Direct practice implementation	• meets identified nursing care needs of less-complex clients with predictable outcomes, including health teaching • meets current identified client care needs using a systematic framework for providing care (e.g., nursing process or theory) • selects from a known range of options • performs nursing interventions for which she/he can manage the client during and after the intervention or has access to resources • works in consultation with RNs and others to meet care needs of more complex clients • provides elements of care for highly complex clients when in close consultation with the RN directing that client's care	• meets a wide range of nursing care needs of clients regardless of complexity and predictability, including health teaching • meets immediate and anticipated long-term client needs, drawing from a comprehensive assessment and range of options • selects from a wide range of options • manages multiple nursing interventions simultaneously in rapidly changing situations • directs plans of care for highly complex clients
Direct practice evaluation	• collaborates with client to evaluate overall goal achievement and modifies plans of care for less-complex clients • identifies expected outcomes of specific interventions and modifies plan of care in collaboration with client • recognizes deviations from predicted client response(s) and consults appropriately	• collaborates with client to evaluate overall goal achievement and modifies plan of care • identifies and anticipates a multiplicity of outcomes and modifies plan of care in collaboration with client • recognizes, analyzes and interprets deviations from predicted client response(s); modifies plan of care autonomously
Direct practice consultation	• consults with RNs and other health care team members about identified client needs	• consults with other health care team members about a broad range of client needs • acts as a resource for RPNs to meet client needs
Direct practice (other)	• delivers elements of established health programs	• designs, coordinates and implements health programs

Nurse Factors	RPN	RN
Leadership	• represents nursing and nursing care issues (e.g., participates in committees, workgroups, union/ regulatory activities) • acts as a preceptor to students and novice nurses • directs unregulated care providers, as appropriate • Provides leadership through formal and informal roles	• assumes role of leader within interprofessional team • provides leadership through formal and informal roles • acts as a preceptor to students and novice nurses • directs unregulated care providers, as appropriate • leads team effort to develop plans of care to achieve identified client goals when overall care requirements are more complex
Resource management	• contributes to appropriate resource utilization	• makes decisions about and allocates resources at program/ unit/organizational level
Research	• participates in data collection for research • uses research to inform practice (e.g., practice guidelines)	• critically evaluates theoretical and research-based approaches for application to practice • appraises the value of evidence, incorporates research into practice, develops research questions and participates on research teams • integrates theoretical and research-based approaches to design care and implement change

Environment factors

Environment factors include practice supports, consultation resources and the stability/ predictability of the environment. Practice supports and consultation resources support nurses in clinical decision-making.

The less stable these factors are, the greater the need for RN staffing. The less available the practice supports and consultation resources are, the greater the need for more in-depth nursing competencies and skills in the areas of clinical practice, decision-making, critical thinking, leadership, research utilization and resource management.

Environment Continuum

More stable environment — Less stable environment

Autonomous RPN or RN practice — RN Practice

Increasing need for RN consultation and collaboration

Environment Factors	More Stable	Less Stable
Practice supports	• clear and identified procedures, policies, medical directives, protocols, plans of care, care pathways and assessment tools • high proportion of expert nurses or low proportion of novice nurses • high proportion of nurses familiar with the environment	• unclear or unidentified procedures, policies, medical directives, protocols, plans of care, care pathways and assessment tools • low proportion of expert nurses or high proportion of novice nurses and unregulated staff • low proportion of nurses familiar with the environment
Consultation resources	• many consultation resources available to manage outcomes	• few consultation resources available to manage outcomes
Stability and predictability of the environment	• low rate of client turnover • few unpredictable events	• high rate of client turnover • many unpredictable events

Conclusion

The more complex the client situation and the more dynamic the environment, the greater the need for the RN to provide the full range of care, assess changes, reestablish priorities and determine the need for additional resources. The technical and cognitive aspects of nursing practice cannot be separated. Decisions about utilizing an RN or RPN are made after considering client care requirements and the nurse's cognitive and technical expertise in a given environment. By considering the client, nurse and environment factors, nurses and key stakeholders can determine which category of nursing is appropriate for specific roles in client care. The application of the three-factor framework will help decision-makers determine which roles and activities are not appropriate for autonomous RPN practice. Examples include, but are not limited to, the following:

• triage nurse
• circulating nurse
• administering conscious sedation or monitoring sedated clients (includes deep sedation and general anaesthesia).

Appendix

Quality Practice Settings

A quality practice setting is a workplace that supports nursing practice, fosters professional development and promotes the delivery of quality care. As partners in the effort to achieve quality care, nurses and employers have a shared responsibility to create practice environments that support competent nurses in providing quality outcomes for clients. To create quality practice settings that support effective utilization of nurses, the College encourages employers and nurses to consider incorporating the following strategies.

Care delivery processes

These factors support the delivery of nursing care/services and include the care/program delivery model, staffing ratios and staffing mix, standards of care, accountability and ongoing quality improvement measures. There is a growing body of research about the link between staff mix and nursing-sensitive client outcomes. This research points to the need for decision-makers to consider the appropriate utilization of RNs and RPNs in the practice setting. An appropriate mix is key to providing quality care.

Possible strategies include:
- an evidence-based nursing care delivery model that takes into consideration relevant best practices, client complexity and the practice expectations for the typical nurse, and facilitates quality nursing practices
- considering client complexity, staffing mix and ratios, and the nurses' roles in coordinating resources when addressing staffing issues
- clear accountability to ensure support for nurses who report gaps between their individual competencies (practice limitations) and practice expectations
- a continual quality improvement process, led by nurses in collaboration with other members of the team, to facilitate regular review of nursing roles and expectations.

Communication systems

These systems support the sharing of information and decisions about client care and services. Factors affecting the quality of communication systems include communication with clients and families, professional communications, information systems and technology, communication within and between programs, and conflict resolution mechanisms.

Possible strategies include:
- developing mechanisms ensuring that major changes to nursing roles and practice expectations are communicated in a timely manner
- engaging nurses in discussions regarding current or changing roles and practice expectations within the organization
- creating communication systems that promote and support the exchange of information between RN or RPNs and the health care team to facilitate the delivery of quality client care.

Leadership

Leadership occurs at all levels within an organization. It is the process of supporting others to improve client care and services by promoting professional practice. Effective leadership is demonstrated by staff participation in decision-making, the philosophy of the organization and the style of individual leaders within the organization.

Possible strategies include:
- developing a nursing governance structure to address all nursing practice issues
- providing opportunities for nurses to enhance their individual leadership skills within a defined role
- creating mechanisms to help nurses manage professional role conflict effectively, as it arises, on a one-to-one and collective basis.

Organizational supports

Organizations support the delivery of client care, services and programs through their policies, procedures, norms and values. Organizational supports include the organization's philosophy, policies and procedures, health and safety requirements, and recruitment and retention strategies.

Possible strategies include:
- having mission, value and philosophy statements that support and recognize the need for interprofessional and intraprofessional collaborative practice
- having a collaborative practice model within the organization that guides professional practice expectations
- developing evidence-based policies and/or guidelines that outline:
  - role expectations, limitations and responsibilities of nurses
  - accountabilities of all health care team members associated with collaborative professional practice
  - circumstances requiring nurses to consult and collaborate with other members of the health care team
  - situations that threaten client safety
- collaborative decisions and actions taken to ensure client safety; examine the appropriateness of those decisions given the professional practice model, the College's standards and the agency-specific practice expectations.

Professional development systems

The way in which staff members are hired, oriented and encouraged to maintain competence affects the care they provide. Professional development systems include an orientation program, preceptorship, promotion of continuing education and professional quality assurance, training, promoting a learning environment, performance management process and professional practice activities.

Possible strategies include:
- orientation for new staff members that includes information about roles and practice expectations
- access to preceptors or mentors
- ongoing educational opportunities designed to reinforce the principles and decision-making factors associated with demands of a changing environment.

Response systems to external demands

Nurses' ability to provide care is affected by the time in which an organization responds to changes in legislation, consumer demands and health care trends. The indicators include responses to legislated and regulatory requirements, client and community relations, accreditation, and health and safety requirements.

Possible strategies include:
- establishing mechanisms to address changes in legislation and regulations that influence the roles of nurses (such as, the *Regulated Health Professions Act, 1991*).

Facilities and equipment

The physical environment and access to equipment can support and increase the efficiency and effectiveness of client care, services and programs. Indicators of a supportive physical environment include availability of equipment and supplies that meet client needs, reliability of equipment and regular maintenance of equipment.

Possible strategies include:
- having sufficient access to equipment to support professional practice
- involving nurses in facility improvement planning
- involving nurses in equipment selection.

Glossary

Application of knowledge. The use of knowledge in practice. It includes assessment, planning, implementation, evaluation of outcomes and application of research. Application of knowledge encompasses decision-making and leadership.

Autonomous practice. The ability to carry out nursing responsibilities independently.

Client. The client is the person or persons with whom the nurse is engaged in a professional therapeutic relationship. The client may include family members of and/or substitute decision-makers for the individual client. The client may also be a family, group, community or **population**.

Collaboration. Working together with one or more members of the health care team, each of whom makes a unique contribution toward achieving a common goal. Collaboration is an ongoing process that requires effective communication between the members of the health care team and a clear understanding of the roles of the individuals involved in the collaboration process. Nurses collaborate with clients, other nurses and other members of the health care team in the interest of client care.

Community. A group of people living in one place, neighbourhood or district, or sharing common characteristics or interests, or having common health needs. Nursing practice aimed at the community involves helping communities identify, articulate and successfully manage their health concerns. It is concerned primarily with care that is continuing, rather than episodic. When client care is mentioned in the context of the community, it does not mean providing care to an individual in the community — the focus is on the collective or common good, instead of on an individual's health.

Competence. A nurse's ability to integrate the professional attributes required to perform in a given role, situation or practice setting. Professional attributes include, but are not limited to, knowledge, skill, judgment, attitudes, values and beliefs.

Competencies. Statements describing the expected performance or behaviour that reflects the professional attributes required in a given nursing role, situation or practice setting.

Decision-making. The ability to draw on many modes of thinking in order to select a course of action. It involves understanding and anticipating risks, benefits and outcomes beyond what is obvious, and creating a proactive plan of action based on this analysis. Critical thinking is an important component of effective decision-making.

Group. People who interact and share a common purpose(s). There is no clear distinction between a group and a community except that groups tend to have fewer members than communities. The methods used to plan and provide programs or activities for groups and communities are similar except for scale.

Health care team. An interprofessional group of individuals who are either directly or indirectly involved in a client's care. Depending on the practice environment, the composition of the team will vary. The team includes the client and the family.

Interprofessional care. The provision of comprehensive health services to clients by multiple health caregivers who work collaboratively to deliver quality care within and across settings.

Intraprofessional care. The provision of comprehensive health care services to clients by multiple members of the same profession who work collaboratively to deliver quality care within and across settings.

Leadership. In nursing, leadership includes the ability to facilitate client groups, develop plans of care, teach others, work in teams, lead teams, influence the work environment and advocate for or bring about change. All nurses have the opportunity to develop leadership skills throughout their career.

Population. A collection of individuals who have one or more personal or environmental characteristics in common.

Predictable outcomes. Client health outcomes that can reasonably be expected to follow an anticipated path with respect to timing and nature.

Unpredictable outcomes. Client health outcomes that cannot reasonably be expected to follow an anticipated path with respect to timing and nature.

References

Association of Registered Nurses of Newfoundland/ Council for Licensed Practical Nurses of Newfoundland. (2008). *Collaborative nursing practice-guiding principles.* Retrieved from http:// www.arnnl.ca

Nursing Association of New Brunswick. (2009). *Working Together: A Framework for the Registered Nurse and Licensed Practical Nurse:* Retrieved from http://www.nanb.nb.ca

Canadian Nurses Association. (2005). Nursing staff mix: *A key link to patient safety. Nursing Now:* Issues and Trends in Canadian Nursing, 19, 1-6.

Canadian Nurses Association. (2005). *Evaluation framework to determine the impact of nursing staff mix decisions.* Retrieved from http://www.cna-aiic.ca

The Community Health Nurses Association of Canada. (2008). *Canadian Community Health Nursing Standards of Practice.* Retrieved from http://www.chnc.ca *Canadian Community Health Nursing Standards of Practice* pg. 16

College of Licensed Practical Nurses of British Columbia/College of Registered Nurses of British Columbia. (2008). *RNs and LPNs Working Together for Client Safety.* Burnaby, BC: Author.

College of Nurses of Ontario. (2011). *Entry-to-Practice Competencies for Ontario Registered Practical Nurses.* Toronto, ON: Author.

College of Nurses of Ontario. (2009). *National Competencies in the Context of Entry-Level Registered Nurse Practice.* Toronto, ON: Author.

Health Force Ontario (2007). Interprofessional Care: A Blueprint for Action in Ontario. Retrieved July 14, 2009, from www. healthforceontario.ca.

Kenney, P. (2001). Maintaining quality care during a nursing shortage using licensed practical nurses in acute care. *Journal of Nursing Care Quality,* 15(4), pp. 60–68.

Lamond, D. & Thompson, C. (2000). Intuition and analysis in decision-making and choice. *Journal of Nursing Scholarship,* 33(2), pp. 411–414.

LeClerc, C.M., Doyon, J., Gravelle, D., Hall, B. & Roussel, J. (2008). The autonomous-collaborative care model: Meeting the future head on. *Nursing Leadership,* 21(2).

Licensed Practical Nurses Association of Prince Edward Island/The Association of Registered Nurses of Prince Edward Island/PEI Health Sector Council. (2009). *Exemplary Care: Registered Nurses and Licensed Practical Nurses Working Together.* Retrieved from www.peihsc.ca

Royle, J., Dicenso, A., Boblin-Cummings, B., Blythe, J. & Mallette, C. (2000). RN and RPN decision-making across settings. *Canadian Journal of Nursing Leadership,* 13(4), pp. 11–18.

(Stanhope & Lancaster, 2002, p. 24) taken from *Canadian Community Health Nursing Standards of Practice* pg. 17 http://www.chnc.ca/documents/ chn_standards_of_practice_mar08_english.pdf

Notes:

Notes:

Sphere of Nursing Advocacy Model

Robert G. Hanks, RNC, BSN, MSN, FNP-C

The Sphere of Nursing Advocacy (SNA) model explains and depicts nursing advocacy on behalf of a client. The SNA model views the client as continually protected from the external environment by a semipermeable sphere of nursing advocacy that allows clients to self advocate if the client is emotionally and physically able or to be advocated for by the nurse if the patient is unable to advocate for him- or herself. The SNA model can be used to guide research or it can provide the basis for instruction on the subject of nursing advocacy.

Search terms: *Nursing, patient advocacy*

Robert G. Hanks, RNC, BSN, MSN, FNP-C, is an instructor at the University of Texas Medical Branch, School of Nursing, Galveston, Texas.

Introduction

Advocacy for clients is an important aspect in current professional nursing care and is considered to be a fundamental value of professional nursing by several nursing scholars. Nursing has not always practiced advocacy; rather, advocacy is a relatively new role for nursing, emerging in the United States in the 1980s (Hamric, 2000).

For the purposes of this article, the basis of nursing advocacy is formulated from the philosophical work of Curtin (1979), Gadow (1980), and Kohnke (1982). These authors provide definitions and models that have shaped current nursing advocacy. Curtin bases her philosophy of nursing advocacy on the belief that the humanity of each individual comes forth from human needs. The nurse, according to Curtin, provides a supportive atmosphere for the client's decision-making process, which is the basis of all other nursing activities. As human advocates, nurses assist clients to discover the significance of their life processes (Curtin, 1979).

Gadow (1980) has a similar philosophy of nursing advocacy, which she calls existential advocacy. Gadow describes existential advocacy as the nurse's assistance to clients in exercising the client's right of self-determination, utilizing judgments that realize the complexity of the client's values. She argues that only the client can decide what is in his or her own best interest, and that the nurse is entirely engaged in assisting the client in this process.

Gadow (1989) also has explored advocacy for the vulnerable client, concluding that nurses have a moral commitment in regards to enhancing a patient's autonomy. She believes that nurses are in a unique position to assist the vulnerable client through advocacy and that nurses need to be able to understand the patient's needs and speak for the patient.

Kohnke (1982) views the role of nurse advocate as having two functions: that of an informer to the client and as a supporter of the client's decision. Both functions of nurse advocacy carry the risk of alienating the nurse advocate in regards to other healthcare professionals (Kohnke). Kohnke reveals that for a nurse to be proficient as a nurse advocate, the nurse must have an adequate knowledge base in areas such as ethics, social law, and politics.

Development of the Model

The Sphere of Nursing Advocacy (SNA) model was developed using a grounded-theory approach in which three case studies from the author's acute-care experiences were analyzed. Analysis of the three cases resulted in common themes that in turn led to delineation of the concept of the SNA and the assumptions and propositions of the SNA model.

Assumptions

The resounding theme of the assumptions is nursing advocacy for the client (Table 1).

Clients have the need for advocacy when the client is unable to advocate for him- or herself and nurses need to provide this advocacy. Nurses should not let prejudices interfere with advocacy or doubt their own

Table 1. Assumptions of Sphere of Nursing Advocacy Model

Clients need advocacy when they are unable to advocate for themselves.
Nurses need to advocate for clients.
Nurses should not doubt their actions when advocating for clients.
Nurses should not allow prejudices to interfere with advocating for clients.
Nurses should allow clients to self advocate when clients are able to do so.
Nurses should provide a sphere of advocacy for the client.

actions when advocating for clients. By providing a protective barrier of advocacy for their clients, nurses are surrounding their clients in a sphere of advocacy.

Propositions

The propositions of the SNA model were formulated after analysis of the case studies and the resulting assumptions (Table 2). These propositions provide a verbal depiction of the schematic diagram (Figure 1). The nurse provides a semipermeable sphere of advocacy between the client and the client's environment, allowing the client to freely self advocate through the pores of the sphere. The SNA model also provides a protective

Table 2. Propositions From the Sphere of Nursing Advocacy Model

Nursing advocacy provides a protective shield for the client in vulnerable situations where the client may have varying degrees of belief in his/her own ability to self advocate within the external environment/circumstances.

Nurses provide a semipermeable sphere of advocacy between their client and the client's external environment, allowing for protection of the client yet allowing the client to self advocate.

The client and the nurse can be simultaneously acting as advocates: the nurse may be advocating on the client's behalf, and the client may be self advocating through the open areas of the nurse's sphere of advocacy called pores.

If the nurse provides a protective shield of advocacy for the client, then the client is protected from the external environment.

If the client is able to self advocate, then the client will be able to work through the pores in the nurse's sphere of advocacy to interact with the external environment regardless of setting.

Figure 1. Sphere of Nursing Advocacy Model

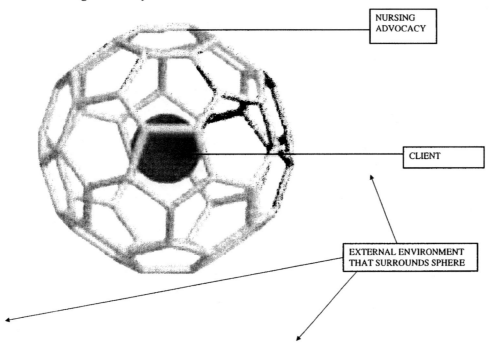

NURSING ADVOCACY

CLIENT

EXTERNAL ENVIRONMENT THAT SURROUNDS SPHERE

shield for the client in vulnerable situations when the client is not able to self advocate. The client and the nurse can be simultaneously acting as advocates on the client's behalf; that is, the client is advocating for self through the pores and the nurse is providing the protective sphere of advocacy at the same time.

Related Nursing Theory

The concept of nursing advocacy providing a protection for the client from the external environment is depicted by the SNA model. This is reflective of Florence Nightingale's concept of physical and emotional environmental manipulation for the betterment of client outcomes (Pfettscher, 2002). Nightingale (1970) also wrote of modifying the client's emotional environment by providing hope and caring for the

client. By advocating for clients, nurses are providing a modified barrier between the client and the client's external environment that is a modification of the client's emotional environment.

Betty Neuman's Systems model utilizes broken lines around a core structure that are lines of resistance and flexible lines of defense that assist a client when challenged with a stressor (Freese, 2002). Although the SNA model has similar pores, Neuman's structure is related to resource factors and the ability to resist a stressor, not advocacy (Freese, 2002).

Utilization

The SNA model can be used in the practice setting to visually depict the concept of advocacy for clients on the part of the practicing nurse. This model also

23

could be utilized in the educational setting as a model to teach student nurses about client decision making and client advocacy.

Further Development

The SNA model provides a basis for inquiry into nurses' perceptions of client advocacy and the meaning of client advocacy to the nurse providing the advocacy. The model can also be used as a source for inquiry into the client's perception of nursing advocacy and the meaning of the advocacy provided by nurses for the client.

Author contact: rghanks@utmb.edu, with a copy to the Editor: cooperconsulting@socal.rr.com

References

Curtin, L. (1979). The nurse as advocate: A philosophical foundation for nursing. *Advances in Nursing Science, 1*(3), 1–10.

Freese, B.T. (2002). Betty Neuman systems model. In A.M. Tomey & M.R. Alligood (Eds.), *Nursing theorists and their work* (5th ed., pp. 299–317). St. Louis, MO: Mosby.

Gadow, S. (1980). Existential advocacy: Philosophical foundation of nursing. In S. Spicker & S. Gadow (Eds.), *Nursing: Images and ideals* (pp. 79–101). New York: Springer Publishing Company.

Gadow, S. (1989). Clinical subjectivity advocacy with silent patients. *Nursing Clinics of North America, 24*(2), 535–541.

Hamric, A. (2000). What is happening to advocacy? *Nursing Outlook, 48*(3), 103–104.

Kohnke, M.F. (1982). *Advocacy: Risk and reality.* St. Louis, MO: CV Mosby.

Nightingale, F. (1970). *Notes on nursing.* London: Brandon Systems Press.

Pfettscher, S.A. (2002). Florence Nightingale modern nursing. In A.M. Tomey & M.R. Alligood (Eds.), *Nursing theorists and their work* (5th ed., pp. 65–83). St. Louis, MO: Mosby.

The process of labour and birth involves more than the birth of a newborn. Numerous physiologic and psychological events occur that ultimately result in the birth of a newborn and the creation or expansion of the family.

This chapter describes labour and birth as a process. It addresses initiation of labour, the premonitory signs of labour, including true and false labour, critical factors affecting labour and birth, maternal and fetal response to the labouring process, and the four stages of labour. The chapter also identifies critical factors related to each stage of labour: the "10 P's" of labour.

Initiation of Labour

Labour is a complex, multifaceted interaction between the mother and the fetus. It is a series of processes by which the fetus is expelled from the uterus. It is difficult to determine exactly why labour begins and what initiates it. Although several theories have been proposed to explain the onset and maintenance of labour, none of these have been proved scientifically. It is widely believed that labour is influenced by a combination of factors, including uterine stretch, progesterone withdrawal, increased oxytocin sensitivity, and increased release of prostaglandins.

One theory suggests that labour is initiated by a change in the estrogen-to-progesterone ratio. During the last trimester of pregnancy, estrogen levels increase and progesterone levels decrease. This change leads to an increase in the number of myometrium gap junctions. Gap junctions are proteins that connect cell membranes and facilitate coordination of uterine contractions and myometrial stretching (Cunningham et al., 2010).

Although physiologic evidence for the role of oxytocin in the initiation of labour is inconclusive, the number of oxytocin receptors in the uterus increases at the end of pregnancy. This creates an increased sensitivity to oxytocin. Estrogen, the levels of which are also rising, increases myometrial sensitivity to oxytocin. With the increasing levels of oxytocin in the maternal blood in conjunction with fetal production, initiation of uterine contractions can occur. Oxytocin also aids in stimulating prostaglandin synthesis through receptors in the decidua. Prostaglandins lead to additional contractions, cervical softening, gap junction induction, and myometrial sensitization, thereby leading to a progressive cervical **dilation** (the opening or enlargement of the external cervical os) (Martin & Kennedy, 2009b).

Prostaglandins are produced in the decidua and fetal membranes and have a central role in the initiation of labour. Prostaglandin levels increase late during pregnancy secondary to elevated estrogen levels. Prostaglandins stimulate smooth muscle contraction of the uterus.

An increase in prostaglandins leads to myometrial contractions and a reduction in cervical resistance. Subsequently, the cervix softens, thins out, and dilates during labour.

Premonitory Signs of Labour

Before the onset of labour, a pregnant woman's body undergoes several changes in preparation for the birth of the newborn. The changes that occur often lead to characteristic signs and symptoms that suggest that labour is near. These premonitory signs and symptoms can vary, and not every woman experiences every one of them.

Cervical Changes

Before labour begins, cervical softening and possible cervical dilation with descent of the presenting part into the pelvis occur. These changes can occur 1 month to 1 hour before actual labour begins.

As labour approaches, the cervix changes from an elongated structure to a shortened, thinned segment. Cervical collagen fibres undergo enzymatic rearrangement into smaller, more flexible fibres that facilitate water absorption, leading to a softer, more stretchable cervix. These changes occur secondary to the effects of prostaglandins and pressure from Braxton Hicks contractions (Murray & Huelsmann, 2009).

Lightening

Lightening occurs when the fetal presenting part begins to descend into the maternal pelvis. The uterus lowers and moves into a more anterior position. The shape of the abdomen changes as a result of the change in the uterus. With this descent, the woman usually notes that her breathing is much easier. However, she may complain of increased pelvic pressure, cramping, and low back pain. She may notice an increase in vaginal discharge and more frequent urination. Also, edema of the lower extremities may occur as a result of the increased stasis of pooling blood. In primigravidas, lightening can occur 2 weeks or more before labour begins; among multigravidas, it may not occur until labour (Ward & Hisley, 2009).

Increased Energy Level

Some women report a sudden increase in energy before labour. This is sometimes referred to as nesting, because many women will focus this energy toward childbirth preparation by cleaning, cooking, preparing the nursery, and spending extra time with other children in the household. The increased energy level usually occurs 24 to 48 hours before the onset of labour.

Bloody Show

At the onset of labour, the mucous plug that fills the cervical canal during pregnancy is expelled as a result of cervical softening and increased pressure of the presenting part. These ruptured cervical capillaries release a small amount of blood that mixes with mucus, resulting in the pink-tinged secretions known as bloody show.

Braxton Hicks Contractions

Braxton Hicks contractions, which the woman may have been experiencing throughout the pregnancy, may become stronger and more frequent. Braxton Hicks contractions are typically felt as a tightening or pulling sensation of the top of the uterus. They occur primarily in the abdomen and groin and gradually spread downward before relaxing. In contrast, true labour contractions are more commonly felt in the lower back. These contractions aid in moving the cervix from a posterior position to an anterior position. They also help in ripening and softening the cervix. However, the contractions are irregular and can be decreased by walking, voiding, eating, increasing fluid intake, or changing position.

Braxton Hicks contractions usually last about 30 seconds but can persist for as long as 2 minutes. As birth draws near and the uterus becomes more sensitive to oxytocin, the frequency and intensity of these contractions increase. However, if the contractions last longer than 30 seconds and occur more often than four to six times an hour, advise the woman to contact her health care provider so that she can be evaluated for possible preterm labour, especially if she is less than 38 weeks pregnant.

> ▷ Take NOTE!
>
> An infant born between 34 and 36 completed weeks of gestation is identified as "late preterm" and experiences many of the same health issues as other preterm birth infants (Association of Women's Health, Obstetric and Neonatal Nurses [AWHONN], 2007).

Spontaneous Rupture of Membranes

Spontaneous rupture of membranes precedes contractions in 10% of term pregnancies and in 40% of preterm pregnancies (Murray & Huelsmann, 2009). The rupture of membranes can result in either a sudden gush or a steady leakage of amniotic fluid. Although much of the amniotic fluid is lost when the rupture occurs, a continuous supply is produced to ensure protection of the fetus until birth.

After the amniotic sac has ruptured, the barrier to infection is gone and an ascending infection is possible. In addition, there is a danger of cord prolapse if engagement has not occurred with the sudden release of fluid and pressure with rupture. Due to the possibility of these complications, advise women to notify their health care provider and go in for an evaluation.

▶ Consider THIS!

I always pictured myself a dignified woman and behaved in ways to demonstrate that, for that was the way I was raised. My mother and grandmother always stressed that you should look good, dress well, and do nothing to embarrass yourself in public. I did a fairly good job of living up to their expectations until I become pregnant. I recall I was overdue according to my dates and was miserable in the summer heat. I decided to go to the store for some ice cream. As I waddled down the grocery aisles, all of a sudden my water broke and came pouring down my legs all over the floor. Not wanting to make a spectacle of myself and remembering what my mother always said about being dignified at all times in public, I quickly reached up onto the grocery shelf and "accidentally" knocked off a large jar of pickles right where my puddle was. As I walked hurriedly away from that mess without my ice cream, I heard on the store loudspeaker, "Clean-up on aisle 13!"

Thoughts: we tend to live by what we are taught, and in this case, this woman needed to save face from her ruptured membranes. Many women experience ruptured membranes before the onset of labour, so it is not out of the ordinary for this to happen in public. What risks can occur when membranes do rupture? What action should this woman take now to minimize these risks? How will the nurse validate this woman's ruptured membranes?

True Versus False Labour

False labour is a condition occurring during the latter weeks of some pregnancies in which irregular uterine contractions are felt, but the cervix is not affected. In contrast, true labour is characterized by contractions occurring at regular intervals that increase in frequency, duration, and intensity. True labour contractions bring about progressive cervical dilation and effacement. Table 13.1 summarizes the differences between true and false labour. False labour, prodromal labour, and Braxton Hicks contractions are all names for contractions that do not contribute in a measurable way toward the goal of birth.

Many women fear being sent home from the hospital with "false labour." All women feel anxious when they feel contractions, but they should be informed that labour could be a long process, especially if it is their first pregnancy. Encourage the woman to think of false labour or "pre-labour signs" as positive, as they are part of the

TABLE 13.1   DIFFERENCES BETWEEN TRUE AND FALSE LABOUR

Parameters	True Labour	False Labour
Contraction timing	Regular, becoming closer together, usually 4–6 min apart, lasting 30–60 s	Irregular, not occurring close together
Contraction strength	Become stronger with time, vaginal pressure is usually felt	Frequently weak, not getting stronger with time or alternating (a strong one followed by weaker ones)
Contraction discomfort	Starts in the back and radiates around toward the front of the abdomen	Usually felt in the front of the abdomen
Any change in activity	Contractions continue no matter what positional change is made	Contractions may stop or slow down with walking or making a position change
Stay or go?	Stay home until contractions are 5 min apart, last 45–60 s, and are strong enough so that a conversation during one is not possible—then go to the hospital or birthing centre.	Drink fluids and walk around to see if there is any change in the intensity of the contractions; if the contractions diminish in intensity after either or both—stay home.

Source: Cunningham et al. (2010). *Williams obstetrics* (23rd ed.). New York: McGraw-Hill.

entire labour continuum. With first pregnancies, the cervix can take up to 20 hours to dilate completely (Cunningham et al., 2010). In clinical care, it is difficult to differentiate between prolonged latent phase and false labour (McDonald, 2010). There is no consensus on how long latent labour should last and it is important to watch and wait for labour.

Remember Kathy and Chuck, the anxious couple who came to the hospital too early? Kathy felt sure she was in labour and is now confused. What explanations and anticipatory guidance should be offered to this couple? What term would describe her earlier contractions?

Factors Affecting the Labour Process

In many references, the critical factors that affect the process of labour and birth are outlined as the "five P's":

1. Passageway (birth canal)
2. Passenger (fetus and placenta)
3. Powers (contractions)
4. Position (maternal)
5. Psychological response

These critical factors are commonly accepted and discussed by health care professionals. However, five additional "P's" can also affect the labour process:

1. Philosophy (low tech, high touch)
2. Partners (support caregivers)
3. Patience (natural timing)

4. Patient preparation (childbirth knowledge base)
5. Pain control (comfort measures)

These five additional "P's" are helpful in planning care for the labouring family. These patient-focused factors are an attempt to foster labour that can be managed through the use of high touch, patience, support, knowledge, and pain management.

Passageway

The birth passageway is the route through which the fetus must travel to be born vaginally. The passageway consists of the maternal pelvis and soft tissues. Of the two, however, the maternal bony pelvis is more important because it is relatively unyielding (except for the coccyx). Typically the pelvis is assessed and measured during the first trimester, often at the first visit to the health care provider, to identify any abnormalities that might hinder a successful vaginal birth. As the pregnancy progresses, the hormones relaxin and estrogen cause the connective tissues to become more relaxed and elastic and cause the joints to become more flexible to prepare the mother's pelvis for birth. Additionally, the soft tissues usually yield to the forces of labour.

Bony Pelvis

The maternal bony pelvis can be divided into the true and false portions. The false (or greater) pelvis is composed of the upper flared parts of the two iliac bones with their concavities and the wings of the base of the sacrum. The false pelvis is divided from the true pelvis by an imaginary line drawn from the sacral prominence at the back to the superior aspect of the symphysis pubis at the front of the pelvis. This imaginary line is called

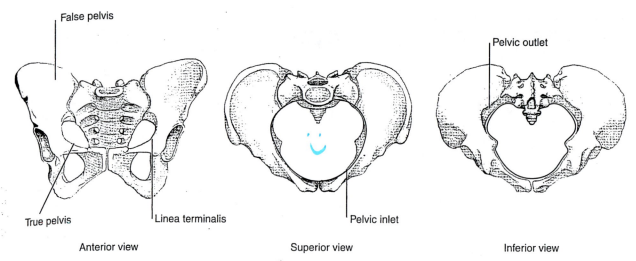

False pelvis

True pelvis   Linea terminalis   Pelvic inlet

Pelvic outlet

Anterior view   Superior view   Inferior view

FIGURE 13.1 The bony pelvis.

linea terminalis. The false pelvis lies above this imaginary line; the true pelvis lies below it (Fig. 13.1). The true pelvis is the bony passageway through which the fetus must travel. It is made up of three planes: the inlet, the midpelvis (cavity), and the outlet.

Pelvic Inlet

The pelvic inlet allows entrance to the true pelvis. It is bounded by the sacral prominence in the back, laterally by the lineal terminalis, and by the superior aspect of the symphysis pubis in the front (Cunningham et al., 2010). The pelvic inlet is wider in the transverse aspect (sideways) than it is from front to back.

Midpelvis

The midpelvis (cavity) occupies the space between the inlet and the outlet. It is through this snug, curved space that the fetus must travel to reach the outside. As the fetus passes through this small area, its chest is compressed, causing lung fluid and mucus to be expelled. This expulsion removes the space-occupying fluid so that air can enter the lungs with the newborn's first breath.

Pelvic Outlet

The pelvic outlet is bound by the ischial tuberosities, the lower rim of the symphysis pubis, and the tip of the coccyx. In comparison with the pelvic inlet, the outlet is wider from front to back. For the fetus to pass through the pelvis, the outlet must be large enough.

To ensure the adequacy of the pelvic outlet for vaginal birth, the following pelvic measurements are assessed:

• Diagonal conjugate of the inlet (distance between the anterior surface of the sacral prominence and the anterior surface of the inferior margin of the symphysis pubis)
• Transverse or ischial tuberosity diameter of the outlet (distance at the medial and lowest aspect of the ischial

tuberosities, at the level of the anus; a known hand span or clenched-fist measurement is generally used to obtain this measurement)
• True or obstetric conjugate (distance estimated from the measurement of the diagonal conjugate; 1.5 cm is subtracted from the diagonal conjugate measurement)

For more information about pelvic measurements, see Chapter 12.

If the diagonal conjugate measures at least 11.5 cm and the true or obstetric conjugate measures 10 cm or more (1.5 cm less than the diagonal conjugate, or about 10 cm), then the pelvis is large enough for a vaginal birth of what would be considered a normal-size newborn.

Pelvic Shape

In addition to size, the shape of a woman's pelvis is a determining factor for a vaginal birth. The pelvis is divided into four main shapes: gynecoid, anthropoid, android, and platypelloid (Fig. 13.2).

The gynecoid pelvis is considered the true female pelvis, occurring in about 50% of all women (Martin & Kennedy, 2009a). Vaginal birth is most favourable with this type of pelvis because the inlet is round and the outlet is roomy. This shape offers the optimal diameters in all three planes of the pelvis. This type of pelvis allows early and complete fetal internal rotation during labour.

The anthropoid pelvis is common in men and occurs in 25% of women (Martin & Kennedy, 2009a). The pelvic inlet is oval and the sacrum is long, producing a deep pelvis (wider front to back [anterior to posterior] than side to side [transverse]). Vaginal birth is more favourable with this pelvic shape compared with the android or platypelloid shape (Ward & Hisley, 2009).

The android pelvis is considered the male-shaped pelvis and is characterized by a funnel shape. It occurs in approximately 20% of women (Martin & Kennedy, 2009a). The pelvic inlet is heart-shaped and the posterior

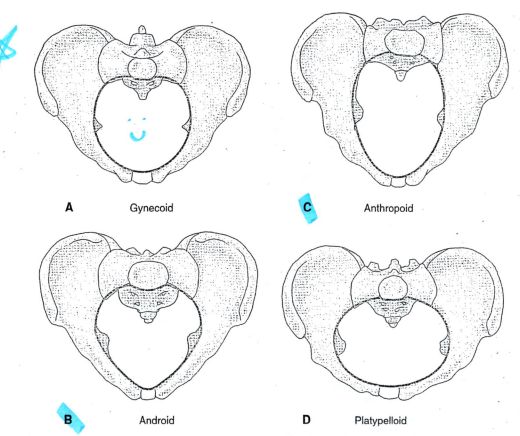

FIGURE 13.2 Pelvic shapes. (**A**) Gynecoid. (**B**) Android. (**C**) Anthropoid. (**D**) Platypelloid.

segments are reduced in all pelvic planes. Descent of the fetal head into the pelvis is slow, and failure of the fetus to rotate is common. The prognosis for labour is poor, subsequently leading to cesarean birth.

The platypelloid or flat pelvis is the least common type of pelvic structure among men and women, with an approximate incidence of 5% (Martin & Kennedy, 2009a). The pelvic cavity is shallow but widens at the pelvic outlet, making it difficult for the fetus to descend through the midpelvis. It is not favourable for a vaginal birth unless the fetal head can pass through the inlet. Women with this type of pelvis usually require cesarean birth.

An important principle is that most pelves are not purely defined but occur in nature as mixed types. Many women have a combination of these four basic pelvis types, with no two pelves being exactly the same. Regardless of the shape, the newborn will be born if size and positioning remain compatible. The narrowest part of the fetus attempts to align itself with the narrowest pelvic dimension (e.g., biparietal to interspinous diameters, which means the fetus generally tends to rotate to the most ample portion of the pelvis).

Soft Tissues

The soft tissues of the passageway consist of the cervix, the pelvic floor muscles, and the vagina. Through **effacement**, the cervix effaces (thins) and dilates (opens) to allow the presenting fetal part to descend into the vagina.

 ▶ **Take** NOTE!

Cervical effacement and dilation are similar to pulling a turtleneck sweater over your head.

The pelvic floor muscles help the fetus to rotate anteriorly as it passes through the birth canal. The soft tissues of the vagina expand to accommodate the fetus during birth.

Passenger

The fetus (with placenta) is the passenger. The fetal head (size and presence of moulding), fetal attitude (degree of body flexion), fetal lie (relationship of body parts), fetal presentation (first body part), fetal position (relationship to maternal pelvis), fetal station, and fetal engagement are all important factors that have an impact on the ultimate outcome in the birthing process.

Fetal Head

The fetal head is the largest and least compressible fetal structure, making it an important factor in relation to labour and birth. Considerable variation in the size and diameter of the fetal skull is often seen.

Compared with an adult, the fetal head is large in proportion to the rest of the body (Ward & Hisley, 2009). The bones that make up the face and cranial base are fused and essentially fixed. However, the bones that make up the rest of the cranium (two frontal bones, two parietal bones, and the occipital bone) are not fused; rather, they are soft and pliable, with gaps between the plates of bone. These gaps, which are membranous spaces between the cranial bones, are called sutures, and the intersections of these sutures are called fontanels. Sutures are important because they allow the cranial bones to overlap in order for the head to adjust in shape (elongate) when pressure is exerted on it by uterine contractions or the maternal bony pelvis. Some diameters shorten whereas others lengthen as the head is moulded during the labour and birthing process. This malleability of the fetal skull may decrease fetal skull dimensions (Cunningham et al., 2010). After birth, the sutures close as the bones grow and the brain reaches its full growth.

The changed (elongated) shape of the fetal skull at birth as a result of overlapping of the cranial bones is known as **moulding**. Along with moulding, fluid can also collect in the scalp (caput succedaneum) or blood can collect beneath the scalp (cephalohematoma), further distorting the shape and appearance of the fetal head. Caput succedaneum can be described as edema of the scalp at the presenting part. This swelling crosses suture lines and disappears within 3 to 4 days. Cephalohematoma is a collection of blood between the periosteum and the bone. It does not cross suture lines and is generally reabsorbed over weeks or months (Cunningham et al., 2010).

▷ **Take** NOTE!

Parents may become concerned about the distortion of their newborn's head. However, reassurance that the oblong shape is only temporary is usually all that is needed to reduce their anxiety.

Sutures also play a role in helping to identify the position of the fetal head during a vaginal examination. Figure 13.3 shows a fetal skull. The coronal sutures are located between the frontal and parietal bones and extend transversely on both sides of the anterior fontanels. The frontal suture is located between the two frontal bones. The lambdoidal sutures are located between the occipital bone and the two parietals, extending transversely on either side of the posterior fontanels. The sagittal suture is located between the parietal bones and divides the skull into the right and left halves. During a pelvic examination, palpation of these sutures by the examiner reveals the position of the fetal head and the degree of rotation that has occurred.

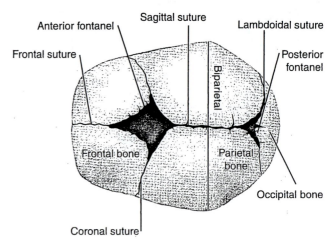

FIGURE 13.3 Fetal skull.

The anterior and posterior fontanels are also useful in helping to identify the position of the fetal head, and they allow for moulding. In addition, the fontanels are important when evaluating the newborn. The anterior fontanel is the famous "soft spot" of the newborn's head. It is diamond-shaped and measures about 2 to 3 cm. It remains open up to 18 months after birth to allow for growth of the brain (Davidson, London, & Ladewig, 2008). The posterior fontanel corresponds to the anterior one but is located at the back of the fetal head; it is triangular. This one closes within 8 to 12 weeks after birth and measures, on average, 0.5 to 1 cm at its widest diameter (Kenner & Lott, 2007).

The diameter of the fetal skull is an important consideration during the labour and birth process. Fetal skull diameters are measured between the various landmarks of the skull. Diameters include occipitofrontal, occipitomental, suboccipitobregmatic, and biparietal (Fig. 13.4). The two most important diameters that can affect the birth process are the suboccipitobregmatic (approximately 9.5 cm at term) and the biparietal (approximately 9.25 cm at term) diameters. The suboccipitobregmatic

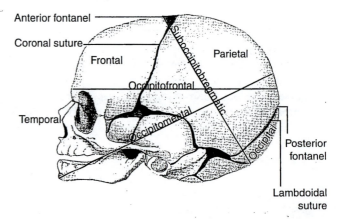

FIGURE 13.4 Fetal skull diameters.

diameter, measured from the base of the occiput to the centre of the anterior fontanel, identifies the smallest anteroposterior diameter of the fetal skull. The biparietal diameter measures the largest transverse diameter of the fetal skull: the distance between the two parietal bones. In a cephalic (headfirst) presentation, which occurs in 95% of all term births, if the fetus presents in a flexed position in which the chin is resting on the chest, the optimal or smallest fetal skull dimensions for a vaginal birth are demonstrated. If the fetal head is not fully flexed at birth, the anteroposterior diameter increases. This increase in dimension might prevent the fetal skull from entering the maternal pelvis.

Fetal Attitude

Fetal attitude is another important consideration related to the passenger. Fetal **attitude** refers to the posturing (flexion or extension) of the joints and the relationship of fetal parts to one another. The most common fetal attitude when labour begins is with all joints flexed—the fetal back is rounded, the chin is on the chest, the thighs are flexed on the abdomen, and the legs are flexed at the knees (Fig. 13.5). This normal fetal position is most favourable for vaginal birth, presenting the smallest fetal skull diameters to the pelvis.

When the fetus presents to the pelvis with abnormal attitudes (no flexion or extension), the diameter can increase the diameter of the presenting part as it passes through the pelvis, increasing the difficulty of birth. An attitude of extension tends to present larger fetal skull diameters, which may make birth difficult.

Fetal Lie

Fetal **lie** refers to the relationship of the long axis (spine) of the fetus to the long axis (spine) of the mother. There are two primary lies: longitudinal (which is the most common) and transverse (Fig. 13.6).

A longitudinal lie occurs when the long axis of the fetus is parallel to that of the mother (fetal spine to maternal spine side-by-side). A transverse lie occurs when the long axis of the fetus is perpendicular to the long axis of

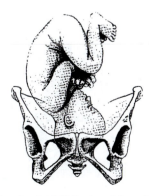

FIGURE **13.5** Fetal attitude: full flexion. Note that the smallest diameter presents to the pelvis.

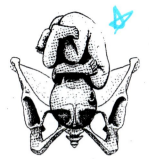

A. Longitudinal lie

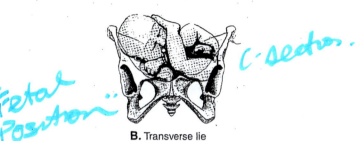

B. Transverse lie

FIGURE **13.6** Fetal lie.

the mother (fetus spine lies across the maternal abdomen and crosses her spine). A fetus in a transverse lie position cannot be delivered vaginally (Cunningham et al., 2010).

Fetal Presentation

Fetal **presentation** refers to the body part of the fetus that enters the pelvic inlet first (the "presenting part"). This is the fetal part that lies over the inlet of the pelvis or the cervical os. Knowing which fetal part is coming first at birth is critical for planning and initiating appropriate interventions.

The three main fetal presentations are cephalic (head first), breech (pelvis first), and shoulder (scapula first). The majority of term newborns enter the world in a cephalic presentation; breech and shoulder presentations are uncommon. In a cephalic presentation, the presenting part is usually the occiput portion of the fetal head (Fig. 13.7). This presentation is also referred to as a vertex presentation. Variations in a vertex presentation include the military, brow, and face presentations.

Breech presentation occurs when the fetal buttocks or feet enter the maternal pelvis first and the fetal skull enters last. This abnormal presentation poses several challenges at birth. Primarily, the largest part of the fetus (skull) is born last and may become "hung up" or stuck in the pelvis. In addition, the umbilical cord can become compressed between the fetal skull and the maternal pelvis after the fetal chest is born because the head is the last to exit. Moreover, unlike the hard fetal skull, the buttocks are soft and are not as effective as a cervical dilator during labour compared with a cephalic presentation

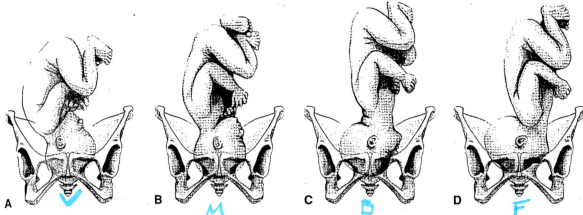

FIGURE **13.7** Fetal presentation: cephalic presentations. (**A**) Vertex. (**B**) Military. (**C**) Brow. (**D**) Face.

Finally, there is the possibility of trauma to the head as a result of the lack of opportunity for moulding.

The types of breech presentations are determined by the positioning of the fetal legs (Fig. 13.8). In a frank breech (50% to 70%), the buttocks present first with both legs extended up toward the face. In a full or complete breech (5% to 10%), the fetus sits cross-legged above the cervix. In a footling or incomplete breech (10% to 30%), one or both legs are presenting. Breech presentations are associated with hydramnios, oligohydramnios, prematurity, placenta previa, multiparity, previous breech delivery, uterine abnormalities (fibroids), multiple fetuses, and some congenital anomalies such as hydrocephaly (Cunningham et al., 2010). A frank breech can result in a vaginal birth, but complete and footling (incomplete) breech presentations generally necessitate a cesarean birth.

A shoulder presentation occurs when the fetal shoulders present first, with the head tucked inside. The fetus is in a transverse lie with the shoulder as the presenting part. Conditions associated with shoulder presentation include placenta previa, multiple gestation, or fetal anomalies. A cesarean birth is typically necessary (Cunningham et al., 2010).

Fetal Position

Fetal **position** describes the relationship of a given point on the presenting part of the fetus to a designated point of the maternal pelvis (Cunningham et al., 2010). The landmark fetal presenting parts include the occipital bone (**O**), which designates a vertex presentation; the chin (mentum [**M**]), which designates a face presentation; the buttocks (sacrum [**S**]), which designate a breech presentation; and the scapula (acromion process [**A**]), which designates a shoulder presentation.

In addition, the maternal pelvis is divided into four quadrants: right anterior, left anterior, right posterior, and left posterior. These quadrants designate whether the presenting part is directed toward the front, back, left, or right side of the pelvis. Fetal position is determined first by identifying the presenting part and then

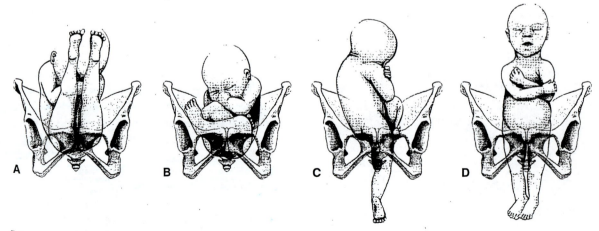

FIGURE **13.8** Breech presentations. (**A**) Frank breech. (**B**) Complete breech. (**C**) Single footling breech. (**D**) Double footling breech.

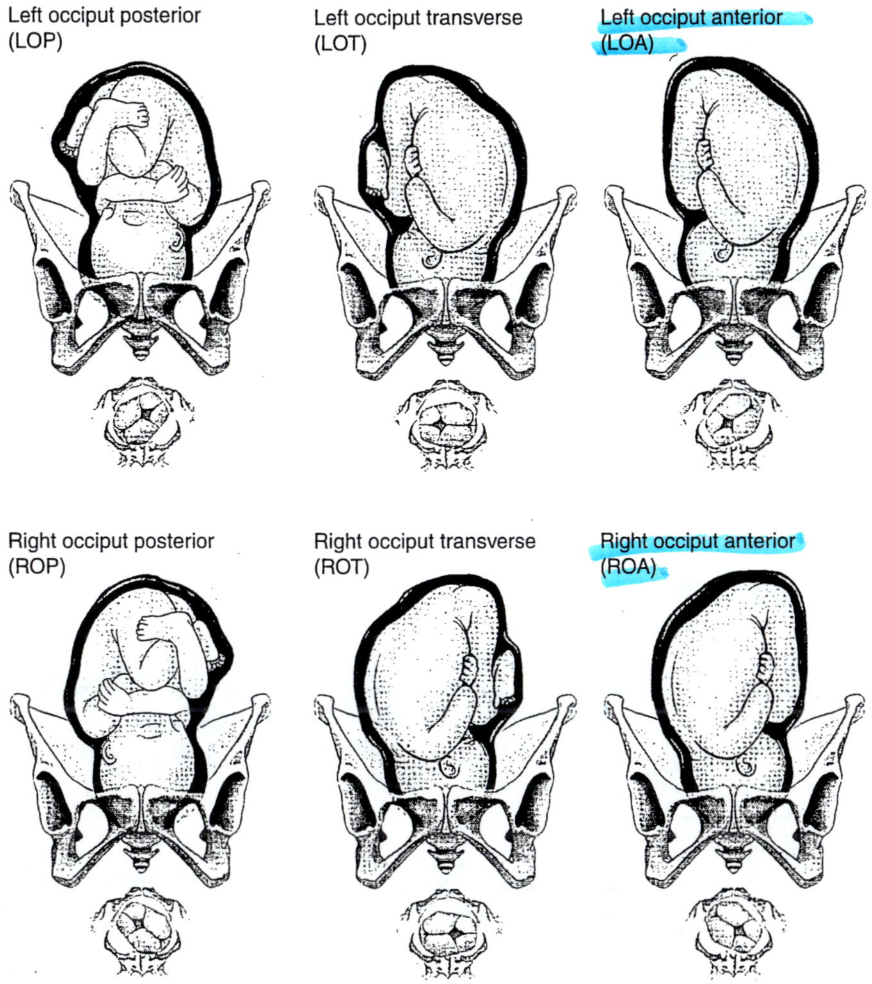

Left occiput posterior
(LOP)

Left occiput transverse
(LOT)

Left occiput anterior
(LOA)

Right occiput posterior
(ROP)

Right occiput transverse
(ROT)

Right occiput anterior
(ROA)

FIGURE 13.9 Examples of fetal positions in a vertex presentation. The lie is longitudinal for each illustration. The attitude is one of flexion. Notice that the view of the top illustration is seen when facing the pregnant woman. The bottom view is that seen with the woman in a dorsal recumbent position.

the maternal quadrant the presenting part is facing (Fig. 13.9). Position is indicated by a three-letter abbreviation as follows:

- The first letter defines whether the presenting part is tilted toward the left (L) or the right (R) side of the maternal pelvis.
- The second letter represents the particular presenting part of the fetus: O for occiput, S for sacrum (buttocks), M for mentum (chin), A for acromion process, and D for dorsal (refers to the fetal back) when denoting the fetal position in shoulder presentations (Cunningham et al., 2010).
- The third letter defines the location of the presenting part in relation to the anterior (A) portion of the maternal pelvis or the posterior (P) portion of the maternal pelvis. If the presenting part is directed to the side of the maternal pelvis, the fetal presentation is designated as transverse (T).

For example, if the occiput is facing the left anterior quadrant of the pelvis, then the position is termed left occipitoanterior and is recorded as LOA. LOA is the most common (and most favourable) fetal position for birthing today, followed by right occipitoanterior (ROA).

The positioning of the fetus allows the fetal head to contour to the diameters of the maternal pelvis. LOA and ROA are optimal positions for vaginal birth. An occiput posterior position may lead to a long and difficult birth, and other positions may or may not be compatible with vaginal birth.

Fetal Station

Station refers to the relationship of the presenting part to the level of the maternal pelvic ischial spines. Fetal station is measured in centimetres and is referred to as a minus or plus, depending on its location above or below the ischial spines. Typically, the ischial spines are the narrowest part of the pelvis and are the natural measuring point for the birth progress.

Zero (0) station is designated when the presenting part is at the level of the maternal ischial spines. When the presenting part is above the ischial spines, the distance is recorded as minus stations. When the presenting part is below the ischial spines, the distance is recorded as plus stations. For instance, if the presenting part is above the ischial spines by 1 cm, it is documented as being a –1 station; if the presenting part is below the ischial spines by 1 cm, it is documented as being a +1 station. An easy way to understand this concept is to think in terms of meeting the goal, which is the birth. If the fetus is descending downward (past the ischial spines) and moving toward meeting the goal of birth, then the station is positive and the centimetre numbers grow bigger from +1 to +4. If the fetus is not descending past the ischial spines, then the station is negative and the centimetre numbers grow bigger from –1 to –4. The farther away the presenting part from the outside, the larger the negative number (–4 cm). The closer the presenting part of the fetus is to the outside, the larger the positive number (+4 cm). Figure 13.10 shows stations of presenting part.

Fetal Engagement

Engagement signifies the entrance of the largest diameter of the fetal presenting part (usually the fetal head) into the smallest diameter of the maternal pelvis (Cunningham et al., 2010). The fetus is said to be "engaged" in the pelvis when the presenting part reaches 0 station. Engagement is determined by pelvic examination.

The largest diameter of the fetal head is the biparietal diameter. It extends from one parietal prominence to the other. It is an important factor in the navigation through the maternal pelvis. Engagement typically occurs in primigravidas 2 weeks before term, whereas multigravidas may experience engagement several weeks before the onset of labour or not until labour begins.

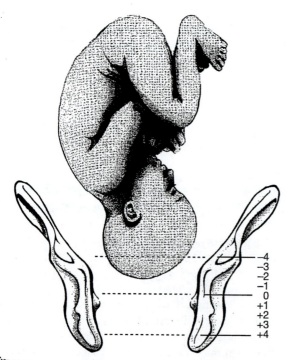

−4
−3
−2
−1
0
+1
+2
+3
+4

FIGURE 13.10 Fetal stations.

▶ Take NOTE!

The term floating is used when engagement has not occurred, because the presenting part is freely movable above the pelvic inlet.

Cardinal Movements of Labour

The fetus goes through many positional changes as it travels through the passageway. These positional changes are known as the cardinal movements of labour. They are deliberate, specific, and very precise movements that allow the smallest diameter of the fetal head to pass through a corresponding diameter of the mother's pelvic structure. Although cardinal movements are conceptualized as separate and sequential, the movements are typically concurrent (Fig. 13.11).

Engagement

Engagement occurs when the greatest transverse diameter of the head in vertex (biparietal diameter) passes through the pelvic inlet (usually 0 station). The head usually enters the pelvis with the sagittal suture aligned in the transverse diameter.

Descent

Descent is the downward movement of the fetal head until it is within the pelvic inlet. Descent occurs intermittently with contractions and is brought about by one or more of the following forces:

• Pressure of the amniotic fluid
• Direct pressure of the fundus on the fetus' buttocks or head (depending on which part is located in the top of the uterus)
• Contractions of the abdominal muscles (second stage)
• Extension and straightening of the fetal body

Descent occurs throughout labour, ending with birth. During this time, the mother experiences discomfort, but she is unable to isolate this particular fetal movement from her overall discomfort.

Flexion

Flexion occurs as the vertex meets resistance from the cervix, the walls of the pelvis, or the pelvic floor. As a result, the chin is brought into contact with the fetal thorax and the presenting diameter is changed from occipitofrontal to suboccipitobregmatic (9.5 cm), which achieves the smallest fetal skull diameter presenting to the maternal pelvic dimensions.

Internal Rotation

After engagement, as the head descends, the lower portion of the head (usually the occiput) meets resistance from one side of the pelvic floor. As a result, the head

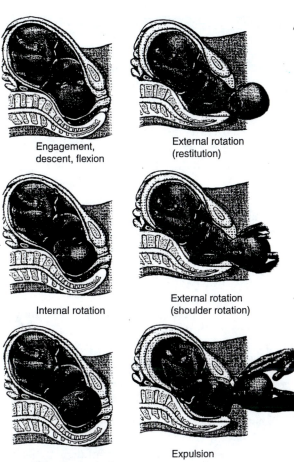

Engagement, descent, flexion

External rotation (restitution)

Internal rotation

External rotation (shoulder rotation)

Extension beginning (rotation complete)

Expulsion

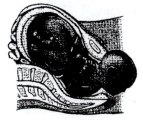

Extension complete

FIGURE 13.11 Cardinal movements of labour.

rotates about 45 degrees anteriorly to the midline under the symphysis. This movement is known as internal rotation. Internal rotation brings the anteroposterior diameter of the head in line with the anteroposterior diameter of the pelvic outlet. It aligns the long axis of the fetal head with the long axis of the maternal pelvis. The widest portion of the maternal pelvis is the anteroposterior diameter, and thus the fetus must rotate to accommodate the pelvis.

Extension

With further descent and full flexion of the head, the nucha (the base of the occiput) becomes impinged under the symphysis. Resistance from the pelvic floor causes the fetal head to extend so that it can pass under the pubic arch. Extension occurs after internal rotation is complete. The head emerges through extension under the symphysis pubis along with the shoulders. The anterior fontanel, brow, nose, mouth, and chin are born successively.

External Rotation (Restitution)

After the head is born and is free of resistance, it untwists, causing the occiput to move about 45 degrees back to its original left or right position (restitution). The sagittal suture has now resumed its normal right-angle relationship to the transverse (bisacromial) diameter of the shoulders (i.e., the head realigns with the position of the back in the birth canal). External rotation of the fetal head allows the shoulders to rotate internally to fit the maternal pelvis.

Expulsion

Expulsion of the rest of the body occurs more smoothly after the birth of the head and the anterior and posterior shoulders (Cunningham et al., 2010).

Powers

The primary stimulus powering labour is uterine contractions. Contractions cause complete dilation and effacement of the cervix during the first stage of labour. The secondary powers in labour involve the use of intraabdominal pressure (voluntary muscle contractions) exerted by the woman as she pushes and bears down during the second stage of labour.

Uterine Contractions

Uterine contractions are involuntary and therefore cannot be controlled by the woman experiencing them, regardless of whether they are spontaneous or induced. Uterine contractions are rhythmic and intermittent, with a period of relaxation between contractions. This pause allows the woman and the uterine muscles to rest. In addition, this pause restores blood flow to the uterus and placenta, which is temporarily reduced during each uterine contraction.

Uterine contractions are responsible for thinning and dilating the cervix, and they thrust the presenting part toward the lower uterine segment. With each uterine contraction, the upper segment of the uterus becomes shorter and thicker, whereas the lower passive segment and the cervix become longer, thinner, and more distended. The division between the contractile upper portion (fundus) of the uterus and the lower portion is described as the physiologic retraction ring. Longitudinal traction on the cervix by the fundus as it contracts and retracts leads to cervical effacement and dilation. Uterine contractions cause the upper uterine segment to shorten, making the cervix paper-thin when it becomes fully effaced.

The cervical canal reduces in length from 2 cm to a paper-thin entity and is described in terms of percentages from 0% to 100%. In primigravidas, effacement typically starts before the onset of labour and usually begins before dilation; in multigravidas, however, neither effacement nor dilation may start until labour ensues (Nettina, 2010). On clinical examination, the following may be assessed:

- Cervical canal 2 cm in length would be described as 0% effaced.
- Cervical canal 1 cm in length would be described as 50% effaced.
- Cervical canal 0 cm in length would be described as 100% effaced.

Dilation is dependent on the pressure of the presenting part and the contraction and retraction of the uterus. The diameter of the cervical os increases from less than 1 cm to approximately 10 cm to allow for birth. When the cervix is fully dilated, it is no longer palpable on vaginal examination. Descriptions may include the following:

- External cervical os closed: 0 cm dilated
- External cervical os half open: 5 cm dilated
- External cervical os fully open: 10 cm dilated

During early labour, uterine contractions are described as mild, they last about 30 seconds, and they occur about every 5 to 7 minutes. As labour progresses, contractions last longer (60 seconds), occur more frequently (2 to 3 minutes apart), and are described as being moderate to high in intensity.

Each contraction has three phases: increment (build-up of the contraction), acme (peak or highest intensity), and decrement (descent or relaxation of the uterine muscle fibres; Fig. 13.12).

Uterine contractions are monitored and assessed according to three parameters: frequency, duration, and intensity.

1. **Frequency** refers to how often the contractions occur and is measured from the increment of one contraction to the increment of the next contraction.

2. **Duration** refers to how long a contraction lasts and is measured from the beginning of the increment to the end of the decrement for the same contraction.

3. **Intensity** refers to the strength of the contraction determined by manual palpation or measured by an internal intrauterine pressure catheter (IUPC). The catheter is positioned in the uterine cavity through the cervix after the membranes have ruptured. It reports intensity by measuring the pressure of the amniotic fluid inside the uterus in millimetres of mercury (Murray & Huelsmann, 2009).

Intra-Abdominal Pressure

Increased intra-abdominal pressure (voluntary muscle contractions) compresses the uterus and adds to the power of the expulsion forces of the uterine contractions (Murray & Huelsmann, 2009). Coordination of these forces in unison promotes birth of the fetus and expulsion of the fetal membranes and placenta from the uterus. Interference with these forces (such as when a woman is highly sedated or extremely anxious) can compromise the effectiveness of these powers.

Psychological Response

Childbearing can be one of the most life-altering experiences for a woman. The experience of childbirth goes beyond the physiologic aspects: it influences her self-confidence, self-esteem, and view of life, relationships, and children. Her state of mind (psyche) throughout the entire process is critical to bring about a positive outcome for her and her family. Factors promoting a positive birth experience include:

- Clear information about procedures
- Support; not being alone
- Sense of mastery, self-confidence
- Trust in staff caring for her
- Positive reaction to the pregnancy

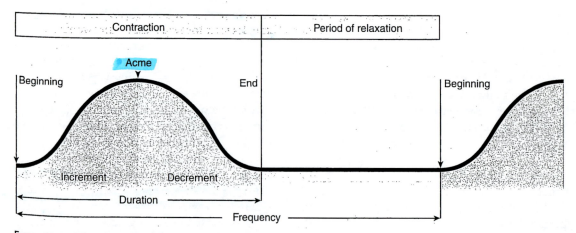

FIGURE 13.12 The three phases of a uterine contraction.

- Personal control over breathing
- Preparation for the childbirth experience

Having a strong sense of self and meaningful support from others can often help women manage labour well. Feeling safe and secure typically promotes a sense of control and ability to withstand the challenges of the childbearing experience. Anxiety and fear, however, decrease a woman's ability to cope with the discomfort of labour. Maternal catecholamines secreted in response to anxiety and fear can inhibit uterine blood flow and placental perfusion. In contrast, relaxation can augment the natural process of labour (Murray & Huelsmann, 2009). Preparing mentally for childbirth is important so that the woman can work with, rather than against, the natural forces of labour.

Position (Maternal)

Maternal positioning during labour has only recently been the subject of well-controlled research. Scientific evidence has shown that nonmoving, back-lying positions during labour are not healthy (Zwelling, 2010). However, despite this evidence to the contrary, most women continue to lie flat on their backs during labour. Some of the reasons why this practice continues include the following:

- Belief that labouring women need to conserve their energy and not tire themselves
- Belief that nurses cannot keep track of the whereabouts of ambulating women
- Belief that the supine position facilitates vaginal examinations and external belt adjustment
- Belief that a bed is "where one is supposed to be" in a hospital setting
- Belief that the position is more convenient for the delivering health professional
- Belief that labouring women are "connected to things" that impede movement (Zwelling, 2010)

Although many labour and birthing facilities claim that all women are allowed to adopt any position of comfort during their labouring experience, the great majority of women spend their time on their backs during labour and birth.

▶ Take NOTE!

If the only furniture provided is a bed, this is what the woman will use. Furnishing rooms with comfortable chairs, beanbags, and other birth props allows a woman to choose from a variety of positions and to be free to move during labour.

Changing positions and moving around during labour and birth offer several benefits. Maternal position can influence pelvic size and contours. Changing position

and walking affect the pelvic joints, which may facilitate fetal descent and rotation. Squatting enlarges the pelvic outlet by approximately 25%, whereas a kneeling position removes pressure on the maternal vena cava and helps to rotate the fetus in the posterior position (Zwelling, 2010). The use of any upright or lateral position, compared with supine or lithotomy positions, may

- Reduce the length of the first stage of labour
- Reduce the duration of the second stage of labour
- Reduce the number of assisted deliveries (vacuum and forceps)
- Reduce episiotomies and perineal tears
- Contribute to fewer abnormal fetal heart rate patterns
- Increase comfort/reduce requests for pain medication
- Enhance a sense of control by the mother
- Alter the shape and size of the pelvis, which assists in descent
- Assist gravity to move the fetus downward (Zwelling, 2010)

Using the research available can bring better outcomes, heightened professionalism, and evidence-based practice to childbearing practices.

Philosophy

Not everyone views childbirth in the same way. A philosophical continuum exists that extends from viewing labour as a disease process to a normal process. One philosophy assumes that women cannot manage the birth experience adequately and therefore need constant expert monitoring and management. The other philosophy assumes that women are capable, reasoning individuals who can actively participate in their birth experience.

The health care system in Canada today appears to be leaning toward the former philosophy, applying technological interventions to most mothers who enter the hospital system. For many women in the 21st century, giving birth in a hospital has become "intervention intensive"—designed to start, continue, and end labour through medical management rather than allowing the normal process of birth to unfold. Advances in medical care have improved safety for women with high-risk pregnancies. However, the routine use of intravenous therapy, electronic fetal monitoring, augmentation, and epidural anesthesia are not supported by national or global practice guidelines (Chalmers et al., 2009). Perhaps a middle-of-the-road philosophy for intervening when circumstances dictate, along with weighing the risks and benefits before doing so, may be appropriate.

During the 1970s, family-centred maternity care was developed in response to consumer reaction to the depersonalization of birth. The hope was to shift the philosophy from "technologization" to personalization to humanize childbirth. The term "family-centred birthing" is more appropriate today to denote the low-tech, high-touch approach requested by many childbearing women, who view childbirth as a normal process. In Canada, there have been positive improvements to family-centred maternity care but more change is needed to assist women and families to achieve positive birthing experiences (Jimenez, Klein, Hivon, & Mason, 2010).

Registered midwives are champions of family-centred birthing, and their participation in the childbirth process is associated with fewer unnecessary interventions when compared with participation by obstetricians. Registered midwives subscribe to a normal birth process in which the woman uses her own instincts and bodily signs during labour. In short, midwives empower women within the birthing environment (Leap, Sandall, Buckland, & Huber, 2010).

No matter what philosophy is held, it is ideal if everyone involved in the particular birth process—from the health care provider to the mother—shares the same philosophy toward the birth process.

Partners

Women desire attentive care during labour and birth from partners who can convey emotional support by offering their continued presence and words of encouragement. Partners can play an important role in providing this comfort (Hanson, Hunter, Bormann, & Sobo, 2009), although they may experience fear related to their role at birth. Although the presence of the baby's father at the birth provides special emotional support, a partner can be anyone who is present to support the woman throughout the experience. See Evidence-based Practice 13.1.

Worldwide, women usually support other women in childbirth. Hodnett, Gates, Hofmeyr, & Sakala (2011) reported that the continuous presence of a trained female support person (**doula**) reduced the need for medication for pain relief, the use of vacuum or forceps delivery, and the need for cesarean births. Continuous support was also associated with a slight reduction in the length of labour. The doula, who is an experienced labour companion, provides the woman and her partner with emotional and physical support and information throughout the entire labour and birth experience.

Given the many benefits of intrapartum support, labouring women should always have the option to receive partner support, whether from nurses, doulas, significant others, or family. Whoever the support partner is, he or she should provide the mother with continuous presence and hands-on comfort and encouragement.

Patience

The birth process takes time. If more time were allowed for women to labour naturally without intervention, the cesarean birth rate would most likely be reduced (Chalmers et al., 2010; Romano & Lothian, 2008; Wilson, Effkren, & Butler, 2010). The literature suggests that delaying interventions can give a woman enough time to

EVIDENCE-BASED PRACTICE 13.1
Continuous Support for Women During Childbirth

● Study

Historically, women have been attended and supported by other women during labour. However, in recent decades in hospitals worldwide, continuous support during labour has become the exception rather than the rule. Concerns about the consequent dehumanization of the birth experience have led to calls for a return to continuous support by women for women during labour.

This review of studies included 16 trials from 11 countries, involving more than 13,000 women in a wide range of settings and circumstances. The primary goal of the review was to assess the effects, on mothers and their babies, of continuous, one-to-one intrapartum support compared with usual care. The secondary goal was to determine whether the effects of continuous support are influenced by (1) routine practices and policies in the birth environment that may affect a woman's autonomy, freedom of movement, and ability to cope with labour; (2) whether the caregiver is a member of the staff of the institution; and (3) whether the continuous support begins early or later in labour.

▲ Findings

Women who received continuous labour support were more likely to give birth "spontaneously" (vaginally, without vacuum or forceps). They were less likely to use pain medications, were more likely to be satisfied with their experience, and had slightly shorter labours. In general, labour support appeared to be more effective when it was provided by women who were not part of the hospital staff. It also appeared to be more effective when started early in labour. No adverse effects were identified.

▣ Nursing Implications

Knowing the results of this evidence-based study, all nurses should strive to be a real "presence" for all of their labouring couples. Based on the findings, continuous nursing support promotes positive birthing outcomes and fewer technical/surgical interventions. Both maternal and fetal well-being is preserved when nurses are present and involved during the childbirth experience.

Hodnett, E. D., Gates, S., Hofmeyr, G. J., & Sakala, C. (2011). Continuous support for women during childbirth. *Cochrane Database of Systematic Reviews, 2*, CD003766. doi: 10.1002/14651858. CD003766.pub3 progress in labour and reduce the need for surgical intervention (Romano & Lothian, 2008).

The current cesarean birth rate in Canada was reported to be 25.6 per 100 hospital deliveries in 2004 and 2005, yet the World Health Organization (WHO) recommends a rate of 10% to 15% (Chalmers et al., 2010; Public Health Agency of Canada [PHAC], 2008). Cesarean birth is associated with increased morbidity and mortality for both mother and infant as well as increased in-patient length of stay and health care costs (Society of Obstetricians and Gynaecologists of Canada [SOGC], 2008). The elective/other category of cesarean births represented 6.7 per 100 hospital births (PHAC, 2008).

It is difficult to predict how any given labour will progress and therefore equally difficult to determine how long a woman's labour will last. There is no way to estimate the likely strength and frequency of uterine contractions, the extent to which the cervix will soften and dilate, and how much the fetal head will mould to fit the birth canal. We cannot know beforehand whether the complex fetal rotations needed for an efficient labour will take place properly. All of these factors are unknowns when a woman starts labour.

There is a trend in health care, however, to attempt to manipulate the process of labour through medical means such as artificial rupture of membranes and augmentation of labour with oxytocin (Chalmers et al., 2010). In Canada, the labour induction rate ranges from 21.6% to 52.5% and the labour augmentation rate ranges from 16.1% to 40.6% (Chalmers et al., 2009). An amniotomy (artificial rupture of the fetal membranes) may be performed to augment or induce labour when the membranes have not ruptured spontaneously. Doing so allows the fetal head to have more direct contact with the cervix in order to dilate it. This procedure is performed with the fetal head at –2 station or lower, with the cervix dilated to at least 3 cm. Synthetic oxytocin (Syntocinon) is also used to induce or augment labour by stimulating uterine contractions. It is administered piggybacked into the primary intravenous line with an infusion pump titrated to uterine activity.

There is compelling evidence that elective induction of labour significantly increases the risk of cesarean birth, especially for nulliparous women (Murray & Huelsmann, 2009). The belief is that many cesarean births could be avoided if women were allowed to labour longer and if the natural labour process were allowed to complete the job. The longer wait (using the intervention of patience) usually results in less intervention.

The Society of Obstetricians and Gynaecologists of Canada (SOGC) suggests that induction should be offered at 41 to 42 weeks' gestation based on evidence that suggests decreased perinatal mortality without an increased rate of cesarean section (Delaney & Roggensack, 2008). Determination of gestational age should be based on ultrasound in the first trimester. Sweeping of the membranes should be offered between 38 and 41 weeks based on a discussion of the risks and benefits. There are medical indications for inducing labour, such as premature rupture of membranes and when labour does not start; a pregnancy more than 41 weeks' gestation; maternal hypertension, diabetes, or a uterine infection; or fetal demise (Dunne, Da Silva, Schmidt, & Natale, 2009). However, more women today are requesting induction for reasons of convenience.

When the labouring woman feels the urge to bear down, pushing begins. Most women respond extremely well to messages from their body without being directed by the nurse. A more natural, undirected approach allows the woman to wait and bear down when she feels the urge to push. Having patience and letting nature take its course will reduce the incidence of physiologic stress in the mother, resulting in less trauma to her perineal tissue.

Patient Preparation

Basic prenatal education can help women manage their labour process and feel in control of their birthing experience. The literature indicates that if a woman is prepared before the labour and birth experience, the labour is more likely to remain normal or natural (without the need for medical intervention) (Leap et al., 2010). An increasing body of evidence also indicates that the well-prepared woman, with good labour support, is less likely to need analgesia or anesthesia and is unlikely to require cesarean birth (Barrett & Stark, 2010).

Prenatal education teaches the woman about the childbirth experience and increases her sense of control. She is then able to work as an active participant during the labour and birth experience (International Childbirth Education Association, n.d.). Research also suggests that prenatal preparation may affect intrapartum and postpartum psychosocial outcomes. For example, prenatal education covering parenting communication classes had a significant effect on postpartum anxiety and adjustment. Prenatal education should be viewed as an opportunity to strengthen families by providing anticipatory guidance and improving their life skills. In short, prenatal education helps to promote healthy families during the transition to parenthood and beyond (International Childbirth Education Association, n.d.).

> **▶ Take NOTE!**
>
> *Learning about labour and birth allows women and couples to express their needs and preferences, enhances their confidence, and improves communication between themselves and the staff.*

Pain Management

Labour and birth, although a normal physiologic process, can produce significant pain. Pain during labour is a nearly universal experience. Controlling the pain without harm to the fetus or labour process is the major focus of pain management during childbirth.

Pain is a subjective experience involving a complex interaction of physiologic, spiritual, sensory, behavioural, cognitive, psychosocial, and cultural influences (Murray & Huelsmann, 2009). Cultural values and learned behaviours influence perception and response to pain, as do anxiety and fear, both of which tend to heighten the sense of pain (Murray & Huelsmann, 2009). The challenge for health care providers is to find the right combination of pain management methods to keep the pain manageable while being mindful of the maternal and fetal outcomes. Chapter 14 presents a full discussion of pain management during labour and birth.

Physiologic Responses to Labour

Labour is the physiologic process by which the uterus expels the fetus and placenta from the body. During pregnancy, progesterone secreted from the placenta suppresses the spontaneous contractions of a typical uterus, keeping the fetus within the uterus. In addition, the cervix remains firm and noncompliant. At term, however, changes that occur in the cervix make it softer. In addition, uterine contractions become more frequent and regular, signalling the onset of labour.

The labour process involves a series of rhythmic, involuntary, usually quite uncomfortable uterine muscle contractions. They bring about a shortening of muscle fibres that causes effacement and dilation of the cervix and a bursting of the fetal membranes. Then, accompanied by both reflex and voluntary contractions of the abdominal muscles (pushing), the uterine contractions result in the birth of the baby (Murray & Huelsmann, 2009). During labour, the mother and fetus make several physiologic adaptations.

Maternal Responses

The labour process stresses several of the woman's body systems, which react through numerous compensatory mechanisms. As the woman progresses through childbirth, numerous physiologic responses occur that help her adapt to the labouring process:

- Heart rate increases by 10 to 20 bpm.
- Cardiac output increases by 10% to 15% during the first stage of labour and by 30% to 50% during the second stage of labour.
- Blood pressure increases by 10 to 30 mm Hg during uterine contractions in all labour stages.
- White blood cell count increases by 25,000 to 30,000 cells/mm³, perhaps as a result of tissue trauma.
- Respiratory rate increases and more oxygen is consumed related to the increase in metabolism.

- Gastric motility and food absorption decrease, which may increase the risk of nausea and vomiting during the transition stage of labour.
- Gastric emptying and gastric pH decrease, increasing the risk for vomiting with aspiration.
- Temperature rises slightly, possibly due to an increase in muscle activity.
- Muscular aches/cramps occur as a result of the stressed musculoskeletal system.

A woman's ability to adapt to the stress of labour is influenced by her psychological and physical state. Among the many factors that affect her coping ability are:

- Previous birth experiences and their outcomes
- Current pregnancy experience (planned versus unplanned, discomforts experienced, age, risk status of pregnancy, chronic illness, weight gain)
- Cultural considerations (values and beliefs about health status)
- Support system (presence and support of a valued partner during labour)
- Childbirth preparation (attended childbirth classes and has practiced paced breathing techniques)
- Exercise during pregnancy
- Expectations of the birthing experience
- Anxiety level
- Fear of labour and loss of control
- Fatigue and weariness (Murray & Huelsmann, 2009)

Fetal Responses

Although the focus during labour may be on assessing the mother's adaptations, several physiologic adaptations occur in the fetus as well. The fetus is experiencing labour along with the mother. If the fetus is healthy, the stress of labour usually has no adverse effects. The nurse needs to be alert to any abnormalities in the fetus' adaptation to labour. Fetal responses to labour include:

- Periodic fetal heart rate accelerations and slight decelerations related to fetal movement, fundal pressure, and uterine contractions
- Decrease in circulation and perfusion to the fetus secondary to uterine contractions (a healthy fetus is able to compensate for this drop)
- Increase in arterial carbon dioxide pressure (PCO_2)
- Decrease in fetal breathing movements throughout labour

▶ *Take NOTE!*

Respiratory changes during labour help to prepare the fetus for extrauterine respiration immediately after birth.

Stages of Labour

Labour is typically divided into four stages: dilation, expulsive, placental, and restorative. Table 13.2 summarizes the major events of each stage.

The first stage is the longest: it begins with the first true contraction and ends with full dilation (opening) of the cervix. Because this stage lasts so long, it is divided into three phases, each corresponding to the progressive dilation of the cervix.

Stage two of labour, or the expulsive stage, begins when the cervix is completely dilated and ends with the birth of the newborn. The expulsive stage can last from minutes to hours.

The third stage, or the placental stage, starts after the newborn is born and ends with the separation and birth of the placenta. Continued uterine contractions typically cause the placenta to be expelled within 5 to 30 minutes.

The fourth stage, or the restorative stage, lasts from 1 to 4 hours after birth. This period is when the mother's

TABLE 13.2 STAGES AND PHASES OF LABOUR

	First Stage	Second Stage	Third Stage	Fourth Stage
Description	From 0 to 10 cm dilation; consists of three phases	From complete dilation (10 cm) to birth of the newborn; lasts up to 1 h	Separation and delivery of the placenta	1–4 h after the birth of the newborn; time of maternal physiologic adjustment
Phases	**Latent phase** (0–3 cm dilation) • Cervical dilation from 0 to 3 cm • Cervical effacement from 0% to 40% • Nullipara, lasts up to 6 h; multigravida, lasts up to 4.5 h • Contraction frequency every 5–10 min • Contraction duration 30–45 s • Contraction intensity mild to palpation **Active phase** (4–7 cm dilation) • Cervical dilation from 4 to 7 cm • Cervical effacement from 40% to 80% • Nullipara, averages 9 h; multigravida averages 6.5 h • Contraction frequency every 2–5 min • Contraction duration 45–60 s • Contraction intensity moderate to palpation **Transition phase** (8–10 cm dilation) • Cervical dilation from 8 to 10 cm • Cervical effacement from 80% to 100% • Nullipara lasts up to 3 h; multigravida, lasts up to 1 h • Contraction frequency every 1–2 min • Contraction duration 60–90 s • Contraction intensity strong by palpation	**Pelvic phase** (period of fetal descent) **Perineal phase** (period of active pushing) • Nullipara, lasts up to 1 h; multigravida, lasts up to 30 min • Contraction frequency every 2–3 min or less • Contraction duration 60–90 s • Contraction intensity strong by palpation • Strong urge to push during the later perineal phase	**Placental separation:** detaching from uterine wall **Placental expulsion:** coming outside the vaginal opening	

body begins to stabilize after the hard work of labour and the loss of the products of conception.

First Stage

During the first stage of labour, the fundamental change underlying the process is progressive dilation of the cervix. Cervical dilation is gauged subjectively by vaginal examination and is expressed in centimetres. The first stage ends when the cervix is dilated to 10 cm in diameter and is large enough to permit the passage of a fetal head of average size. The fetal membranes, or bag of waters, usually rupture during the first stage, but they may have burst earlier or may even remain intact until birth. For the primigravida, the first stage of labour lasts about 12 hours. However, this time can vary widely: for the multiparous woman, it is usually only half that.

During the first stage of labour, women usually perceive the visceral pain of diffuse abdominal cramping and uterine contractions. Pain during the first stage of labour is primarily a result of the dilation of the cervix and lower uterine segment and the distention (stretching) of these structures during contractions. The first stage is divided into three phases: latent or early phase, active phase, and transition phase.

Latent or Early Phase

The latent or early phase gives rise to the familiar signs and symptoms of labour. This phase begins with the start of regular contractions and ends when rapid cervical dilation begins. Cervical effacement occurs during this phase, and the cervix dilates from 0 to 3 cm.

Contractions usually occur every 5 to 10 minutes, last 30 to 45 seconds, and are described as mild by palpation. Effacement of the cervix is from 0% to 40%. Most women are very talkative during this period, perceiving their contractions to be similar to menstrual cramps. Women may remain at home during this phase, contacting their health care professional about the onset of labour.

For the nulliparous woman, the latent phase typically lasts about 6 hours; in the multiparous woman, it lasts about 4.5 hours (Pillitteri, 2010). During this phase, women are apprehensive but excited about the start of labour after their long gestational period.

*T*hink back to the couple who were sent home from the hospital birthing centre. Three days later Kathy awoke with a wet sensation and intense discomfort in her back, spreading around to her abdomen. She decided to go for a walk, but her contractions didn't diminish; instead, they continued to occur every few minutes and grew stronger in intensity. She and Chuck decided to go back to the hospital birthing centre. Was there a difference in the location of Kathy's discomfort this time? What changes will the admission nurse find in Kathy if this is true labour?

Active Phase

Cervical dilation begins to occur more rapidly during the active phase. The cervix usually dilates from 4 to 7 cm, with 40% to 80% effacement taking place. This phase can last about 9 hours for the nulliparous woman and 6.5 hours for the multiparous woman (Varney, Kriebs, & Gegor, 2004). The fetus descends farther in the pelvis. Contractions become more frequent (every 2 to 5 minutes) and increase in duration (45 to 60 seconds). The woman's discomfort intensifies (moderate to strong by palpation). She becomes more intense and inwardly focused, absorbed in the serious work of her labour. She limits interactions with those in the room. If she and her partner have attended childbirth education classes, she will begin to use the relaxation and paced breathing techniques that they learned to cope with the contractions. The typical dilation rate for the nulliparous woman is 1.2 cm/hour; for the multiparous woman, it is 1.5 cm/hour (Cunningham et al., 2010).

Transition Phase

The transition phase is the last phase of the first stage of labour. During this phase, dilation slows, progressing from 8 to 10 cm, with effacement from 80% to 100%. The transition phase is the most difficult and, fortunately, the shortest phase for the woman. During transition, the contractions are stronger (hard by palpation), more painful, and more frequent (every 1 to 2 minutes), and they last longer (60 to 90 seconds). The average rate of fetal descent is 1 cm/hour in nulliparous women and 2 cm/hour in multiparous women. Pressure on the rectum is great and there is a strong desire to contract the abdominal muscles and push.

Other maternal features during the transitional phase include nausea and vomiting, trembling extremities, backache, increased apprehension and irritability, restless movement, increased bloody show from the vagina, inability to relax, diaphoresis, feelings of loss of control, and being overwhelmed (the woman may say, "I can't take it anymore"). This phase should not last longer than 3 hours for nulliparas and 1 hour for multigravidas (Cunningham et al., 2010).

*I*n assessing Kathy, the nurse finds she is 4 cm dilated and 50% effaced with ruptured membranes. In what stage and phase of labour would this assessment finding place Kathy?

Second Stage

The second stage of labour begins with complete cervical dilation (10 cm) and effacement and ends with the birth of the newborn. Although the previous stage of labour primarily involved the thinning and opening of the cervix, this stage involves moving the fetus through

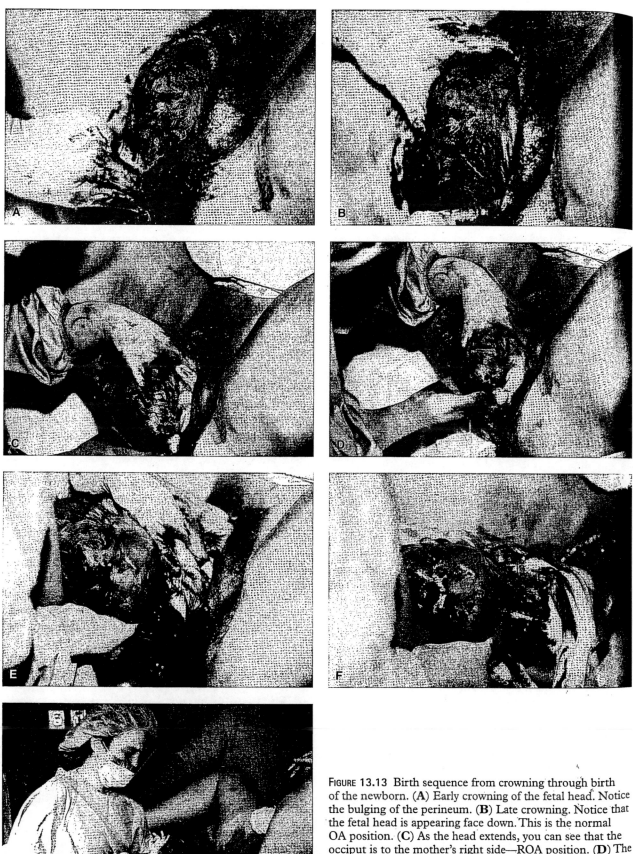

FIGURE 13.13 Birth sequence from crowning through birth of the newborn. (**A**) Early crowning of the fetal head. Notice the bulging of the perineum. (**B**) Late crowning. Notice that the fetal head is appearing face down. This is the normal OA position. (**C**) As the head extends, you can see that the occiput is to the mother's right side—ROA position. (**D**) The cardinal movement of extension. (**E**) The shoulders are born. Notice how the head has turned to line up with the shoulders—the cardinal movement of external rotation. (**F**) The body easily follows the shoulders. (**G**) The newborn is held for the first time! (© B. Proud.)

43

the birth canal and out of the body. The cardinal movements of labour occur during the early phase of passive descent in the second stage of labour.

Contractions occur every 2 to 3 minutes, last 60 to 90 seconds, and are described as strong by palpation. The average length of the second stage of labour in a nullipara is approximately 1 hour and less than half that time for the multigravida (Fig. 13.13). During this expulsive stage, the mother usually feels more in control and less irritable and agitated. She is focused on the work of pushing. Traditionally, women have been taught to hold their breath to the count of 10, inhale again, push again, and repeat the process several times during a contraction. This sustained, strenuous style of pushing has been shown to lead to hemodynamic changes in the mother and interfere with oxygen exchange between the mother and the fetus. In addition, it is associated with pelvic floor damage: the longer the push, the more damage to the pelvic floor (Cooke, 2010). The newest protocol from Association of Women's Health, Obstetric and Neonatal Nurses (AWHONN) recommends an open-glottis method in which air is released during pushing to prevent the build-up of intrathoracic pressure. Doing so also supports mother's involuntary bearing-down efforts (Roberts, Gonzalez, & Sampselle, 2007).

During the second stage of labour, pushing can either follow the mother's spontaneous urge or be directed by the caregiver. Much debate still exists between spontaneous and directed pushing during the second stage of labour. Although directed pushing is common practice in hospitals, there is evidence to suggest that directed pushing should be avoided. Research seems to support spontaneous pushing—when the woman is allowed to follow her own instincts (Hanson, 2009). Evidence is mounting that the management of the second stage, particularly pushing, is a modifiable risk factor in long-term perinatal outcomes. Valsalva (holding breath) bearing down and supine maternal position are linked to negative maternal–fetal hemodynamics and outcomes. The adoption of a physiologic, woman-directed approach to bearing down is advocated (Cooke, 2010).

Evidence-based practice focuses on a physiologic approach to the second stage of labour. Behaviours demonstrated by labouring women during this time include pushing at the onset of the urge to bear down, using their own pattern and technique of bearing down in response to sensations they experience, using open-glottis bearing down with contractions, pushing with variations in strength and duration, pushing down with progressive intensity, and using multiple positions to increase progress and comfort. This approach is in stark contrast to management by arbitrary time limits and the directed bearing-down efforts seen in practice today (Martin, 2009).

Labouring down (promotion of passive descent) is an alternative strategy for second-stage management in women with epidurals. Using this approach, the fetus descends and is born without coached maternal pushing.

The second stage of labour has two phases (pelvic and perineal) related to the existence and quality of the maternal urge to push and to obstetric conditions related to fetal descent. The early phase of the second stage is called pelvic phase because it is during this phase that the fetal head is negotiating the pelvis, rotating, and advancing in descent. The later phase is called perineal phase because at this point the fetal head is lower in the pelvis and is distending the perineum. The occurrence of a strong urge to push characterizes the later phase of the second stage and has also been called phase of active pushing (Hanson, 2009).

The later perineal phase occurs when the mother feels a tremendous urge to push as the fetal head is lowered and is distending the perineum. The perineum bulges and there is an increase in bloody show. The fetal head becomes apparent at the vaginal opening but disappears between contractions. When the top of the head no longer regresses between contractions, it is said to have crowned. The fetus rotates as it manoeuvres out (Fig. 13.13).

Third Stage

The third stage of labour begins with the birth of the newborn and ends with the separation and birth of the placenta. It consists of two phases: placental separation and placental expulsion.

Placental Separation

After the infant is born, the uterus continues to contract strongly and can now retract, decreasing markedly in size. These contractions cause the placenta to pull away from the uterine wall. The following signs of separation indicate that the placenta is ready to deliver:

- The uterus rises upward.
- The umbilical cord lengthens.
- A sudden trickle of blood is released from the vaginal opening.
- The uterus changes its shape to globular.

Spontaneous birth of the placenta occurs in one of two ways: the fetal side (shiny grey side) presenting first (called Schultz's mechanism or, more commonly, "shiny Schultz's") or the maternal side (red raw side) presenting first (termed Duncan's mechanism or "dirty Duncan").

Placental Expulsion

After separation of the placenta from the uterine wall, continued uterine contractions cause the placenta to be expelled within 2 to 30 minutes unless there is gentle external traction to assist. After the placenta is expelled, the uterus is massaged briefly by the attending physician or midwife until it is firm so that uterine blood vessels constrict, minimizing the possibility of hemorrhage. Normal blood loss is approximately 500 to 600 mL for a vaginal birth and 1,000 mL for a cesarean birth (Cunningham et al., 2010).

If the placenta does not spontaneously deliver, the health care professional assists with its removal by manual extraction. On expulsion, the placenta is inspected for its intactness by the health care professional and the nurse to make sure that all sections are present. If any piece is still attached to the uterine wall, it places the woman at risk for postpartum hemorrhage because it becomes a space-occupying object that interferes with the ability of the uterus to contract fully and effectively.

Fourth Stage

The fourth stage begins with completion of the expulsion of the placenta and membranes and ends with the initial physiologic adjustment and stabilization of the mother (1 to 4 hours after birth). This stage initiates the postpartum period. The mother usually feels a sense of peace and excitement, is wide awake, and is very talkative initially. The attachment process begins with her inspecting her newborn and desiring to cuddle and breastfeed him or her. The mother's fundus should be firm and well contracted. Typically it is located at the midline between the umbilicus and the symphysis, but it then slowly rises to the level of the umbilicus during the first hour after birth (Ward & Hisley, 2009). If the uterus becomes boggy, it is massaged to keep it firm. The lochia (vaginal discharge) is red, mixed with small clots, and of moderate flow. If the woman has had an episiotomy during the second stage of labour, it should be intact, with the edges approximated and clean and no redness or edema present.

The focus during this stage is to monitor the mother closely to prevent hemorrhage, bladder distention, and venous thrombosis. Usually the mother is thirsty and hungry during this time and may request food and drink. Her bladder is hypotonic and thus she has limited sensation to acknowledge a full bladder or to void. Vital signs, the amount and consistency of the vaginal discharge (lochia), and the uterine fundus are usually monitored every 15 minutes for at least 1 hour. The woman will be feeling cramp-like discomfort during this time due to the contracting uterus.

∎∎∎ Key Concepts

- ▢ Labour is a complex, multifaceted interaction between the mother and the fetus. Thus, it is difficult to determine exactly why labour begins and what initiates it.
- ▢ Before the onset of labour, a pregnant woman's body undergoes several changes in preparation for the birth of the newborn, often leading to characteristic signs and symptoms that suggest that labour is near. These changes include cervical changes, lightening, increased energy level, bloody show, Braxton Hicks contractions, and spontaneous rupture of membranes.
- ▢ False labour is a condition seen during the latter weeks of some pregnancies in which irregular uterine contractions are felt, but the cervix is not affected.
- ▢ The critical factors in labour and birth are designated as the 10 P's: passageway (birth canal), passenger (fetus and placenta), powers (contractions), psychological response, maternal position, philosophy (low tech, high touch), partners (support caregivers), patience (natural timing), patient preparation (childbirth knowledge base), and pain control (comfort measures).
- ▢ The size and shape of a woman's pelvis are determining factors for a vaginal birth. The female pelvis is classified according to four main groups: anthropoid, android, gynecoid, and platypelloid.
- ▢ The labour process comprises of a series of rhythmic, involuntary, usually quite uncomfortable uterine muscle contractions that bring about a shortening (effacement) and opening (dilation) of the cervix and a bursting of the fetal membranes. Important parameters of uterine contractions are frequency, duration, and intensity.
- ▢ The diameters of the fetal skull vary considerably, with some diameters shortening and others lengthening as the head is moulded during the labour and birth process.
- ▢ Pain during labour is a nearly universal experience for childbearing women. Having a strong sense of self and meaningful support from others can often help women manage labour well and reduce their sensation of pain.
- ▢ Preparing mentally for childbirth is important for women to enable them to work with the natural forces of labour and not against them.
- ▢ As the woman experiences and progresses through childbirth, numerous physiologic responses occur that assist her adaptation to the labouring process.
- ▢ Labour is typically divided into four stages that are unequal in length.
- ▢ During the first stage of labour, the fundamental change underlying the process is progressive dilation of the cervix. It is further divided into three phases: latent phase, active phase, and transition.
- ▢ The second stage of labour begins with complete cervical dilation (10 cm) and effacement and ends with the birth of the infant.
- ▢ The third stage of labour is that of separation and birth of the placenta. It consists of two phases: placental separation and placental expulsion.
- ▢ The fourth stage of labour begins after the birth of the placenta and membranes and ends with the initial physiologic adjustment and stabilization of the mother (1 to 4 hours).

REFERENCES

Association of Women's Health, Obstetric and Neonatal Nurses. (2007). *AWHONN late preterm infant initiative: What parents of late preterm (near-term) infants need to know.* Retrieved February 10, 2012 from http://www.awhonn.org/awhonn/content.do?name=02_PracticeResources/2C3_Focus_NearTermInfant.htm

Barrett, S. J., & Stark, M. A. (2010). Factors associated with labour support behaviors of nurses. *Journal of Perinatal Education, 19*(1), 12–18.

Chalmers, B., Kaczorowski, J., Darling, E., Heaman, M., Fell, D. B., O'Brien, B., & Lee, L. (2010). Cesarean and vaginal birth in Canadian women: A comparison of experiences. *Birth, 37*(1), 44–49.

Chalmers, B., Kaczorowski, J., Levitt, C., Dzakpasu, S., O'Brien, B., Lee, L., Boscoe, M., & Young, D. (2009). Use of routine interventions in vaginal labour and birth: Findings from the Maternity Experiences Survey. *Birth, 36*(1), 13–25.

Cooke, A. (2010). When will we change practice and stop directing pushing in labour? *British Journal of Midwifery, 18*(2), 76–81.

Cunningham, F. G., Leveno, K. J., Bloom, S. L., Hauth, J. C., Rouse, D. J., & Spong, C. Y. (2010). *Williams obstetrics* (23rd ed.). New York: McGraw-Hill.

Davidson, M. R., London, M. L., Ladewig, P. A. W. (2008). *Olds' maternal–newborn nursing and women's health across the lifespan.* Upper Saddle River, NJ: Pearson/Prentice Hall.

Delaney, M., & Roggensack, A. (2008). Guidelines for the management of pregnancy at 41 + 0 to 42 + 0 weeks. *Journal of Obstetrics and Gynaecology Canada, 214,* 800–810.

Dunne, C., Da Silva, O., Schmidt, G., & Natale, R. (2009). outcomes of elective labour induction and elective caesarean section in low-risk pregnancies between 37 and 41 weeks' gestation. *Journal of Obstetrics and Gynaecology Canada, 31*(12), 1124–1130.

Hanson, L. (2009). Second-stage labour care: Challenges in spontaneous bearing down. *Journal of Perinatal and Neonatal Nursing, 23*(1), 31–39.

Hanson, S., Hunter, L. P., Bormann, J. R., & Sobo, E. J. (2009). Paternal fears of childbirth: A literature review. *Journal of Perinatal Education, 18*(4), 12–20.

Hodnett, E. D., Gates, S., Hofmeyr, G. J., & Sakala, C. (2011). Continuous support for women during childbirth. *Cochrane Database of Systematic Reviews, 2,* CD003766. doi: 10.1002/14651858. CD003766.pub3

International Childbirth Education Association. (n.d.). *Mission and philosophy.* Retrieved February 10, 2012 from www.icea.org/content/mission

Jimenez, V., Klein, M., Hivon, M., & Mason, C. (2010). A mirage of change: Family-centered maternity care in practice. *Birth, 37*(2), 160–167.

Kenner, C., & Lott, J. W. (2007). *Comprehensive neonatal care: An interdisciplinary approach* (4th ed.). St. Louis, MO: Saunders Elsevier.

Leap, N., Sandall, J., Buckland, S., & Huber, U. (2010). Journey to confidence: Women's experiences of pain in labour and relational continuity of care. *Journal of Midwifery and Women's Health, 55*(3), 234–242.

Martin, C. J. H. (2009). Effects of Valsalva manoeuvre on maternal and fetal wellbeing. *British Journal of Midwifery, 17*(5), 279–285.

Martin, E. J., & Kennedy, B. B. (2009a). Maternal and fetal response to labor. In B. B. Kennedy, D. J. Ruth, & E. J. Martin (Eds.), *Intrapartum management modules* (pp. 17–45). Philadelphia: Wolters Kluwer.

Martin, E. J., & Kennedy, B. B. (2009b). Overview of labour. In B. B. Kennedy, D. J. Ruth, & E. J. Martin (Eds.), *Intrapartum management modules.* Philadelphia: Wolters Kluwer.

McDonald, G. (2010). Diagnosing the latent phase of labour: Use of the partogram. *British Journal of Midwifery, 18*(10), 630–637.

Murray, M. L., & Huelsmann, G. M. (2009). *Labor and delivery nursing: A guide to evidence-based practice.* New York: Springer.

Nettina, S. M. (2010). *Lippincott manual of nursing practice.* Philadelphia: Lippincott.

Pillitteri, A. (2010). *Maternal & child health nursing: Care of the childbearing & childrearing family* (6th ed.). Philadelphia: Wolters Kluwer.

Public Health Agency of Canada. (2008). *Canadian perinatal health report, 2008 edition.* Retrieved February 10, 2012 from www.publichealth.gc.ca/cphr/

Roberts, J. M., Gonzalez, C. B., & Sampselle, C. (2007). Why do supportive birth attendants become directive of maternal bearing-down efforts in second-stage labor? *Journal of Midwifery and Women's Health, 52*(2), 134–141.

Romano, A. M., & Lothian, J. A. (2008). Promoting, protecting, and supporting normal birth: A look at the evidence. *Journal of Obstetric, Gynecologic, & Neonatal Nursing, 37*(1), 94–105.

Society of Obstetricians and Gynaecologists of Canada. (2008). *Rising C-section rates add risks during childbirth and place excess strain on the healthcare system, warn Canadian obstetricians.* Retrieved February 10, 2012 from www.sogc.org/media/pdf/advisories/ACM_June2008_C-Sections_e.pdf

Varney, H., Kriebs, J. M., & Gegor, C. L. (2004). *Varney's midwifery* (4th. ed.). Boston: Jones and Bartlett.

Ward, S., & Hisley, S. (2009). *Maternal-child nursing care.* Philadelphia: F.A. Davis.

Wilson, B. L., Effkren, J., & Butler, R. J. (2010). Relationship between cesarean section and labor induction. *Journal of Nursing Scholarship, 42*(2), 130–138.

Zwelling, E. (2010). Overcoming the challenges: Maternal movement. *The American Journal of Maternal/Child Nursing, 35*(2), 72–78.

The labouring and birthing process is a life-changing event for many women. Nurses need to be respectful, available, encouraging, supportive, and professional in dealing with all women. A recent study by Bryanton, Gagnon, Johnston, et al. (2008) demonstrated that nurses can promote a positive birth experience by responding to the needs of the labouring woman through appropriate nursing interventions.

The health of mothers and their infants is of critical importance, both as a reflection of the current health status of a large segment of our population and as a predictor of the health of the next generation. The Society of Obstetricians and Gynaecologists of Canada (SOGC) established a National Birthing Initiative in 2008 with the overall goal of ensuring that all Canadian women have access to quality maternity care that is centred around women and family. The framework for this initiative arose from the Multidisciplinary Collaborative Primary Maternity Care Project (MCP²), which produced national guidelines in 2006 for collaborative models of care in Canada (SOGC, 2008a).

This chapter provides information about nursing management during labour and birth. First, the essentials for in-depth assessment of maternal and fetal status during labour and birth are discussed. This is followed by a thorough description of the major methods of promoting comfort and providing pain management. The chapter concludes by putting all the information together with a discussion of the nursing care specific to each stage of labour, including the necessary data to be obtained with the admission assessment, methods to evaluate labour progress during the first stage of labour, and key nursing measures that focus on maternal and fetal assessments and pain relief for all stages of labour.

Maternal Assessment During Labour and Birth

During labour and birth, various techniques are used to assess maternal status. These techniques provide an ongoing source of data to determine the woman's response and her progress in labour. Assess maternal vital signs, including temperature, blood pressure, pulse, respiration, and pain, which are primary components of the physical examination and ongoing assessment. Also review the prenatal record to identify risk factors that may contribute to a decrease in uteroplacental circulation during labour. If there is no vaginal bleeding on admission, a vaginal examination is performed to assess cervical dilation, after which it is monitored periodically as necessary to identify progress. Evaluate maternal pain and the effectiveness of pain-management strategies at regular intervals during labour and birth.

Vaginal Examination

Although not all nurses perform vaginal examinations on labouring women in all practice settings, most nurses working in community hospitals do so because physicians are not routinely present in labour and birth suites. Nurses care for women and attend almost every birth in Canada. It is not uncommon for the nurse to be the only health care provider present, in the absence of a physician or midwife. Thus appropriate educational preparation for nurses in these settings is imperative as new models of interprofessional collaborative care come into play (SOGC, 2008a).

> ▶ **Take** NOTE!
>
> *A vaginal examination is an assessment skill that takes time and experience to develop; only by doing it frequently in clinical practice can the practitioner's skill level improve.*

The purpose of performing a vaginal examination is to assess the amount of cervical dilation, the percentage of cervical effacement, and the fetal membrane status and to gather information on presentation, position, station, degree of fetal head flexion, and presence of fetal skull swelling or molding (Fig. 14.1). Prepare the woman by informing her about the procedure, what information will be obtained from it, how she can assist with the procedure, how it will be performed, and who will be performing it.

The woman is typically on her back during the vaginal examination. The vaginal examination is performed gently, with concern for the woman's comfort. If it is the

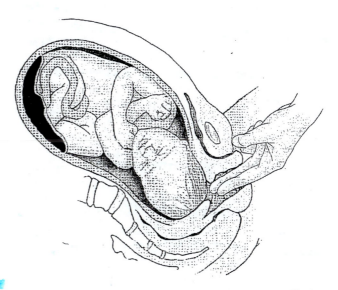

FIGURE **14.1** Vaginal examination to determine cervical dilation and effacement.

initial vaginal examination to check for membrane status, water is used as a lubricant. If the membranes have already ruptured, an antiseptic solution is used to prevent an ascending infection. After donning sterile gloves, the examiner inserts his or her index and middle fingers into the vaginal introitus. Next, the cervix is palpated to assess dilation, effacement, and position (e.g., posterior or anterior). If the cervix is open to any degree, the presenting fetal part, fetal position, station, and presence of molding can be assessed. In addition, the membranes can be evaluated and described as intact, bulging, or ruptured.

At the conclusion of the vaginal examination, the findings are discussed with the woman and her partner to bring them up to date about labour progress. In addition, the findings are documented either electronically or in writing and reported to the primary health care professional in charge of the case.

Cervical Dilation and Effacement

The amount of cervical dilation and the degree of cervical effacement are key areas assessed during the vaginal examination as the cervix is palpated with the gloved index finger. Although this finding is somewhat subjective, experienced examiners typically come up with similar findings. The width of the cervical opening determines dilation, and the length of the cervix assesses effacement. The information yielded by this examination serves as a basis for determining which stage of labour the woman is in and what her ongoing care should be.

Fetal Descent and Presenting Part

In addition to cervical dilation and effacement findings, the vaginal examination can also determine fetal descent (station) and presenting part. During the vaginal examination, the gloved index finger is used to palpate the fetal skull (if vertex presentation) through the opened cervix or the buttocks in the case of a breech presentation. Station is assessed in relation to the maternal ischial spines and the presenting fetal part. These spines are not sharp protrusions but rather blunted prominences at the midpelvis. The ischial spines serve as landmarks and have been designated as zero station. If the presenting part is palpated higher than the maternal ischial spines, a negative number is assigned; if the presenting fetal part is felt below the maternal ischial spines, a plus number is assigned, denoting how many centimetres below zero station.

Progressive fetal descent (–5 to +4) is the expected norm during labour—moving downward from the negative stations to zero station to the positive stations in a timely manner. If progressive fetal descent does not occur, a disproportion between the maternal pelvis and the fetus might exist and needs to be investigated.

Rupture of Membranes

The integrity of the membranes can be determined during the vaginal examination. Typically, if intact, the membranes will be felt as a soft bulge that is more prominent during a contraction. If the membranes have ruptured, the woman may have reported a sudden gush of fluid. Membrane rupture also may occur as a slow trickle of fluid. When membranes rupture, the priority focus should be on assessing fetal heart rate (FHR) first to identify a deceleration, which might indicate cord compression secondary to cord prolapse. If the membranes are ruptured when the woman comes to the hospital, it is important to ascertain when it occurred. Prolonged ruptured membranes increase the risk of infection as a result of ascending vaginal organisms for both mother and fetus. Signs of intrauterine infection to be alert for include maternal fever, fetal and maternal tachycardia, foul odour of vaginal discharge, and an increase in white blood cell count.

To confirm that membranes have ruptured, a sample of fluid is taken from the vagina and tested with nitrazine paper to determine the fluid's pH. Vaginal fluid is acidic, whereas amniotic fluid is alkaline and turns nitrazine paper blue. Sometimes, however, false-positive results may occur, especially in women experiencing a large amount of bloody show, because blood is alkaline. The membranes are most likely intact if the nitrazine test tape remains yellow to olive green, suggesting an acidic pH from 5 to 6. The membranes are probably ruptured if the nitrazine test tape turns a blue-green to deep blue, suggesting an alkaline pH from 6.5 to 7.5 (Evans, Evans, Brown, et al., 2010; Ladewig, London, & Davidson, 2009; Moldenhauer, 2008).

If the nitrazine test is inconclusive, an additional test, called the fern test, can be used to confirm rupture of membranes. With this test, a sample of fluid is obtained, applied to a microscope slide, and allowed to dry. Using a microscope, the slide is examined for a characteristic fern pattern that indicates the presence of amniotic fluid.

Assessing Uterine Contractions

The primary power of labour is uterine contractions, which are involuntary. Uterine contractions increase intrauterine pressure, causing tension on the cervix. This tension leads to cervical dilation and thinning, which in turn eventually forces the fetus through the birth canal. Normal uterine contractions have a contraction (systole) and a relaxation (diastole) phase. The contraction resembles a wave, moving downward to the cervix and upward to the fundus of the uterus. Each contraction starts with a building up (increment), gradually reaching an acme (peak intensity), and then a letting down (decrement). Each contraction is followed by an interval of rest, which ends when the next contraction begins. At the acme (peak) of the contraction, the entire uterus is contracting, with the greatest intensity in the fundal area. The relaxation phase follows and occurs simultaneously throughout the uterus.

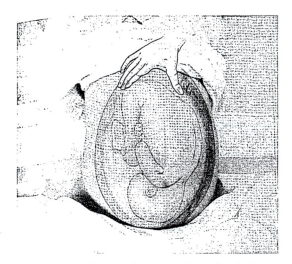

FIGURE 14.2 Nurse palpating the woman's fundus during a contraction.

Uterine contractions during labour are monitored by palpation, external fetal monitoring (tocodynamometer), or internal monitoring (intrauterine pressure catheter [IUPC]). Assessment of the contractions includes frequency, duration, intensity, and uterine resting tone. The type of information obtained is determined by the method selected (Kennedy, Ruth, & Martin, 2009). (See Chapter 13 for a more detailed discussion.) To palpate the fundus for contraction intensity, place the pads of your fingers on the fundus and describe how it feels: like the tip of the nose (mild), like the chin (moderate), or like the forehead (strong). Palpation of intensity is a subjective judgment of the indentability of the uterine wall; a descriptive term is assigned (mild, moderate, or strong) (Fig. 14.2).

> ▷ **Take** NOTE!
>
> *Frequent clinical experience is needed to gain accuracy in assessing the intensity of uterine contractions.*

The second method used to assess the intensity of uterine contractions is electronic fetal monitoring (EFM). EFM can be done either externally or internally, although internal monitoring provides a more accurate measurement of intensity than external monitoring (Matsuo, Scanlon, Atlas, et al., 2008). When using the tocodynamometer, contraction intensity must also be assessed by palpation (Kennedy et al., 2009).

For women at risk for preterm birth, home uterine activity monitoring can be used to screen for prelabour uterine contractility so that escalating contractility can be identified, allowing earlier intervention to prevent preterm birth. The home uterine activity monitor consists of a pressure sensor attached to a belt that is held against the abdomen and a recording/storage device that is carried on a belt or hung from the shoulder. Uterine activity is typically recorded by the woman for 1 hour twice daily, while she is performing routine activities. The stored data are transmitted via telephone to a perinatal nurse, and a receiving device prints out the data. The woman is contacted if there are any problems.

There is no consensus in the literature to show that home monitoring improves outcomes for high-risk mothers and fetuses (Currell, Urquhart, Harlow, et al., 2009). Iams, Romero, Culhane, et al. (2008) reviewed the literature to identify what primary, secondary, or tertiary approaches work best to reduce the morbidity and mortality associated with preterm birth from early contractions. They found that even when high-risk women met daily with health care professionals, their rates of preterm birth did not change. The most successful efforts identified thus far have been from active tertiary treatment to stop contractions with, for example, the use of tocolytics. The SOGC (2007) recommends that the frequency of antenatal fetal testing should be individualized to reflect the risk factor(s) present.

Performing Leopold's Manoeuvres

Leopold's manoeuvres are a method for determining the presentation, position, and lie of the fetus through the use of four specific steps (Pillitteri, 2010). This method involves inspection and palpation of the maternal abdomen as a screening assessment for malpresentation. A longitudinal lie is expected, and the presentation can be cephalic, breech, or shoulder. Each manoeuvre answers a question:

- What fetal part (head or buttocks) is located in the fundus (top of the uterus)?
- On which maternal side is the fetal back located? (Fetal heart tones are best auscultated through the back of the fetus.)
- What is the presenting part?
- Is the fetal head flexed and engaged in the pelvis?

Leopold's manoeuvres are described in Nursing Procedure 14.1.

Fetal Assessment During Labour and Birth

A fetal assessment identifies well-being or signs that indicate compromise. The character of the amniotic fluid is assessed, but the fetal assessment focuses primarily on determining the FHR pattern. Fetal scalp sampling, fetal pulse oximetry (FPO), and fetal stimulation are additional assessments performed as necessary in the case of questionable FHR patterns.

Nursing Procedure 14.1

PERFORMING LEOPOLD'S MANOEUVRES

Purpose: To Determine Fetal Presentation, Position, and Lie

1. Place the woman in the supine position and stand beside her.
2. Perform the first manoeuvre to determine presentation.
   a. Facing the woman's head, place both hands on the abdomen to determine fetal position in the uterine fundus.
   b. Feel for the buttocks, which will feel soft and irregular (indicates vertex presentation); feel for the head, which will feel hard, smooth, and round (indicates a breech presentation).

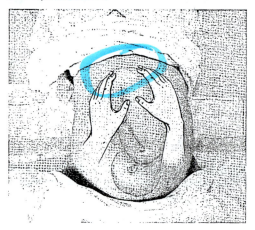

3. Complete the second manoeuvre to determine position.
   a. While still facing the woman, move hands down the lateral sides of the abdomen to palpate on which side the back is located (feels hard and smooth).
   b. Continue to palpate to determine on which side the limbs are located (irregular nodules with kicking and movement).

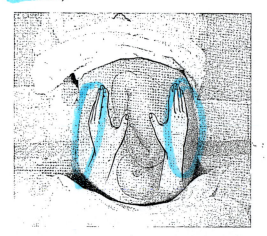

4. Perform the third manoeuvre to confirm presentation.
   a. Move hands down the sides of the abdomen to grasp the lower uterine segment and palpate the area just above the symphysis pubis.

   b. Place thumb and fingers of one hand apart and grasp the presenting part by bringing fingers together.
   c. Feel for the presenting part. If the presenting part is the head, it will be round, firm, and ballottable; if it is the buttocks, it will feel soft and irregular.

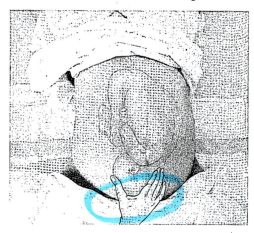

5. Perform the fourth manoeuvre to determine attitude.
   a. Turn to face the client's feet and use the tips of the first three fingers of each hand to palpate the abdomen.
   b. Move fingers toward each other while applying downward pressure in the direction of the symphysis pubis. If you palpate a hard area on the side opposite the fetal back, the fetus is in flexion, because you have palpated the chin. If the hard area is on the same side as the back, the fetus is in extension, because the area palpated is the occiput.

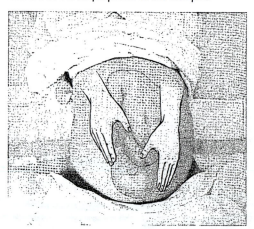

Also, note how your hands move. If the hands move together easily, the fetal head is not descended into the woman's pelvic inlet. If the hands do not move together and stop because of resistance, the fetal head is engaged into the woman's pelvic inlet (Lowdermilk et al., 2010).

Analysis of Amniotic Fluid

Amniotic fluid should be clear when the membranes rupture, either spontaneously or artificially through an amniotomy (a disposable plastic hook [Amnihook] is used to perforate the amniotic sac). Cloudy or foul-smelling amniotic fluid indicates infection. Green fluid may indicate that the fetus has passed meconium secondary to transient hypoxia; however, it is considered a normal occurrence if the fetus is in a breech presentation. If it is determined that meconium-stained amniotic fluid is due to fetal hypoxia, the maternity and pediatric teams work together to prevent meconium aspiration syndrome. This would necessitate suctioning after the head is born before the infant takes a breath and perhaps direct tracheal suctioning after birth if the Apgar score is low. In some cases, an amnioinfusion (introduction of warmed, sterile normal saline or Ringer's lactate solution into the uterus) is used to dilute moderate to heavy meconium released in utero to assist in preventing meconium aspiration syndrome.

Analysis of the FHR

Analysis of the FHR is one of the primary evaluation tools used to determine fetal oxygen status indirectly. FHR assessment can be done intermittently using a fetoscope (a modified stethoscope attached to a headpiece) or a Doppler (ultrasound) device, or continuously with an electronic fetal monitor applied externally or internally.

Intermittent FHR Monitoring

FHR monitoring through intermittent auscultation involves the use of a fetoscope or a hand-held Doppler device that uses ultrasound waves that bounce off the fetal heart, producing echoes or clicks that reflect the rate of the fetal heart (Fig. 14.3). The SOGC (2007) recommends the use of intermittent auscultation as the preferred method of intrapartum fetal surveillance in low-risk women in the active phase of labour.

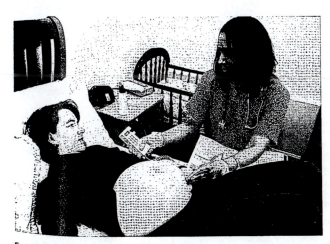

FIGURE 14.3 Auscultating fetal heart rate.

> ▷ **Take** *NOTE!*
>
> *Intermittent auscultation is less invasive, inexpensive, easy to use, and does not restrict movement (Lowdermilk, Perry, & Cashion, 2010; SOGC, 2007), whether in hospital or community-based settings. Studies show little difference in fetal or neonatal outcomes when intermittent auscultation is used as an alternative to EFM (Lavender, Hart, & Smyth, 2008; Steer, 2008.)*

Intermittent FHR monitoring allows the woman to be mobile in the first stage of labour. She is free to move around and change position at will since she is not attached to a stationary electronic fetal monitor. However, intermittent monitoring does not provide a continuous FHR recording and does not document how the fetus responds to the stress of labour (unless listening is done during the contraction). The best way to assess fetal well-being would be to start listening to the FHR at the end of the contraction (not after one) so that late decelerations can be detected. However, the pressure of the device during a contraction is uncomfortable and can distract the woman from using her paced-breathing patterns.

Intermittent FHR auscultation can be used to detect FHR baseline and rhythm and changes from baseline. However, it cannot be used to assess variability and transient changes as no visual record is available to assess FHR patterns (Tucker, Miller, & Miller, 2009). During intermittent auscultation to establish a baseline, the FHR is assessed for a full minute after a contraction. From then on, unless there is a problem, listening for 30 seconds and multiplying the value by two is sufficient. The FHR should be assessed regularly to ensure that it is in the same range after the contraction as it was in the previous assessments. If not, assess possible causes for the change (SOGC, 2007). If the woman experiences a change in condition during labour, auscultation assessments should be more frequent. The SOGC (2007) also recommends checking the FHR after any invasive procedure, rupture of membranes, vaginal examinations, and administration of medications. The FHR is heard most clearly at the fetal back. In a cephalic presentation, the FHR is best heard in the lower quadrant of the maternal abdomen. In a breech presentation, it is heard at or above the level of the maternal umbilicus (Fig. 14.4). As labour progresses, the FHR location will change accordingly as the fetus descends into the maternal pelvis for the birthing process. To ensure that the maternal heart rate is not confused with the FHR, palpate the client's radial pulse simultaneously while the FHR is being auscultated through the abdomen.

The procedure for using a fetoscope or Doppler device to assess FHR is similar (see Nursing Procedure 12.1

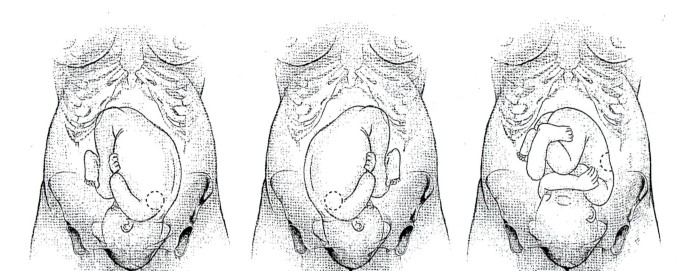

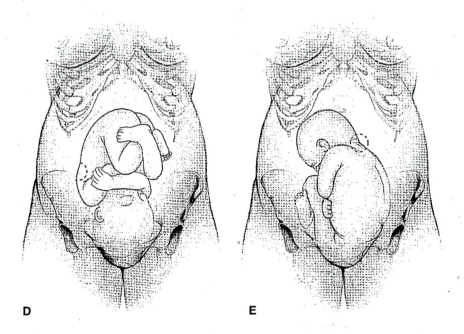

FIGURE 14.4 Locations for auscultating fetal heart rate based on fetal position. (**A**) Left occiput anterior (LOA). (**B**) Right occiput anterior (ROA). (**C**) Left occiput posterior (LOP). (**D**) Right occiput posterior (ROP). (**E**) Left sacral anterior (LSA).

in Chapter 12). The main difference is that a small amount of water-soluble gel is applied to the woman's abdomen or ultrasound device before auscultation with the Doppler device to promote sound wave transmission. This gel is not needed when a fetoscope is used. Usually the FHR is best heard in the woman's lower abdominal quadrants; if it is not found quickly, it may help to locate the fetal back by performing Leopold's manoeuvres.

Although the intermittent method of FHR assessment allows the client to move about during labour, the information obtained fails to provide a complete picture of the well-being of the fetus moment to moment. This leads to the question of what the fetal status is during the times that are not assessed. For women who are considered at low risk for complications, this period of non-assessment is not a problem. However, for the undiagnosed high-risk woman, it might prove ominous.

The SOGC is the leading national obstetric professional organization in Canada and provides guidelines for evidence-based obstetric care, including guidelines for assessment during labour and delivery. Comprising gynaecologists, obstetricians, family physicians, nurses, midwives, and allied health professionals, the SOGC works collaboratively with several other national maternity health care providers: the College of Family Physicians of Canada (CFP), the Canadian Association of Midwives (CAM), the Canadian Association of Perinatal and Women's Health Nurses (CAPWHN), and the Society of Rural Physicians of Canada (SRPC), all of whom help inform the clinical practice guidelines and support the initiatives of the SOGC. The SOGC cautions that the information it provides should not dictate an exclusive course of treatment/procedure and should not substitute for the advice of a physician.

Intermittent auscultation is the recommended fetal surveillance method during labour for healthy women without identified risk factors for adverse perinatal outcome (SOGC, 2007, 2008b). The following guidelines are recommended for assessing FHR by intermittent auscultation:

• Admission fetal heart tracings are not recommended for healthy women at term in labour in the absence of risk factors for adverse perinatal outcome, as there is no evident benefit.
• Intensive fetal surveillance by intermittent auscultation or EFM requires the continuous presence of nursing or midwifery staff.
  • Assess FHR on admission and every hour in the latent phase of the first stage of labour.
  • Assess FHR every 15 to 30 minutes during the active phase of the first stage of labour.
  • Assess FHR every 5 minutes during the active second stage of labour.

The SOGC recommendation of having the continuous presence of a nurse or nurse midwife suggests that adequate staffing is essential with intermittent FHR monitoring to ensure optimal outcomes for mother and fetus. The overall goal of these guidelines is to contribute to the best possible fetal outcomes while maintaining the lowest possible rates of intervention (SOGC, 2007).

Continuous Electronic Fetal Monitoring (Cardiotocography)

Electronic fetal monitoring is a term used interchangeably with **cardiotocography (CTG),** which uses an external monitor to record changes in the FHR with an aim to identify babies who may be short of oxygen

(hypoxic) (Alfirevic, Devane, & Gyte, 2008; SOGC, 2007). The monitor produces a sound with each heartbeat and provides a visual graphic record of the FHR pattern. CTG is considered by some to be a more precise term than EFM because it also monitors the mother's contractions. In addition, other forms of fetal monitoring are also considered electronic, such as electrocardiography and FPO (Alfirevic et al., 2008). The purpose of FHR monitoring is to identify fetal hypoxemia and acidemia in order to allow early intervention in an effort to prevent fetal morbidity and mortality (ICSI, 2011).

In a recent review of randomized controlled trials, Alfirevic et al. (2008) found insufficient evidence to identify specific situations in which continuous EFM might result in better outcomes when compared with intermittent auscultation. However, continuous EFM is associated with an increase in cesarean section and instrumental vaginal births. Nevertheless, SOGC guidelines (2007) state that women with risk factors for adverse perinatal outcomes should receive EFM. However, with an identified normal tracing, maternal stability, and no increase in the rate of oxytocin infusions, mothers can be allowed up to ambulate for periods of up to 30 minutes.

Current methods of continuous EFM were introduced in Canada and the United States during the 1960s specifically for use in clients whose babies were considered to be at high risk for hypoxemia. However, the use of these methods gradually increased and they eventually came to be used in non–high risk cases as well. This increased use is now the centre of controversy as continuous EFM is known to be associated with the steadily increasing rates of cesarean births in Canada and abroad (Low, 2009; Menacker & Martin, 2009; Public Health Agency of Canada [PHAC], 2008; SOGC, 2008c). Additional studies also suggest that the use of intrapartum EFM increases the number of preterm and surgical births with no significant effect on reducing the incidence of intrapartum death or long-term neurologic injury (Alfirevic et al., 2008; ICSI, 2011). With EFM, there is a continuous record of the FHR: no gaps exist, as they do with intermittent auscultation. The concept of hearing and evaluating every beat of the fetus's heart to allow for early intervention seems logical. On the downside, however, continuous monitoring can limit maternal movement and encourages the woman to lie in the supine position, which reduces placental perfusion and potentially contributes to problems. Despite the criticisms, EFM remains an accurate method for determining fetal health status by providing moment-to-moment information about FHR status. However, FHR readings are dynamic and transient and require frequent reassessment and interpretation (Macones, Hankins, Spong, et al., 2008).

Various groups within the medical community have criticized the use of continuous fetal monitoring for all pregnant clients, whether high risk or low risk. Concerns about the efficiency and safety of routine EFM in labour have led expert panels in Canada to recommend that such monitoring be limited to high-risk pregnancies (SOGC, 2008d). Continuous EFM can be performed externally (indirectly), with the equipment attached to the maternal abdominal wall, or internally (directly), with the equipment attached to the fetus. Both methods provide a continuous printout of the FHR, but they differ in their specificity. The efficacy of EFM depends on the accurate interpretation of the tracings, not necessarily which method (external versus internal) is used.

Continuous External Monitoring

In external or indirect monitoring, two ultrasound transducers, each of which is attached to a belt, are applied around the woman's abdomen. They are similar to the hand-held Doppler device. One transducer, which is pressure sensitive, is called a tocodynamometer. It is placed over the uterine fundus in the area of greatest contractility to monitor and record uterine contractions (Evans et al., 2010). The other ultrasound transducer records the baseline FHR, long-term variability, accelerations, and decelerations. It is positioned on the maternal abdomen in the midline between the umbilicus and the symphysis pubis. The diaphragm of the ultrasound transducer is moved to either side of the abdomen to obtain a stronger sound and is then attached to the second elastic belt. This transducer converts the fetal heart movements into beeping sounds and records them on graph paper (Fig. 14.5).

Good continuous data are provided on the FHR. External monitoring can be used while the membranes are still intact and the cervix is not yet dilated. It is non-invasive and can detect relative changes in abdominal pressure between uterine resting tone and contractions. External monitoring also measures the approximate duration and frequency of contractions, providing a permanent record of FHR (Tucker et al., 2009).

However, external monitoring can restrict the mother's movements. It also cannot detect short-term

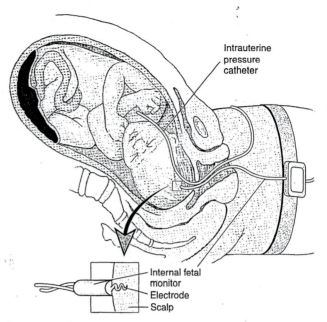

Intrauterine pressure catheter

Internal fetal monitor
Electrode
Scalp

FIGURE 14.6 Continuous internal electronic fetal monitoring.

variability. Signal disruptions can occur due to maternal obesity, fetal malpresentation, and fetal movement, as well as by artefact. **Artefact** describes irregular variations or the absence of FHR on the fetal monitor record that result from mechanical limitations of the monitor or electrical interference. For instance, the monitor may pick up transmissions from CB radios used by truck drivers on nearby roads and translate them into a signal. Additionally, gaps in the monitor strip can occur periodically without explanation.

Continuous Internal Monitoring

Continuous internal monitoring is usually indicated for women or fetuses considered to be at high risk. Possible conditions might include multiple gestation, decreased fetal movement, abnormal FHR on auscultation, intrauterine growth restriction (IUGR), maternal fever, pre-eclampsia, dysfunctional labour, preterm birth, or medical conditions such as diabetes or hypertension. It involves the placement of a spiral electrode on the fetal presenting part, usually the head, to assess FHR and a pressure transducer placed internally within the uterus to record uterine contractions (Fig. 14.6). The fetal spiral electrode is considered the most accurate method of detecting fetal heart characteristics and patterns because it involves receiving a signal directly from the fetus (Menihan & Kopel, 2008). Trained labour and birth nurses can place the spiral electrode on the fetal head when the membranes rupture in some health care facilities, but they do not place the IUPC in the uterus. Internal monitoring does not have to include both an IUPC and a scalp electrode. A fetal scalp electrode can be used to monitor the fetal heartbeat without monitoring the maternal intrauterine pressure.

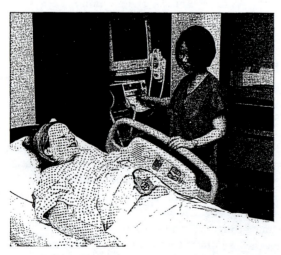

FIGURE 14.5 Continuous external electronic fetal monitoring device applied to the woman in labour.

Both the FHR and the duration and interval of uterine contractions are recorded on the graph paper. This method permits evaluation of baseline heart rate and changes in rate and pattern.

Four specific criteria must be met for this type of monitoring to be used:

- Ruptured membranes
- Cervical dilation of at least 2 cm
- Presenting fetal part low enough to identify correctly and allow placement of the scalp electrode
- Skilled practitioner available to insert spiral electrode (Ladewig et al., 2009)

Compared with external monitoring, continuous internal monitoring can accurately detect both short-term (moment-to-moment) changes and long-term variability (fluctuations within the baseline) as well as FHR dysrhythmias. In addition, maternal position changes and movement do not interfere with the quality of the tracing.

Determining FHR Patterns

It is imperative for all obstetric nurses, midwives, and physicians who deliver newborns to achieve competence in FHR monitoring and analysis (Macones et al., 2008; SOGC, 2007). FHR patterns provide information on the current acid–base status of the fetus and, although they may fluctuate from time to time, require prompt ongoing evaluation (Macones et al., 2008; SOGC, 2007). Assessment parameters of the FHR are classified as baseline rate, baseline variability, and periodic changes in the rate (accelerations and decelerations). To effectively care for women during labour and birth, the nurse must accurately interpret FHR tracings to determine if the pattern is normal (indicating fetal well-being), atypical or indeterminate (necessitating continued surveillance and re-evaluation), or abnormal (indicating the need for immediate intervention) (Macones et al., 2008; SOGC, 2007). The National Institute of Child Health & Human Development (NICHD) and the Institute for Clinical Systems Improvement (ICSI), both United States-based organizations, recently recommended a three-tier system for the categorization of FHR patterns that is very similar to the Canadian guidelines (ICSI, 2011; Macones et al., 2008).

Table 14.1 summarizes these patterns.

Baseline FHR

Baseline fetal heart rate refers to the average FHR that occurs during a 10-minute segment that excludes periodic or episodic rate changes (such as tachycardia or bradycardia) and periods of marked variability. It is assessed when the woman has no contractions. The normal baseline FHR ranges between 110 and 160 beats/minute (Alfirevic et al., 2008) and can be obtained by auscultation, ultrasound, Doppler, or an internal fetal spiral electrode.

TABLE 14.1   INTERPRETING FHR PATTERNS

Normal FHR signs	• Normal baseline (110–160 beats/min) • Moderate bradycardia (100–110 beats/min); good variability • Good beat-to-beat variability and fetal accelerations
Atypical signs	• Fetal tachycardia (>160 beats/min) • Moderate bradycardia (100–110 beats/min); lost variability • Absent beat-to-beat variability • Marked bradycardia (90–100 beats/min) • Moderate variable decelerations
Abnormal signs	• Fetal tachycardia with loss of variability • Prolonged marked bradycardia (<90 beats/min) • Severe variable decelerations (<70 beats/min) • Persistent late decelerations

Sources: Institute for Clinical Systems Improvement. (2011). *Health care guideline: Management of labor* (4th ed.). Retrieved February 22, 2012 from http://www.icsi.org/labor/labor__management_of__full_version__2.html; Macones, G. A., Hankins, G. D. V., Spong, C. Y., Hauth, J., & Moore, T. (2008). The 2008 National Institute of Child Health and Human Development workshop report on electronic fetal monitoring: Update on definitions, interpretation, and research guidelines. *Journal of Obstetric, Gynecologic, & Neonatal Nursing*, 37(5), 510–515; & Society of Obstetricians and Gynecologists of Canada. (2007). *SOGC clinical practice guidelines: Fetal health surveillance: Antepartum and intrapartum consensus guideline. Journal of Obstetrics and Gynecology in Canada*, 29(9), S3–S56. Retrieved February 22, 2012 from http://www.sogc.org/guidelines/documents/gui197CPG0709.pdf.

Fetal bradycardia occurs when the FHR is below 110 beats/minute and lasts 10 minutes or longer (Tucker et al., 2009). It can be the initial response of a healthy fetus to asphyxia. Causes of fetal bradycardia might include fetal hypoxia, prolonged maternal hypoglycemia, fetal acidosis, viral infections, administration of drugs to the mother, maternal hypothermia, maternal hypotension, prolonged umbilical cord compression, and fetal congenital heart block (SOGC, 2007; Tucker et al., 2009). Bradycardia may be benign if it is an isolated event, but it is considered an ominous sign when accompanied by a decrease in long-term variability and late decelerations.

Fetal tachycardia is a baseline FHR greater than 160 beats/minute that lasts for 10 minutes or longer (SOGC, 2007; Tucker et al., 2009). It can represent an early fetal compensatory response to asphyxia and can be maternal or fetal in nature (Tucker et al., 2009). Maternal causes such as fever, medication, and dehydration are amenable to interventions. Other causes include fetal hypoxia/acidosis, maternal anxiety, thyroid disease, fetal heart failure, and fetal arrhythmias (Tucker et al., 2009). Fetal tachycardia is considered an ominous sign if it is accompanied by a decrease in variability and late decelerations (Lowdermilk et al., 2010).

Baseline Variability

Baseline variability is defined as normal physiologic variations in the time intervals that elapse between each fetal heartbeat observed along the baseline in the absence of contractions, decelerations, and accelerations (Menihan & Kopel, 2008). It represents the interplay between the parasympathetic and sympathetic nervous systems producing moment-to-moment changes in the FHR. Because variability is in essence the combined result of autonomic nervous system branch function, its presence implies that both branches are working and receiving adequate oxygen (Tucker et al., 2009). Thus, variability is one of the most important characteristics of the FHR.

Variability is described in three ways: minimal or absent, moderate, and marked. Minimal or absent variability typically is caused by uteroplacental insufficiency, cord compression, maternal hypotension, uterine hyperstimulation (tachysystole), abruptio placentae, or a fetal dysrhythmia. Interventions to improve uteroplacental blood flow and perfusion through the umbilical cord include lateral positioning of the mother, increasing the IV fluid rate to improve maternal circulation, administering oxygen at 8 to 10 L/min by mask, considering internal fetal monitoring, documenting findings, and reporting to the health care provider. Preparation for a surgical birth may be necessary if no changes occur after attempting the interventions.

Moderate variability indicates that the autonomic and central nervous systems of the fetus are well developed and well oxygenated. It is considered a good sign of fetal well-being and correlates with the absence of significant metabolic acidosis (Fig. 14.7).

Marked variability occurs when there are more than 25 beats of fluctuation in the FHR baseline. Causes of this include cord prolapse or compression, maternal hypotension, uterine hyperstimulation (tachysystole), and abruptio placentae. Interventions include determining the cause, if possible, lateral positioning, increasing the IV fluid rate, administering oxygen at 8 to 10 L/min by mask, discontinuing oxytocin infusion, observing for changes in tracing, considering internal fetal monitoring, communicating an abnormal pattern to the health care provider, and preparing for a surgical birth if no change in pattern is noted (Menihan & Kopel, 2008).

FHR variability is an important clinical indicator that is predictive of fetal acid–base balance and cerebral tissue perfusion (Tucker et al., 2009). As the central nervous system is desensitized by hypoxia and acidosis, FHR decreases until a smooth baseline pattern appears. Loss of variability may be associated with a poor outcome. Some causes of decreased variability include fetal hypoxia/acidosis, drugs that depress the central nervous system, congenital abnormalities, fetal sleep, prematurity, and fetal tachycardia (Tucker et al., 2009).

> ▶ **Take** NOTE!
>
> *External EFM cannot assess short-term variability. Therefore, if external monitoring shows a baseline that is smoothing out, use of an internal spiral electrode should be considered to gain a more accurate picture of the fetal health status.*

Periodic Baseline Changes

Periodic baseline changes are temporary, recurrent changes made in response to a stimulus such as a contraction. The FHR can demonstrate patterns of acceleration or deceleration in response to most stimuli. Fetal **accelerations** are transitory increases in the FHR above the baseline associated with sympathetic nervous stimulation. They are visually apparent, with elevations of FHR of more than 15 beats/minute above the baseline, and their duration is less than 2 minutes (Macones et al., 2008). They are generally considered transient and require no interventions. Accelerations denote fetal movement and fetal well-being and are the basis for non-stress testing.

A **deceleration** is a transient fall in FHR caused by stimulation of the parasympathetic nervous system. Decelerations are described by their shape and association with a uterine contraction. They are classified as early, late, variable, and prolonged (Fig. 14.8).

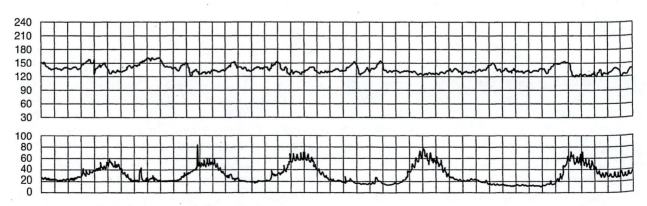

FIGURE 14.7 Long-term variability (average or moderate).

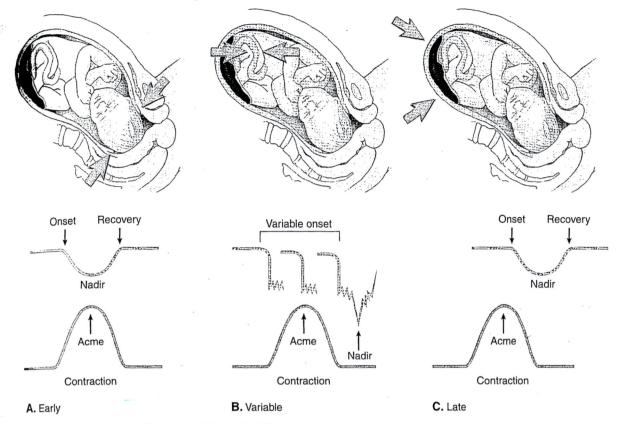

Onset Recovery

Nadir

Acme

Contraction

A. Early

Variable onset

Nadir

Acme

Nadir

Contraction

B. Variable

Onset Recovery

Nadir

Acme

Contraction

C. Late

FIGURE 14.8 Decelerations. (**A**) Early. (**B**) Variable. (**C**) Late.

Early decelerations are characterized by a gradual decrease in the FHR in which the nadir (lowest point) occurs at the peak of the contraction. They rarely decrease more than 30 to 40 beats/minute below the baseline. Typically, the onset, nadir, and recovery of the deceleration occur at the same time as the onset, peak, and recovery of the contraction. They are most often seen during the active stage of any normal labour, during pushing, crowning, or vacuum extraction. They are thought to be a result of fetal head compression that results in a reflex vagal response with a resultant slowing of the FHR during uterine contractions. Early decelerations are not indicative of fetal distress and do not require intervention.

Late decelerations are transitory decreases in FHR that occur after a contraction begins. The FHR does not return to baseline levels until well after the contraction has ended. In most cases, the onset, nadir, and recovery of the deceleration occur after the beginning, peak, and ending of the contraction, respectively (Macones et al., 2008). Late decelerations are associated with uteroplacental insufficiency, causing hypoxemia from inadequate placental perfusion during contractions. Conditions that may decrease uteroplacental perfusion with resultant decelerations include maternal hypotension, gestational hypertension, placental aging secondary to diabetes and postmaturity, uterine hyperstimulation (tachysystole) via oxytocin infusion, maternal smoking, anemia, and cardiac disease. Repetitive late decelerations and late decelerations with decreasing baseline variability are ominous signs (Tucker et al., 2009). Box 14.1 highlights interventions for decelerations. When decelerations are repetitive, the fetal scalp pH should be obtained if clinically appropriate and prepare for delivery (SOGC, 2007).

Variable decelerations present as visually apparent abrupt decreases in FHR below baseline and have an unpredictable shape on the FHR baseline, possibly demonstrating no consistent relationship with uterine contractions. Variable decelerations are usually associated with cord compression. These are usually uncomplicated variable decelerations. However, they can also be complicated and abnormal when the FHR decreases to less than 70 beats/minute, persists at that level for at least 60 seconds, and is repetitive (SOGC, 2007). The pattern of variable deceleration consistently related to the contractions with a slow return to FHR baseline may also be indicative of hypoxemia.

Prolonged decelerations are gradual or abrupt FHR declines of at least 15 beats/minute that last longer than 2 minutes but less than 10 minutes (Macones et al., 2008). The rate usually drops to less than 90 beats/minute. These decelerations are caused by some disruption to the oxygen supply. Many factors are associated with this pattern, including prolonged cord compression,

BOX 14.1   Interventions for Atypical Decelerations

If a patient develops an atypical deceleration pattern such as late or variable decelerations:

- Notify the health care provider about the pattern and obtain further orders, making sure to document all interventions and their effects on the FHR pattern.
- Reduce or discontinue oxytocin as dictated by the facility's protocol, if it is being administered.
- Provide reassurance that interventions are being done to effect a pattern change.

Additional interventions specific for a late deceleration FHR pattern would include:

- Turning the client on her left side to increase placental perfusion
- Administering oxygen by mask to increase fetal oxygenation
- Increasing the IV fluid rate to improve intravascular volume
- Assessing the client for any underlying contributing causes
- Providing reassurance that interventions are to effect pattern change

Specific interventions for a variable deceleration FHR pattern would include:

- Changing the client's position to relieve compression on the cord
- Providing reassurance that interventions are to effect pattern change
- Giving oxygen and IV fluids as ordered

---

abruptio placentae, cord prolapse, and supine maternal position (Lowdermilk et al., 2010). Prolonged decelerations can be remedied by identifying the underlying cause and correcting it.

Other Fetal Assessment Methods

In situations suggesting the possibility of fetal compromise, such as inconclusive or atypical FHR patterns, further ancillary testing such as fetal scalp sampling, FPO, and fetal stimulation may be used to validate the FHR findings and assist in planning interventions.

Fetal Scalp Blood Sampling

Fetal scalp blood sampling was developed as a means of measuring fetal distress in conjunction with EFM to make critical decisions about the management of labour and to prevent unnecessary operative interventions resulting from the use of EFM alone. Abnormal FHR patterns may not necessarily indicate fetal hypoxia or acidosis. Therefore, assessing fetal acid–base status through fetal scalp blood sampling may help to prevent unnecessary surgical intervention.

A sample of fetal scalp blood is obtained to measure the pH. In order to carry out the test, the woman must have ruptured membranes, have met a requirement for cervical dilation, and have a vertex presentation (Lowdermilk et al., 2010). The test procedure is complicated, and there is often a need for repetitive tests and interpretations (Lowdermilk et al., 2010; SOGC, 2007). Although seldom used today (Lowdermilk et al., 2010), the procedure is still recommended by the SOGC (2007) to assess fetal acid–base balance when gestational age is greater than 34 weeks, delivery is not imminent, and the FHR tracing is considered atypical or abnormal.

▶ **Take** NOTE!

During the past decade, the use of fetal scalp sampling has decreased, being replaced by less invasive techniques that yield similar information.

Fetal Oxygen Saturation Monitoring (Fetal Pulse Oximetry)

FPO measures fetal oxygen saturation directly and in real time. It can be used with EFM as an adjunct method of assessment when the FHR pattern is abnormal or atypical. A soft sensor is introduced through the dilated cervix and placed on the cheek, forehead, or temple of the fetus. It is held in place by the uterine wall. The sensor then is attached to a special adapter on the fetal monitor that provides a real-time recording that is displayed on the uterine activity panel of the tracing. FPO is a non-invasive and safe method for assessing fetal oxygenation. However, recent research shows that FPO has not proven to be clinically useful in determining fetal status (American College of Obstetricians and Gynecologists [ACOG], 2009; East, Chan, Colditz, et al., 2007) or reducing overall cesarean section rates. Based on earlier evidence, the SOGC (2007) does not recommend routine use of FPO during intrapartum care.

Fetal Stimulation

An indirect method used to evaluate fetal oxygenation and acid–base balance to identify fetal hypoxia is fetal scalp stimulation and vibroacoustic stimulation. If the fetus does not have adequate oxygen reserves, carbon dioxide builds up, leading to acidemia and hypoxemia. These metabolic states are reflected in abnormal FHR patterns as well as fetal inactivity. Fetal stimulation is performed to promote fetal movement with the hope that FHR accelerations will accompany the movement.

Fetal movement can be stimulated with a vibroacoustic stimulator (artificial larynx) applied to the woman's lower abdomen and turned on for a few seconds to produce sound and vibration or by tactile stimulation via pelvic examination and stimulation of the fetal scalp with the gloved fingers. A well-oxygenated fetus will respond when stimulated (tactile or by noise) by moving in conjunction with an acceleration of 15 beats/minute above the baseline heart rate that lasts at least 15 seconds. This FHR acceleration reflects a pH of more than 7 and a fetus with an intact central nervous system. However, the absence of a response does not necessarily indicate fetal compromise (SOGC, 2007; Tucker et al., 2009). The SOGC recommends the use of digital fetal scalp stimulation in response to atypical electronic fetal heart tracings.

Promoting Comfort and Pain Management During Labour

Pain during labour is a universal experience, although the intensity of the pain may vary. Although labour and childbirth are viewed as natural processes, both can produce significant pain and discomfort. The acute pain of labour is primarily physical in nature, has a fixed duration, and can often be relieved by non-pharmacologic methods (Evans et al., 2010).

Pain is uniquely personal, and the pain of labour can be influenced by personality traits, cultural expectations, anxiety, access to social and emotional support, social status, environment, and past experiences (Wolf, 2009). Therefore, techniques used to manage labour pain vary according to geography and culture. At the beginning of regular-onset uterine contractions, the appearance of bloody show, or membrane rupture, for example, Orthodox Jewish women observe the law of *niddah*. At this point, the husband will no longer touch his wife but may remain in the room providing spiritual support. He may or may not look at his wife during the birth (Berkowitz, 2008). Korean women do not express pain outwardly for fear of shaming the family, and silence is valued by the Chinese (Ladewig et al., (2009). Canada has a substantial Aboriginal population for whom childbirth is a sacred event that traditionally involved the family and community as a whole (National Aboriginal Health Organization, 2008). Many Aboriginals today not only need to leave their communities to experience the birth alone but also they are limited in the number of support people who are allowed to attend the birth. This can create anxiety for the mother, potentially increasing pain, lengthening the labour, and contributing to complications.

Culturally diverse childbearing families present to the labour and birth suites with the same needs and desires of all families. Regardless of the expression of pain, it is imperative for nurses to explore with labouring mothers their perception of the pain and how best to support them. Give them and their families the same respect and sense of welcome shown to all families. Make sure they have a high-quality birth experience by upholding their religious, ethnic, and cultural values and integrating them into care. Today, women have many safe non-pharmacologic and pharmacologic choices for the management of pain during labour and birth, which may be used separately or in combination with one another.

Nurses are in an ideal position to provide childbearing women with balanced, clear, concise information about effective non-pharmacologic and pharmacologic measures to relieve pain. It is important for nurses to be knowledgeable about the most recent scientific research on labour pain-relief modalities, to make sure that accurate and unbiased information about effective pain-relief measures is available to labouring women, to be sure that the woman determines what is an acceptable labour pain level for her, and to allow the woman the choice of pain-relief method.

Non-pharmacologic Measures

Non-pharmacologic measures may include continuous labour support, hydrotherapy, ambulation and position changes, acupuncture and acupressure, attention focusing and imagery, therapeutic touch and massage, breathing techniques, and effleurage. Most of these methods are based on the "gate control" theory of pain, which proposes that local physical stimulation can interfere with pain stimuli by closing a hypothetical gate in the spinal cord, thus blocking pain signals from reaching the brain (Lowdermilk et al., 2010). It has long been a standard of care for labour nurses to first provide or encourage a variety of non-pharmacologic measures before moving to the pharmacologic interventions.

Reynolds (2010) reviewed the role of pain, stress, and loss of maternal control on the development of progressive fetal metabolic acidosis. Unmanaged increased stress leads to the release of cortisol and catecholamines, prolonging labour and impairing fetal blood flow. In addition, maternal hyperventilation can lead to fetal respiratory alkalosis and metabolic acidosis. This supports the need for the labouring mother to gain control through one or a combination of non-pharmacologic measures that are usually simple, safe, and inexpensive. Many of these measures are taught in childbirth classes and should be practiced for best results with the partner/coach before the onset of labour. The nurse's role is to provide support and encouragement for the woman and her partner during this time. Although women can't consciously direct the labour contractions, they can control how they respond to the contractions, thereby enhancing their feelings of control.

Continuous Labour Support

Continuous labour support involves offering a sustained presence to the labouring woman by providing emotional support, comfort measures, advocacy, information and advice, and support for the partner. A woman's family, a midwife, a nurse, a doula, or anyone else close to the woman can provide this continuous presence (Adams & Bianchi, 2008; Leap, Sandall, Buckland, et al., 2010;

Simkin, 2008). A support person can assist the woman to ambulate, reposition herself, and use breathing techniques. A support person can also aid with the use of acupressure, massage, music therapy, or therapeutic touch. During the natural course of childbirth, a labouring woman's functional ability is limited secondary to pain, and she often has trouble making decisions. The support person can help her make decisions based on his or her knowledge of the woman's birth plan and personal wishes.

A recent *Cochrane* review concluded that women who received continuous labour support were more likely to give birth spontaneously (vaginally), had shorter labours, were less likely to use pain medications, and expressed more satisfaction with the birth experience (Hodnett, Gates, Hofmeyr, et al., 2009a). The SOGC (2007) and Association of Women's Health, Obstetric, and Neonatal Nurses (2011) both stress the importance of having continuous labour support from a registered nurse or other trained personnel for the labouring woman and her family.

> ▶ *Take* NOTE!
>
> *The human presence is of immeasurable value in making the labouring woman feel secure.*

Hydrotherapy

Hydrotherapy is a non-pharmacologic measure in which the woman immerses herself in warm water for relaxation and relief of discomfort. The warm water releases endorphins and provides better circulation and oxygenation (Lowdermilk et al., 2010). Contractions are usually less painful in warm water because the warmth and buoyancy of the water have a relaxing effect.

Hydrotherapy may shorten the length of labour and enhance coping by encouraging an upright position and increased movements (Stark, Rudell, & Haus, 2008).

Evidence indicates that water immersion in the first stage of labour reduces pain and the use of epidural/spinal analgesia (Cluett & Burns, 2009). There is no evidence of increased adverse outcomes for the fetus, neonate, or woman from labouring in water. Immersion during the second stage of labour needs further investigation (Cluett & Burns, 2009), but at present, there is no clear evidence to support or not support a woman's decision to give birth in water. The Royal Australian and New Zealand College of Obstetricians and Gynaecologists (2008) cautions against the consequences of unintended water birth, while the SOGC has not issued any position statement to date on hydrotherapy.

A wide range of hydrotherapy options is available, from ordinary bathtubs to whirlpool baths and showers,

combined with low lighting and music. Many hospitals provide showers and whirlpool baths for labouring women for pain relief. However, hydrotherapy is more commonly practiced in birthing centres managed by midwives.

Hydrotherapy is an effective pain-management option for many women. Women who are experiencing a healthy pregnancy can be offered this option.

Ambulation and Position Changes

Ambulation and position changes during labour are another extremely useful comfort measure. The medical profession traditionally has influenced women to assume a recumbent position throughout labour but without evidence to demonstrate its appropriateness (Lawrence, Lewis, Hofmeyr, et al., 2009). Changing position frequently (every 30 minutes or so)—sitting, walking, kneeling, standing, lying down, getting on hands and knees, and using a birthing ball—helps relieve pain (Fig. 14.9). Walking, moving around, and changing positions throughout labour make use of gravity to facilitate movement of the baby downward, helping to increase pelvic diameter and promote fetal rotation, thereby shortening the length of the first stage of labour (Lawrence et al., 2009). Supine and sitting positions for prolonged time should be avoided because they may interfere with the progress of labour and can cause compression of the vena cava and decreased blood return to the heart.

A recent pilot study in Canada demonstrated favourable outcomes for women who laboured in an "ambient room," where the hospital bed was removed and additional equipment was added to promote relaxation, mobility, and a calm atmosphere. Sixty-two participants were allocated to either a standard birthing room or the "ambient room." The women in the ambient group spent 50% or less time labouring in bed, and the need for artificial oxytocin infusions was reduced (Hodnett, Stremler, Weston, et al., 2009b).

Swaying from side to side, rocking, or other rhythmic movements may also be comforting. If labour is progressing slowly, ambulating may speed it up again. Upright positions such as walking, kneeling forward, or doing the lunge on the birthing ball give most women a greater sense of control and active movement than just lying down. Table 14.2 highlights some of the more common positions that can be used during labour and birth.

Acupuncture and Acupressure

Acupuncture and acupressure can be used to relieve pain during labour. Acupuncture involves stimulating key trigger points with needles. This form of Chinese medicine has been practiced for approximately 3,000 years. Classic Chinese teaching holds that throughout the body there are meridians or channels of energy (*qi*) that when in balance regulate body functions. Pain

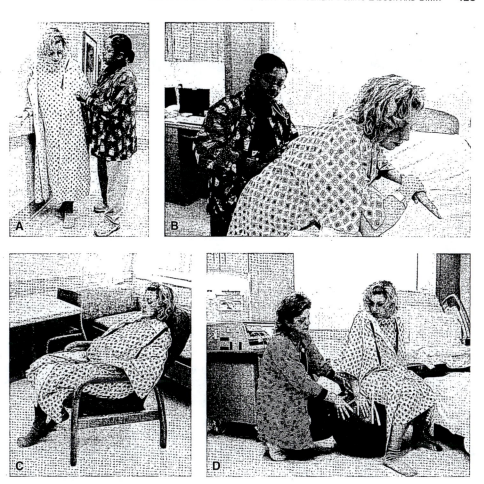

FIGURE 14.9 Various positions for use during labour. (**A**) Ambulation. (**B**) Leaning forward. (**C**) Sitting in a chair. (**D**) Using a birthing ball.

reflects an imbalance or obstruction of the flow of energy. Stimulating the trigger points causes the release of endorphins, reducing the perception of pain. Although controlled research studies are limited, Smith et al. (2006) found that acupuncture may be helpful for pain management during labour. In addition, a recent large randomized controlled trial of more than 600 Danish women demonstrated that acupuncture reduced the need for pharmacologic and invasive methods during delivery and was a good supplement to existing pain relief methods (Borup, Wurlitzer, Hedegaard, et al., 2009).

Acupressure involves the application of a firm finger or massage at the same trigger points to reduce the pain sensation. The amount of pressure is important. The intensity of the pressure is determined by the needs of the woman. Holding and squeezing the hand of a woman in labour may trigger the point most commonly used for both techniques. Acupressure points are found along the spine, neck, shoulder, toes, wrists, lower back (including sacral points), hips, below kneecaps, ankles, and along the toenails (Lowdermilk et al., 2010). A recent *Cochrane* review found that while acupressure does significantly shorten the length of labour, evidence regarding its effectiveness in pain management is insufficient and further research is required (Smith et al., 2009).

Attention Focusing and Imagery

Attention focusing or distraction and imagery use many of the senses and the mind to focus on stimuli. Distraction entails the use of specific activities such as the use of a visual focal point, guided imagery, visualization, hypnosis, or rituals (Adams & Bianchi, 2008). The woman can focus on tactile stimuli such as touch, massage, or stroking. She may focus on auditory stimuli such as music, humming, or verbal encouragement. Guided imagery supports distraction by visually allowing the mind to create a pleasant image and enhance relaxation in early labour, such as by imagining a beach scene (Adams & Bianchi, 2008) or revisiting a happy memory. Breathing, relaxation, positive thinking, and positive visualization work well for mothers in labour and are examples of labour support behaviours (Adams & Bianchi, 2008). Practicing these behaviours with maternal clients in labour will positively affect birth experiences. Adams & Bianchi (2008) states that a call to action is necessary to design and implement a certification program that would lend importance and credibility to these concepts.

TABLE 14.2 Common Positions for Use During Labour and Birth

Position	Potential Advantages
Standing	• Takes advantage of gravity during and between contractions • Makes contractions feel less painful and be more productive • Helps fetus line up with angle of maternal pelvis • Helps to increase urge to push in second stage of labour
Walking	• Has the same advantages as standing • Causes changes in the pelvic joints, helping the fetus move through the birth canal
Standing and leaning forward on partner, bed, birthing ball	• Has the same advantages as standing • Is a good position for a backrub • May feel more restful than standing • Can be used with electronic fetal monitor
Slow dancing (standing with woman's arms around partner's neck, head resting on his chest or shoulder, with his hands rubbing woman's lower back; sway to music and breathe in rhythm if it helps)	• Has the same advantages as walking • Back pressure helps relieve back pain • Rhythm and music help woman relax and provide comfort
Lunge (having a straight chair to side of the labouring woman with one foot on the seat with knee and foot to the side; woman bends raised knee and hip and lunges sideways repeatedly during a contraction, holding each lunge for 5 seconds; partner holds chair and helps with balance)	• Widens one side of the pelvis (the side toward lunge) • Encourages rotation of baby • Can also be done in a kneeling position
Sitting upright	• Helps promote rest • Has more gravity advantage than lying down • Can be used with electronic fetal monitor
Semi-sitting (setting the head of the bed at a 45-degree angle with pillows used for support)	• Has the same advantages as sitting upright • Is an easy position if on a bed
Sitting on toilet or commode	• Has the same advantages as sitting upright • May help relax the perineum for effective bearing down
Rocking in a chair	• Has the same advantages as sitting upright • May help speed labour (rocking movement)
Sitting, leaning forward with support	• Has the same advantages as sitting upright • Is a good position for a backrub
On all fours, on hands and knees	• Helps relieve backache • Assists rotation of baby in posterior position • Allows for pelvic rocking and body movement • Relieves pressure on hemorrhoids • Allows for vaginal examinations • Is sometimes preferred as a pushing position by women with back labour
Kneeling, leaning forward with support on a chair seat, the raised head of the bed, or on a birthing ball	• Has the same advantages as all-fours position • Puts less strain on wrists and hands
Side-lying	• Is a very good position for resting and convenient for many kinds of medical interventions • Helps lower elevated blood pressure • May promote progress of labour when alternated with walking • Is useful to slow a very rapid second stage • Takes pressure off hemorrhoids • Facilitates relaxation between contractions

Position	Potential Advantages
Squatting	• May relieve backache • Takes advantage of gravity • Requires less bearing-down effort • Widens pelvic outlet • May help fetus turn and move down in a difficult birth • Helps if the woman feels no urge to push • Allows freedom to shift weight for comfort • Offers an advantage when pushing, since upper trunk presses on the top of the uterus
Supported squat (leaning back against partner, who supports woman under the arms and takes the entire woman's weight; standing up between contractions)	• Requires great strength in partner • Lengthens trunk, allowing more room for fetus to manoeuvres into position • Lets gravity help
Dangle (partner sitting high on bed or counter with feet supported on chairs or footrests and thighs spread; woman leaning back between partner's legs, placing flexed arms over partner's thighs; partner gripping sides with his thighs; woman lowering herself and allowing partner to support her full weight; standing up between contractions)	• Has the same advantages of a supported squat • Requires less physical strength from the partner than with supported squat position

Sources: Adams, E. D., & Bianchi, A. L. (2008). A practical approach to labor support. *Journal of Obstetric, Gynecologic, & Neonatal Nursing, 37,* 106–115; Lowdermilk, D. L., Perry, S. E., & Cashion, K. (2010). *Maternity nursing* (8th ed.). Maryland Heights, MO: Mosby Elsevier; & Rice Simpson, K., & Creehan, P. A. (2008). *Perinatal nursing.* Philadelphia: AWHONN & Lippincott Williams & Wilkins.

Therapeutic Touch and Massage

Touch is an integral part of human nature and is used in many ways in health and illness, including assessment, diagnosis, and healing (Rose, 2009). Both therapeutic touch and massage can serve to relax patients and distract them from discomfort (Evidence-based Practice 14.1).

Therapeutic touch is an intentionally directed process of energy exchange that uses the hands to promote relaxation and reduce pain and anxiety without actually

---

EVIDENCE-BASED PRACTICE 14.1
The Effects of Complementary and Alternative Therapies for Pain Management in Labour on Maternal and Perinatal Morbidity

● Study

The pain of labour can be intense, with tension, anxiety, and fear making it worse. Many women would like to labour without using drugs and turn to alternatives to manage pain. These alternative methods include acupuncture, mind–body techniques, massage, reflexology, herbal medicines or homeopathy, hypnosis, and music. This review examined currently available evidence supporting the use of alternative and complementary therapies for pain management during labour. Fourteen trials were reviewed, with data reporting on 1,537 women using different modalities of pain management; 1,448 women were included in the meta-analysis.

▲ Findings

There is insufficient evidence regarding the benefits of music, massage, relaxation, white noise, acupressure, and

aromatherapy and no evidence about the effectiveness of massage or other complementary therapies. Acupuncture and hypnosis may be beneficial for the management of pain during labour; however, the number of women studied has been small. Few other complementary therapies have been subjected to proper scientific study.

▦ Nursing Implications

Although this study didn't offer conclusive evidence that alternative therapies for pain management work better than pharmacologic or invasive methods, they should not be discounted. Many women wish to avoid artificial means to control the discomfort of labour. The nurse should be supportive and open-minded about a woman's efforts to meet her pain management goals.

Source: Smith, C. A., Collins, C. T., Cyna, A. M., & Crowther, C. A. (2006). Complementary and alternative therapies for pain management in labour. *Cochrane Database of Systematic Reviews, 4,* CD003521.

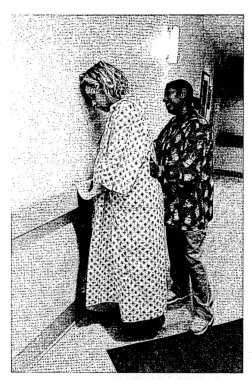

FIGURE 14.10 Nurse massaging the client's back during a contraction while she ambulates during labour.

touching the physical body of the patient (Monroe, 2009; Therapeutic Touch International Association [TTIA], 2010). In order to perform therapeutic touch correctly, the technique must be learned and practiced (TTIA, 2010). Therapeutic touch is often used in conjunction with massage for women during labour.

During massage, some women prefer a light touch while others find a firmer touch more soothing. Massage of the neck, shoulders, back, thighs, feet, and hands can be very comforting. The use of firm counterpressure in the lower back or sacrum is especially helpful for back pain during contractions (Fig. 14.10). Problems with the skin, such as skin rashes, varicose veins, bruises, or infections, are contraindications for massage. In a study of 93 labouring women in Taiwan, most considered massage for low back pain to provide effective pain relief but a few thought massage made the labour even worse (Tzeng & Su, 2008). Thus an individualized approach to massage during labour is recommended. While performing this intervention, nurses should assess the reaction of the woman in order to provide individualized nursing care.

Effleurage is a form of massage that uses light, stroking, superficial touch of the abdomen in rhythm with breathing during contractions. Like traditional massage and therapeutic touch, effleurage is used as a relaxation technique and a distraction from discomfort. However, external fetal monitor belts may interfere with the ability to perform effleurage properly.

Breathing Techniques

Breathing techniques are effective in producing relaxation and pain relief through the use of distraction. If the woman is concentrating on slow-paced rhythmic breathing, she isn't likely to fully focus on contraction pain. Breathing techniques are often taught in childbirth education classes (see Chapter 12 for additional information).

Breathing techniques use controlled breathing to reduce the pain experienced through a stimulus-response conditioning. The woman selects a focal point within her environment to stare at during the first sign of a contraction. This focus creates a visual stimulus that goes directly to her brain. The woman takes a deep cleansing breath, which is followed by rhythmic breathing. Verbal commands from her partner supply an ongoing auditory stimulus to her brain. Effleurage can be combined with the breathing to provide a tactile stimulus, all blocking pain sensations to her brain. There are many benefits to breathing exercises during labour:

- Increased confidence
- Enhanced sense of control
- Distraction from pain
- Enhanced relaxation
- An even flow of oxygen and carbon dioxide
- Prevention of breath holding during contractions
- Relief of labour pain (Adams & Bianchi, 2008; Simkin, 2010)

In their childbirth education classes, many couples learn some form of rhythmic breathing for use during labour. Various patterns may be taught, but each begins and ends with a cleansing breath that involves inhaling through the nose with the shoulders relaxed and exhaling through the mouth and releasing all tension.

In the first pattern, also known as slow-paced breathing, the breathing rate is half the number of breaths normally taken per minute. Following the cleansing breath, the woman inhales through the nose to a count of four and then exhales through the mouth to a count of four, repeating until the end of the contraction when another cleansing breath is taken. In the second pattern, modified-paced breathing, the breathing rate is slightly faster than normal but not more than twice the resting rate. Following the cleansing breath, inhalation and exhalation are done to the count of two following the procedure for slow-paced breathing. The third pattern, pant blow breathing, uses the same rate as with modified-paced breathing except that the breathing is punctuated every few breaths by blowing softly through pursed lips. The pant is an in-breath and an out-breath (touching the tip of the tongue to the roof of the mouth to keep the mouth moist). Patterns may vary: pant-2-3-4-blow or pant-2-3-blow (Perinatal Education Associates, Inc., 2010).

Many childbirth educators do not recommend specific breathing techniques or trying to teach parents the "right" way to breathe during labour and birth. Couples are encouraged to find breathing styles that enhance their relaxation and use them. There are numerous benefits to controlled and rhythmic breathing in childbirth, and many women choose these techniques to manage their discomfort during labour.

Pharmacologic Measures

With varying degrees of success, generations of women have sought ways to relieve the pain of childbirth. Pharmacologic pain relief during labour includes systemic analgesia and regional or local anesthesia. Women have seen dramatic changes in pharmacologic pain management options over the years. Methods have evolved from biting down on a stick to a more complex pharmacologic approach such as epidural/intrathecal analgesia. Systemic analgesia and regional analgesia/anesthesia have become less common, while newer neuraxial analgesia/anesthesia techniques involving minimal motor blockade have become more popular. **Neuraxial analgesia/anesthesia** is the administration of analgesic (opioids) or anesthetic (medication capable of producing a loss of sensation in an area of the body) agents, either continuously or intermittently, into the epidural or intrathecal space to relieve pain. Low-dose and ultra-low-dose epidural analgesia, spinal analgesia, and combined spinal-epidural (CSE) analgesia have replaced the traditional epidural for labour (Simmons, Cyna, Dennis, et al., 2009). This shift in pain management allows a woman to be an active participant in labour.

> ▷ **Take** NOTE!
>
> *Regardless of which approach is used during labour, the woman has the right to choose the methods of pain control that will best suit her and meet her needs.*

Systemic Analgesia

Systemic analgesia involves the use of one or more drugs administered orally, intramuscularly, or intravenously (IV); they become distributed throughout the body via the circulatory system. Depending on which administration method is used, the therapeutic effect of pain relief can occur within minutes and last for several hours. The most important complication associated with the use of this class of drugs is respiratory depression. Therefore, women given these drugs require careful monitoring. Opioids given close to the time of birth can cause central nervous system depression in the newborn, necessitating the administration of naloxone (Narcan) to reverse the depressant effects of the opioids.

> ▶ **Consider** THIS!
>
> *When I was expecting my first child, I was determined to put my best foot forward and do everything right. I was an experienced OB nurse, and in my mind doing everything right was expected behaviour. I was already 2 weeks past my calculated due date and I was becoming increasingly worried. That particular day I went to work with a backache but felt no contractions.*
>
> *I managed to finish my shift but felt completely wiped out. As I walked to my car outside the hospital, my water broke and I felt the warm fluid run down my legs. I went back inside to be admitted for this much-awaited event.*
>
> *Although I had helped thousands of women go through their childbirth experience, I was now the one in the bed and not standing alongside it. My husband and I had practiced our breathing techniques to cope with the discomfort of labour, but this "discomfort" in my mind was more than I could tolerate. So despite my best intentions of doing everything right, within an hour I begged for a painkiller to ease the pain. While the medication took the edge off my pain, I still felt every contraction and truly now appreciate the meaning of the word "labour." Although I wanted to use natural childbirth without any medication, I know that I was a full participant in my son's birthing experience, and that is what "doing everything right" was for me!*
>
> *Thoughts: doing what is right varies for each individual, and as nurses we need to support whatever that is. Having a positive outcome from the childbirth experience is the goal; the means it takes to achieve it is less important. How can nurses support women in making their personal choices to achieve a healthy outcome? Are any women "failures" if they ask for pain medication to tolerate labour? How can nurses help women overcome this stigma of being a "wimp"?*

Several drug categories may be used for systemic analgesia:

- Opioids, such as butorphanol (Stadol), nalbuphine (Nubain), meperidine (Demerol), or fentanyl (Sublimaze)
- Ataractics, such as hydroxyzine (Vistaril) or promethazine (Phenergan)
- Benzodiazepines, such as diazepam (Valium) or midazolam (Versed)
- Barbiturates, such as secobarbital (Seconal) or pentobarbital (Nembutal)

Drug Guide 14.1 highlights some of the major drugs used for systemic analgesia.

DRUG GUIDE 14.1 COMMON AGENTS USED FOR SYSTEMIC ANALGESIA

Type	Drug	Comments
Opioids	Morphine 2–5 mg IV	May be given IV, intrathecally, or epidurally Rapidly crosses the placenta Can cause maternal and neonatal CNS depression Decreases uterine contractions May be given IV or epidurally with maximal fetal uptake 2–3 hours after administration Can cause fetal CNS depression
	Meperidine (Demerol) 25–50 mg IV[a]	Decreases fetal variability Naloxone does not reverse and may even worsen fetal neurotoxicity Is given IV Is rapidly transferred across the placenta Causes neonatal respiratory depression Is given IV
	Butorphanol (Stadol) 1 mg IV q3–4h	Causes less maternal nausea and vomiting Causes decreased FHR variability, fetal bradycardia, and respiratory depression Is given IV or epidurally
	Nalbuphine (Nubain) 10 mg IV	Can cause maternal hypotension, maternal and fetal respiratory depression Rapidly crosses placenta Rapid action and short duration of 1–2 hours
	Fentanyl (Sublimaze) 25–50 mcg IV	
Ataractics	Hydroxyzine (Vistaril) 50 mg IM	Does not relieve pain but reduces anxiety and potentiates opioid analgesic effects Is used to decrease nausea and vomiting Is used for antiemetic effect when combined with opioids
	Promethazine (Phenergan) 25 mg IV	Causes sedation and reduces apprehension May contribute to maternal hypotension and neonatal depression
Benzodiazepines	Diazepam (Valium) 2–5 mg IV	Is given to enhance pain relief of opioid and cause sedation May be used to stop eclamptic seizures Decreases nausea and vomiting Can cause newborn depression; therefore, lowest possible dose should be used Is not used for analgesic but amnesia effect Is used as adjunct for anesthesia Is excreted in breast milk
	Midazolam (Versed) 1–5 mg IV	
Barbiturates	Secobarbital (Seconal) 100 mg PO/IM	Causes sedation Is used in very early labour to alter a dysfunctional pattern Is not used for pain relief in active labour
	Pentobarbital (Nembutal) 100 mg PO/IM	Crosses placenta and is secreted in breast milk

[a]Not recommended.

Sources: British Columbia Perinatal Health Program. (2009). *Core competencies: Management of labour in an institutional setting if the primary maternal care provider is absent. Guidelines for registered nurses.* Vancouver, BC: BC Perinatal Health Program. Retrieved February 22, 2012 from http://www. perinatalservicesbc.ca/sites/bcrcp/files/FHS/Linked_Core_Competencies_with_DST.pdf; Datta, S., Kodali, B. S., & Segal, S. (2009). *Obstetric anesthesia handbook* (5th ed.). New York: Springer; deglin, J. H., Vallerand, A. H., & Sanoski, C. A. (2011). *Davis's drug guide for nurses* (12th ed.). Philadelphia: FA Davis Company; & The Merck Manual. (2007). *Management of normal labor.* Retrieved February 22, 2012 from http://www.merck.com/mmpe/sec18/ch260/ch260d.html#sec18-ch260-ch260d-1073.

Systemic analgesics are typically administered parenterally, usually through an existing IV line. Maternal analgesia during labour often directly affects the baby because of placental transfer of drugs administered to the mother; the baby is also affected indirectly by the secondary physiologic or biochemical changes experienced by the mother (Evans et al., 2010; Reynolds, 2010). Historically, opioids have been administered by nurses, but in the past decade there has been increasing use of client-controlled IV analgesia (patient-controlled analgesia [PCA]). With this system, the woman is given a button connected to a computerized pump on the IV line. When the woman desires analgesia, she presses the button and the pump delivers a preset amount of medication. This system provides the woman with a sense of control over her own pain management and active participation in the childbirth process.

Opioids

Opioids are morphine-like medications that are most effective for the relief of moderate to severe pain. Opioids typically are administered IV. Meperidine [Demerol] was once the most commonly used of all the synthetic opioids (others include butorphanol [Stadol], nalbuphine [Nubain], fentanyl [Sublimaze]) for the management of pain during labour. However, many hospitals are now reconsidering this standard because meperidine metabolizes to normeperidine, leading to neurobehavioural depression in many women lasting for several days (British Columbia Perinatal Health Program, 2009; Rice Simpson & Creehan, 2008; The Merck Manual, 2007). Opioids can impact early breastfeeding (Reynolds, 2010) and are associated with newborn respiratory depression, yet they do not achieve adequate maternal analgesia (Akerman & Dresner, 2009; Reynolds, 2010).

All opioids are considered good analgesics. However, respiratory depression can occur in both mother and fetus depending on the dose given. They may also cause a decrease in FHR variability identified on the fetal monitor strip. This FHR pattern change is usually transient. Other systemic side effects include nausea, vomiting, pruritus, delayed gastric emptying, drowsiness, hypoventilation, and newborn respiratory depression. To reduce the incidence of newborn respiratory depression, birth should occur within 1 hour or after 4 hours of administration to prevent the fetus from receiving the peak concentration (Deglin, Vallerand, & Sanoski, 2011). Opioid antagonists such as naloxone (Narcan) are given to reverse the effects of the central nervous system depression, including respiratory depression, caused by opioids. Nurses need to be aware of the fact that the duration of naloxone's effect is very short, and they should therefore be alert for a potential return of respiratory depression and the need for repeated doses (Evans et. al., 2010). Opioid antagonists also are used to reverse the side effects of neuraxial opioids, such as pruritus (Deglin et al., 2011).

Ataractics

The ataractic group of medications is used in combination with an opioid to decrease nausea and vomiting and lessen anxiety. These adjunct drugs potentiate the effectiveness of the opioid so that a lesser dose can be given. They may also be used to increase sedation.

Benzodiazepines

Benzodiazepines are used for minor tranquilizing and sedative effects. Diazepam (Valium) is given IV to stop seizures due to pregnancy-induced hypertension. However, it is not used during labour itself. It can be administered to calm a woman who is out of control, thereby enabling her to relax enough so that she can participate effectively during her labour process rather than fighting against it. Lorazepam (Ativan) can also be used for its tranquilizing effect, but increased sedation is experienced with this medication (Deglin et al., 2011). Midazolam (Versed), also given IV, produces amnesia but no analgesia. It is most commonly used as an adjunct for anesthesia but is given in small doses and should be used cautiously due to its amnesic effect (Datta, Kodali, & Segal, 2009). Diazepam and midazolam cause central nervous system depression in both the woman and the newborn (Deglin et al., 2011).

Barbiturates

Barbiturates are used only in early labour to promote sleep when birth is unlikely for 12 to 24 hours. The goal is to promote therapeutic rest for a few hours to enhance the woman's ability to cope with active labour. These drugs cross the placenta and cause central nervous system depression in the newborn (Rice Simpson & Creehan, 2008).

Regional Analgesia/Anesthesia

Regional techniques, also referred to as neuraxial analgesia/anesthesia, provide unrivaled pain relief in labour with minimal side effects. The drugs are administered into a specific region, the lower neuraxis. Only small doses are needed as this technique provides a local effect in blocking pain pathways.

The routes for regional pain relief include epidural block, CSE block, local infiltration, pudendal block, and intrathecal (spinal) analgesia/anesthesia (Grant, 2010). Local and pudendal routes are used during birth for episiotomies; epidural and intrathecal routes are used for pain relief during active labour and birth. The major advantage of regional pain-management techniques is that the woman can participate in the birthing process and still have good pain control.

Epidural Block

While the rates of epidural use during labour vary among provinces and territories in Canada, nationally there has been a significant overall increase. Approximately two-thirds of all vaginal deliveries in Quebec (69%) and

Ontario (60%), were preceded by an epidural. Rates have continued to climb in six of the remaining eight provinces and in two of the three territories (Canadian Institute for Health Information, 2010). Over just a 2-year period, from 2006–2007 to 2008–2009, the largest increases noted were in Nova Scotia (increasing by 6.2% for a total of 54.6%) and Prince Edward Island (increasing by 9.3% for a total of 39.5%). The Canadian Anesthesiologists' Society [CAS], (2010) has developed consensus-based guidelines for acute pain management using neuraxial analgesia (intrathecal or epidural administration of opioids and/or local anesthetics). Among these are the availability of an anesthesiologist at all times and appropriate education of nurses involved in the care of patients in receipt of this treatment (CAS, 2010). Despite the rising rates of epidural use, many rural Canadian communities are unable to offer this service to their clients during labour based on these guidelines.

An epidural block involves the injection of a drug into the epidural space, which is located outside the dura mater between the dura and the spinal canal. The epidural space is typically entered through the third and fourth lumbar vertebrae with a needle, and a catheter is threaded into the epidural space. The needle is removed and the catheter is left in place to allow for continuous infusion or intermittent injections of medicine (Fig. 14.11). An epidural block provides analgesia and anesthesia and can be used for both vaginal and cesarean births. It has evolved from a regional block producing total loss of sensation to analgesia with minimal blockade. The effectiveness of epidural analgesia depends on the technique and medications used. It is usually started after labour is well established, typically when cervical dilation is greater than 5 cm.

Theoretically, epidural local anesthetics could block all labour pain if used in large volumes and high concentrations. However, pain relief is balanced against other goals such as walking during the first stage of labour, pushing effectively in the second stage, and minimizing maternal and fetal side effects.

An epidural is contraindicated for women with a previous history of spinal surgery or spinal abnormalities, coagulation defects, infections, and hypovolemia. It also is contraindicated for the woman who is receiving anticoagulation therapy.

Complications may include nausea and vomiting, hypotension, fever, pruritus, intravascular injection, and respiratory depression (*Childbirth: An epidural*, 2011). Effects on the fetus during labour include fetal distress secondary to maternal hypotension (British Columbia Perinatal Health Program, 2009). Ensuring that the woman avoids a supine position after an epidural catheter has been placed will help to minimize hypotension.

Changes in epidural drugs and techniques have been made to optimize pain control while minimizing side effects. Today many women receive a continuous lumbar epidural infusion of a local anesthetic as well as an opioid (Rice Simpson & Creehan, 2008). The addition of

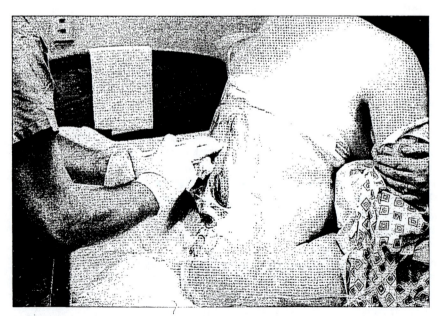

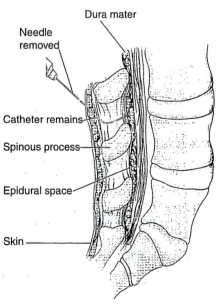

A
B

FIGURE 14.11 Epidural catheter insertion. (**A**) A needle is inserted into the epidural space. (**B**) A catheter is threaded through the needle into the epidural space; the needle is then removed. The catheter allows medication to be administered intermittently or continuously to relieve pain during labour and childbirth.

opioids, such as fentanyl or morphine, to the local anesthetic helps decrease the amount of motor block obtained (Reynolds, 2010). Continuous infusion pumps are often used to administer the epidural analgesia, allowing the woman to be in control and administer a bolus dose on demand (Akerman & Dresner, 2009).

Spinal (Intrathecal) Analgesia/Anesthesia

The spinal (intrathecal) pain-management involves the injection of an anesthetic "caine" agent, with or without opioids, into the subarachnoid space to provide pain relief during labour or cesarean birth. The contraindications are similar to those for the epidural block. Potential adverse reactions for the woman include hypotension and spinal headache.

Combined Spinal–Epidural Analgesia

Another epidural technique is CSE analgesia. This technique involves inserting the epidural needle into the epidural space and subsequently inserting a small-gauge spinal needle through the epidural needle into the subarachnoid space. An opioid, without a local anesthetic, is injected into this space. The spinal needle is then removed and an epidural catheter is inserted for later use.

CSE is advantageous because of its rapid onset of pain relief (within 3 to 5 minutes) that can last up to 3 hours. In a recent review of CSE analgesia studies, Cheng & Caughey (2012) found this method to offer superior pain control. In their review of 19 randomized, controlled trials involving close to 3,000 women, Simmons and colleagues (2009) concluded that CSE had a faster onset of action and was associated with less pruritus than with epidurals; however, there was no difference in the woman's ability to mobilize or in the obstetric or neonatal outcomes. Although women can theoretically walk with CSE, they often choose not to because of poor mobility and leg weakness (Simmons et al., 2009).

Ambulating during labour provides several benefits: it may help control pain better, shorten the first stage of labour, increase the intensity of the contractions, and decrease the possibility of an operative vaginal or cesarean birth. However, nurses need to be cognizant of the potential for injury in patients using CSE analgesia if the client is verbalizing or demonstrating poor mobility or weakness.

Other complications include maternal hypotension, which can lead to fetal distress; postdural puncture headache (Alam, Raheen, Iqbal, et al., 2011); inadequate or failed block (Evans et al., 2010); pruritus; and urinary retention (Akerman & Dresner, 2009). In addition, the procedure is known to slow down the first stage or labour and/or extend the second stage (Evans et al., 2010; Klein, Kaczorowski, Hall, et al., 2009). Hypotension and associated FHR changes are managed with maternal positioning (semi-Fowler's, left lateral tilt), intravenous hydration, and supplemental oxygen (Evans et al., 2010). The patient may need a urinary catheter to either prevent (inserted during labour) or relieve urinary retention postpartum (Akerman & Dresner, 2009; Evans et al., 2010). Itching and rash may occur secondary to the anesthetic and is often easily managed with diphenhydramine hydrochloride (Benadryl).

Patient-Controlled Epidural Analgesia

Epidural PCA involves the use of an indwelling epidural catheter with an infusion of medication and a programmed pump that allows the woman to control the dosing. This method allows the woman to have a sense of control over her pain and reach her own individually acceptable analgesia level. Studies have shown that women report high levels of satisfaction with both CSE and epidural PCA, but they appear to prefer controlling their pain with the push of a button (Landau, 2009).

With epidural PCA, the woman uses a hand-held device connected to an analgesic agent that is attached to an epidural catheter. When she pushes the button, a bolus dose of agent is administered via the catheter to reduce her pain. This method allows the woman to manage her pain at will without having to ask a staff member to provide pain relief.

Local Infiltration

Local infiltration involves the injection of a local anesthetic, such as lidocaine, into the superficial perineal nerves to numb the perineal area. This technique is done by the physician or midwife just before performing an episiotomy (surgical incision into the perineum to facilitate birth) or before suturing a laceration. Local infiltration does not alter the pain of uterine contractions, but it does numb the immediate area of the episiotomy or laceration. Local infiltration does not cause side effects for the woman or her newborn.

Pudendal Nerve Block

A pudendal nerve block refers to the injection of a local anesthetic agent (e.g., bupivacaine, ropivacaine) into the pudendal nerves near each ischial spine. It provides pain relief in the lower vagina, vulva, and perineum (Fig. 14.12).

A pudendal block is used for the second stage of labour, an episiotomy, or an operative vaginal birth with outlet forceps or vacuum extractor. It must be administered about 15 minutes before it is needed to ensure its full effect. A transvaginal approach is generally used to inject an anesthetic agent at or near the pudendal nerve branch. Neither maternal nor fetal complications are common.

General Anesthesia

General anesthesia is typically reserved for emergency cesarean births when there is not enough time to provide

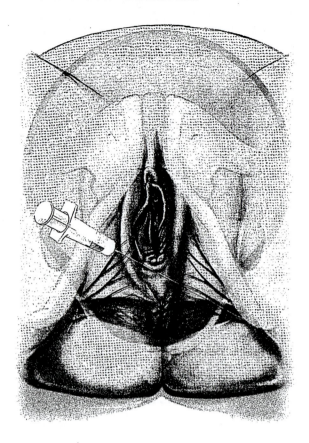

FIGURE 14.12 Pudendal nerve block.

spinal or epidural anesthesia or if the woman has a contraindication to the use of regional anesthesia. It can be started quickly and causes a rapid loss of consciousness. General anesthesia can be administered by IV injection, inhalation of anesthetic agents, or both. Commonly, thiopental, a short-acting barbiturate, is given IV to produce unconsciousness. This is followed by administration of a muscle relaxant. After the woman is intubated, nitrous oxide and oxygen are administered.

All anesthetic agents cross the placenta and affect the fetus. The primary complication with general anesthesia is fetal depression, along with uterine relaxation and potential maternal vomiting and aspiration.

Although the anesthesiologist or nurse anesthetist administers the various general anesthesia agents, the nurse needs to be knowledgeable about the pharmacologic aspects of the drugs used and must be aware of airway management. Ensure that the woman is NPO and has a patent IV. In addition, administer a nonparticulate (clear) oral antacid (e.g., Bicitra or sodium citrate) or a proton pump inhibitor (Protonix) as ordered to reduce gastric acidity. Assist with placement of a wedge under the woman's right hip to displace the gravid uterus and prevent vena cava compression in the supine position. Once the newborn has been removed from the uterus, assist the perinatal team in providing supportive care.

Nursing Care During Labour and Birth

WATCH&LEARN

Childbirth, a physiologic process that is fundamental to all human existence, is one of the most significant cultural, psychological, spiritual, and behavioural events in a woman's life. Although the act of giving birth is a universal phenomenon, it is a unique experience for each woman. Continuous evaluation and appropriate intervention for women during labour are the keys to promoting a positive outcome for the family.

The nurse's role in childbirth is to ensure a safe environment for the mother and her newborn. Nurses begin evaluating the mother and fetus during the admission procedures at the health care agency and continue to do so throughout labour. It is critical to provide anticipatory guidance and explain each procedure (fetal monitoring, IV therapy, medications given, and expected reactions) and what will happen next. This will prepare the woman for the upcoming physical and emotional challenges, thereby helping to reduce her anxiety. Acknowledging her support systems (family or partner) helps allay their fears and concerns, thereby assisting them in carrying out their supportive role. Knowing how and when to evaluate a woman during the various stages of labour is essential for all labour and birth nurses to ensure a positive maternal experience and a healthy newborn.

A major focus of care for the woman during labour and birth is assisting her with maintaining control over her pain, emotions, and actions while being an active participant. Nurses can help and support women to be actively involved in their childbirth experience by allowing time for discussion, offering companionship, listening to worries and concerns, paying attention to the woman's emotional needs, and offering information to help her understand what is happening in each stage of labour.

Nursing Care During the First Stage of Labour

Depending on how far advanced the woman's labour is when she arrives at the facility, the nurse will determine assessment parameters of maternal–fetal status and plan care accordingly. The nurse will provide high-touch, low-tech supportive nursing care during the first stage of labour when admitting the woman and orienting her to the labour and birth suite. Nursing care during this stage will include taking an admission history (reviewing the prenatal record); checking the results of routine laboratory tests and any special tests such as chorionic villi sampling, amniocentesis, genetic studies, and biophysical profile done during pregnancy; asking the woman about her childbirth preparation (birth plan, classes taken, coping skills); and completing a physical assessment of the woman to establish a baseline of values for future comparison.

Key nursing interventions include:

• Identifying the estimated date of birth from the client and the prenatal chart
• Validating the client's prenatal history to determine fetal risk status
• Determining fundal height to validate dates and fetal growth
• Performing Leopold's manoeuvres to determine fetal position, lie, and presentation
• Checking FHR
• Performing a vaginal examination (as appropriate) to evaluate effacement and dilation progress
• Instructing the client and her partner about monitoring techniques and equipment
• Assessing fetal response and FHR against contractions and recovery time
• Interpreting fetal monitoring strips
• Checking FHR baseline for accelerations, variability, and decelerations
• Repositioning the client to obtain an optimal FHR pattern
• Recognizing FHR problems and initiating corrective measures
• Checking amniotic fluid for meconium staining, odour, and amount
• Comforting the client throughout the testing period and labour
• Supporting the client's decisions regarding intervention or avoidance of intervention
• Assessing the client's support system and coping status frequently

In addition to these interventions to promote optimal outcomes for the mother and fetus, the nurse must document care accurately and in a timely fashion. The purpose of the health record is to communicate the health status of the mother to other members of the team. In addition, accurate and timely documentation of the care provided and the responses shown will be critical in potential cases of litigation (Rice Simpson & Creehan, 2008), which is prevalent in the childbirth arena. In addition to following provincial and agency policies, guidelines for recording care include the following:

• Ensure that only factual and objective information on care provided is recorded
• Include all communication with other health care team members (direct or indirect)
• Document only clinically relevant information
• Include comprehensive data about maternal–fetal status
• Record nursing interventions and patient response

The SOGC (2007) stresses the importance of good, clear, effective communication and accurate documentation pertaining to fetal health assessments. In particular, specific required documentation inclusions are listed as they pertain to intermittent auscultation and EFM.

Assessing the Woman Upon Admission

The nurse usually first comes in contact with the woman either by phone or in person. It is important to ascertain whether the woman is in true or false labour and whether she should be admitted or sent home. Upon admission to the labour and birth suite, the highest priorities include assessing FHR, assessing cervical dilation/effacement, and determining whether membranes have ruptured or are intact. These assessment data will guide the critical thinking in planning care for the patient.

If the initial contact is by phone, establish a therapeutic relationship with the woman. Speaking in a calm, caring tone facilitates this. When completing a phone assessment, include questions about the following:

• Estimated date of birth, to determine if term or preterm
• Fetal movement (frequency in the past few days)
• Other premonitory signs of labour experienced
• Parity, gravida, and previous childbirth experiences
• Time from start of labour to birth in previous labours
• Characteristics of contractions, including frequency, duration, and intensity
• Appearance of any vaginal bloody show
• Membrane status (ruptured or intact)
• Presence of supportive adult in household or if she is alone

When speaking with the woman over the telephone, review the signs and symptoms that denote true versus false labour, and suggest various positions she can assume to provide comfort and increase placental perfusion. Also suggest walking, massage, and taking a warm shower to promote relaxation. Outline what foods and fluids are appropriate for oral intake in early labour. Throughout the phone call, listen to the woman's concerns and answer any questions clearly.

Rice Simpson and Creehan (2008) advise against telephone triage; they advise nurses simply to instruct women to call their primary health care provider or come to the hospital to be evaluated. Ruling out true labour and possible maternal–fetal complications cannot be done accurately over the phone.

Additional nursing responsibilities associated with a phone assessment include:

• Consulting the woman's prenatal record for parity status, estimated date of birth, and untoward events
• Calling the health care provider to inform him or her of the woman's status
• Preparing for admission to the perinatal unit to ensure adequate staff assignment
• Notifying the admissions office of a pending admission

If the nurse's first encounter with the woman is in person, an assessment is completed to determine whether she should be admitted to the perinatal unit or sent home until her labour advances. Entering a facility is often an intimidating and stressful event for women since it is an unfamiliar environment. Giving birth for the first time is a pivotal event in the lives of most women. Therefore, demonstrate respect when addressing the client; listen carefully and express interest and concern. As part of the National Birthing Initiative for Canada, the SOGC (2008a) recognizes the importance of ensuring that maternity care is patient centred and empowering for women and identifies listening to women's voices as the highest priority. Inviting the labouring woman to share her birth plan and making her a part of the decisions that affect her care demonstrates respect and will enhance her sense of self-control.

An admission assessment includes maternal health history, physical assessment, fetal assessment, laboratory studies, and assessment of psychological status. Usually the facility has a form that can be used throughout labour and birth to document assessment findings (Fig. 14.13).

Maternal Health History

A maternal health history should include typical biographical data such as the woman's name and age and the name of the delivering health care provider. Other information that is collected includes the prenatal record data, including the estimated date of birth, a history of the current pregnancy, and the results of any laboratory and diagnostic tests, such as blood type, Rh status, and group B streptococcal status; past pregnancy and obstetric history; past health history and family history; prenatal education; list of medications; risk factors such as diabetes, hypertension, and use of tobacco, alcohol, or illicit drugs; reason for admission, such as labour, cesarean birth, or observation for a complication; history of potential domestic violence; history of previous preterm births; allergies; time of last food ingestion; method chosen for infant feeding; name of birth attendant and pediatrician; and pain management plan.

Ascertaining this information is important so that an individualized plan of care can be developed for the woman. If, for example, the woman's due date is still 2 months away, it is important to establish this information so interventions can be initiated to arrest the labour immediately or notify the intensive perinatal team to be available. In addition, if the woman is a diabetic, it is critical to monitor her glucose levels during labour, to prepare for a surgical birth if dystocia of labour occurs, and to alert the newborn nursery of potential hypoglycemia in the newborn after birth. By collecting important information about each woman they care for, nurses can help improve the outcomes for all concerned.

Be sure to observe the woman's emotions, support system, verbal interaction, body language and posture, perceptual acuity, and energy level. Also note her cultural background and language spoken. This psychosocial information provides cues about the woman's emotional state, culture, and communication systems. For example, if the woman arrives at the labour and birth suite extremely anxious, alone, and unable to communicate in English, how can the nurse meet her needs and plan her care appropriately? It is only by assessing each woman physically and psychosocially that the nurse can make astute decisions regarding proper care. In this case, an interpreter would be needed to assist in the communication process between the staff and the woman to initiate proper care.

It is important to acknowledge and try to understand the cultural differences in women with cultural backgrounds different from that of the nurse. Attitudes toward childbirth are heavily influenced by the culture in which the woman has been raised. As a result, within every society, specific attitudes and values shape the woman's childbearing behaviours. Be aware of what these are. When carrying out a cultural assessment during the admission process, ask questions (Box 14.2) to help plan culturally competent care during labour and birth.

Physical Examination

The physical examination typically includes a generalized assessment of the woman's body systems, including hydration status, vital signs, auscultation of heart and lung sounds, and measurement of height and weight.

BOX 14.2 Questions for Providing Culturally Competent Care During Labour and Birth

- Where were you born? How long have you lived in Canada?
- What languages do you speak and read?
- Who are your major support people?
- What are your religious practices?
- How do you view childbearing?
- Are there any special precautions or restrictions that are important?
- Is birth considered a private or a social experience?
- Are there any practices in your culture related to the birth of your child that are important?
- Are there any practices in your culture related to your newborn that are important, such as a naming ceremony?
- How would you like to manage your labour discomfort?
- Who will provide your labour support?

Source: D'Avanzo, C. E. (2008). *Cultural health assessment* (4th ed.). St. Louis, MO: Mosby Elsevier.

ADMISSION ASSESSMENT OBSTETRICS

▲ PATIENT IDENTIFICATION ▲

ADMISSION DATA

Date	Time	Via
		☐ Ambulatory ☐ Wheelchair ☐ Stretcher

Grav.	Term	Pre-term	Ab.	Living	EDC	LMP	GA

Prev. adm. date _____ Reason _____

Obstetrician _____ Pediatrician _____

Ht._____ Wt. _____ Wt. gain _____

Allergies (meds/food) ☐ None _____ ☐ Hx latex sensitivity

BP _____ T _____ P _____ R _____

FHR _____ Vag exam _____

Reason for Admission

☐ Labor / SROM   ☐ Induction _____

☐ Primary C/S _____ ☐ Repeat C/S

☐ Observation _____

☐ OB / Medical complication _____

Onset of labor: ☐ Not in labor

Date _____ Time _____

Membranes: ☐ Intact

☐ Ruptured / Date _____ Time _____

☐ Clear   ☐ Meconium   ☐ Bloody   ☐ Foul

Vaginal bleeding: ☐ None

☐ Normal show   ☐ _____

Current Pregnancy Labs   ☐ NPC

☐ POL   ☐ PPROM   ☐ Cerclage

☐ PIH   ☐ Chr. HTN   ☐ Other _____

☐ Diabetes _____ Diet _____

☐ Insulin _____

☐ Amniocentesis _____ Results _____

Bld type / RH____Date Rhogam____

Antibody screen ☐ Neg ☐ Pos

Rubella ☐ Non-immune ☐ Immune

Diabetic screen ☐ Normal ☐ Abnormal

Recent exposure to chick pox ☐

Current meds:_____

_____

	Pos	Neg	Tested
Hepatitis B	☐	☐	☐ No
HIV	☐	☐	☐ No
Group B strep	☐	☐	☐ No
GC	☐	☐	☐ No
Chlamydia	☐	☐	☐ No
RPR	☐	☐	☐ No

Previous OB History

☐ POL   ☐ Multiple gestation

☐ Prev C/S type _____ Reason _____

☐ PIH   ☐ Chronic HTN   ☐ Diabetes _____

☐ Stillbirth/demise   ☐ Neodeath   ☐ Anomalies

☐ Precipitous labor (<3 H)   ☐ Macrosomia

☐ PP Hemorrhage

☐ Hx Transfusion reaction   ☐ Yes   ☐ No

☐ Other _____

Latest risk assessment   ☐ None

1. _____ 3. _____

2. _____ 4. _____

Signature _____ Date _____ Time _____

NEUROLOGICAL

☐ WNL

Variance: ☐ HA

☐ Scotoma / visual changes

Reflexes ☐ < 2 +   ☐ > 2 +

☐ Clonus ___ bts

☐ Numbness   ☐ Tingling

☐ Hx Seizures

☐

RESPIRATORY

☐ WNL

Variance: ☐ Hx Asthma ☐ URI

Respirations: ☐ < 12 ☐ > 24

Effort: ☐ SOB

☐ Shallow ☐ Labored

Auscultation:

☐ Diminished ☐ Crackles

☐ Wheezes ☐ Rhonchi

	No	Yes
Cough for greater than 2 weeks?	☐	☐
Is the cough productive?	☐	☐
Blood in the sputum?	☐	☐
Experiencing any fever or night sweats?	☐	☐
Ever had TB in the past?	☐	☐
Recent exposure to TB?	☐	☐
Weight loss in last 3 weeks?	☐	☐

If the patient answers yes to any three of the above questions implement policy and procedure # 5725-0704.

GASTROINTESTINAL

☐ WNL

Variance: ☐ Heartburn

☐ Epigastric pain   Nausea

☐ Vomiting ☐ Diarrhea

☐ Constipation ☐ Pain

☐ Wt. Gain < 2lbs / month**

☐ Recent change in appetite of < 50% of usual intake for > 5 days

INTEGUMENTARY

☐ WNL

Variance: ☐ Rash ☐ Lacerations

☐ Abrasion ☐ Swelling

☐ Uticaria ☐ Bruising

☐ Diaphoretic/hot

☐ Clammy/cold

☐ Scars

☐

FETAL ASSESSMENT

☐ WNL

Variance:

☐ NRFS

FHR ☐ < 110   ☐ > 160

LTV ☐ Absent ☐ Minimal

☐ Increased

STV Absent

Decelerations: _____

☐ Decreased fetal movement

☐ IUGR

☐

			Amt
Tobacco use	☐ Denies	☐ Yes	
Alcohol use	☐ Denies	☐ Yes	Amt
Drug use	☐ Denies	☐ Yes	Amt type
Primary language	☐ English	☐ Spanish	☐

CARDIOVASCULAR

☐ WNL

Variance:

☐ MVP

Heart rate: ☐ < 60 ☐ > 100

B/P: Systolic: ☐ < 90 ☐ > 140

Diastolic: ☐ < 50 ☐ > 90

☐ Edema _____

☐ Chest pain / palpitations

☐

MUSCULOSKELETAL

☐ WNL

Variance:

☐ Numbness   ☐ Tingling

☐ Paralysis   ☐ Deformity

☐ Scoliosis

☐

GENITOURINARY

☐ WNL

Variance: ☐ Albumin _____

Output: ☐ < 30 cc/Hr.

☐ UTI   ☐ Rx   ☐ Frequency

☐ Dysuria   ☐ Hematuria

☐ CVA Tenderness

☐ Hx STD _____

☐ Vag. discharge _____

☐ Rash   ☐ Blisters

☐ Warts   ☐ Lesions

☐

EARS, NOSE, THROAT, AND EYES

☐ WNL

Variance:

☐ Sore throat   ☐ Eyeglasses

☐ Runny nose   ☐ Contact lenses

☐ Nasal congestion

☐

PSYCHOSOCIAL

☐ WNL

Variance: ☐ Hx depression

☐ Yes   ☐ No

☐ Emotional behavioral care

Affect: ☐ Flat   ☐ Anxious

☐ Uncooperative   ☐ Combative

Living will   ☐ Yes   ☐ No

☐ On chart

Healthcare surrogate ☐ Yes   ☐ No

☐ On chart

Are you being hurt, hit, frightened by anyone at home or in your life? ☐ Yes   ☐ No

Religious preference _____

PAIN ASSESSMENT

1. Do you have any ongoing pain problems?   ☐ No   ☐ Yes

2. Do you have any pain now?   ☐ No   ☐ Yes

3. If any of the above questions are answered yes, the patient has a positive pain screening.

4. Patient to be given pain management education material. Complete pain / symptom assessment on flowsheet.

5. Please proceed to complete pain assessment.

FIGURE 14.13 Sample documentation form used for admission to the perinatal unit. (Used with permission. Briggs Corporation, 2001.)

The physical examination also includes the following assessments:

- Fundal height measurement
- Uterine activity, including contraction frequency, duration, and intensity
- Status of membranes (intact or ruptured)
- Cervical dilation and degree of effacement
- Fetal status, including heart rate, position, and station
- Pain level

These assessment parameters form a baseline against which the nurse can compare all future values throughout labour. The findings should be similar to those of the woman's prepregnancy and pregnancy findings, with the exception of her pulse rate, which might be elevated secondary to her anxious state with beginning labour.

Laboratory Studies

On admission, laboratory studies typically are done to establish a baseline. Although the exact tests may vary among facilities, they usually include a urinalysis via clean-catch urine specimen and complete blood count (CBC). Blood typing and Rh factor analysis may be necessary if the results of these are unknown or unavailable. In addition, if the following test results are not included in the maternal prenatal history, it may be necessary to perform them at this time. They include syphilis screening, hepatitis B surface antigen (HBsAg) screening, group B streptococcus (GBS) testing, human immunodeficiency virus (HIV) testing (if the woman gives consent), and possible drug screening if the history is positive.

GBS is a gram-positive organism that is present in the vaginal and gastrointestinal tract of 15% to 45% of women (Woods & Levy, 2011). These women are asymptomatic carriers but can cause GBS disease of the newborn through vertical transmission. The mortality rate of infected newborns varies according to time of onset (early or late). Risk factors for GBS include maternal intrapartum fever, prolonged ruptured membranes, previous birth of an infected newborn, and GBS bacteriuria in the present pregnancy.

In 2004, the SOGC issued guidelines that advised universal screening of pregnant women at 35 to 37 weeks' gestation for GBS and intrapartum antibiotic therapy for GBS carriers. In addition, women at term whose membranes ruptured more than 18 hours previously should receive treatment (SOGC, 2004a). Maternal infections associated with GBS include acute chorioamnionitis, endometritis, and urinary tract infection. Neonatal clinical manifestations include pneumonia and sepsis. Identified GBS carriers receive IV antibiotic prophylaxis (penicillin G or ampicillin) at the onset of labour or when membranes rupture.

The SOGC (2001) recommends elective cesarean section at 38 weeks for HIV-positive women who meet one of the following criteria: women who have not received any anti-retroviral therapy, women receiving anti-retroviral monotherapy regardless of the viral load, women with detectable viral load regardless of the amount of therapy received, women with unknown viral load status, and women who have received no prenatal care. Read and Newell's (2009) findings in a *Cochrane* review support elective cesarean section for women not taking anti-retrovirals or for those only in receipt of zidovudine. However, they say the relationship between mother to child transmission is less clear when HIV-positive women have low viral loads and recommend further study in this area. Additional interventions to reduce the transmission risk include avoiding use of a scalp electrode for fetal monitoring or doing a scalp blood sampling for fetal pH, delaying amniotomy, and avoiding invasive procedures such as forceps or vacuum-assisted delivery. The nurse stresses the importance of all interventions and the goal to reduce transmission of HIV to the newborn.

Continuing Assessment During the First Stage of Labour

After the admission assessment is complete, assessment continues for changes that would indicate that labour is progressing as expected. Assess the woman's knowledge, experience, and expectations of labour. Typically, blood pressure, pulse, and respirations are assessed every hour during the latent phase of labour unless the clinical situation dictates that vital signs be taken more frequently. During the active and transition phases, they are assessed every 30 minutes. The temperature is taken every 4 hours throughout the first stage of labour unless the clinical situation dictates more frequent measurement (maternal fever).

Vaginal examinations are performed periodically to track labour progress. This assessment information is shared with the woman to reinforce that she is making progress toward the goal of birth. Uterine contractions are monitored for frequency, duration, and intensity every 30 to 60 minutes during the latent phase, every 15 to 30 minutes during the active phase, and every 15 minutes during transition. Note the changes in the character of the contractions as labour progresses, and inform the woman of her progress. Continually determine the woman's level of pain and her ability to cope and use relaxation techniques effectively.

When the fetal membranes rupture, spontaneously or artificially, assess the FHR and check the amniotic fluid for colour, odour, and amount. Assess the FHR intermittently or continuously via electronic monitoring. During the latent phase of labour, assess the FHR every 30 to 60 minutes; in the active phase, assess FHR at least every 15 to 30 minutes. Also, be sure to assess the FHR before ambulation, prior to any procedure, and before administering analgesia or anesthesia to the mother. Table 14.3 summarizes assessments for the first stage of labour.

TABLE 14.3   SUMMARY OF ASSESSMENTS DURING THE FIRST STAGE OF LABOUR

Assessments	Latent Phase (0–3 cm)	Active Phase (4–7 cm)	Transition (8–10 cm)
Vital signs (blood pressure, pulse, respirations)	Every 30–60 min	Every 30 min	Every 15–30 min
Temperature	Every 4 hours	Every 4 hours	Every 4 hours
Contractions (frequency, duration, intensity)	Every 30–60 min by palpation or continuously by electronic fetal monitoring (EFM)	Every 15–30 min by palpation or continuously by EFM	Every 15 min by palpation or continuously by EFM
Fetal heart rate	Every hour by Doppler or continuously by EFM	Every 30 min by Doppler or continuously by EFM	Every 15–30 min by Doppler or continuously by EFM
Vaginal examination	Initially on admission to determine phase and as needed based on maternal cues to document labour progression	As needed to monitor labour progression	As needed to monitor labour progression
Behaviour/psychosocial	With every client encounter: talkative, excited, anxious	With every client encounter: self-absorbed in labour; intense and quiet now	With every client encounter: discouraged, irritable, feels out of control, declining coping ability

*The frequency of assessments is dictated by the health status of the woman and fetus and can be altered if either one of their conditions changes.

*R*emember Sheila from the chapter-opening scenario? What is the nurse's role with Sheila in active labour? What additional comfort measures can the labour nurse offer Sheila?

Nursing Interventions

Nursing interventions during the admission process should include:

- Asking about the client's expectations of the birthing process
- Providing information about labour, birth, pain-management options, and relaxation techniques
- Presenting information about fetal monitoring equipment and the procedures needed
- Monitoring FHR and identifying patterns that need further intervention
- Monitoring the mother's vital signs to obtain a baseline for later comparison
- Reassuring the client that her labour progress will be monitored closely and nursing care will focus on ensuring fetal and maternal well-being throughout

As the woman progresses through the first stage of labour, nursing interventions include:

- Encouraging the woman's partner to participate
- Keeping the woman and her partner up to date on the progress of the labour
- Orienting the woman and her partner to the labour and birth unit and explaining all of the birthing procedures
- Providing clear fluids (e.g., ice chips) as needed or requested
- Maintaining the woman's parenteral fluid intake at the prescribed rate if she has an IV
- Initiating or encouraging comfort measures, such as backrubs, cool cloths to the forehead, frequent position changes, ambulation, showers, slow dancing, leaning over a birth ball, side-lying, or counterpressure on lower back (Teaching Guideline 14.1)
- Encouraging the partner's involvement with breathing techniques
- Assisting the woman and her partner to focus on breathing techniques
- Informing the woman that the discomfort will be intermittent and of limited duration; urging her to rest between contractions to preserve her strength; and encouraging her to use distracting activities to lessen the focus on contractions
- Changing bed linens and gown as needed
- Keeping the perineal area clean and dry

TEACHING GUIDELINE 14.1

Positioning During the First Stage of Labour

- Walking with support from your partner (adds the force of gravity to contractions to promote fetal descent)
- Slow-dancing position with your partner holding you (adds the force of gravity to contractions and promotes support from and active participation of your partner)
- Side-lying with pillows between the knees for comfort (offers a restful position and improves oxygen flow to the uterus)
- Semi-sitting in bed or on a couch leaning against the partner (reduces back pain because fetus falls forward, away from the sacrum)
- Sitting in a chair with one foot on the floor and one on the chair (changes pelvic shape)
- Leaning forward by straddling a chair, a table, or a bed or kneeling over a birth ball (reduces back pain, adds the force of gravity to promote descent; possible pain relief if partner can apply sacral pressure)
- Sitting in a rocking chair or on a birth ball and shifting weight back and forth (provides comfort because rocking motion is soothing; uses the force of gravity to help fetal descent)
- Lunge by rocking weight back and forth with foot up on chair during contraction (uses force of gravity by being upright; enhances rotation of fetus through rocking)

Sources: Adams, E. D., & Bianchi, A. L. (2008). A practical approach to labor support. *Journal of Obstetric, Gynecologic, & Neonatal Nursing, 37*, 106–115; Evans, R. J., Evans, M. K., Brown, Y. M. R., & Orshan, S. A. (2010). *Canadian maternity, newborn, & women's health nursing.* Philadelphia: Lippincott Williams & Wilkins; Lawrence, A., Lewis, L., Hofmeyr, G. J., Dowswell, T., & Styles, C. (2009). Maternal positions and mobility during first stage labour. *Cochrane Database of Systematic Reviews, 2,* CD003934; Lowdermilk, D. L., Perry, S. E., & Cashion, K. (2010). *Maternity nursing* (8th ed.). Maryland Heights, MO: Mosby Elsevier; & Schilling, T. (2009). *Healthy birth practices from Lamaze International: #2 Walk, move around, and change positions throughout labor.* Retrieved February 22, 2012 from http://www.lamaze.org/Portals/0/carepractices/CarePractice2.pdf.

- Supporting the woman's decisions about pain management
- Monitoring maternal vital signs frequently and reporting any abnormal values
- Ensuring that the woman takes deep cleansing breaths before and after each contraction to enhance gas exchange and oxygen to the fetus
- Educating the woman and her partner about the need for rest and helping them plan strategies to conserve strength
- Monitoring FHR for baseline, accelerations, variability, and decelerations

- Checking on bladder status and encouraging voiding at least every 2 hours to make room for birth
- Repositioning the woman as needed to obtain optimal heart rate pattern
- Communicating requests from the woman to appropriate personnel
- Respecting the woman's sense of privacy by covering her when appropriate
- Offering human presence by being present with the woman, not leaving her alone for long periods
- Being patient with the natural labour pattern to allow time for change
- Reporting any deviations from normal to the health care professional so that interventions can be initiated early to be effective (SOGC, 2007).

See Nursing Care Plan 14.1.

*R*emember Sheila, who was admitted in active labour? She has progressed to the transition phase (8 cm dilated) and is becoming increasingly more uncomfortable. She is using a patterned-paced breathing pattern now but thrashing around in the hospital bed.

Nursing Management During the Second Stage of Labour

Nursing care during the second stage of labour focuses on supporting the woman and her partner with interventions such as assisting with positioning and breathing techniques and providing instruction and assistance as needed. Research suggests that delaying pushing in the second stage of labour reduces the time spent in this stage, decreases the need for instrument-assisted delivery, and lessens postpartum fatigue, which ultimately affect both mother and newborn (Man-Lung, Kuan-Chia, Hsin Yang, et al., 2009). Shortening the phase of active pushing and lengthening the early phase of passive descent can be achieved by encouraging the woman not to push until she has a strong desire to do so and until the descent and rotation of the fetal head are well advanced. Berghella, Baxter, & Chauhan. (2008), in a review of evidence-based interventions, found upright positions such as sitting, semi-recumbency, kneeling, and squatting to be associated with shorter birth intervals, less pain and perineal damage, and fewer operative births.

Perineal lacerations or tears can occur during the second stage when the fetal head emerges through the vaginal introitus. The extent of the laceration is defined by depth: a first-degree laceration extends through the skin; a second-degree laceration extends through the muscles of the perineal body; a third-degree laceration continues through the anal sphincter muscle; and a

Nursing Care Plan 14.1

OVERVIEW OF THE WOMAN IN THE ACTIVE PHASE OF THE FIRST STAGE OF LABOUR

Candice, a 23-year-old gravida 1, para 0 (G1,P0) is admitted to the labour and birth suite at 39 weeks' gestation having contractions of moderate intensity every 5 to 6 minutes. A vaginal examination reveals her cervix is 80% effaced and 5 cm dilated. The presenting part (vertex) is at 0 station and her membranes ruptured spontaneously 4 hours ago at home. She is admitted and an IV is started for hydration and vascular access. An external fetal monitor is applied. FHR is 140 beats/minute and regular. Her partner is present at her bedside. Candice is now in the active phase of the first stage of labour, and her assessment findings are as follows: cervix dilated 7 cm, 80% effaced; moderate to strong contractions occurring regularly, every 3 to 5 minutes, lasting 45 to 60 seconds; at 0 station on pelvic examination; FHR auscultated loudest below umbilicus at 140 beats/minute; vaginal show—pink or bloody vaginal mucus; currently apprehensive, inwardly focused, with increased dependency; voicing concern about ability to cope with pain; limited ability to follow directions.

NURSING DIAGNOSIS: Anxiety related to labour and birth process and fear of the unknown related to client's first experience

Outcome Identification and Evaluation

Client will remain calm and in control as evidenced by ability to make decisions and use positive coping strategies.

Interventions: Promoting Positive Coping Strategies

- Provide instruction regarding the labour process *to allay anxiety.*
- Reorient the woman to the physical environment and equipment as necessary *to keep her informed of events.*
- Encourage verbalization of feelings and concerns *to reduce anxiety.*
- Listen attentively to woman and partner *to demonstrate interest and concern.*
- Inform woman and partner of standard procedures/processes *to ensure adequate understanding of events and procedures.*
- Frequently update woman of progress and labour status *to provide positive reinforcement for actions.*
- Reinforce relaxation techniques and provide instruction if needed *to aid in coping.*
- Encourage participation of the partner in the coaching role; role-model to facilitate partner participation in labour process *to provide support and encouragement to the client.*
- Provide a presence and remain with woman as much as possible *to provide comfort and support.*

NURSING DIAGNOSIS: Pain related to effects of contractions and cervical dilation and events of labour

Outcome Identification and Evaluation

Client will maintain a tolerable level of pain and discomfort as evidenced by statements of pain relief, pain rating of 2 or less on pain rating scale, and absence of adverse effects in client and fetus from analgesia or anesthesia.

Interventions: Providing Pain Relief

- Monitor vital signs, observe for signs of pain, and have client rate pain on a scale of 0 to 10 *to provide baseline for comparison.*
- Encourage client to void every 1 to 2 hours *to decrease pressure from a full bladder.*
- Assist woman to change positions frequently *to increase comfort and promote labour progress.*
- Encourage use of distraction *to reduce focus on contraction pain.*
- Suggest pelvic rocking, massage, or back counterpressure *to reduce pain.*
- Assist with use of relaxation and breathing techniques *to promote relaxation.*
- Use touch appropriately (backrub) when desired by the woman *to promote comfort.*
- Integrate use of non-pharmacologic measures for pain relief, such as warm water, birthing ball, or other techniques *to facilitate pain relief.*
- Administer pharmacologic agents as ordered when requested *to control pain.*
- Provide reassurance and encouragement between contractions *to foster self-esteem and continued participation in labour process.*

(continued)

Nursing Care Plan 14.1 (continued)

NURSING DIAGNOSIS: Risk of infection related to vaginal examinations following rupture of membranes

Outcome Identification and Evaluation

Client will remain free of infection as evidenced by absence of signs and symptoms of infection, vital signs and FHR within acceptable parameters, lab test results within normal limits, and clear amniotic fluid without odour.

Interventions: Preventing Infection

- Monitor vital signs (every 1 to 2 hours after rupture of membranes) and FHR frequently as per protocol *to allow for early detection of problems;* report fetal tachycardia (early sign of maternal infection) *to ensure prompt treatment.*
- Provide frequent perineal care and pad changes *to maintain good perineal hygiene.*
- Change linens and woman's gown as needed *to maintain cleanliness.*
- Ensure that vaginal examinations are performed only when needed *to prevent introducing pathogens into the vaginal vault.*
- Monitor lab test results such as white blood cell count *to assess for elevations indicating infection.*
- Use aseptic technique for all invasive procedures *to prevent infection transmission.*
- Carry out good handwashing techniques before and after procedures and use standard precautions as appropriate *to minimize risk of infection transmission.*
- Document amniotic fluid characteristics—colour, odour—*to establish baseline for comparison.*

---

fourth-degree laceration also involves the anterior rectal wall. Third- and fourth-degree lacerations need to be repaired carefully to retain fecal continence (Lowdermilk et al., 2010). The primary care provider should repair any lacerations during the third stage of labour.

An **episiotomy** is an incision made in the perineum to enlarge the vaginal outlet and theoretically to shorten the second stage of labour. An episiotomy can be either midline or mediolateral. There is insufficient evidence to determine which type of incision is better (Carroli & Mignini, 2009). Figure 14.14 shows episiotomy locations.

Registered midwives can perform and repair episiotomies, but they frequently use alternative measures if possible. Alternative measures such as warm compresses and continual massage with oil have been successful in stretching the perineal area to prevent cutting it. The routine use of episiotomies as compared with a needed (restrictive) approach has been studied for several years; conclusions support use of a restrictive approach, which yields many benefits for the recipients (Carroli & Mignini, 2009). The use of restrictive episiotomy results in less pain postpartum, better sexual function later, and less relaxation of pelvic musculature (Schuurmans, Senikas, & Lalonde, 2009).

Despite the lack of evidence supporting the routine use of episiotomies (PHAC, 2000; SOGC, 2004b, 2010), the Canadian Maternity Experiences Survey reported that one in five women has undergone one. Women who

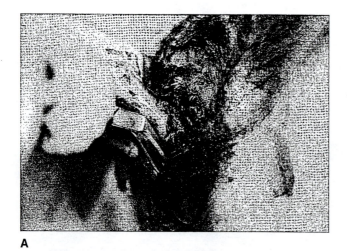
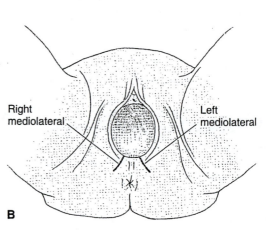

Right mediolateral

Left mediolateral

A

B

FIGURE 14.14 Location of an episiotomy. (**A**) Midline episiotomy. (**B**) Right and left mediolateral episiotomies.

TABLE 14.4   SUMMARY OF ASSESSMENTS DURING THE SECOND, THIRD, AND FOURTH STAGES OF LABOUR

Assessments	Second Stage of Labour (Birth of Neonate)	Third Stage of Labour (Placenta Expulsion)	Fourth Stage of Labour (Recovery)
Vital signs (blood pressure, pulse, respirations)	Every 5–15 min	Every 15 min	Every 15 min
Fetal heart rate	Every 5–15 min by Doppler or continuously by electroinc fetal monitoring (EFM)	Apgar scoring at 1 and 5 min	Newborn—complete head-to-toe assessment; vital signs every 15 min until stable
Contractions/ uterus	Palpate every one	Observe for placental separation	Palpate for firmness and position every 15 min for first hour
Bearing down/ pushing	Assist with every effort	None	None
Vaginal discharge	Observe for signs of descent—bulging of perineum, crowning	Assess bleeding after expulsion *lochia*	Assess every 15 min with fundus firmness check
Behaviour/ psychosocial	Observe every 15 min: cooperative, focus is on work of pushing newborn out	Observe every 15 min: often feelings of relief after hearing newborn crying; calmer	Observe every 15 min: usually excited, talkative, awake; needs to hold newborn, be close, and inspect body

•The frequency of assessments is dictated by the health status of the woman and fetus and can be altered if either one of their conditions changes.

have episiotomies are more likely than women who do not have episiotomies to experience more severe perineal trauma, more suturing, more pain, and more healing complications (Carroli & Mignini, 2009).

Assessment

Assessment is continuous during the second stage of labour. Hospital policies dictate the specific type and timing of assessments, as well as the way in which they are documented. Assessment involves identifying the signs typical of the second stage of labour, including:

• Increase in apprehension or irritability
• Spontaneous rupture of membranes
• Sudden appearance of sweat on upper lip
• Increase in blood-tinged show
• Low grunting sounds from the woman
• Complaints of rectal and perineal pressure
• Beginning of involuntary bearing-down efforts

Other ongoing assessments include the contraction frequency, duration, and intensity; maternal vital signs every 5 to 15 minutes; fetal response to labour as indicated by FHR monitor strips; amniotic fluid for colour, odour, and amount when membranes are ruptured; and the coping status of the woman and her partner (Table 14.4).

Assessment also focuses on determining the progress of labour. Associated signs include bulging of the perineum, labial separation, advancing and retreating of the newborn's head during and between bearing-down efforts, and **crowning** (fetal head is visible at vaginal opening; Fig. 14.15).

A vaginal examination is completed to determine if it is appropriate for the woman to push. Pushing is appropriate if the cervix has fully dilated to 10 cm and the woman feels the urge to do so.

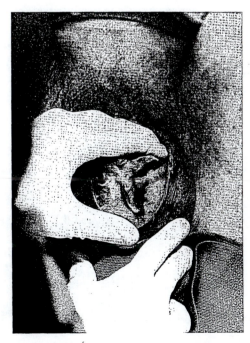

FIGURE 14.15 Crowning.

Nursing Interventions

Nursing interventions during this stage focus on motivating the woman, encouraging her to put all her efforts to pushing this newborn to the outside world, and giving her feedback on her progress. If the woman is pushing and not making progress, suggest that she keep her eyes open during the contractions and look toward where the infant is coming out. Changing positions every 20 to 30 minutes will also help in making progress. Positioning a mirror so the woman can visualize the birthing process and how successful her pushing efforts are can help motivate her.

The benefits of upright positioning during the second stage of labour are related to gravity with less aortovagal compression, improved fetal alignment, and larger anterior–posterior and transverse pelvic outlets (Berghella et al., 2008). Some suggestions for positions in the second stage include:

- Lithotomy with feet up in stirrups: most convenient position for caregivers
- Semi-sitting with pillows underneath knees, arms, and back
- Lateral/side-lying with curved back and upper leg supported by partner
- Sitting on birthing stool: opens pelvis, enhances the pull of gravity, and helps with pushing
- Squatting/supported squatting: gives the woman a sense of control
- Kneeling with hands on bed and knees comfortably apart

Other important nursing interventions during the second stage include:

- Providing continuous comfort measures such as mouth care, position changes, changing bed linen and under-pads, and providing a quiet, focused environment
- Instructing the woman on the following bearing-down positions and techniques:
  - Pushing only when she feels an urge to do so
  - Using abdominal muscles when bearing down
  - Using short pushes of 6 to 7 seconds
  - Focusing attention on the perineal area to visualize the newborn
  - Relaxing and conserving energy between contractions
  - Pushing several times with each contraction (Lowdermilk et al., 2010)
- Continuing to monitor contraction and FHR patterns to identify problems
- Providing brief, explicit directions throughout this stage
- Continuing to provide psychosocial support by reassuring and coaching
- Facilitating the upright position to encourage the fetus to descend

- Continuing to assess blood pressure, pulse, respirations, uterine contractions, bearing-down efforts, FHR, coping status of the client and her partner
- Providing pain management if needed
- Providing a continuous nursing presence
- Offering praise for the client's efforts
- Preparing for and assisting with delivery by:
  - Notifying the health care provider of the estimated time frame for birth
  - Preparing the delivery bed and positioning the client
  - Preparing the perineal area according to the facility's protocol
  - Offering a mirror and adjusting it so the woman can watch the birth
  - Explaining all procedures and equipment to the client and her partner
  - Setting up delivery instruments needed while maintaining sterility
  - Receiving newborn and transporting him or her to a warming environment, or covering the newborn with a warmed blanket on the woman's abdomen
  - Providing initial care and assessment of the newborn (see the Birth section that follows)

*S*heila is completely dilated now and experiencing the urge to push. How can the nurse help Sheila with her pushing efforts? What additional interventions can the labour nurse offer Sheila now?

Birth

The second stage of labour ends with the birth of the newborn. The maternal position for birth varies from the standard lithotomy position to side-lying to squatting to standing or kneeling, depending on the birthing location, the woman's preference, and standard protocols. Once the woman is positioned for birth, cleanse the vulva and perineal areas. The primary health care provider then takes charge after donning protective eyewear, mask, gown, and gloves and performing hand hygiene.

Once the fetal head has emerged, the primary care provider explores the fetal neck to see if the umbilical cord is wrapped around it. If it is, the cord is slipped over the head to facilitate delivery. As soon as the head emerges, the health care provider suctions the newborn's mouth first (because the newborn is an obligate nose breather) and then the nares with a bulb syringe to prevent aspiration of mucus, amniotic fluid, or meconium (Fig. 14.16). The umbilical cord is double-clamped and cut between the clamps. With the first cries of the newborn, the second stage of labour ends.

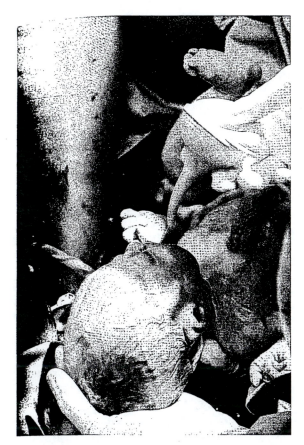

FIGURE 14.16 Suctioning the newborn immediately after birth.

In addition to encouraging Sheila to rest between pushing and offering praise for her efforts, what is the nurse's role during the birthing process?

Immediate Care of the Newborn

Once the infant is born, place him or her under the radiant warmer, dry him or her, assess him or her, wrap him or her in warmed blankets, and place him or her on the woman's abdomen for warmth and closeness. In some health care facilities, the newborn is placed on the woman's abdomen immediately after birth and covered with a warmed blanket. In either scenario, the stability of the newborn dictates the location of aftercare. The nurse can also assist the mother with breastfeeding her newborn for the first time.

Assessment of the newborn begins at the moment of birth and continues until the newborn is discharged. Drying the newborn and providing warmth to prevent heat loss by evaporation is essential to help support thermoregulation and provide stimulation. Placing the newborn under a radiant heat source and putting on a stockinet cap will further reduce heat loss after drying.

Assess the newborn by assigning an Apgar score at 1 and 5 minutes. The Apgar score assesses five parameters—heart rate (absent, slow, or fast), respiratory effort (absent,

weak cry, or good strong yell), muscle tone (limp, or lively and active), response to irritation stimulus, and colour—that evaluate a newborn's cardiorespiratory adaptation after birth. The parameters are arranged from the most important (heart rate) to the least important (colour). The newborn is assigned a score of 0 to 2 in each of the five parameters. The purpose of the Apgar assessment is to evaluate the physiologic status of the newborn; see Chapter 18 for additional information on Apgar scoring.

To verify his or her identity, secure two identification bands on the newborn, one on the wrist and one on the ankle, that match the band on the mother's wrist. This identification process is completed in the birthing suite before anyone leaves the room. Some facilities provide an additional identical band for the father as well (Lowdermilk et al., 2010). The bands should fit snugly to prevent loss.

Other types of newborn security systems can also be used to prevent abduction. Some systems have sensors that are attached to the newborn's identification bracelet or cord clamp. An alarm is set off if the bracelet or clamp activates receivers near exits. Others have an alarm that is activated when the sensor is removed from the newborn (Fig. 14.17). Although newborn abduction is not common in hospitals, additional security measures in maternity wards are now common across Canada and are supported by policies. Visitors are often screened in some way before they are allowed access to the newborn (Evans et al., 2010). Examples include controlled unit access with videos and alarms, family and support people wearing identification bracelets to match baby's, all newborns transported in cribs and those carrying a newborn in their arms are questioned. Parents are educated in the basics of hospital security (Evans et al., 2010).

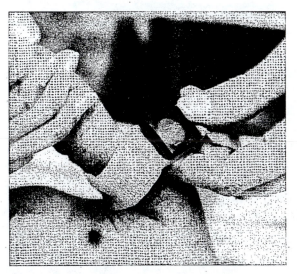

FIGURE 14.17 An example of a security sensor applied to a newborn's arm.

Sheila gave birth to a healthy 7-pound, 7-ounce baby girl (3,500 g). She is eager to hold and nurse her newborn. What is the initial care of the newborn? How can the nurse meet the needs of both the newborn and Sheila, who is exhausted but eager to bond with her newborn?

Nursing Management During the Third Stage of Labour

During the third stage of labour, strong uterine contractions continue at regular intervals under the continuing influence of oxytocin. The uterine muscle fibres shorten, or retract, with each contraction, leading to a gradual decrease in the size of the uterus, which helps shear the placenta away from its attachment site. The third stage is complete when the placenta is delivered. Nursing care during the third stage of labour focuses primarily on immediate newborn care and assessment and being available to assist with the delivery of the placenta and inspecting it for intactness.

Three hormones play important roles in the third stage. During this stage the woman experiences peak levels of oxytocin and endorphins, while the high adrenaline levels that occurred during the second stage of labour to aid with pushing begin falling. The hormone oxytocin causes uterine contractions and helps the woman to enact instinctive mothering behaviours such as holding the newborn close to her body and cuddling the baby.

Skin-to-skin contact immediately after birth and the newborn's first attempt at breastfeeding further augment maternal oxytocin levels, strengthening the uterine contractions that will help the placenta to separate and the uterus to contract to prevent hemorrhage. Endorphins, the body's natural opiates, produce an altered state of consciousness and aid in blocking out pain. In addition, the drop in adrenaline level from the second stage, which had kept the mother and baby alert at first contact, causes most women to shiver and feel cold shortly after giving birth.

▶ *Take NOTE!*

A crucial role for nurses during this time is to protect the natural hormonal process by ensuring unhurried and uninterrupted contact between mother and newborn after birth, providing warmed blankets to prevent shivering, and allowing skin-to-skin contact and breastfeeding.

Assessment

Assessment during the third stage of labour includes:

- Monitoring placental separation by looking for the following signs:
  - Firmly contracting uterus
  - Change in uterine shape from discoid to globular ovoid
  - Sudden gush of dark blood from vaginal opening
  - Lengthening of umbilical cord protruding from vagina
- Examining placenta and fetal membranes for intactness the second time (the health care provider assesses the placenta for intactness the first time) (Fig. 14.18)
- Assessing for any perineal trauma, such as the following, before allowing the birth attendant to leave:
  - Firm fundus with bright-red blood trickling: laceration
  - Boggy fundus with red blood flowing: uterine atony
  - Boggy fundus with dark blood and clots: retained placenta
- Inspecting the perineum for condition of episiotomy, if performed
- Assessing for perineal lacerations and ensuring repair by birth attendant

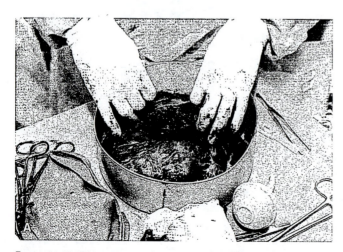 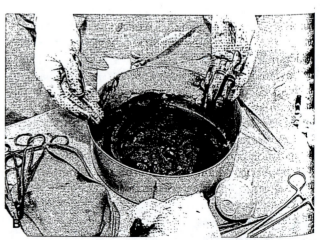

FIGURE 14.18 Placenta. (**A**) Fetal side. (**B**) Maternal side.

Nursing Interventions

Interventions during the third stage of labour include:

- Describing the process of placental separation to the couple
- Instructing the woman to push when signs of separation are apparent
- Administering oxytocin if ordered and indicated after placental expulsion
- Providing support and information about episiotomy and/or laceration
- Cleaning and assisting the client into a comfortable position after birth, making sure to lift both legs out of stirrups (if used) simultaneously to prevent strain
- Repositioning the birthing bed to serve as a recovery bed if applicable
- Assisting with transfer to the recovery area if applicable
- Providing warmth by replacing warmed blankets over the woman
- Applying an ice pack to the perineal area to provide comfort to episiotomy if indicated
- Explaining what assessments will be carried out over the next hour and offering positive reinforcement for actions
- Ascertaining any needs
- Monitoring maternal physical status by assessing:
  - Vaginal bleeding: amount, consistency, and colour
  - Vital signs: blood pressure, pulse, and respirations taken every 15 minutes
  - Uterine fundus, which should be firm, in the midline, and at the level of the umbilicus
- Recording all birthing statistics and securing the primary caregiver's signature
- Documenting birthing event in the birth book (official record of the facility that outlines every birth event), detailing any deviations

Nursing Management During the Fourth Stage of Labour

The fourth stage of labour begins after the placenta is expelled and lasts up to 4 hours after birth, during which time recovery takes place. This recovery period may take place in the same room where the woman gave birth, in a separate recovery area, or in her postpartum room. During this stage, the woman's body is beginning to undergo the many physiologic and psychological changes that occur after birth. The focus of nursing management during the fourth stage of labour involves frequent close observation for hemorrhage, provision of comfort measures, and promotion of family attachment.

Assessment

Assessments during the fourth stage centre on the woman's vital signs, status of the uterine fundus and perineal area, comfort level, lochia amount, and bladder status. During the first hour after birth, vital signs are taken every 15 minutes, then every 30 minutes for the next hour if needed. The woman's blood pressure should remain stable and within normal range after giving birth. A decrease may indicate uterine hemorrhage; an elevation might suggest pre-eclampsia.

The pulse usually is typically slower (60 to 70 beats/minute) than during labour. This may be associated with a decrease in blood volume following placental separation. An elevated pulse rate may be an early sign of blood loss. The blood pressure usually returns to its pre-pregnancy level and therefore is not a reliable early indicator of shock. Fever is indicative of dehydration (<100.4°F or 38°C) or infection (>101°F or 38.3°C), which may involve the genitourinary tract. Respiratory rate is usually between 16 and 24 breaths/minute and regular. Respirations should be unlaboured unless there is an underlying preexisting respiratory condition.

Assess fundal height, position, and firmness every 15 minutes during the first hour following birth. The fundus needs to remain firm to prevent excessive postpartum bleeding. The fundus should be firm (feels like the size and consistency of a grapefruit), located in the midline and below the umbilicus. If it is not firm (boggy), gently massage it until it is firm (see Nursing Procedure 22.1 in Chapter 22 for more information). Once firmness is obtained, stop massaging.

> **▶ Take NOTE!**
>
> *If the fundus is displaced to the right of the midline, suspect a full bladder as the cause.*

The vagina and perineal areas are quite stretched and edematous following a vaginal birth. Assess the perineum, including the episiotomy if present, for possible hematoma formation. Suspect a hematoma if the woman reports excruciating pain or cannot void or if a mass is noted in the perineal area. Also assess for hemorrhoids, which can cause discomfort.

Assess the woman's comfort level frequently to determine the need for analgesia. Ask the woman to rate her pain on a scale of 1 to 10; it should be less than 3. If it is higher, further evaluation is needed to make sure there aren't any deviations contributing to her discomfort.

Assess vaginal discharge (lochia) every 15 minutes for the first hour and every 30 minutes for the next hour. Palpate the fundus at the same time to ascertain its firmness and help to estimate the amount of vaginal discharge. In addition, palpate the bladder for fullness, since many women receiving an epidural block experience limited sensation in the bladder region. Voiding should produce large amounts of urine (diuresis) each time. Palpation of the woman's bladder after each voiding helps to ensure complete emptying. A full bladder will displace the uterus to either side of the midline and potentiate uterine hemorrhage secondary to bogginess.

Nursing Interventions

Nursing interventions during the fourth stage might include:

- Providing support and information to the woman regarding episiotomy repair and related pain-relief and self-care measures
- Applying an ice pack to the perineum to promote comfort and reduce swelling
- Assisting with hygiene and perineal care; teaching the woman how to use the perineal bottle after each pad change and voiding; helping the woman into a new gown
- Monitoring for return of sensation and ability to void (if regional anesthesia was used)
- Encouraging the woman to void by ambulating to bathroom, listening to running water, or pouring warm water over the perineal area with the peri bottle
- Monitoring vital signs and fundal and lochia status every 15 minutes and documenting them
- Promoting comfort by offering analgesia for afterpains and warm blankets to reduce chilling
- Offering fluids and nourishment if desired
- Encouraging parent–infant attachment by providing privacy for the family
- Being knowledgeable about and sensitive to typical cultural practices after birth
- Assisting the mother to nurse, if she chooses, during the recovery period to promote uterine firmness (the release of oxytocin from the posterior pituitary gland stimulates uterine contractions)
- Teaching the woman how to assess her fundus for firmness periodically and to massage it if it is boggy
- Describing the lochia flow and normal parameters to observe for postpartum
- Teaching safety techniques to prevent newborn abduction
- Demonstrating the use of the portable sitz bath as a comfort measure for her perineum if she had a laceration or an episiotomy repair
- Explain comfort/hygiene measures and when to use them
- Assisting with ambulation when getting out of bed for the first time
- Providing information about the routine on the mother–baby unit or nursery for her stay
- Assessing for signs of early parent–infant attachment: provides touch at times other than during feedings, meets all of baby's physical needs (Rice Simpson & Creehan, 2010)

□▨■ Key Concepts

- A nurse provides physical and emotional support during the labour and birth process to assist a woman to achieve her goals.
- When a woman is admitted to the labour and birth area, the admitting nurse must assess and evaluate the risk status of the pregnancy and initiate appropriate interventions to provide optimal care for the client.
- Completing an admission assessment includes taking a maternal health history; performing physical assessment on the woman and fetus, including her emotional and psychosocial status; and obtaining the necessary laboratory studies.
- The nurse's role in fetal assessment for labour and birth includes determining fetal well-being and interpreting signs and symptoms of possible compromise. Determining the FHR pattern and assessing amniotic fluid characteristics are key.
- FHR can be assessed intermittently or continuously. Although the intermittent method allows the client to move about during labour, the information obtained intermittently does not provide a complete picture of fetal well-being from moment to moment.
- Assessment parameters of the FHR are classified as baseline rate, baseline variability (long-term and short-term), and periodic changes in the rate (accelerations and decelerations).
- The nurse monitoring the labouring client needs to be knowledgeable about which parameters are normal, atypical, and abnormal so that appropriate interventions can be instituted.
- For an atypical FHR pattern, the nurse should notify the health care provider about the pattern and obtain further orders, making sure to document all interventions and their effects on the FHR pattern.
- In addition to interpreting assessment findings and initiating appropriate inventions for the labouring client, accurate and timely documentation must be carried out continuously.
- Today's women have many safe non-pharmacologic and pharmacologic choices for the management of pain during childbirth. They may be used individually or in combination to complement one another.
- Nursing management for the woman during labour and birth includes comfort measures, emotional support, information and instruction, advocacy, and support for the partner.
- Nursing care during the first stage of labour includes taking an admission history (reviewing the prenatal record), checking the results of routine laboratory work and special tests done during pregnancy, asking the woman about her childbirth preparation (birth plan, classes taken, coping skills), and completing a physical assessment of the woman to establish a baseline of values for future comparison.

■ Nursing care during the second stage of labour focuses on supporting the woman and her partner in making decisions about her care and labour management, implementing strategies to prolong the early passive phase of fetal descent, supporting involuntary bearing-down efforts, providing instruction and assistance, and encouraging the use of maternal positions that can enhance descent and reduce the pain.

■ Nursing care during the third stage of labour primarily focuses on immediate newborn care and assessment and being available to assist with the delivery of the placenta and inspecting it for intactness.

■ The focus of nursing management during the fourth stage of labour involves frequently observing the mother for hemorrhage, providing comfort measures, and promoting family attachment.

REFERENCES

Adams, E. D., & Bianchi, A. L. (2008). A practical approach to labor support. *Journal of Obstetric, Gynecologic, and Neonatal Nursing, 37*, 106–115.

Akerman, N., & Dresner, M. (2009). The management of breakthrough pain during labour. *CNS Drugs, 23*(8), 669–679.

Alam, R., Raheen, M. R., Iqbal, K. M., & Chowdhury, R. A. (2011). Headache following spinal anaesthesia: A review on recent update. *Journal of Bangladesh College of Physicians and Surgeons, 29*(1), 32–40.

Alfirevic, Z., Devane, D., & Gyte, G. M. L. (2008). Continuous cardiotocography (CTG) as a form of electronic fetal monitoring (EFM) for fetal assessment during labour. *Cochrane Database of Systematic Reviews, 3*, CD006066.

American College of Obstetricians and Gynecologists. (2009). *Intrapartum fetal heart rate monitoring: Nomenclature, interpretation, and general management principles. ACOG Practice Bulletin No. 106.* Washington, DC: Author.

Association of Women's Health, Obstetric, and Neonatal Nurses. (2011). *Nursing support of laboring women [Clinical Position Statement].* Washington, DC: Author. Retrieved from http://www.awhonn.org/awhonn/content.do?name=05_HealthPolicyLegislation/5H_PositionStatements.htm

Berghella, V., Baxter, J. K., & Chauhan, S. K. (2008). Evidence-based labor and delivery management. *American Journal of Obstetrics and Gynecology, 100*(5), 445–454.

Berkowitz, B. (2008). Cultural aspects in the care of the orthodox Jewish woman. *Journal of Midwifery and Women's Health, 53*(1), 62–67.

Borup, L., Wurlitzer, W., Hedegaard, M., Kesmodel, U., & Hvidman, L. (2009). Acupuncture as pain relief during delivery: a randomized controlled trial. *Birth: Issues in Perinatal Care, 36*(1), 5–12.

British Columbia Perinatal Health Program. (2009). *Core competencies: Management of labour in an institutional setting if the primary maternal care provider is absent. Guidelines for registered nurses.* Vancouver, BC: BC Perinatal Health Program. Retrieved February 22, 2012 from http://www.viha.ca/NR/rdonlyres/A20CC622-1C76-4ADA-9CE5-06A464AD99F3/0/mol_linked_core_competencies_with_dst_june_2010.pdf

Bryanton, J., Gagnon, A., Johnston, C., & Hatem, M. (2008). Predictor of women's perceptions of the childbirth experience. *Journal of Obstetric, Gynecologic, and Neonatal Nursing, 37*(1), 24–34.

Canadian Anesthesiologists' Society. (2010). *Guidelines for acute pain management using neuraxial analgesia.* Retrieved September 4, 2010 from http://www.cas.ca/members/

Canadian Institute for Health Information. (2010). *Highlights of 2008-2009 selected indicators describing the birthing process in Canada.* Retrieved February 22, 2012 from http://secure.cihi.ca/cihiweb/products/childbirth_highlights_2010_05_18_e.pdf

Carroli, G., & Mignini, L. (2009). Episiotomy for vaginal birth. *Cochrane Database of Systematic Reviews, 1*, CD000081.

Cheng, Y., & Caughey, A. B. (2012). *Normal labor and delivery.* Retrieved February 20, 2012 from http://emedicine.medscape.com/article/260036-print

Childbirth: An epidural. (2011). Retrieved September 4, 2010 from http://womenshealthmatters.info/centres/pregnancy/childbirth/epidural.html

Cluett, E. R., & Burns, E. (2009). Immersion in water in labour and birth. *Cochrane Database of Systematic Reviews, 2*, CD000111.

Currell, R., Urquhart, C., Harlow, F., & Callow, L. (2009). Home uterine monitoring for detecting preterm labour. *Cochrane Database of Systematic Reviews, 1*, CD006172.

D'Avanzo, C. E. (2008). *Cultural health assessment* (4th ed.). St. Louis, MO: Mosby Elsevier.

Datta, S., Kodali, B. S., & Segal, S. (2009). *Obstetric anesthesia handbook* (5th ed.). New York: Springer.

Deglin, J. H., Vallerand, A. H., & Sanoski, C. A. (2011). *Davis's drug guide for nurses* (12th ed.). Philadelphia: FA Davis Company.

East, C. E., Chan, F. Y., Colditz, P. B., & Begg, L. (2007). Fetal pulse oximetry for fetal assessment in labour. *Cochrane Database of Systematic Reviews, 2*, CD004075.

Evans, R. J., Evans, M. K., Brown, Y. M. R., & Orshan, S. A. (2010). *Canadian maternity, newborn, & women's health nursing.* Philadelphia: Lippincott Williams & Wilkins.

Grant, G. J. (2010). Neuraxial analgesia and anesthesia for labor and delivery: Drugs. Retrieved February 22, 2012 from http://www.uptodate.com/patients/content/topic.do?topicKey=~.vo.0WZNfzauWD

Hodnett, E. D., Gates, S., Hofmeyr, G. J., & Sakala, C. (2009a). Continuous support for women during childbirth. *Cochrane Database of Systematic Reviews, 3*, CD003766.

Hodnett, E. D., Stremler, R., Weston, J. A., & McKeever, P. (2009b). Re-conceptualizing the hospital labor room: The PLACE (Pregnant and Laboring in an Ambient Clinical Environment) pilot trial. *Birth, 36*(2), 159–166 DOI: 10.1111/j.1523-536X.2009.00311.x

Iams, J. D., Romero, R., Culhane, J. F., & Goldenberg, R. L. (2008). Primary, secondary, and tertiary interventions to reduce the morbidity and mortality of preterm birth. *Lancet, 37*(9607), 164–175.

Institute for Clinical Systems Improvement. (2011). *Health care guideline: Management of labor* (4th ed.). Retrieved February 22, 2012 from http://www.icsi.org/labor/labor_management_of_full_version_2.html

Kennedy, B. B., Ruth, D. J., & Martin, E. J. (2009). *Intrapartum management modules: A perinatal education program* (4th ed.). Philadelphia: Lippincott Williams & Wilkins.

Klein, M. C., Kaczorowski, J., Hall, W. A., et al. (2009). The attitudes of Canadian maternity care practitioners towards labour and birth: Many differences but important similarities. *Journal of Obstetrics and Gynaecology Canada, 31*(9), 827–840.

Ladewig, P. A., London, M. L., & Davidson, M. R. (2009). *Contemporary maternal-newborn nursing care* (7th ed.). Upper Saddle River, NJ: Pearson.

Landau, R. (2009). What's new in obstetric anesthesia. *International Journal of Obstetric Analgesia, 18*, 368–372.

Lavender, T., Hart, A., & Smyth, R. M. D. (2008). Effect of partogram use on outcomes for women in spontaneous labour at term. *Cochrane Database of Systematic Reviews, 4*, CD005461.

Lawrence, A., Lewis, L., Hofmeyr, G. J., Dowswell, T., & Styles, C. (2009). Maternal positions and mobility during first stage labour. *Cochrane Database of Systematic Reviews, 2*, CD003934.

Leap, N., Sandall, J., Buckland, S., & Huber, U. (2010). Journey to confidence: Women's experiences of pain in labour and relational continuity of care. *Journal of Midwifery and Women's Health, 55*(3), 234–242.

Low, J. (2009). Operative delivery: Yesterday and today. *Journal of Obstetrics and Gynaecology Canada, 29*(2), 132–141.

Lowdermilk, D. L., Perry, S. E., & Cashion, K. (2010). *Maternity nursing* (8th ed.). Maryland Heights, MO: Mosby Elsevier.

Macones, G. A., Hankins, G. D. V., Spong, C. Y., Hauth, J., & Moore, T. (2008). The 2008 National Institute of Child Health and Human Development workshop report on electronic fetal monitoring: Update on definitions, interpretation, and research guidelines. *Journal of Obstetric, Gynecologic, and Neonatal Nursing, 37*(5), 510–515.

Man-Lung, L., Kuan-Chia, L., Hsin Yang, L., Kuang-Shing, S., & Meei-Ling, G. (2009). Effects of delayed pushing during the second stage of labor on postpartum fatigue and birth outcomes in nulliparous women. *Journal of Nursing Research, 17*(1), 62–72.

Matsuo, K., Scanlon, J. T., Atlas, R. O., & Kopelman, J. N. (2008). Staircase sign: A newly described uterine contraction pattern seen in rupture of unscarred gravid uterus. *Journal of Obstetrics and Gynaecological Research, 34*(1), 100–104.

Menacker, F., & Martin, J. (2009). BirthStats: rates of cesarean delivery, and unassisted and assisted vaginal delivery, United States, 1996, 2000, and 2006. *Birth: Issues in Perinatal Care, 36*(2), 167.

Menihan, C. A., & Kopel, E. (2008). *Fetal monitoring: Concepts and applications.* Philadelphia: Lippincott Williams & Wilkins.

Moldenhauer, J. S. (2008). Premature rupture of membranes (PROM). *The Merck Manual for Healthcare Professionals.* Retrieved February 20, 2012 from http://www.merck.com/mmpe/sec18/ch264/ch264j.html

Monroe, C. M. (2009). The effects of therapeutic touch on pain. *Journal of Holistic Nursing, 27*(2), 84–92.

National Aboriginal Health Organization. (2008). *Celebrating birth: Aboriginal midwifery in Canada.* Ottawa, ON: Author. Retrieved February 20, 2012 from http://www.naho.ca/documents/naho/english/midwifery/celebratingBirth/Midwiferypaper_English.pdf

Perinatal Education Associates, Inc. (2010). *Breathing.* Retrieved February 20, 2012 from http://www.birthsource.com/scripts/article.asp?articleid=211

Pillitteri, A. (2010). *Maternal & child health nursing: Care of the childbearing & childrearing family.* Philadelphia: Wolters Kluwer.

Public Health Agency of Canada. (2000). *Family-centred maternity and newborn care: National Guidelines.* Retrieved February 20, 2012 from http://www.phac-aspc.gc.ca/hp-ps/dca-dea/publications/fcm-smp/index-eng.php

Public Health Agency of Canada. (2008). *Canadian perinatal health report, 2008 edition.* Retrieved February 20, 2012 from http://www.publichealth.gc.ca/cphr/

Read, J. S., & Newell, M. L. (2009). Efficacy and safety of cesarean delivery for prevention of mother-to-child transmission of HIV-1. *Cochrane Database of Systematic Reviews, 1,* 1–15.

Reynolds, F. (2010). The effects of maternal labour analgesia on the fetus. *Best Practice and Research: Clinical Obstetrics and Gynaecology, 24*(3), 289–302.

Rice Simpson, K., & Creehan, P. A. (2008). *Perinatal nursing.* Philadelphia: AWHONN & Lippincott Williams & Wilkins.

Rose, M. K. (2009). *Comfort touch: Massage for the elderly and the ill.* Philadelphia: Lippincott Williams & Wilkins.

Royal Australian and New Zealand College of Obstetricians and Gynaecologists. (2008). *Warm water immersion during labour and birth: College statement C-Obs 24.* Retrieved February 22, 2012 from http://www.ranzcog.edu.au/womens-health/statements-a-guidelines/college-statements/424-warm-water-immersion-in-labour-and-birth-c-obs-24.html

Schilling, T. (2009). *Healthy birth practices from Lamaze International: #2 Walk, move around, and change positions throughout labor.* Retrieved February 22, 2012 from http://www.lamaze.org/Portals/0/carepractices/CarePractice2.pdf

Schuurmans, N., Senikas, V., & Lalonde, A. B. (2009). *Healthy beginnings* (4th ed.). Mississauga: Wiley.

Simkin, P. (2008). *The birth partner: A complete guide to childbirth for dads, doulas, and all other labor companions* (3rd ed.). Boston, MA: The Harvard Common Press.

Simkin, P. (2010). Ten ways to relieve labor pain. *Pregnancy Birth and Beyond: Lamaze International.* Retrieved February 22, 2012 from http://magazine.lamaze.org/Birth/ComfortZone/tabid/195/Default.aspx

Simmons, S. W., Cyna, A. M., Dennis, A. T., & Hughes, D. (2009). Combined spinal-epidural versus epidural analgesia in labour. *Cochrane Database of Systematic Reviews, 1,* CD003401.

Smith, C. A., Collins, C. T., Cyna, A. M., & Crowther, C. A. (2006). Complementary and alternative therapies for pain management in labour. *Cochrane Database of Systematic Reviews, 4,* CD003521.

Society of Obstetricians and Gynaecologists of Canada. (2008a). *National Birthing Initiative for Canada.* Retrieved February 22, 2012 from http://www.sogc.org/projects/birthing-strategy_e.asp

Society of Obstetricians and Gynaecologists of Canada. (2008b). Joint policy statement on normal childbirth. *Journal of Obstetrics and Gynecology in Canada, 30*(12), 1163–1165. Retrieved February 22, 2012 from http://www.sogc.org/guidelines/documents/gui221PS0812.pdf

Society of Obstetricians and Gynaecologists of Canada. (2008c). *Media advisories: Rising C-section rates add risks during childbirth and place excess strain on the healthcare system, warn Canadian obstetricians.* Retrieved February 22, 2012 from http://www.sogc.org/media/advisories-20080625_e.asp

Society of Obstetricians and Gynaecologists of Canada. (2008d). Joint policy statement on normal childbirth. *Journal of Obstetrics and Gynaecology Canada, 30*(12), 1163–1165.

Society of Obstetricians and Gynecologists of Canada. (2001). SOGC clinical practice guidelines: Mode of delivery for pregnant women infected by the human immunodeficiency virus. *Journal of Obstetrics and Gynaecology Canada, 23*(4), 348–350. Retrieved February 22, 2012 from http://www.sogc.org/guidelines/public/101E-CPG-April2001.pdf

Society of Obstetricians and Gynecologists of Canada. (2004a). SOGC clinical practice guidelines: The prevention of early-onset neonatal group B streptococcal disease. *Journal of Obstetrics and Gynaecology Canada, 26*(9), 826–832. Retrieved February 22, 2012 from http://www.sogc.org/guidelines/public/149E-CPG-September2004.pdf

Society of Obstetricians and Gynecologists of Canada. (2004b). SOGC clinical practice guidelines: Guidelines for operative vaginal birth. *Journal of Obstetrics and Gynaecology Canada, 26*(8), 747–753. Retrieved February 22, 2012 from http://www.sogc.org/guidelines/public/148E-CPG-August2004.pdf

Society of Obstetricians and Gynecologists of Canada. (2007). SOGC clinical practice guidelines: Fetal health surveillance: Antepartum and intrapartum consensus guideline. *Journal of Obstetrics and Gynecology in Canada, 29*(9), S3–S56. Retrieved February 22, 2012 from http://www.sogc.org/guidelines/documents/gui197CPG0709.pdf

Stark, M. A., Rudell, B., & Haus, G. (2008). Observing position and movements in hydrotherapy: A pilot study. *Journal of Obstetric, Gynecologic, and Neonatal Nursing, 37*(1), 116–122.

Steer, P. J. (2008). Has electronic fetal heart rate monitoring made a difference. *Seminars in Fetal and Neonatal Medicine, 13*(1), 2–3.

The Merck Manual. (2007). *Management of normal labor.* Retrieved February 22, 2012 from http://www.merck.com/mmpe/sec18/ch260/ch260d.html#sec18-ch260-ch260d-1073

Therapeutic Touch International Association. (2010). *Therapeutic touch policy and procedure for health care professionals.* Retrieved February 22, 2012 from http://www.therapeutic-touch.org/newsarticle.php?newsID=6

Tucker, S. M., Miller, L. A., & Miller, D. A. (2009). *Mosby's pocket guide to fetal monitoring: A multidisciplinary approach* (6th ed.). St. Louis, MO: Mosby.

Tzeng, Y., & Su, T. (2008). Low back pain during labor and related factors. *Journal of Nursing Research, 16*(3), 231–240.

Wolf, J. H. (2009). *Deliver me from pain: Anesthesia and Birth in America.* Baltimore, MD: The Johns Hopkins University Press.

Woods, C. J., & Levy, C. S. (2011). *Streptococcus group B infections.* Retrieved September 4, 2010 from http://emedicine.medscape.com/article/229091-overview

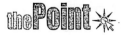 **For additional learning materials, including Internet Resources, go to http://thePoint.lww.com/Chow1e.**

The postpartum period is a time of major adjustments and adaptations not just for the mother but for all members of the family. It is during this time that parenting starts and a relationship with the newborn begins. A positive, loving relationship between parents and their newborn promotes the emotional well-being of all. This relationship endures and has profound effects on the child's growth and development.

> ▶ **Take** NOTE!
>
> *Parenting is a skill that is often learned by trial and error, with varying degrees of success. Successful parenting, a continuous and complex interactive process, requires the parents to learn new skills and to integrate the new member into the family.*

Once the infant is born, each system in the mother's body takes several weeks to return to its non-pregnant state. The physiologic changes in women during the postpartum period are dramatic. Nurses should be aware of these changes and should be able to make observations and assessments to validate normal occurrences and detect any deviations.

In addition to physical assessment and care of the woman in the postpartum period, strong social support is vital to help her integrate the baby into the family. In today's mobile society, extended families may live far away and may be unable to help care for the new family. As a result, many new parents turn to health care professionals for information as well as physical and emotional support during this adjustment period. Nurses can be an invaluable resource by serving as mentors, teaching about self-care measures and baby care basics, and providing emotional support. Nurses can "mother" the new mother by offering physical care, emotional support, and information and practical help. The nurse's support and care through this critical time can increase the new parents' confidence, giving them a sense of accomplishment in their parenting skills.

One important intervention during the postpartum period is the promotion of breastfeeding. All women require individualized assessment and support around infant feeding decisions. Women also require attention and support for breastfeeding challenges (Breastfeeding Committee for Canada [BCC], 2011).

As in all nursing care, nurses should provide culturally competent care during the postpartum period. The nurse should engage in ongoing cultural self-assessment to ensure that appropriate understanding exists around the concepts of race, ethnicity, and the need to avoid stereotyping (London, Ladewig, Ball, et al., 2011). Providing culturally competent nursing care during the postpartum

period requires time, open-mindedness, and patience. To promote positive outcomes, the nurse should be sensitive to the woman's and family's culture, religion, and ethnic influences (see Providing Optimal Cultural Care in the Nursing Interventions section).

Remember the couple introduced at the beginning of the chapter? When the postpartum nurse comes to examine Raina, her husband quickly leaves the room and returns a short time later after the examination is complete. How do you interpret his behaviour toward his wife? What might you communicate to this couple?

This chapter describes the nursing management of the woman and her family during the postpartum period. It outlines physical assessment parameters for new mothers and newborns. It also focuses on bonding and attachment behaviours; nurses need to be aware of these behaviours so they can perform appropriate interventions. Steps to address physiologic needs such as comfort, self-care, nutrition, and contraception are described. Ways to help the woman and her family adapt to the birth of the newborn are also discussed (Fig. 16.1).

Nursing management during the postpartum period focuses on assessing the woman's ability to adapt to the physiologic and psychological changes occurring at this time (see Chapter 15 for a detailed discussion of these adaptations). Family members are also assessed to determine how well they are making the transition to this new stage. Based on the assessment findings, the nurse plans and implements care to address the family's needs. Because of today's shortened lengths of hospital stay, the nurse may be able to focus only on priority needs and may need to arrange for follow-up in the home to ensure that all the family's needs are met.

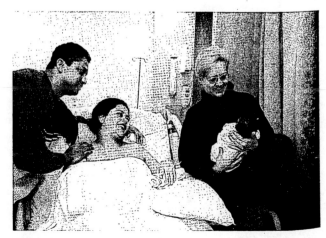

FIGURE 16.1 Parents and grandmother interacting with the newborn.

Assessment

Comprehensive nursing assessment begins within an hour after the woman gives birth and continues through discharge.

▷ *Take* NOTE!

Nurses need a firm grasp of normal findings so that they can recognize abnormal findings and intervene appropriately.

This assessment includes vital signs and physical and psychosocial assessments. Although the exact protocol may vary among facilities, postpartum assessment typically is performed at 5- to 15-minute intervals during the initial recovery period as needed. After that, vital signs should be taken:

• Every 30 minutes for 1 hour
• Every hour for 2 hours
• Every 4 to 8 hours (London et al., 2011)

During each assessment, keep in mind risk factors that may lead to complications, such as infection or hemorrhage, during the recovery period (Box 16.1). Early identification is critical to ensure prompt intervention.

As with any assessment, always review the woman's medical record for information about her pregnancy, labour, and birth. Note any preexisting conditions; any complications that occurred during pregnancy, labour, birth, and immediately afterward; and any treatments provided. This information is usually recorded on the labour record and any documents that were completed on admission as well as on the antenatal record that is provided by the physician. Postpartum assessment of the mother typically includes vital signs, pain level, and a systematic head-to-toe review of body systems. The acronym BUBBLE-EE—breasts, uterus, bladder, bowels, lochia, episiotomy/perineum, extremities, and emotional status—can be used as a guide for this head-to-toe review (Evans, Evans, Brown, et al., 2010). While assessing the woman and her family during the postpartum period, be alert for danger signs (Box 16.2). Notify the primary health care provider immediately if any are noted.

Postpartum assessment also includes assessing the parents and other family members, such as siblings and grandparents, for attachment and bonding with the newborn.

Vital Signs

Obtain vital signs and compare them with the previous values, noting and reporting any deviations. Vital sign changes can be an early indicator of complications.

BOX 16.1 Factors Increasing the Woman's Risk for Postpartum Complications

Risk Factors for Postpartum Infection
• Operative procedure (forceps, cesarean birth, vacuum extraction)
• History of diabetes, including gestational-onset diabetes
• Prolonged labour (more than 24 hours)
• Use of indwelling urinary catheter
• Anemia (hemoglobin <120 g/L)
• Multiple vaginal examinations during labour
• Prolonged rupture of membranes (more than 24 hours)
• Manual extraction of placenta
• Compromised immune system (HIV positive)

Risk Factors for Postpartum Hemorrhage
• Precipitous labour (less than 3 hours)
• Uterine atony
• Placenta previa or abruptio placentae
• Labour induction or augmentation
• Operative procedures (vacuum extraction, forceps, cesarean birth)
• Retained placental fragments
• Prolonged third stage of labour (more than 30 minutes)
• Multiparity, more than three births closely spaced
• Uterine overdistention (large infant, twins, hydramnios)

Temperature

Use a consistent measurement technique (oral, axillary, or tympanic) to get the most accurate readings. Typically, the new mother's temperature during the first 24 hours postpartum is within the normal range. Some women experience a slight fever, up to 38°C (100.4°C), during the first 24 hours as a result of the exertion of labour and the possibility of dehydration that subsequently occurs. Temperature should be normal after 24 hours with replacement of fluids lost during labour

---

BOX 16.2 Postpartum Danger Signs

• Fever higher than 38°C (100.4 °F)
• Foul-smelling lochia or an unexpected change in colour or amount
• Visual changes, such as blurred vision or spots, or headaches
• Calf pain with dorsiflexion of the foot
• Swelling, redness, or discharge at the episiotomy site
• Dysuria, burning, or incomplete emptying of the bladder
• Shortness of breath or difficulty breathing
• Depression or extreme mood swings

and birth (London et al., 2011). A temperature above 38°C (100.4°F) at any time or an abnormal temperature after the first 24 hours may indicate infection and must be reported. Abnormal temperature readings warrant continued monitoring until an infection can be ruled out through cultures or blood studies.

Pulse

Because of the changes in blood volume and cardiac output after delivery, relative bradycardia may be noted. The woman's pulse rate may range from 50 to 70 beats/minute as a decreased cardiac output takes hold following the expulsion of the placenta and the body adjusts to decreased circulating blood volume and a subsequent increased stroke volume. Pulse usually stabilizes to pre-pregnancy levels within 10 days (London et al., 2011).

Tachycardia in the postpartum woman can suggest anxiety, excitement, fatigue, pain, excessive blood loss, infection, or underlying cardiac problems. Further investigation is warranted to rule out complications.

Respirations

Respiratory rates in the postpartum woman should be within the normal range of 16 to 20 breaths/minute. Any change in respiratory rate out of the normal range might indicate respiratory infection, pulmonary edema, atelectasis, or pulmonary embolism and must be reported. Lungs should be clear on auscultation.

Blood Pressure

Assess the woman's blood pressure and compare it with her usual range. Report any deviation from this range. Elevations in blood pressure from baseline might suggest pregnancy-induced hypertension; decreases may suggest dehydration or excessive blood loss. A diastolic blood pressure reading of 90 to 95 mm Hg is suggestive of pregnancy-induced hypertension and needs to be reported.

Blood pressure also may vary based on the woman's position, so assess blood pressure with the woman in the same position every time. Be alert for orthostatic hypotension, which can occur when the woman moves rapidly from a lying or sitting position to a standing one. This potential is especially significant after childbirth, since there has been a significant change in body fluid volume and blood loss (London et al., 2011). Consider mobilizing the woman initially with the assistance of another nurse in case of fainting.

Pain

Pain, the fifth vital sign, is assessed along with the other four parameters. Question the woman about the type of pain and its location and severity. Have the woman rate the pain using a numeric scale from 0 to 10 points.

Many postpartum orders will have the nurse pre-medicate the woman routinely for afterbirth pains rather than wait for her to experience them first. The goal of pain management is to have the woman's pain scale rating maintained between 0 and 2 points at all times, especially after breastfeeding. This can be accomplished by assessing the woman's pain level frequently and preventing pain by administering analgesics. Comfort measures such as warm showers, deep breathing, reassurance, and a calm environment can also be helpful in preventing and alleviating postpartum discomfort. If the woman has severe pain in the perineal region despite use of physical comfort measures, check for a hematoma by inspecting and palpating the area. If one is found, notify the health care provider immediately.

Breasts

Inspect the breasts for size, contour, asymmetry, engorgement, or erythema. Check the nipples for cracks, redness, fissures, or bleeding, and note whether they are erect, flat, or inverted. Flat or inverted nipples can make breastfeeding challenging for both mother and infant. Cracked, blistered, fissured, bruised, or bleeding nipples in the breastfeeding woman are generally indications that the baby is improperly positioned on the breast. Palpate the breasts lightly to ascertain if they are soft, filling, or engorged, and document your findings. For women who are not breastfeeding, use a gentle, light touch to avoid breast stimulation, which will exacerbate engorgement. As milk is starting to come in, the breasts become firmer; this is charted as "filling." Engorged breasts are hard, tender, and taut. Ask the woman if she is having any nipple discomfort. Palpate the breasts for any nodules, masses, or areas of warmth, which may indicate a plugged duct that may progress to **mastitis** if not treated promptly. Any discharge from the nipple should be described and documented if it is not colostrum (creamy yellow) or foremilk (bluish white).

Uterus

Assess the fundus (top portion of the uterus) to determine the degree of uterine involution. If possible, have the woman empty her bladder before assessing the fundus. If the patient has had a cesarean birth and has a patient-controlled anesthesia pump, instruct her to self-medicate prior to fundal assessment to decrease her discomfort. Using a two-handed approach with the woman in the supine position and the bed in a flat position or as low as possible, palpate the abdomen gently, feeling for the top of the uterus while the other hand is placed on the lower segment of the uterus to stabilize it (Fig. 16.2).

The fundus should be midline and should feel firm. A boggy or relaxed uterus is a sign of uterine atony. This can be the result of bladder distention, which displaces the uterus upward and to the right, or retained placental fragments. Either situation predisposes the woman to

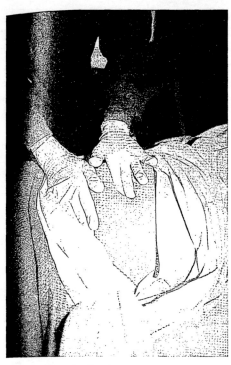

FIGURE 16.2 Palpating the fundus.

hemorrhage. Once the fundus is located, place your index finger on the fundus and count the number of fingerbreadths between the fundus and the umbilicus (one fingerbreadth is approximately equal to 1 cm). One to two hours after birth, the fundus typically is between the umbilicus and the symphysis pubis. Approximately 6 to 12 hours after birth, the fundus usually is at the level of the umbilicus (U/U).

Normally, the fundus progresses downward at a rate of one fingerbreadth (or 1 cm) per day after childbirth (London et al., 2011). On the first postpartum day, the top of the fundus is located 1 cm below the umbilicus and is recorded as U-1. Similarly, on the second postpartum day, the fundus would be 2 cm below the umbilicus and should be recorded as U-2, and so on. If the fundus is not firm, gently massage the uterus using a circular motion until it becomes firm.

Bladder

Considerable diuresis (called "puerperal diuresis")—as much as 3,000 mL—may follow for several days after childbirth as the woman's body adjusts its fluid balance to its pre-pregnant state. This heightened state of diuresis begins during the first 12 to 24 hours after delivery (London et al., 2011). However, many postpartum women do not sense the need to void even if their bladder is full. Women who received regional anesthesia during labour are at risk for bladder distention and for difficulty voiding until sensation returns within several hours after birth. Impediments to normal voiding could also be attributed to the tissue trauma that may have occurred during the birthing process (especially in the case of a large baby, use of forceps during delivery, or a prolonged second stage of labour). It is important to consider the possibility of urethral edema, which has the potential to make the passage of urine difficult.

Assess for voiding problems by asking the woman the following questions:

• Have you (passed your water, urinated, gone to the bathroom) yet?
• Have you noticed any burning or discomfort with urination?
• Do you have any difficulty passing your urine?
• Do you feel that your bladder is empty when you finish urinating?
• Do you have any signs of infection such as urgency, frequency, or pain?
• Are you able to control the flow of urine by squeezing your muscles?
• Have you noticed any leakage of urine when you cough, laugh, or sneeze?

Assess the bladder for distention and adequate emptying after efforts to void. Palpate the area over the symphysis pubis. If empty, the bladder is not palpable. Palpation of a rounded mass suggests bladder distention. Also percuss the area: a full bladder is dull to percussion. If the bladder is full, lochia drainage will be more than normal because the uterus cannot contract to suppress the bleeding. The nurse must review the fluid intake and output (including blood loss) measurements during labour and into the postpartum period in order to evaluate for dehydration as a possible reason for low urine output.

▷ **Take** NOTE!

Note the location and condition of the fundus; a full bladder tends to displace the uterus up and to the right.

After the woman voids, palpate and percuss the area again to determine adequate emptying of the bladder. If the bladder remains distended, the woman may be retaining urine in her bladder, and measures such as urinary catheterization should be instituted in order to ensure that the bladder has been emptied. Be alert for signs of infection, including infrequent or insufficient voiding, fever, chills, nausea, discomfort, burning, urgency, or foul-smelling urine (Potter & Perry, 2010). Document urine output.

Bowels

Spontaneous bowel movements may not occur for 2 to 3 days after giving birth because of a decrease in muscle tone in the intestines during labour or because of bowel evacuation during delivery. Women with lacerations or an episiotomy or those who have undergone a cesarean birth may be reluctant to bear down to achieve a bowel movement; these women may benefit from stool softeners (London et al., 2011).

Inspect the woman's abdomen for distention, auscultate for bowel sounds in all four quadrants, and palpate for tenderness. The abdomen typically is soft, nontender, and nondistended. Bowel sounds are present in all four quadrants. Ask the woman if she has had a bowel movement or has passed gas since giving birth because constipation is a common problem during the postpartum period (especially following cesarean birth) and most women do not offer this information unless asked about it. Normal assessment findings are active bowel sounds, passing gas, and a nondistended abdomen.

Lochia

Assess lochia in terms of amount, colour, odour, and change with activity and time. To assess how much a woman is bleeding, ask her how many perineal pads she has used in the past 1 to 2 hours and how much drainage was on each pad. For example, did she saturate the pad completely, or was only half of the pad covered with drainage? Ask about the colour and odour of the drainage as well as the presence of any clots. Lochia has a definite musky scent, with an odour similar to that of menstrual flow without any large clots. Foul-smelling lochia suggests an infection, and large clots suggest poor uterine involution, necessitating additional intervention.

To determine the amount of lochia, observe the amount of lochia saturation on the perineal pad and relate it to time (Fig. 16.3). Lochia flow will increase when the woman gets out of bed (lochia pools in the vagina and the uterus while she is lying down) and when

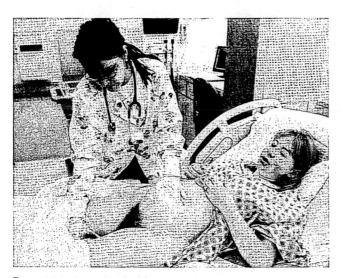

FIGURE 16.3 Assessing lochia.

she breastfeeds (oxytocin release causes uterine contractions). A woman who saturates a perineal pad within 30 to 60 minutes is bleeding much more than one who saturates a pad in 2 hours. Typically, the amount of lochia is described as follows:

- Scant: a 2.5 to 5 cm (1- to 2-inch) lochia stain on the perineal pad
- Light or small: an approximately 10 cm (4-inch) stain
- Moderate: a 10 to 15 cm (4- to 6-inch) stain
- Large or heavy: the pad is saturated within 1 hour

For more accurate assessment of blood loss, perineal pads can be weighed, with each millilitre of blood loss equating to 1 g of weight on the pad (London et al., 2011).

The total volume of lochia is approximately 240 to 270 mL (8 to 9 oz), and the amount decreases daily (London et al., 2011). Check under the woman to make sure there isn't additional blood hidden and not absorbed on her perineal pad. An estimated blood loss of 500 to 1,000 mL or more constitutes a hemorrhage.

Report any abnormal findings, such as heavy, bright-red lochia with large tissue fragments or a foul odour. If excessive bleeding occurs, the first step would be to massage the boggy fundus until it is firm to reduce the flow of blood. Document all findings.

Women who had a cesarean birth will usually have less lochia discharge than those who had a vaginal birth, but stages and colour changes remain the same. There is also a risk for postpartum hemorrhage among women who give birth by cesarean section, and it is important to assess for excessive bleeding according to the same guidelines used following a vaginal birth. Although the woman's abdomen will be tender after surgery, the nurse must palpate the fundus and assess the lochia to make sure they are within the normal range and that there is no excessive bleeding. Administering analgesic prior to the assessment is helpful when possible.

Anticipatory guidance to give the woman at discharge should include information about lochia and the expected changes. Urge the woman to notify her health care provider if lochia rubra returns after the serosa and alba transitions have taken place. This is abnormal and may indicate subinvolution or that the woman is too active and needs to rest more. Lochia is an excellent medium for bacterial growth. Explain to the woman that frequent changing of perineal pads, continued use of her peri bottle for rinsing the perineal area, and handwashing before and after pad changes are important infection control measures.

Episiotomy and Perineum

To assess the episiotomy and perineal area, position the woman on her side with her top leg flexed upward at the knee and drawn up toward her waist. If necessary, use a penlight to provide adequate lighting during the

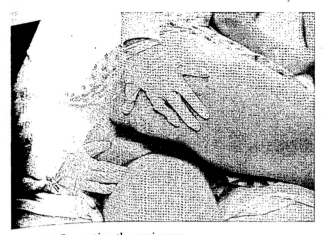

FIGURE 16.4 Inspecting the perineum.

assessment. Wearing gloves and standing at the woman's side with her back to you, gently lift the upper buttock to expose the perineum and anus (Fig. 16.4). Inspect the episiotomy for irritation, ecchymosis, tenderness, or hematomas. Assess for hemorrhoids and their condition.

During the early postpartum period, the perineal tissue surrounding the episiotomy is typically edematous and slightly bruised. The normal episiotomy site should not have redness, discharge, or edema. The majority of healing takes place within the first 2 weeks, but it may take 4 to 6 months for the episiotomy to heal completely (London et al., 2011). Lacerations to the perineal area sustained during the birthing process that were identified and repaired also need to be assessed to determine their healing status. Lacerations are classified based on their severity and tissue involvement:

• First-degree laceration—involves only skin and superficial structures above muscle
• Second-degree laceration—extends through perineal muscles
• Third-degree laceration—extends through the anal sphincter muscle
• Fourth-degree laceration—continues through anterior rectal wall

Assess the episiotomy and any lacerations at least every 8 hours to detect hematomas or signs of infection. Large areas of swollen, bluish skin with complaints of severe pain in the perineal area indicate pelvic or vulvar hematomas. Redness, swelling, increasing discomfort, or purulent drainage may indicate infection. Both findings need to be reported immediately.

A white line the length of the episiotomy is a sign of infection, as is swelling or discharge. Severe, intractable pain, perineal discolouration, and ecchymosis indicate a perineal hematoma, a potentially dangerous condition. Report any unusual findings. Ice can be applied to relieve discomfort and reduce edema; sitz baths also can promote comfort and perineal healing (see Promoting Comfort in the Nursing Interventions section).

Extremities

During pregnancy, the state of hypercoagulability protects the mother against excessive blood loss during childbirth and placental separation. However, this hypercoagulable state can increase the risk of thromboembolic disorders during pregnancy and postpartum. Three factors predispose women to thromboembolic disorders during pregnancy: stasis (compression of the large veins because of the gravid uterus), altered coagulation (state of pregnancy), and localized vascular damage (may occur during birthing process). All of these increase the risk of clot formation.

> ▶ **Take** *NOTE!*
>
> *Changes in coagulation during pregnancy, in combination with compression of the common iliac vein because of the pregnant uterus, increase the risk for thromboembolic disease in pregnant and postpartum women. Approximately 1 in 500 to 700 women experience superficial vein thrombosis.*

Pulmonary embolus is a potentially life-threatening event that occurs when thrombi originating from the extremities travel to the pulmonary artery and obstruct the flow of blood to the lungs. Risk factors associated with thromboembolic conditions include:

• Anemia
• Diabetes mellitus
• Cigarette smoking
• Obesity
• Pre-eclampsia secondary to exaggeration of hypercoagulable state
• Hypertension
• Varicose veins
• Pregnancy
• Oral contraceptive use or hormone replacement therapy
• Cesarean birth
• Previous thromboembolic disease
• Multiparity
• Inactivity
• Advanced maternal age (London et al., 2011)

Because of the subtle presentation of thromboembolic disorders, the physical examination may not be enough to detect them. The woman may report lower extremity tightness or aching when ambulating that is relieved with rest and elevation of the leg. Edema in the affected leg (typically the left), along with warmth and tenderness, may also be noted. Diagnosis is dependent on a variety of factors and tests, including client history, physical examination, and venous ultrasonography or occlusive impedance plethysmography. Women at increased risk for this condition during the postpartum period should wear antiembolism stockings or use sequential compression devices to reduce their risk for thrombophlebitis. Encouraging the client to ambulate after childbirth reduces the incidence of thrombophlebitis. Heparin therapy is used for deep vein thrombosis (London et al., 2011).

Emotional Status

Assess the woman's emotional status by observing how she interacts with her family, her level of independence, energy levels, eye contact with her infant (within a cultural context), posture and comfort level while holding the newborn, and sleep and rest patterns. Be alert for mood swings, irritability, or crying episodes.

*R*emember Raina and her "quiet" husband, the Muslim couple? The postpartum nurse informs Raina that her doctor, Nancy Schultz, has been called away for emergency surgery and won't be available the rest of the day. The nurse explains that Dr. Robert Nappo will be making rounds for her. Raina and her husband become upset. Why? Is culturally competent care being provided to this couple?

Bonding and Attachment

Nurses can be instrumental in promoting attachment by assessing attachment behaviours (positive and negative) and intervening appropriately if needed. Nurses must be able to identify any family discord that might interfere with the attachment process. Remember, however, that mothers from different cultures may behave differently from what is expected in your own culture. Use of herbal remedies after childbirth, for example, may be common among women of Aboriginal or Chinese descent (London et al., 2011). Don't assume that different behaviour is wrong. Engaging in conversation with the woman regarding different practices can be helpful for both the nurse and the patient in order to deepen cultural awareness.

Meeting their newborn for the first time after birth can be an exhilarating experience for parents. Although the mother has spent many hours dreaming of her unborn child and how he or she will look, it is not until after birth that they meet face to face. They both need to get to know one another and to develop feelings for one another.

Bonding is the close emotional attraction to a newborn by the parents that optimally develops during the first 30 to 60 minutes after birth. It is unidirectional, from parent to infant. It is thought that optimal bonding of the parents to a newborn requires a period of close contact within the first few minutes to a few hours after birth (Society of Obstetricians and Gynaecologists of Canada [SOGC], 2010). The mother initiates bonding when she caresses her infant and exhibits certain behaviours typical of a mother tending her child. Skin-to-skin contact, wherein the unclothed baby is next to the mother's skin, is encouraged as soon after the birth as is feasible (BCC, 2011). The infant's responses to the initial contact with the mother, including body and eye movements, are thought to be a necessary part of the process. During this initial period, the infant is in a quiet, alert state, looking directly at the holder.

▷ **Take** NOTE!

The length of time necessary for bonding depends on the health of the infant and mother as well as the circumstances surrounding the labour and birth (London et al., 2011).

Immediately after the birth of a newborn, all parents are faced with the task of learning and understanding as much as possible about caring for this new family member, even if the parents already have other children. In their new or expanded role as parents, they will face many demands and challenges. For most, this is a wonderful, exciting time filled with many discoveries and much information. Promoting a collaborative, enabling relationship with the family can enhance their experience.

Parents learn as they watch the nurse interacting with and caring for their newborn. This care should be individualized and family-centred as nurses play a major role in teaching parents about typical newborn characteristics and about ways to foster optimal growth and development. This role is even more important today because of limited hospital stays.

The newborn has come from a dark, small, enclosed space in the mother's uterus into the bright, cold extrauterine environment. Nurses can easily forget that they are caring for a small human being who is experiencing his or her first taste of human interaction outside the uterus. The newborn period is an extremely important and vulnerable one, and health goals and guidelines have been developed to address this critical period (Health Canada, 2000).

It is also easy to overlook the intensity with which parents, family members, and other visitors observe the actions of nurses as they care for their new family member. Nurses need to serve as a model for giving nurturing care to newborns and play a profound role at the time of birth in facilitating attachment between mothers and newborns as well as family closeness. Therefore, the mother and her newborn, within the context of their family or personal support, should be viewed as a unit.

This chapter provides information about assessment and interventions in the period immediately following the birth of a newborn and during the early newborn period. For the purposes of this chapter, information is presented within the context of hospital birth, but it is important to note that an increasing number of births in Canada occur at home or in a birth centre setting. The information in this chapter is also general in nature. Most provinces and territories, as well as Health Canada, have developed a number of guidelines related to the care of newborns. It is important to be aware of the recommendations that are followed in each practice setting. Finally, although the term *parents* is used frequently throughout the chapter, it is important to note that there is great diversity in our population in family structures and cultural practices related to birth and the many roles that mothers, fathers, aunts, uncles, other relatives, foster families, adoptive families, and friends play in raising children in our society.

Nursing Management During the Immediate Newborn Period

The period of transition from intrauterine to extrauterine life occurs during the first several hours after birth. During this time, the newborn is undergoing numerous adaptations, many of which are occurring simultaneously (see Chapter 17 for more information on the newborn's adaptation). The neonate's temperature, respiration, and cardiovascular dynamics stabilize during this period. Close observation of the newborn's status is essential. Careful examination of the newborn at birth can detect anomalies, birth injuries, and disorders that can compromise adaptation to extrauterine life. Problems that occur during this critical time can have a lifelong impact.

Assessment

The initial newborn assessment is completed in the birthing area, with the uncompromised baby placed directly on the mother's chest to remain warm and to complete transition. A more thorough assessment can be done within the first 2 to 4 hours, once the parents have had time to bond with their newborn. In addition to ongoing vital sign and physical assessment, a third and more thorough assessment is completed before discharge. The purpose of these assessments is to determine whether the baby is transitioning effectively into the extrauterine environment, to identify apparent physical abnormalities, and to provide parents with information and health teaching (Fraser & Cooper, 2009).

During the initial newborn assessment, look for signs that might indicate a problem, including:

- Nasal flaring
- Chest retractions
- **Grunting** on exhalation
- Laboured breathing
- Generalized cyanosis
- Abnormal breath sounds: rhonchi, crackles (rales), wheezing, stridor
- Abnormal respiratory rate (**tachypnea**, more than 60 breaths/minute; bradypnea, less than 25 breaths/minute)
- Flaccid body posture
- Abnormal heart rate (**tachycardia**, more than 160 beats/minute; bradycardia, less than 100 beats/minute)
- Abnormal newborn size: small or large for gestational age

If any of these findings are noted, medical intervention may be necessary. The US-based Neonatal Resuscitation Program (NRP) provides recommendations for nurses and physicians to manage complications that arise at or shortly after birth. A subcommittee of the Canadian NRP Program Steering Committee was convened to review the textbook as they may apply within the health care system and culture of care in Canada (Canadian Pediatric Society [CPS], n.d.).

Apgar Scoring

The **Apgar score**, introduced in 1952 by Dr. Virginia Apgar, is used to evaluate newborns at 1 minute and 5 minutes after birth. An additional Apgar assessment is done at 10 minutes if the 5-minute score is less than 7 points or if resuscitation is prolonged (Kattwinkel, 2011; Kliegman, Behrman, Jenson, et al., 2011). Assessment of the newborn at 1 minute provides data about the newborn's initial adaptation to extrauterine life. Assessment at 5 minutes provides a clearer indication of the newborn's overall central nervous system status.

Five parameters are assessed with Apgar scoring. A quick way to remember the parameters of Apgar scoring is as follows:

- A = appearance (colour)
- P = pulse (heart rate)
- G = grimace (reflex irritability)
- A = activity (muscle tone)
- R = respiratory (respiratory effort)

Each parameter is assigned a score ranging from 0 to 2 points. A score of 0 indicates an absent or poor response; a score of 2 indicates a normal response (Table 18.1). A normal newborn's score should be 8 to 10 points. It is rare for an infant to receive a score of 10 on the Apgar because pink hands and feet are usually not seen (acrocyanosis) in the newborn in the first few minutes of life. The higher the score, the better the condition of the newborn. If the Apgar score is 8 or higher, no intervention is needed other than supporting normal respiratory efforts and maintaining thermoregulation. Scores of 4 to 7 signify moderate difficulty, and scores of 0 to 3 represent severe distress in adjusting to extrauterine life. The Apgar score is influenced by a variety of factors, including the presence of maternal medications, infection, and fetal malformations (Cunningham, Leveno, Bloom, et al., 2010).

When the newborn experiences physiologic depression, the Apgar score characteristics disappear in a predictable manner: first the pink colouration is lost, next the respiratory effort, and then the tone, followed by reflex irritability and, finally, heart rate (Cunningham et al., 2010).

> ▶ **Take** NOTE!
>
> Although Apgar scoring is done at 1 and 5 minutes, it also can be used as a guide during the immediate newborn period to evaluate the newborn's status for any changes because it focuses on critical parameters that must be assessed throughout the early transition period.

Length and Weight

Parents are eager to know their newborn's length and weight. Accurate measurements of these characteristics are important as they will provide a foundation for assessment of growth and development and will be needed if the infant requires fluids or medications during his or her

TABLE 18.1 **APGAR SCORING FOR NEWBORNS**

Parameter (Assessment Technique)	0 Point	1 Point	2 Points
Heart rate (auscultation of apical heart rate for 1 full min)	Absent	Slow (<100 beats/min)	>100 beats/min
Respiratory effort (observation of the volume and vigour of the newborn's cry; auscultation of depth and rate of respirations)	Apneic	Slow, irregular, shallow	Regular respirations (usually 30–60 breaths/min), strong, good cry
Muscle tone (observation of extent of flexion in the newborn's extremities and newborn's resistance when the extremities are pulled away from the body)	Limp, flaccid	Some flexion, limited resistance to extension	Tight flexion, good resistance to extension with quick return to flexed position after extension
Reflex irritability (flicking of the soles of the feet or suctioning of the nose with a bulb syringe)	No response	Grimace or frown when irritated	Sneeze, cough, or vigorous cry
Skin colour (inspection of trunk and extremities with the appropriate colour for ethnicity appearing within minutes after birth)	Cyanotic or pale	Appropriate body colour; blue extremities (acrocyanosis)	Completely appropriate colour (pink on both trunk and extremities)

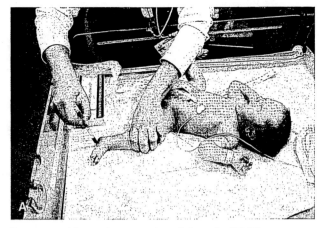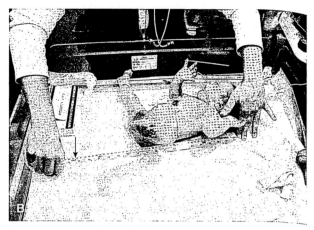

FIGURE 18.1 Measuring a newborn's length. (**A**) The nurse extends the newborn's leg and marks the pad at the heel. (**B**) The nurse measures from the newborn's head to the heel mark.

stay in the hospital. These measurements are taken within the first 1 to 2 hours after birth. A disposable tape measure or a built-in measurement board located on the side of the scale can be used. Obtaining an accurate length measurement is challenging with a moving infant; research has shown that measuring with calibrated equipment such as a board is more accurate (Fraser & Cooper, 2009). Length is measured from the head of the newborn to the heel with the newborn unclothed (Fig. 18.1). Because of the flexed position of the newborn after birth, place the newborn in a supine position and extend the leg completely when measuring the length. The expected length of a full-term newborn is usually 48 to 53 cm (19 to 21 inches). Molding can affect measurement (Kliegman et al., 2011; Tappero & Honeyfield, 2009).

Most often, newborns are weighed using a digital scale that reads the weight in grams. First, balance the scale if it is not balanced. Place a warmed protective cloth or paper as a barrier on the scale to prevent heat loss by conduction; recalibrate the scale to zero after applying the barrier. Next, place the unclothed newborn in the centre of the scale. Keep a hand above the newborn for safety (Fig. 18.2).

Typically, the term newborn weighs 2,500 to 4,000 g (5.5 to 8.5 lb). In 2006, the World Health Organization developed updated child growth standards based on breastfed infants and appropriately fed infants of different ethnic origins. Birth weights less than 10% or more than 90% on a growth chart are outside the normal range and need further investigation. Weights taken at later times are compared with previous weights and are documented with regard to gain or loss on a nursing flow sheet. Newborns typically lose approximately 10% of their initial birth weight by 3 to 4 days of age secondary to loss of meconium and extracellular fluid as well as limited food intake. This weight is usually regained by the 10th day of life (Kliegman et al., 2011). Weight loss may also be influenced by the method of feeding; infants who are breastfed normally lose weight over a longer period of time and take

longer to regain initial weight loss. It is important to keep this in mind when assessing the adequacy of feeding.

Newborns can be classified by their birth weight regardless of their gestational age (Canadian Perinatal Surveillance System, 2008) as follows:

- Low birth weight: <2,500 g (<5.5 lb)
- Very low birth weight: <1,500 g (<3.5 lb)
- Extremely low birth weight: <1,000 g (<2.5 lb)

Vital Signs

Heart rate and respiratory rate are assessed immediately after birth with Apgar scoring. Heart rate, obtained by

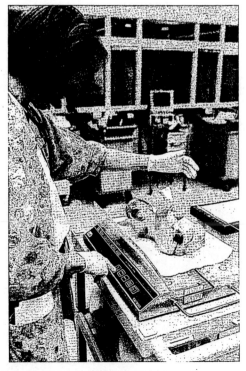

FIGURE 18.2 Weighing a newborn. Note how the nurse guards the newborn from above to prevent injury.

taking an apical pulse for 1 full minute, typically is 120 to 160 beats/minute. Some term newborns may have a resting heart rate as low as 80 beats/minute depending on their level of arousal (Acute Care of at-Risk Newborns [ACoRN] Neonatal Society, 2010). Newborns' respirations are assessed when they are quiet or sleeping. Place a stethoscope on the right side of the chest and count the breaths for 1 full minute to identify any irregularities. The normal newborn respiratory rate is 40 to 60 breaths/minute with symmetric chest movement.

All babies are at risk for temperature instability because their ability to regulate body temperature has not yet fully developed. Maintaining a neutral thermal environment is one of the key physiologic challenges a newborn faces after delivery; the risk for hypothermia is real and potentially dangerous (Soll, 2008). Maintaining temperature within the normal range by providing warmth and minimizing heat loss is an important component of newborn care (ACoRN Neonatal Society, 2010). When there are no contraindications, skin-to-skin thermal management should be encouraged. This has been shown to improve axillary temperature 90 minutes after birth and improved abdominal temperature within the first 21 minutes after birth (Soll, 2008). The normal axillary temperature for a term newborn is 36.5° to 37.5°C (97.9° to 99.7°F). Although mild variations from normal are common, wider variations can be detrimental. If the baby's temperature falls outside this normal range, readings should be done more frequently (every 15 to 30 minutes) until the temperature is normalized. Rectal temperatures are no longer taken because of the risk for perforation (Blackburn, 2007). The thermometer or temperature probe is held in the midaxillary space according to manufacturer's directions and hospital protocol.

Blood pressure is not usually assessed as part of a newborn examination unless there is a clinical indication or low Apgar scores. If assessed, an oscillometer (electronic blood pressure monitor) is used. The typical range is 50 to 75 mm Hg (systolic) and 30 to 45 mm Hg (diastolic). Crying, moving, and late clamping of the umbilical cord will increase systolic pressure (Tappero & Honeyfield, 2009). The proper-size cuff must be used when measuring blood pressure; the most common cause of a hypertensive measurement is a cuff that is too small. It is recommended that the cuff width should be 40% to 50% of the circumference of the extremity or 25% to 55% wider than the diameter of the extremity being measured, and that the bladder should entirely circle the extremity without overlapping (Tappero & Honeyfield, 2009). Typical values for newborn vital signs are provided in Table 18.2.

Gestational Age Assessment

To determine a newborn's **gestational age** (the stage of maturity), physical signs and neurologic characteristics are assessed. Typically, gestational age is determined by

TABLE 18.2 NEWBORN VITAL SIGNS

Newborn Vital Signs	Ranges of values
Temperature	36.5°–37.5°C (97.9°–99.7°F)
Heart rate (pulse)	120–160 beats/min; can increase to 180 during crying
Respirations	30–60 breaths/min at rest; will increase with crying
Blood pressure	50–75 mm Hg systolic, 30–45 mm Hg diastolic

using a tool such as the Dubowitz/Ballard or New Ballard Score system (Fig. 18.3). This scoring system provides an objective estimate of gestational age by scoring the specific parameters of physical and neuromuscular maturity. Points are given for each assessment parameter, with a low score of −1 or −2 points for extreme immaturity to 4 or 5 points for postmaturity. The scores from each section are added together to correspond to a specific gestational age in weeks.

The physical maturity section of the examination is done during the first 2 hours after birth. The physical maturity assessment section of the Ballard examination evaluates physical characteristics that appear different at different stages depending on a newborn's gestational maturity. Newborns who are physically mature have higher scores than those who are not. The areas assessed on the physical maturity examination include:

- Skin texture—typically ranges from sticky and transparent to smooth, with varying degrees of peeling and cracking, to parchment-like or leathery with significant cracking and wrinkling
- **Lanugo**—soft downy hair on the newborn's body, which is absent in preterm newborns, appears with maturity, and then disappears again with postmaturity
- Plantar creases—creases on the soles of the feet, which range from absent to covering the entire foot, depending on maturity (the greater the number of creases, the greater the newborn's maturity)
- Breast tissue—the thickness and size of breast tissue and areola (the darkened ring around each nipple), which range from being imperceptible to full and budding
- Eyes and ears—eyelids can be fused or open and ear cartilage and stiffness determine the degree of maturity (the greater the amount of ear cartilage with stiffness, the greater the newborn's maturity)
- Genitals—in males, evidence of testicular descent and appearance of scrotum (which can range from smooth to covered with rugae) determine maturity; in females, appearance and size of clitoris and labia determine maturity (a prominent clitoris with flat labia suggests

NEUROMUSCULAR MATURITY

NEUROMUSCULAR MATURITY SIGN	SCORE							RECORD SCORE HERE
	−1	0	1	2	3	4	5	
POSTURE								
SQUARE WINDOW (Wrist)	>90°	90°	60°	45°	30°	0°		
ARM RECOIL		180°	140°–180°	110°–140°	90°–110°	<90°		
POPLITEAL ANGLE	180°	160°	140°	120°	100°	90°	<90°	
SCARF SIGN								
HEEL TO EAR								
						TOTAL NEUROMUSCULAR MATURITY SCORE		

SCORE

Neuromuscular ___
Physical ___
Total ___

MATURITY RATING

Score	Weeks
−10	20
−5	22
0	24
5	26
10	28
15	30
20	32
25	34
30	36
35	38
40	40
45	42
50	44

PHYSICAL MATURITY

PHYSICAL MATURITY SIGN	SCORE							RECORD SCORE HERE
	−1	0	1	2	3	4	5	
SKIN	sticky, friable, transparent	gelatinous, red, translucent	smooth, pink, visible veins	superficial peeling and/or rash, few veins	cracking pale areas, rare veins	parchment, deep cracking, no vessels	leathery, cracked, wrinkled	
LANUGO	none	sparse	abundant	thinning	bald areas	mostly bald		
PLANTAR SURFACE	heel-toe 40–50 mm:−1 <40 mm:−2	>50 mm no crease	faint red marks	anterior transverse crease only	creases ant. 2/3	creases over entire sole		
BREAST	imperceptible	barely perceptible	flat areola no bud	stippled areola 1–2 mm bud	raised areola 3–4 mm bud	full areola 5–10 mm bud		
EYE-EAR	lids fused loosely: −1 tightly: −2	lids open pinna flat stays folded	sl. curved pinna; soft; slow recoil	well-curved pinna; soft but ready recoil	formed and firm instant recoil	thick cartilage, ear stiff		
GENITALS (Male)	scrotum flat, smooth	scrotum empty, faint rugae	testes in upper canal, rare rugae	testes descending, few rugae	testes down, good rugae	testes pendulous, deep rugae		
GENITALS (Female)	clitoris prominent and labia flat	prominent clitoris and small labia minora	prominent clitoris and enlarging minora	majora and minora equally prominent	majora large, minora small	majora cover clitoris and minora		
						TOTAL PHYSICAL MATURITY SCORE		

FIGURE 18.3 Gestational age assessment tool. (Source: Ballard, J. L., Khoury, J. C., Wedig, K., et al. [1991]. New Ballard Score, expanded to include extremely premature infants. *Journal of Pediatrics, 119*[3], 417–423.)

prematurity, whereas a clitoris covered by labia suggests greater maturity)

The neuromuscular maturity section typically is completed within 24 hours after birth. Six activities or manoeuvres that the newborn performs with various body parts are evaluated to determine the newborn's degree of maturity:

1. Posture—how does the newborn hold his or her extremities in relation to the trunk? The greater the degree of flexion, the greater the maturity. For example, extension of arms and legs is scored as 0 point and full flexion of arms and legs is scored as 4 points.
2. Square window—how far can the newborn's hands be flexed toward the wrist? The angle is measured

and scored from more than 90 degrees to 0 degree to determine the maturity rating. As the angle decreases, the newborn's maturity increases. For example, an angle of more than 90 degrees is scored as −1 point and an angle of 0 degree is scored as 4 points.

3. Arm recoil—how far do the newborn's arms "spring back" to a flexed position? This measure evaluates the degree of arm flexion and the strength of recoil. The reaction of the arm is then scored from 0 to 4 points based on the degree of flexion as the arms are returned to their normal flexed position. The higher the points assigned, the greater the neuromuscular maturity (for example, recoil less than a 90-degree angle is scored as 4 points).

4. Popliteal angle—how far will the newborn's knees extend? The angle created when the knee is extended is measured. An angle less than 90 degrees indicates greater maturity. For example, an angle of 180 degrees is scored as −1 point and an angle of less than 90 degrees is scored as 5 points.

5. Scarf sign—how far can the elbows be moved across the newborn's chest? An elbow that does not reach midline indicates greater maturity. For example, if the elbow reaches or nears the level of the opposite shoulder, this is scored as −1 point; if the elbow does not cross the proximate axillary line, it is scored as 4 points.

6. Heel to ear—how close can the newborn's feet be moved to the ears? This manoeuvre assesses hip flexibility: the lesser the flexibility, the greater the newborn's maturity. The heel-to-ear assessment is scored in the same manner as the scarf sign.

After the scoring is completed, the 12 scores are totalled and then compared with standardized values to determine the appropriate gestational age in weeks. Scores range from very low in preterm newborns to very high for mature and postmature newborns.

Typically newborns are also classified according to gestational age as:

- Preterm or premature—born before 37 weeks' gestation, regardless of birth weight
- Term—born between 38 and 42 weeks' gestation
- Postterm or postdates—born after completion of week 42 of gestation
- Postmature—born after 42 weeks and demonstrating signs of placental aging

Using the information about gestational age and then considering birth weight, newborns can also be classified as follows:

- Small for gestational age (SGA)—weight less than the 10th percentile on standard growth charts (usually <5.5 lb)
- Appropriate for gestational age (AGA)—weight between 10th and 90th percentiles on standard growth charts
- Large for gestational age (LGA)—weight more than the 90th percentile on standard growth charts (usually >9 lb)

Chapter 23 describes these variations in birth weight and gestational age in greater detail.

▶ **Take** NOTE!

Gestational age assessment is important because it allows the nurse to plot growth parameters and to anticipate problems related to prematurity, postmaturity, and growth abnormalities. Most provincial and territorial birth forms have reference charts to document gestational age assessment as well as growth parameters.

Nursing Interventions

During the immediate newborn period, care focuses on helping the newborn to make the transition to extrauterine life. Nursing interventions include maintaining airway patency, promoting skin-to-skin contact, ensuring proper identification, administering prescribed medications, and maintaining thermoregulation.

Maintaining Airway Patency

Once the baby has been delivered and placed on the mother's chest, the nurse can continue to assess the need for resuscitation by noting respiratory effort, heart rate, and skin colour. If excessive secretions are noted that the newborn is unable to clear on his or her own, consider oral and nasal suctioning and turn the baby's head to the side. Turning the newborn's head "will allow secretions to collect in the cheek where they can be removed more easily" (Kattwinkel, 2011, p. 46). Typically, the newborn's mouth is suctioned gently first with a bulb syringe to remove debris and then the nose is suctioned. Suctioning in this manner helps to prevent aspiration of fluid into the lungs by an unexpected gasp. Routine suctioning of the newborn's oral and nasal passages is no longer recommended in the vigorous infant (Kattwinkel, 2011).

When suctioning a newborn with a bulb syringe, compress the bulb before placing it into the oral or nasal cavity. Release the bulb slowly, making sure the tip is placed away from the mucous membranes to draw up the excess secretions. Remove the bulb syringe from the mouth or nose and then, while holding the bulb syringe tip over an emesis basin lined with paper towel or tissue, compress the bulb to expel the secretions. Repeat the procedure gently as needed until all secretions are removed.

> ▶ **Take** NOTE!
>
> *Always keep a bulb syringe near the newborn in case he or she develops sudden choking or a blockage in the nose.*

> ▶ **Take** NOTE!
>
> *It make take several minutes for the newborn to transition and for his or her colour to improve. Continued assessment can take place while the baby is on his or her mother's chest.*

Skin-to-Skin Contact

Early skin-to-skin contact ideally begins immediately after birth and involves placing the naked newborn, covered with a warm blanket, on the mother's bare chest. This practice between mother and baby has been shown to reduce maternal bleeding, improve oxygenation, stabilize the baby's glucose, reduce crying, improve mother–baby interaction, maintain thermoregulation, and assist with successful breastfeeding (Caruana, 2008). If the newborn is healthy and stable, wipe the newborn from head to toe with a dry cloth and place him or her skin-to-skin on the mother's abdomen. Then cover the newborn and mother with another warmed blanket to hold in the warmth. Immediate mother–newborn contact takes advantage of the newborn's natural alertness after a vaginal birth and fosters bonding. Skin-to-skin care can also be modified for those parents who are not comfortable with immediate full skin-to-skin care, and can also be done with the father or other caregivers.

Initiating Breastfeeding

Helping mother breastfeed immediately after birth is gradually becoming the norm instead of attending immediately to what have become routine delivery room interventions. Since infants are the most alert within the first 60 to 90 minutes following birth, it is an ideal time to initiate breastfeeding. Helping mothers initiate breastfeeding within half an hour of birth is one of the World Health Organization's 10 Steps to Successful Breastfeeding (La Leche League International, 2010).

Left alone on the mother's abdomen, a healthy newborn moves upward, pushing with the feet, pulling with the arms, and bobbing the head until finding and latching on to the mother's nipple. A newborn's sense of smell is highly developed, which also helps in finding the nipple. As the newborn moves to the nipple, the mother produces high levels of oxytocin, which contracts the uterus, thereby minimizing bleeding. Oxytocin also causes the breasts to release colostrum when the newborn sucks on the nipple. Colostrum is rich in antibodies and thus provides the newborn with his or her "first immunization" against infection.

Ensuring Proper Identification

Starting at birth and throughout the hospital stay, attention to the safety and security of the newborn is important. The newborn commonly receives two ID bracelets, one on a wrist and one on an ankle. The mother receives a matching one, usually on her wrist. Four-band systems are also available. The ID bands usually state the infant's name, sex, date and time of birth, and identification number. The same identification number is on the bracelets of all the family members. If there are twins, each baby will have his or her own set of bracelets that will also identify birth order (Twin A for the first born and Twin B for the second born).

These ID bracelets provide for the safety of the newborn and must be secured before the mother and newborn leave the birthing area. The ID bracelets are checked by all nurses to validate that the correct newborn is brought to the right mother if they are separated for any period of time (Fig. 18.4). They also serve as the official newborn identification and are checked before initiating any procedure on that newborn and on discharge from the unit. Taking the newborn's picture within 2 hours after birth with a colour camera or colour video/digital image also helps prevent mix-ups and abduction. Some facilities use electronic devices that sound an alarm if the newborn is removed from the area. Parents are also key partners in safety and are encouraged to ask to see the photo identification of staff before giving their baby to someone (Association of Women's Health, Obstetric and Neonatal Nurses [AWHONN], 2007; Colling & York, 2010).

Although abductions from Canadian hospitals are rare, hospital security staff must always be well prepared to handle such incidents. Local law enforcement officials can be helpful in these situations too, especially if an Amber Alert search and recovery plan is activated. Many

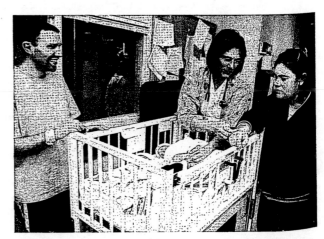

FIGURE **18.4** The nurse checks the newborn's identification band against the mother's.

DRUG GUIDE 18.1 DRUGS FOR THE NEWBORN

Drug	Action/Indication	Nursing Implications
Phytonadione (vitamin K [Aqua-MEPHYTON, Konakion, Mephyton])	Provides the newborn with vitamin K (necessary for production of adequate clotting factors II, VII, IX, and X by the liver) during the first week of birth until newborn can manufacture it Prevents vitamin K deficiency bleeding	• Administer within 1 to 2 h after birth. • Give as an IM injection at a 90-degree angle into the middle third of the vastus lateralis muscle. • Use a 25 gauge, 5/8 in needle for injection. • Hold the leg firmly and inject medication slowly after aspirating. • Adhere to standard precautions. • Assess for bleeding at injection site after administration.
Erythromycin ophthalmic ointment 0.5% or tetracycline ophthalmic ointment 1%	Provides bactericidal and bacteriostatic actions to prevent *Neisseria gonorrhoeae* and *Chlamydia trachomatis* conjunctivitis Prevents ophthalmia neonatorum	• Be alert for chemical conjunctivitis for 1–2 days. • Wear gloves, and open eyes by placing thumb and finger above and below the eye. • Gently squeeze the tube or ampoule to apply medication into the conjunctival sac from the inner canthus to the outer canthus of each eye. • Do not touch the tip to the eye. • Close the eye to make sure the medication permeates. • Wipe off excess ointment after 1 min.

facilities now have protocols and procedures in place for this situation.

Administering Prescribed Medications

During the immediate newborn period, two medications are commonly ordered: vitamin K and eye prophylaxis with either erythromycin or tetracycline ophthalmic ointment (Drug Guide 18.1).

Vitamin K

Vitamin K, a fat-soluble vitamin, promotes blood clotting by increasing the synthesis of prothrombin by the liver. A deficiency of this vitamin would delay clotting and might lead to unexpected bleeding.

Generally, the bacteria of the intestine produce vitamin K in adequate quantities. However, the newborn's bowel is sterile, so vitamin K is not produced in the intestine until after microorganisms are introduced, such as with the first feeding.

The administration of vitamin K to prevent early vitamin K deficiency bleeding has been the standard of care since the early 1960s. CPS recommends that vitamin K be given as a single intramuscular dose of 0.5 mg (birth weight 1,500 g or less) or 1.0 mg (birth weight greater than 1,500 g) to all newborns within the first 6 hours after birth following initial stabilization and an appropriate opportunity for maternal and family interaction (Fig. 18.5) (CPS,

2011b). If parents are not comfortable with intramuscular administration, oral vitamin K is available. Oral administration requires three doses, however, and parents need to be informed that there is an increased risk for late hemorrhagic disease.

Eye Prophylaxis

The CPS (2002) recommends that all newborns, whether delivered vaginally or by cesarean section, receive an instillation of a prophylactic agent in their eyes as soon as

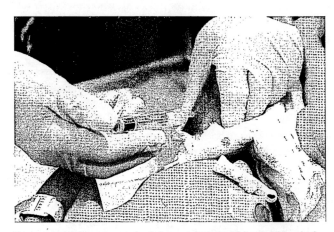

FIGURE 18.5 The nurse administers vitamin K intramuscularly to the newborn.

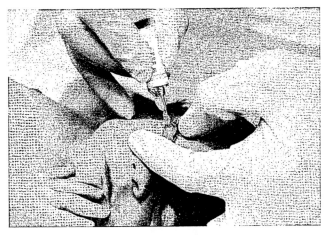

FIGURE 18.6 The nurse administers eye prophylaxis.

possible after birth. This is to prevent **ophthalmia neonatorum** (chlamydia trachomatis is the most common organism) and **gonoccocal ophthalmia**, which can cause neonatal blindness (CDC, 2010). Ophthalmia neonatorum is a hyperacute purulent conjunctivitis occurring during the first 10 days of life. It is usually contracted during birth when the baby comes in contact with infected vaginal discharge of the mother (CDC, 2010). Most often both eyelids become swollen and red with purulent discharge.

Prophylactic agents that are currently recommended include erythromycin 0.5% ophthalmic ointment or tetracycline 1% ophthalmic ointment in a single application; 1% silver nitrate solution was formerly used but has little efficacy in preventing chlamydial eye disease (CDC, 2010). Regardless of which agent is used, the medication should be instilled within 1 hour after birth (Fig. 18.6). (Health Canada, 2000).

Inform all parents about the eye treatment, including why it is recommended, what problems may arise if the treatment is not given, and possible adverse effects of the treatment.

> ▶ *Take NOTE!*
>
> *Parents have the right to refuse this treatment. Ensure this is an informed decision based on accurate information and teaching.*

Maintaining Thermoregulation

Newborns have trouble regulating their temperature, especially during the first few hours after birth (see Chapter 17 for a complete discussion). Therefore, maintaining body temperature is a crucial nursing role.

Remember the potential for heat loss in newborns, and perform all nursing interventions in a way that minimizes heat loss and prevents hypothermia. Thoroughly drying the infant, placing a cap on his or her head, and ensuring skin-to-skin contact with the mother while the infant is covered with a warm blanket all minimize heat loss. Ongoing care to prevent hypothermia involves making sure the newborn is not exposed to cold surfaces or cool drafts and wrapping the newborn in warm blankets when skin-to-skin contact is not possible. If the newborn is to be placed under a heat warmer, unwrap the infant and put a sensor in place to monitor temperature and avoid hyperthermia.

A wide variety of devices are available to measure temperature in newborns; most birthing facilities are now using electronic thermometers. Axillary temperatures are recommended to assess the newborn's body temperature. At one time, rectal thermometers were routinely used to monitor body temperature, but their use is no longer recommended because of the risk for traumatizing the rectal lining (Blackburn, 2007). Axillary temperature should be maintained between 36.3° and 37.0°C (inclusive) and skin temperature between 36.5° and 37.0°C (ACoRN Neonatal Society, 2010). Nursing interventions to help maintain body temperature include:

- Promote skin-to-skin contact with the newborn's mother or another caregiver immediately after birth.
- Dry the newborn immediately after birth to prevent heat loss through evaporation.
- Cover or wrap the baby in warmed blankets to reduce heat loss via convection.
- Use a warmed cover on the scale to weigh the unclothed newborn to prevent heat loss through conduction.
- Warm stethoscopes and hands before examining the baby or providing care.
- Avoid placing newborns in drafts or near air vents to prevent heat loss through convection.
- Delay the initial bath until the baby's temperature has stabilized to prevent heat loss through evaporation.
- Avoid placing cribs near cold outer walls to prevent heat loss through radiation.
- Put a cap on the newborn's head after it is thoroughly dried after birth.
- Place the newborn in an incubator or under a temperature-controlled radiant warmer if other interventions are not effective at improving the temperature (Fig. 18.7).

Most people view pregnancy as a natural process with a positive outcome—the birth of a healthy newborn. Unfortunately, conditions can occur that may result in negative outcomes for the fetus, mother, or both. A **high-risk pregnancy** is one in which a condition exists that jeopardizes the health of the mother, her fetus, or both. The condition may result from the pregnancy, or it may be a condition that was present before the woman became pregnant.

In Canada, approximately 10% of all pregnancies are considered high risk. According to the Canadian Institute for Health Information (2004), "Pregnancies are deemed high-risk if there is a higher-than-average chance of complications developing. For example, women with a history of medical conditions such as gestational diabetes, heart disease, or those carrying more than one child, may be considered high-risk." The risk status of a woman and her fetus can change during the pregnancy, with a number of problems occurring during labour, birth, or afterward, even in women without any known previous antepartal risk. Examples of high-risk conditions include gestational diabetes and ectopic pregnancy. Early identification of the woman at risk is essential to ensure that appropriate interventions are instituted promptly, increasing the opportunity to change the course of events and provide a positive outcome.

The term "risk" may mean different things to different groups. For example, health care professionals may focus on the disease processes and treatments to prevent complications. Nurses may focus on nursing care and on the psychosocial impact on the woman and her family. The woman's attention may be focused on her own needs and those of her family. Together, working as a collaborative team, the ultimate goal of care is to ensure the best possible outcome for the woman, her fetus, and her family.

Risk assessment begins at the first antepartal visit and continues with each subsequent visit because factors may be identified in later visits that were not apparent during earlier visits. For example, as the nurse and client develop a trusting relationship, previously unidentified or unsuspected factors (such as drug abuse or intimate partner violence) may be revealed. Through education and support, the nurse can encourage the client to inform her health care provider of these concerns, and necessary interventions or referrals can be made.

A comprehensive approach to high-risk pregnancy is needed. For example, prenatal stress and distress have been shown to have significant consequences for the mother, child, and family (Reid, Power, & Cheshire, 2009). Risks are grouped into broad categories based on threats to health and pregnancy outcome. Current categories of risk are biophysical, psychosocial, sociodemographic, and environmental (Gilbert, 2010) (Box 19.1).

This chapter describes the major conditions directly related to the pregnancy that can complicate a pregnancy, possibly affecting maternal and fetal outcomes. These include bleeding during pregnancy (spontaneous abortion, ectopic pregnancy, gestational trophoblastic disease (GTD), cervical insufficiency, placenta previa, and abruptio placentae), hyperemesis gravidarum, gestational hypertension, HELLP (hemolysis, elevated liver enzymes, and low platelets) syndrome, gestational diabetes, blood incompatibility, amniotic fluid imbalances (hydramnios and oligohydramnios), multiple gestation, and premature rupture of membranes. Chapter 20 addresses preexisting conditions that can complicate a woman's pregnancy as well as populations that are considered to be at high risk.

Bleeding During Pregnancy

Bleeding at any time during pregnancy is potentially life-threatening. Bleeding can occur early or late in the pregnancy and may result from numerous conditions. Conditions commonly associated with early bleeding (first half of pregnancy) include spontaneous abortion, ectopic pregnancy, GTD, and conditions associated with midtrimester bleeding, such as cervical insufficiency. Conditions associated with late bleeding include placenta previa and abruptio placentae, which usually occur after the 20th week of gestation.

Spontaneous Abortion

An **abortion** is the loss of an early pregnancy, usually before week 20 of gestation. Abortion can be spontaneous or induced. A spontaneous abortion refers to the loss of a fetus resulting from natural causes—that is, not elective or therapeutically induced by a procedure. The term *miscarriage* is often used by nonmedical people to denote an abortion that has occurred spontaneously. A miscarriage can occur during early pregnancy, and many women who miscarry may not even be aware that they are pregnant. About 80% of spontaneous abortions occur within the first trimester.

The overall rate of spontaneous abortion in Canada is reported to be 8% of recognized pregnancies (Einarson, Choi, Einarson, et al., 2009). However, with the development of highly sensitive assays for human chorionic gonadotropin (hCG) levels that detect pregnancies prior to the expected next menses, the incidence of pregnancy loss increases significantly—from 22% to 57% (Stephenson, 2008).

Pathophysiology

The causes of spontaneous abortion are varied and often unknown. The most common cause for first-trimester abortions is fetal genetic abnormalities, usually unrelated to the mother. The major non-genetic causes, at any time

BOX 19.1 Factors Placing a Woman at Risk During Pregnancy

Biophysical Factors
- Genetic conditions
- Chromosomal abnormalities
- Multiple pregnancy
- Defective genes
- Inherited disorders
- ABO incompatibility
- Large fetal size
- Medical and obstetric conditions
- Preterm labour and birth
- Cardiovascular disease
- Chronic hypertension
- Incompetent cervix
- Placental abnormalities
- Infection
- Diabetes
- Maternal collagen diseases
- Pregnancy-induced hypertension
- Asthma
- Postterm pregnancy
- Hemoglobinopathies
- Nutritional status
- Inadequate dietary intake
- Food fads
- Excessive food intake
- Under- or overweight status
- Hematocrit value less than 33%
- Eating disorder

Psychosocial Factors
- Smoking
- Caffeine
- Alcohol
- Drugs
- Inadequate support system
- Situational crisis
- History of violence
- Emotional distress
- Unsafe cultural practices

Sociodemographic Factors
- Poverty status
- Lack of prenatal care
- Age younger than 15 years or older than 35 years
- Parity—all first pregnancies and more than five pregnancies
- Marital status—increased risk for unmarried
- Accessibility to health care
- Ethnicity—increased risk in nonwhite women

Environmental Factors
- Infections
- Radiation
- Pesticides
- Illicit drugs
- Industrial pollutants
- Secondhand cigarette smoke
- Personal stress

Source: Gilbert, E. (2010). *Manual of high-risk pregnancy and delivery* (5th ed.). St. Louis, MO: Mosby.

in the pregnancy, include maternal–fetal infection, including rubella virus, cytomegalovirus, herpes simplex virus, bacterial vaginosis, and toxoplasmosis; obstetric complications, including placental abruption and hemorrhage; and maternal medical conditions, including diabetes, hypertension, hypothyroidism, and chronic nephritis. (Silver, 2009).

Nursing Assessment

When a pregnant woman calls to report vaginal bleeding, she must be seen as soon as possible by a health care professional to ascertain the etiology. Varying degrees of vaginal bleeding, low back pain, abdominal cramping, and passage of products of conception tissue may be reported. Ask the woman about the colour of the vaginal bleeding (bright red is significant) and the amount—for example, question her about the frequency with which she is changing her peripads (saturation of one peripad hourly is significant) and the passage of any clots or tissue. Instruct her to save any tissue or clots passed and bring them with her to the health care facility. Also obtain a description of any other signs and symptoms the

woman may be experiencing, along with a description of their severity and duration. It is important to remain calm and listen to the woman's description.

When the woman arrives at the health care facility, assess her vital signs and observe the amount, colour, and characteristics of the bleeding. Ask her to rate her current pain level, using an appropriate pain assessment tool. Also evaluate the amount and intensity of the woman's abdominal cramping or contractions, and assess the woman's level of understanding about what is happening to her. A thorough assessment helps in determining the type of spontaneous abortion, such as threatened abortion, inevitable abortion, incomplete abortion, complete abortion, missed abortion, and habitual abortion, that the woman may be experiencing (Table 19.1).

Nursing Management

Nursing management of the woman with a spontaneous abortion focuses on providing continued monitoring and psychological support, for the family is experiencing acute loss and grief. An important component of this support is reassuring the woman that spontaneous abortions usually

TABLE 19.1 CATEGORIES OF SPONTANEOUS ABORTION

Category	Assessment Findings	Diagnosis	Therapeutic Management
Threatened abortion	Vaginal bleeding (often slight) early in a pregnancy No cervical dilation or change in cervical consistency Mild abdominal cramping Closed cervical os No passage of fetal tissue	Vaginal ultrasound to confirm whether sac is empty Declining maternal serum hCG and progesterone levels to provide additional information about viability of pregnancy	Conservative supportive treatment Possible reduction in activity in conjunction with nutritious diet and adequate hydration
Inevitable abortion	Vaginal bleeding (greater than that associated with threatened abortion) Rupture of membranes Cervical dilation Strong abdominal cramping Possible passage of products of conception	Ultrasound and hCG levels to indicate pregnancy loss	Vacuum curettage if products of conception are not passed, to reduce risk for excessive bleeding and infection Prostaglandin analogues such as misoprostol to empty uterus of retained tissue (only used if fragments are not completely passed)
Incomplete abortion (passage of some of the products of conception)	Intense abdominal cramping Heavy vaginal bleeding Cervical dilation	Ultrasound confirmation that products of conception are still in uterus	Client stabilization Evacuation of uterus via dilation and curettage (D&C) or prostaglandin analogue
Complete abortion (passage of all products of conception)	History of vaginal bleeding and abdominal pain Passage of tissue with subsequent decrease in pain and significant decrease in vaginal bleeding	Ultrasound demonstrating an empty uterus	No medical or surgical intervention necessary Follow-up appointment to discuss family planning
Missed abortion (nonviable embryo retained in utero for at least 6 weeks)	Absent uterine contractions Irregular spotting Possible progression to inevitable abortion	Ultrasound to identify products of conception in uterus	Evacuation of uterus (if inevitable abortion does not occur): suction curettage during first trimester, dilation and evacuation during second trimester Induction of labour with intravaginal PGE2 suppository to empty uterus without surgical intervention
Habitual abortion	History of three or more consecutive spontaneous abortions Not carrying the pregnancy to viability or term	Validation via client's history	Identification and treatment of underlying cause (possible causes such as genetic or chromosomal abnormalities, reproductive tract abnormalities, chronic diseases or immunologic problems) Cervical cerclage in second trimester if incompetent cervix is the cause

107

result from an abnormality and that her actions did not cause the abortion.

Providing Continued Monitoring

Continued monitoring and ongoing assessments are essential for the woman experiencing a spontaneous abortion. Monitor the amount of vaginal bleeding through pad counts and observe for passage of products of conception tissue. Assess the woman's pain and provide appropriate pain management to address the cramping discomfort.

Assist in preparing the woman for procedures and treatments such as surgery to evacuate the uterus or medications such as misoprostol or prostaglandin E2 (PGE2). If the woman is Rh negative and not sensitized, expect to administer Rh immune globulin (WinRho) within 72 hours after the abortion is complete. Drug Guide 19.1 gives more information about these medications.

Providing Support

A woman's emotional reaction may vary depending on her desire for this pregnancy and her available support network. Provide both physical and emotional support. In addition, prepare the woman and her family for the assessment process, and answer their questions about what is happening.

Explaining some of the causes of spontaneous abortions can help the woman to understand what is happening and may allay her fears and guilt that she did something to cause this pregnancy loss. Most women experience an acute sense of loss and go through a grieving process with a spontaneous abortion. Providing sensitive listening, counselling, and anticipatory guidance to the woman and her family will allow them to verbalize their feelings and ask questions about future pregnancies.

The grieving period may last as long as 2 years after a pregnancy loss, with each person grieving in his or her own way. Encourage friends and family to be supportive but give the couple space and time to work through their loss. Referral to a community support group for parents who have experienced a miscarriage can be very helpful during this grief process.

DRUG GUIDE 19.1 MEDICATIONS USED FOR SPONTANEOUS ABORTIONS

Medication	Action/Indications	Nursing Implications
Misoprostol (Cytotec)	Stimulates uterine contractions to terminate a pregnancy Evacuates the uterus after abortion to ensure passage of all the products of conception	Monitor for side effects such as diarrhea, abdominal pain, nausea, vomiting, dyspepsia. Assess vaginal bleeding and report any increased bleeding, pain, or fever. Monitor for signs and symptoms of shock, such as tachycardia, hypotension, and anxiety.
Mifepristone (RU-486)	Acts as progesterone antagonist, allowing prostaglandins to stimulate uterine contractions; causes the endometrium to slough May be followed by administration of misoprostol within 48 h	Monitor for headache, vomiting, diarrhea, and heavy bleeding. Anticipate administration of antiemetic prior to use to reduce nausea and vomiting. Encourage client to use acetaminophen to reduce discomfort from cramping.
PGE2, dinoprostone (Cervidil, Prepidil Gel, Prostin E2)	Stimulates uterine contractions, causing expulsion of uterine contents Expels uterine contents in fetal death or missed abortion during second trimester Effaces and dilates the cervix in pregnancy at term	Bring gel to room temperature before administering. Avoid contact with skin. Administer using sterile technique. Keep client supine 30 min after administering. Document time of insertion and dosing intervals. Remove insert with retrieval system after 12 h or at the onset of labour. Explain purpose and expected response to client.
Rh(D) immunoglobulin (WinRho, Gamulin, HydroRho-D, RhoGAM)	Suppresses immune response of non-sensitized Rh-negative patients who are exposed to Rh-positive blood Prevents isoimmunization in Rh-negative women exposed to Rh-positive blood after abortions, miscarriages, and pregnancies	Administer intramuscularly in deltoid area. Give only WinRho for abortions and miscarriages <12 weeks unless fetus or father is Rh negative (unless patient is Rh positive, Rh antibodies are present). Educate woman that she will need this after subsequent deliveries if newborns are Rh positive; also check lab study results prior to administering the drug.

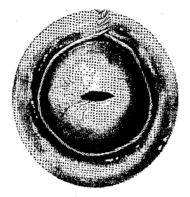

FIGURE 19.3 Cervical cerclage.

Cervical Insufficiency

Cervical insufficiency, also called premature dilation of the cervix, describes a weak, structurally defective cervix that spontaneously dilates in the absence of contractions in the second trimester, resulting in the loss of the pregnancy. The incidence of cervical insufficiency is less than 1%; estimates range from 1 in 500 to 1 in 2,000 pregnancies, accounting for approximately 20% to 25% of midtrimester losses (Fox & Chervenak, 2008).

Pathophysiology

The exact mechanism contributing to cervical insufficiency is not known. Some studies have linked the incompetent cervix with having less collagen and more smooth muscle than the normal cervix, while others have disproven this link (Oxlund, Ørtoft, Brüel, et al., 2010). Several theories have been proposed that focus on damage to the cervix as a key component.

Cervical insufficiency is likely to be the clinical end point of many pathologic processes, such as congenital cervical disorders, deep cervical laceration secondary to prior vaginal or cesarean birth, infection/inflammation, trauma to the cervix (conization, amputation, obstetric laceration, or forced cervical dilation, which may occur during elective pregnancy termination). However, the exact etiology of cervical insufficiency is not known.

Cervical length also has been associated with cervical insufficiency and subsequently preterm birth. Recent studies have examined the association between a short cervical length and the risk for preterm birth. Some have demonstrated a continuum of risk between a shorter cervix on ultrasound and a higher risk for preterm birth, leading to the hypothetical argument that women with a short cervix on ultrasound might benefit from cervical cerclage, but there have been conflicting results (Mancuso & Owen, 2009).

Therapeutic Management

Cervical insufficiency may be treated in a variety of ways: bed rest, pelvic rest, avoidance of heavy lifting, or surgically, via a procedure of cervical cerclage in the second trimester. Cervical cerclage involves using a heavy purse-string suture to secure and reinforce the internal os of the cervix (Fig. 19.3).

According to the Society of Obstetricians and Gynaecologists of Canada (SOGC), to reduce the risk for preterm labour, cervical cerclage should be considered for asymptomatic pregnant women with a history of preterm birth and a cervical measurement of less than 25 mm prior to 24 weeks' gestation (Lim, Butt, & Crane, 2011). Asymptomatic women are defined as those with no signs of infections, are not in labour, and who's membranes are intact.

Nursing Assessment

Nursing assessment focuses on obtaining a thorough history to determine any risk factors that might have a bearing on this pregnancy—previous cervical trauma, preterm labour, fetal loss in the second trimester, or previous surgeries or procedures involving the cervix. History may reveal a previous loss of pregnancy around 20 weeks.

Also be alert for complaints of vaginal discharge or pelvic pressure. Commonly with cervical insufficiency the woman will report a pink-tinged vaginal discharge or an increase in pelvic pressure. Cervical dilation also occurs. If this continues, rupture of the membranes, release of amniotic fluid, and uterine contractions occur, subsequently resulting in delivery of the fetus, often before it is viable.

> ▶ **Take** NOTE!
>
> *The diagnosis of cervical insufficiency remains difficult in many circumstances. The cornerstone of diagnosis is a history of midtrimester pregnancy loss associated with painless cervical dilation without evidence of uterine activity.*

Transvaginal ultrasound typically is done around 20 weeks' gestation to determine cervical length and evaluate for shortening. Cervical shortening occurs from the internal os outward and can be viewed on ultrasound as funnelling. The amount of funnelling can be determined by dividing funnel length by cervical length. The most

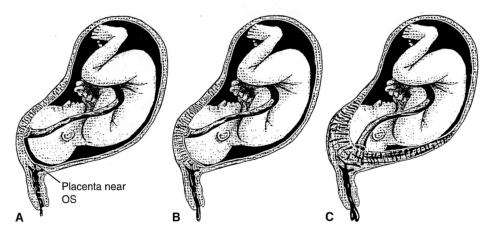

A Placenta near OS

Marginal

B

Partial

C

Complete

FIGURE 19.4 Classification of placenta previa. (**A**) Marginal. (**B**) Partial. (**C**) Complete.

common time at which a short cervix or funnelling develops is 18 to 22 weeks, so ultrasound screening should be performed during this interval (Fox & Chervenak, 2008). A cervical length less than 25 mm is abnormal between 14 and 24 weeks and may increase the risk for preterm labour.

Nursing Management

Nursing management focuses on monitoring the woman very closely for signs of preterm labour: backache, increased vaginal discharge, rupture of membranes, and uterine contractions. Provide emotional support and education to allay the couple's anxiety about the well-being of their fetus. Provide preoperative care and teaching as indicated if the woman will be undergoing cerclage. Teach the client and her family about the signs and symptoms of preterm labour and the need to report any changes immediately. Also reinforce the need for activity restrictions (if appropriate) and continued regular follow-up. Continuing surveillance throughout the pregnancy is important to promote a positive outcome for the family.

Placenta Previa

Placenta previa is a bleeding condition that occurs during the last two trimesters of pregnancy. In placenta previa (literally, "afterbirth first"), the placenta implants over the cervical os. This condition may cause serious morbidity and mortality to the fetus and the mother. It complicates approximately 3.5 to 6 of every 1,000 births and is associated with potentially serious consequences from hemorrhage, abruption (separation) of the placenta, preterm birth, or emergency cesarean birth (Bahar, Abusham, Eskandar, et al., 2009; Joy, Lyon, & Stone, 2010).

Pathophysiology

The exact cause of placenta previa is unknown. It is initiated by implantation of the embryo in the lower uterus.

With placental attachment and growth, the cervical os may become covered by the developing placenta. Placental vascularization is defective, allowing the placenta to attach directly to the myometrium (accreta), invade the myometrium (increta), or penetrate the myometrium (percreta).

Placenta previa is generally classified according to the degree of coverage or proximity to the internal os, as follows (Fig. 19.4):

• Complete placenta previa: the internal cervical os is completely covered by the placenta
• Partial placenta previa: the internal os is partially covered by the placenta
• Marginal placenta previa: the placenta is at the margin or edge of the internal os
• Low-lying placenta previa: the placenta is implanted in the lower uterine segment and is near the internal os but does not reach it

Therapeutic Management

Therapeutic management depends on the extent of bleeding, the amount of placenta over the cervical os, whether the fetus is developed enough to survive outside the uterus, the position of the fetus, the mother's parity, and the presence or absence of labour (Zeltzer, 2011).

If the mother and fetus are both stable, therapeutic management may involve expectant ("wait-and-see") care. This care can be carried out at home or on an antepartal unit in the health care facility. If there is no active bleeding and the client has readily available access to reliable transportation, can maintain bed rest at home, and can comprehend instructions, expectant care at home is appropriate. However, if the client requires continuous care and monitoring and cannot meet the home care requirements, the antepartal unit is the best environment.

Nursing Assessment

Nursing assessment involves a thorough history, including possible risk factors, and physical examination. Evaluate the client closely for these risk factors:

- Advancing maternal age (more than 35 years)
- Previous cesarean birth
- Multiparity
- Uterine insult or injury
- Prior placenta previa
- Multiple gestations
- Previous induced surgical abortion
- Smoking (Ko & Yoon, 2011)

Health History and Physical Examination

Ask the client if she has had any problems associated with bleeding, now or in the recent past. The classic clinical presentation is painless, bright-red vaginal bleeding occurring during the second or third trimester. The initial bleeding usually is not profuse and it ceases spontaneously, only to recur. The first episode of bleeding occurs (on average) at 27 to 32 weeks' gestation. The bleeding is thought to arise secondary to the thinning of the lower uterine segment in preparation for the onset of labour. When the bleeding occurs at the implantation site in the lower uterus, the uterus cannot contract adequately and stop the flow of blood from the open vessels. Typically with normal placental implantation in the upper uterus, minor disruptive placental attachment is not a problem because there is a larger volume of myometrial tissue able to contract and constrict bleeding vessels.

Assess the client for uterine contractions, which may or may not occur with the bleeding. Palpate the uterus; typically it is soft and nontender on examination. Auscultate the fetal heart rate; it commonly is within normal parameters. Fetal distress is usually absent but may occur when cord problems arise, such as umbilical cord prolapse or cord compression, or when the client has experienced blood loss to the extent that maternal shock or placental abruption has occurred (Liston, Sawchuk, & Young, 2007).

Laboratory and Diagnostic Testing

To validate the position of the placenta, a transvaginal ultrasound is done. In addition, magnetic resonance imaging may be ordered when preparing for delivery because it allows identification of placenta accreta (placenta abnormally adherent to the myometrium), increta (placenta accreta with penetration of the myometrium), or percreta (placenta accreta with invasion of the myometrium to the peritoneal covering, causing rupture of the uterus) in addition to placenta previa. These placental abnormalities, although rare, carry a very high morbidity and mortality rate, possibly necessitating a hysterectomy at delivery.

Nursing Management

Whether the care setting is in the client's home or in the health care facility, the nurse focuses on monitoring the maternal–fetal status, including assessing for signs and symptoms of vaginal bleeding and fetal distress, and providing support and education to the client and her family, including what events and diagnostic studies are being performed. For the majority of women, a cesarean birth will be planned. Nursing Care Plan 19.1 discusses the nursing process for the woman with placenta previa.

Monitoring Maternal–Fetal Status

Assess the degree of vaginal bleeding; inspect the perineal area for blood that may be pooled underneath the woman. Estimate and document the amount of bleeding. Perform a peripad count on an ongoing basis, making sure to report any changes in amount or frequency to the health care provider. If the woman is experiencing active bleeding, prepare for blood typing and cross-matching in the event a blood transfusion is needed.

> ▶ **Take** NOTE!
>
> *Avoid performing vaginal examinations in the woman with placenta previa. They may disrupt the placenta and cause hemorrhage.*

Monitor maternal vital signs and uterine contractility frequently for changes. Have the client rate her level of pain using an appropriate pain rating scale.

Assess fetal heart rates via Doppler or electronic monitoring to detect fetal distress. Monitor the woman's cardiopulmonary status, reporting any difficulties in respirations, changes in skin colour, or complaints of difficulty breathing. Have oxygen equipment readily available should fetal or maternal distress develop. Encourage the client to lie on her side to enhance placental perfusion.

If the woman has an intravenous (IV) line inserted, inspect the IV site frequently. Alternately, anticipate the insertion of an intermittent IV access device such as a saline lock, which can be used if quick access is needed for fluid restoration and infusion of blood products. Obtain laboratory tests as ordered, including complete blood count (CBC), coagulation studies, and Rh status if appropriate.

Administer pharmacologic agents as necessary. Give WinRho if the client is Rh negative at 28 weeks' gestation. Monitor tocolytic medication if prevention of preterm labour is needed.

Providing Support and Education

Determine the woman's level of understanding about placenta previa and the associated procedures and treatment plan. Doing so is important to prevent confusion

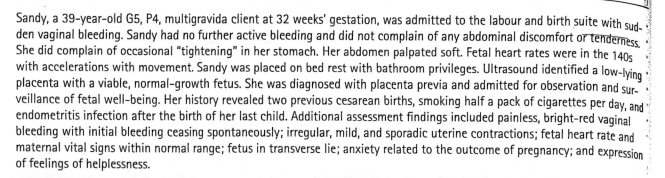

Nursing Care Plan 19.1

OVERVIEW OF THE WOMAN WITH PLACENTA PREVIA

Sandy, a 39-year-old G5, P4, multigravida client at 32 weeks' gestation, was admitted to the labour and birth suite with sudden vaginal bleeding. Sandy had no further active bleeding and did not complain of any abdominal discomfort or tenderness. She did complain of occasional "tightening" in her stomach. Her abdomen palpated soft. Fetal heart rates were in the 140s with accelerations with movement. Sandy was placed on bed rest with bathroom privileges. Ultrasound identified a low-lying placenta with a viable, normal-growth fetus. She was diagnosed with placenta previa and admitted for observation and surveillance of fetal well-being. Her history revealed two previous cesarean births, smoking half a pack of cigarettes per day, and endometritis infection after the birth of her last child. Additional assessment findings included painless, bright-red vaginal bleeding with initial bleeding ceasing spontaneously; irregular, mild, and sporadic uterine contractions; fetal heart rate and maternal vital signs within normal range; fetus in transverse lie; anxiety related to the outcome of pregnancy; and expression of feelings of helplessness.

NURSING DIAGNOSIS: Ineffective tissue perfusion (fetal and maternal) related to blood loss

Outcome Identification and Evaluation

Client will maintain adequate tissue perfusion as evidenced by stable vital signs, decreased blood loss, few or no uterine contractions, normal fetal heart rate patterns and variability, and positive fetal movement

Interventions: Maintaining Adequate Tissue Perfusion

- Establish IV access *to allow for administration of fluids, blood, and medications as necessary.*
- Obtain type and cross-match for at least 2 U of blood products *to ensure availability should bleeding continue.*
- Obtain specimens as ordered for blood studies, such as CBC and clotting studies, *to establish a baseline and use for future comparison.*
- Monitor output *to evaluate adequacy of renal perfusion.*
- Administer IV fluid replacement therapy as ordered *to maintain blood pressure and blood volume.*
- Palpate for abdominal tenderness and rigidity *to determine bleeding and evidence of uterine contractions.*
- Institute bed rest *to reduce oxygen demands.*
- Assess for rupture of membranes *to evaluate for possible onset of labour.*
- Avoid vaginal examinations *to prevent further bleeding episodes.*
- Complete an Rh titer *to identify need for WinRho.*
- Avoid nipple stimulation *to prevent uterine contractions.*
- Continuously monitor for contractions or PROM *to allow for prompt intervention.*
- Administer tocolytic agents as ordered *to stall preterm labour.*
- Monitor vital signs frequently *to identify possible hypovolemia and infection.*
- Assess frequently for active vaginal bleeding *to minimize risk for hemorrhage.*
- Continuously monitor fetal heart rate with electronic fetal monitor *to evaluate fetal status.*
- Assist with fetal surveillance tests as ordered *to aid in determining fetal well-being.*
- Observe for abnormal fetal heart rate patterns, such as loss of variability, decelerations, tachycardia, *to identify fetal distress.*
- Position patient in side-lying position with wedge for support *to maximize placental perfusion.*
- Assess fetal movement *to evaluate for possible fetal hypoxia.*
- Teach woman to monitor fetal movement *to evaluate well-being.*
- Administer oxygen as ordered *to increase oxygenation to mother and fetus.*

NURSING DIAGNOSIS: Anxiety related to threats to self and fetus

Outcome Identification and Evaluation

Client will experience a decrease in anxiety as evidenced by verbal reports of less anxiety, use of effective coping measures, and calm demeanor

Nursing Care Plan 19.1 (continued)

Interventions: Minimizing Anxiety

- Provide factual information about the diagnosis and treatment, and explain interventions and the rationale behind them *to provide client with a clear understanding of her condition.*
- Answer questions about health status honestly *to establish a trusting relationship.*
- Speak calmly to patient and family members *to minimize environmental stress.*
- Encourage the use of past effective techniques for coping *to promote relaxation and feelings of control.*
- Acknowledge and facilitate the woman's spiritual needs *to promote effective coping.*
- Involve the woman and family in the decision-making process *to foster self-confidence and control over situation.*
- Maintain a presence during stressful periods *to allay anxiety.*
- Use the sense of touch if appropriate *to convey caring and concern.*
- Encourage talking as a means *to release tension.*

and gain her cooperation. Provide information about the condition and make sure that all information related is consistent with information from the primary care provider. Explain all assessments and treatment measures as needed. Act as a client advocate in obtaining information for the family.

Teach the woman how to perform and record daily fetal movement. This action serves two purposes. One, it provides valuable information about the fetus. Two, it is an activity that the client can participate in, thereby fostering some feeling of control over the situation.

If the woman will require prolonged hospitalization or home bed rest, assess the physical and emotional impact that this may have on her. Evaluate her coping mechanisms to help determine how well she will be able to adjust to and cooperate with the treatment plan. Allow the client to verbalize her feelings and fears and provide emotional support. Also, provide opportunities for distraction—educational videos or DVDs, arts and crafts, computer games, reading books—and evaluate the client's response.

In addition to the emotional impact of prolonged bed rest, thoroughly assess the woman's skin to prevent skin breakdown and to help alleviate her discomfort secondary to limited physical activity. Instruct the woman in appropriate skin care measures. Encourage her to eat a balanced diet with adequate fluid intake to ensure that adequate nutrition and hydration and prevent complications associated with urinary and bowel elimination secondary to bed rest.

Teach the client and family about any signs and symptoms that should be reported immediately. In addition, prepare the woman for the possibility of a cesarean birth. The woman must notify her health care provider about any bleeding episodes or backaches (may indicate preterm labour contractions) and must adhere to the prescribed bed rest regimen. To ensure compliance and a positive outcome, she needs to be aware of the purpose of all of the observations that need to be made.

Abruptio Placentae

Abruptio placentae is the separation of a normally located placenta after the 20th week of gestation and prior to birth that leads to hemorrhage. It is a significant cause of third-trimester bleeding and carries a high mortality rate. It occurs in about 1% of all pregnancies throughout the world (Deering, 2011), or 1 in 120 pregnancies. The overall fetal mortality rate for placental abruption is 20% to 40%, depending on the extent of the abruption. Maternal mortality is approximately 6% in abruptio placentae and is related to cesarean birth and/or hemorrhage/coagulopathy (Deering, 2011).

Pathophysiology

The etiology of this condition is unknown; however, it has been proposed that abruption starts with degenerative changes in the small maternal arterioles, resulting in thrombosis, degeneration of the decidua, and possible rupture of a vessel. Bleeding from the vessel forms a retroplacental clot. The bleeding causes increased pressure behind the placenta and results in separation (Deering, 2011).

Fetal blood supply is compromised and fetal distress develops in proportion to the degree of placental separation. This is caused by the insult of the abruption itself and by issues related to prematurity when early birth is required to alleviate maternal or fetal distress.

Abruptio placentae is classified according to the extent of separation and the amount of blood loss from the maternal circulation. Classifications include:

- Mild (grade 1): minimal bleeding (less than 500 mL), marginal separation (10% to 20%), tender uterus, no coagulopathy, no signs of shock, no fetal distress
- Moderate (grade 2): moderate bleeding (1,000 to 1,500 mL), moderate separation (20% to 50%), continuous abdominal pain, mild shock
- Severe (grade 3): absent to moderate bleeding (more than 1,500 mL), severe separation (more than 50%),

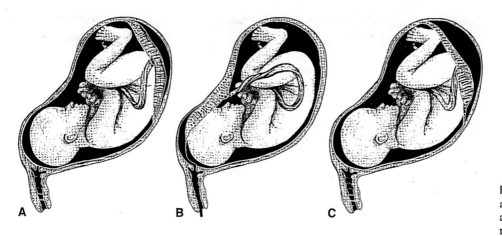

Partial abruption,
concealed hemorrhage

Partial abruption,
apparent hemorrhage

Complete abruption,
concealed hemorrhage

FIGURE 19.5 Classification of abruptio placentae. (**A**) Partial abruption with concealed hemorrhage. (**B**) Partial abruption with apparent hemorrhage. (**C**) Complete abruption with concealed hemorrhage.

profound shock, agonizing abdominal pain, and development of disseminated intravascular coagulopathy (DIC) (Gilbert, 2010)

Abruptio placentae also may be classified as partial or complete, depending on the degree of separation. Alternately, it can be classified as concealed or apparent, by the type of bleeding (Fig. 19.5).

*R*emember Helen, the pregnant woman with severe abdominal pain? Electronic fetal monitoring revealed uterine hypertonicity with absent fetal heart sounds. Palpation of her abdomen revealed rigidity and extreme tenderness in all four quadrants. Her vital signs were as follows—temperature, afebrile; pulse, 94; respirations, 22; blood pressure, 130/90 mm Hg. What might you suspect as the cause of Helen's abdominal pain? What course of action would you anticipate for Helen?

Therapeutic Management

Treatment of abruptio placentae is designed to assess, control, and restore the amount of blood lost; to provide a positive outcome for both mother and newborn; and to prevent coagulation disorders, such as DIC (Box 19.2). Emergency measures include starting two large-bore IV lines with normal saline or lactated Ringer's solution to combat hypovolemia, obtaining blood specimens for evaluating hemodynamic status values and for typing and cross-matching, and frequently monitoring fetal and maternal well-being. After the severity of abruption is determined and appropriate blood and fluid replacement is given, cesarean birth is done immediately if fetal distress is evident. If the fetus is not in distress, close monitoring continues, with delivery planned at the earliest signs of fetal distress. Because of the possibility of fetal blood loss through the placenta, a neonatal intensive care team should be available during the birth process to assess and treat the newborn immediately for shock, blood loss, and hypoxia.

If the woman develops DIC, treatment focuses on determining and correcting the underlying cause. Replacement therapy of the coagulation factors is achieved by

---

BOX 19.2 Disseminated Intravascular Coagulation (DIC)

DIC is a bleeding disorder characterized by an abnormal reduction in the elements involved in blood clotting resulting from their widespread intravascular clotting (Day, Paul, Williams, et al., 2010). This disorder can occur secondary to abruptio placentae.

Simply put, the clinical and pathologic manifestations of DIC can be described as a loss of balance between the clot-forming activity of thrombin and the clot-lysing activity of plasmin. Therefore, too much thrombin tips the balance toward the prothrombic state and the client develops clots. Alternately, too much clot lysis (fibrinolysis) results from plasmin formation and the client hemorrhages. Small clots form throughout the body, and eventually the blood-clotting factors are used up, rendering them unavailable to form clots at sites of tissue injury. Clot-dissolving mechanisms are also increased, which results in bleeding (possibly severe).

DIC can be stimulated by many factors, including sepsis, malignancy, and obstetric conditions such as placental abruption, missed abortion or retained dead fetus, amniotic fluid embolism, and eclampsia.

Laboratory studies that assist in the diagnosis include:
- Decreased fibrinogen and platelets
- Prolonged PT and aPTT
- Positive D-dimer tests and fibrin (split) degradation products (objective evidence of the simultaneous formation of thrombin and plasmin) (Levi & Schmaier, 2011)

transfusion of fresh-frozen plasma along with cryoprecipitate to maintain the circulating volume and provide oxygen to the cells of the body. Anticoagulant therapy (low-molecular-weight heparin), packed red cells, platelet concentrates, antithrombin concentrates, and nonclotting protein-containing volume expanders are also used to combat this serious condition (Levi & Schmaier, 2011). Prompt identification and early intervention are essential for a woman with acute DIC associated with abruptio placentae to treat DIC and possibly save her life.

Nursing Assessment

Abruptio placentae is a medical emergency. The nurse plays a critical role in assessing the pregnant woman presenting with abdominal pain and/or experiencing vaginal bleeding, especially in a concealed hemorrhage, in which the extent of bleeding is not recognized. Rapid assessment is essential to ensure prompt, effective interventions to prevent maternal and fetal morbidity and mortality. Comparison Chart 19.1 compares placenta previa with abruptio placentae.

Health History and Physical Examination

Begin the health history by assessing the woman for risk factors that may predispose her to abruptio placentae, such as maternal smoking, advanced maternal age (over 35 years old), poor nutrition, multiple gestation, excessive intrauterine pressure caused by hydramnios, hypertension, severe trauma (e.g., auto accident, intimate partner violence), cocaine use, alcohol ingestion, and multiparity (Norwitz & Schorge, 2010; Zeltzer, 2011). Ask the woman about her previous pregnancies to determine whether she has experienced a prior abruption. In addition, be alert for other notable risk factors, such as male fetal gender, chorioamnionitis, prolonged ruptured membranes (more than 24 hours), pre-eclampsia, and low socioeconomic status (Deering, 2011).

Assess the woman for bleeding. As the placenta separates from the uterus, hemorrhage ensues. It can be apparent, appearing as vaginal bleeding, or it can be concealed. Vaginal bleeding is present in 80% of women diagnosed with abruptio placentae and may be significant enough to jeopardize both maternal and fetal health within a short time frame. The remaining 20% of abruptions are associated with a concealed hemorrhage and the absence of vaginal bleeding. Monitor the woman's level of consciousness, noting any signs or symptoms that may suggest shock.

▷ **Take** NOTE!

Vital signs can be within normal range, even with significant blood loss, because a pregnant woman can lose up to 40% of her total blood volume without showing signs of shock (Gilbert, 2010).

Assess the woman for complaints of pain, including the type, onset, and location. Ask if she has had any contractions. Palpate the abdomen, noting any contractions, uterine tenderness, tenseness, or rigidity. Ask if she has noticed any changes in fetal movement and activity. Decreased fetal movement may be the presenting complaint, resulting from fetal jeopardy or fetal death (Deering, 2011). Assess fetal heart rate and continue to monitor it electronically.

▷ **Take** NOTE!

Classic manifestations of abruptio placentae include painful, dark-red vaginal bleeding (port wine colour) because the bleeding comes from the clot that was formed behind the placenta; "knife-like" abdominal pain; uterine tenderness; contractions; and decreased fetal movement. Rapid assessment is essential to ensure prompt, effective interventions to prevent maternal and fetal morbidity and mortality.

COMPARISON CHART 19.1   PLACENTA PREVIA VERSUS ABRUPTIO PLACENTAE

Manifestation	Placenta Previa	Abruptio Placentae
Onset	Insidious	Sudden
Type of bleeding	Always visible; slight, then more profuse	Can be concealed or visible
Blood description	Bright red	Dark
Discomfort/pain	None (painless)	Constant; uterine tenderness on palpation
Uterine tone	Soft and relaxed	Firm to rigid
Fetal heart rate	Usually in normal range	Fetal distress or absent
Fetal presentation	May be breech or transverse lie; engagement is absent	No relationship

Laboratory and Diagnostic Testing

Laboratory and diagnostic tests may be helpful in diagnosing the condition and guiding management. These studies may include:

- CBC: determines the current hemodynamic status; however, it is not reliable for estimating acute blood loss
- Fibrinogen levels: typically are increased in pregnancy (hyperfibrinogenemia); thus, a moderate dip in fibrinogen levels might suggest coagulopathy (DIC) and, if profuse bleeding occurs, the clotting cascade might be compromised
- Prothrombin time (PT)/activated partial thromboplastin time (aPTT): determines the client's coagulation status, especially if surgery is planned
- Type and cross-match: determines blood type if a transfusion is needed
- Kleihauer–Betke test: detects fetal red blood cells in the maternal circulation, determines the degree of fetal–maternal hemorrhage, and helps calculate the appropriate dosage of WinRho to give to Rh-negative clients
- Nonstress test: demonstrates findings of fetal jeopardy manifested by late decelerations or bradycardia
- Biophysical profile: aids in evaluating clients with chronic abruption; a low score (less than 6 points) suggests possible fetal compromise (Deering, 2011)

Ultrasound is not useful for making a definitive diagnosis because the clot is sonographically visible in less than 50% of the cases (Zeltzer, 2011).

Nursing Management

Nursing management of the woman with abruptio placentae warrants immediate care to provide the best outcome for both mother and fetus.

Ensuring Adequate Tissue Perfusion

Upon arrival to the facility, place the woman on strict bed rest and in a left lateral position to prevent pressure on the vena cava. This position provides uninterrupted perfusion to the fetus. Expect to administer oxygen therapy via nasal cannula to ensure adequate tissue perfusion. Monitor oxygen saturation levels via pulse oximetry to evaluate the effectiveness of interventions.

Obtain maternal vital signs frequently, as often as every 15 minutes as indicated, depending on the woman's status and amount of blood loss. Observe for changes in vital signs suggesting hypovolemic shock and report them immediately. Also expect to insert an indwelling urinary (Foley) catheter to assess hourly urine output and initiate an IV infusion for fluid replacement using a large-bore catheter.

Assess fundal height for changes. An increase in size would indicate bleeding. Monitor the amount and characteristics of any vaginal bleeding as frequently as every 15 to 30 minutes. Be alert for signs and symptoms of

DIC, such as bleeding gums, tachycardia, oozing from the IV insertion site, and petechiae, and administer blood products as ordered if DIC occurs.

Institute continuous electronic fetal monitoring. Assess uterine contractions and report any increased uterine tenseness or rigidity. Also observe the tracing for tetanic uterine contractions or changes in fetal heart rate patterns suggesting fetal compromise.

Providing Support and Education

A woman diagnosed with abruptio placentae may be filled with a sense of heightened anxiety and apprehension, for her own health as well as that of her fetus. Communicate empathy and understanding of the client's experience, and provide emotional support throughout this frightening time. Remain with the couple, acknowledge their emotions and fears, and address their spiritual and cultural needs. Answer their questions about the status of their fetus openly and honestly, being sure to explain indicators of fetal well-being. Provide information about the various diagnostic tests, treatments, and procedures that may be done, including the possible need for a cesarean birth.

Depending on the client's status, extent of bleeding, and length of gestation, the fetus may not survive. If the fetus does survive, he or she most likely will require neonatal intensive care. Assist the client and family to deal with the loss or with the birth of a newborn in the neonatal intensive care unit.

Although abruptio placentae is not a preventable condition, client education is important to help reduce the risk for a recurrence of this condition. Encourage the woman to avoid drinking, smoking, or using drugs during pregnancy. Urge her to seek early and continuous prenatal care and to receive prompt health care if any signs and symptoms occur in future pregnancies.

Think back to Helen, the pregnant woman described at the beginning of the chapter. She was diagnosed with abruptio placentae and was prepared for an emergency cesarean birth. On exploration, there was almost a 75% abruption, with approximately 800 mL of concealed blood between the uterus and the placenta. In addition, she lost an additional 500 mL during surgery. What in Helen's history may have placed her at increased risk for abruption? What assessments and interventions would be essential during her postpartum recovery secondary to her large blood loss? What psychosocial interventions would be necessary due to her fetal loss?

Gestational Hypertension

Gestational hypertension is characterized by hypertension without proteinuria after 20 weeks of gestation and a return of the blood pressure to normal postpartum. Previously, gestational hypertension was known as pregnancy-induced hypertension or toxemia of pregnancy, but these terms are no longer used. Gestational hypertension is clinically characterized by a blood pressure of 140/90 mm Hg or more on two occasions at least 6 hours apart (Magee, Helewa, Moutquin, et al., 2008). Gestational hypertension can be differentiated from chronic hypertension, which appears before the 20th week of gestation or before the current pregnancy and continues after the woman gives birth. Regardless of its onset, hypertension jeopardizes the well-being of the mother as well as the fetus.

Gestational hypertension with edema and proteinuria is one of the causes of maternal death in Canada (Statistics Canada, 2011). Hypertension complicates 2% to 3% of pregnancies (Carson & Gibson, 2012). The highest rates are in women younger than 20 or older than 40 years of age (Magee et al., 2008). "The classification of the hypertensive disorders of pregnancy is based on the two most common manifestations of pre-eclampsia: hypertension and proteinuria" (Magee et al., 2008, p. 9). The recommended classification of hypertensive disorders in pregnancy is based on guidelines from the SOGC (Magee et al., 2008) (Box 19.3).

Gestational hypertension can be classified as pre-eclampsia or eclampsia, each of which is associated with specific criteria. Pre-eclampsia is further categorized as mild or severe.

Pathophysiology

Gestational hypertension remains an enigma. The condition can be devastating to both the mother and fetus, and yet the etiology remains a mystery to medical science despite decades of research. Many theories exist, but none have truly explained the widespread pathologic changes that result in pulmonary edema, oliguria, seizures, thrombocytopenia, coagulation, abnormal liver function, and abnormal liver enzymes (Lindheimer, Taler,

---

BOX 19.3 **SOGC Hypertension Classifications**

1. Hypertensive disorders of pregnancy should be classified as pre-existing hypertension or gestational hypertension on the basis of different diagnostic and therapeutic factors.
2. The presence or absence of pre-eclampsia must be ascertained, given its clear association with more adverse maternal and perinatal outcomes.
3. In women with pre-existing hypertension, pre-eclampsia should be defined as resistant hypertension, new *or* worsening proteinuria, *or* one or more of the other adverse conditions.*
4. In women with gestational hypertension (blood pressure elevation to 140/90 mm Hg identified after mid-pregnancy without proteinuria), pre-eclampsia should be defined as new-onset proteinuria *or* one or more of the other adverse conditions.*
5. Severe pre-eclampsia should be defined as pre-eclampsia with onset before 34 weeks' gestation, with heavy proteinuria *or* one or more of the other adverse conditions.*
6. The term pregnancy-induced hypertension should be abandoned, as its meaning in clinical practice is unclear.

---

*Other adverse conditions consist of maternal symptoms (persistent or new/unusual headache, visual disturbances, persistent abdominal or right upper quadrant pain, severe nausea or vomiting, chest pain or dyspnea), maternal signs of end-organ dysfunction, abnormal maternal laboratory testing (elevated serum creatinine [according to local laboratory criteria]; elevated AST, ALT or LDH with symptoms; platelet count $<100 \times 10^9/L$; or serum albumin <20 g/L), or fetal morbidity (oligohydramnios, IUGR, absent or reversed end-diastolic flow in the umbilical artery by Doppler velocimetry, or intrauterine fetal death).

Source: Magee, L. A., Helewa, M., Moutquin, J.-M., & von Dadelszen, P. (2008). SOGC clinical practice guidelines: Diagnosis, evaluation and management of the hypertensive disorders of pregnancy. *Journal of Obstetrics and Gynaecology Canada, 30*(3 Suppl. 1), S1–S52. Retrieved March 9, 2012 from http://www.sogc.org/guidelines/documents/gui206CPG0803_001.pdf.

& Cunningham, 2008). Despite the results of several research studies, low-dose aspirin; supplementation with calcium, magnesium, zinc, or antioxidant therapy (vitamin C and E); salt restriction; diuretic therapy; and fish oils have not proven to prevent this destructive condition (Carson & Gibson, 2012; Lindheimer et al., 2008). Only low-dose aspirin and calcium have shown minimal protective effects (Lindheimer et al., 2008). Vitamin C and E supplementation have been shown to have no effect and may be harmful in some high-risk populations.

The underlying mechanisms involved with this disorder are vasospasm and hypoperfusion. In addition, endothelial injury occurs, leading to platelet adherence, fibrin deposition, and the presence of schistocytes (fragment of an erythrocyte).

Generalized vasospasm results in elevation of blood pressure and reduced blood flow to the brain, liver, kidneys, placenta, and lungs. Decreased liver perfusion leads to impaired liver function and subcapsular hemorrhage. This is demonstrated by epigastric pain and elevated liver enzymes in the maternal serum. Decreased brain perfusion leads to small cerebral hemorrhages and symptoms of arterial vasospasm such as headaches, visual disturbances, blurred vision, and hyperactive deep tendon reflexes (DTRs). A thromboxane/prostacyclin imbalance leads to increased thromboxane (potent vasoconstrictor and stimulator of platelet aggregation) and decreased prostacyclin (potent vasodilator and inhibitor of platelet aggregation), which contribute to the hypertensive state. Decreased kidney perfusion reduces the glomerular filtration rate (GFR), resulting in decreased urine output and increased serum levels of sodium, BUN, uric acid, and creatinine, further increasing extracellular fluid and edema. Increased capillary permeability in the kidneys allows albumin to escape, which reduces plasma colloid osmotic pressure and moves more fluid into extracellular spaces; this leads to pulmonary edema and generalized edema. Poor placental perfusion resulting from prolonged vasoconstriction helps to contribute to intrauterine growth restriction (IUGR), premature separation of the placenta (abruptio placentae), persistent fetal hypoxia, and acidosis. In addition, hemoconcentration (resulting from decreased intravascular volume) causes increased blood viscosity and elevated hematocrit (Ross, 2011; Stokes, 2011).

Therapeutic Management

The SOGC recently revised its guidelines for the treatment of hypertension in the pregnant woman (Magee et al., 2008). Management of the woman with gestational hypertension varies depending on the severity of her condition and its effects on the fetus. Typically the woman is managed conservatively if she is experiencing mild symptoms. However, if the condition progresses, management becomes more aggressive.

Management for Mild Pre-Eclampsia

Conservative strategies for mild pre-eclampsia are used if the woman exhibits no signs of renal or hepatic dysfunction or coagulopathy. A woman with mild elevations in blood pressure may be placed on bed rest at home. She is encouraged to rest as much as possible in the lateral recumbent position to improve uteroplacental blood flow, reduce her blood pressure, and promote diuresis. In addition, antepartal visits and diagnostic testing—such as CBC, clotting studies, liver enzymes, and platelet levels—increase in frequency. The woman will be asked to monitor her blood pressure daily (every 4 to 6 hours while awake) and report any increased readings; she will also measure the amount of protein found in her urine

using a dipstick and will weigh herself to detect any weight gain. Daily fetal movement counts also are implemented. If there is any decrease in movement, the woman needs to be evaluated by her health care provider that day. A balanced, nutritional diet with no sodium restriction is advised. In addition, she is encouraged to drink six to eight 8-oz glasses of water daily.

If home management fails to reduce the blood pressure, admission to the hospital is warranted and the treatment strategy is individualized based on the severity of the condition and the gestational age at the time of diagnosis. During the hospitalization, the woman with mild pre-eclampsia is monitored closely for signs and symptoms of severe pre-eclampsia or impending eclampsia (e.g., persistent headache, hyperreflexia). Blood pressure measurements are frequently recorded along with daily weights to detect excessive weight gain resulting from edema. Fetal surveillance is instituted in the form of daily fetal movement counts, nonstress testing, and serial ultrasounds to evaluate fetal growth and amniotic fluid volume to confirm fetal well-being. Expectant management usually continues until the pregnancy reaches term, fetal lung maturity is documented, or complications develop that warrant immediate birth (Han & Norwitz, 2011).

Prevention of disease progression is the focus of treatment during labour. Blood pressure is monitored frequently, and a quiet environment is important to minimize the risk for stimulation and to promote rest. IV magnesium sulphate is infused to prevent any seizure activity, along with antihypertensives if blood pressure values begin to rise. Calcium gluconate is kept at the bedside in case the magnesium level becomes toxic. Continued close monitoring of neurologic status is warranted to detect any signs or symptoms of hypoxemia, impending seizure activity, or increased intracranial pressure. An indwelling urinary (Foley) catheter usually is inserted to allow for accurate measurement of urine output.

Management for Severe Pre-Eclampsia

Severe pre-eclampsia may develop suddenly and bring with it high blood pressure of more than 160/110 mm Hg, proteinuria of more than 5 g in 24 hours, oliguria of less than 400 mL in 24 hours, cerebral and visual symptoms, and rapid weight gain. This clinical picture signals severe pre-eclampsia, and immediate hospitalization is needed.

Treatment is highly individualized and based on disease severity and fetal age. Birth of the infant is the only cure because pre-eclampsia depends on the presence of trophoblastic tissue. Therefore, the exact age of the fetus is assessed to determine viability.

Severe pre-eclampsia is treated aggressively because hypertension poses a serious threat to mother and fetus. The goal of care is to stabilize the mother–fetus dyad and prepare for birth. Therapy focuses on controlling hypertension, preventing seizures, preventing long-term morbidity, and preventing maternal, fetal, or newborn death (Magee et al., 2008). Intense maternal and fetal surveillance starts when the mother enters the hospital and continues throughout her stay.

The woman in labour with severe pre-eclampsia typically receives oxytocin to stimulate uterine contractions and magnesium sulphate to prevent seizure activity. Oxytocin and magnesium sulphate can be given simultaneously via infusion pumps to ensure both are administered at the prescribed rate. The client is evaluated closely for magnesium toxicity. If at all possible, a vaginal delivery is preferable to a cesarean birth. PGE2 gel may be used to ripen the cervix. A cesarean birth may be performed if the client is seriously ill. A pediatrician/neonatologist must be available in the birthing room to care for the newborn. A newborn whose mother received magnesium sulphate needs to be monitored for respiratory depression, hypotension, and hypotonia (Deglin, Vallerand, & Sanoski, 2011).

Management of Eclampsia

In the woman who develops an eclamptic seizure, the convulsive activity begins with facial twitching, followed by generalized muscle rigidity. Respirations cease for the duration of the seizure, resulting from muscle spasms, thus compromising fetal oxygenation. Coma usually follows the seizure activity, with respiration resuming. Eclamptic seizures are life-threatening emergencies and require immediate treatment to decrease maternal morbidity and mortality.

As with any seizure, the initial management is to clear the airway and administer adequate oxygen. Positioning the woman on her left side and protecting her from injury during the seizure are key. Suction equipment must be readily available to remove secretions from her mouth after the seizure is over. IV fluids are administered after the seizure at a rate to replace urine output and additional insensible losses. Fetal heart rate is monitored closely. Magnesium sulphate is administered IV to prevent further seizures. Hypertension is controlled with antihypertensive medications. After the seizures are controlled, the woman's stability is assessed and birth commences via induction or cesarean delivery (Magee et al., 2008).

If the woman's condition remains stable, she will be transferred to the postpartum unit for care. If she becomes unstable after giving birth, she may be transferred to the critical care unit for closer observation.

Nursing Assessment

Preventing complications related to hypertension during pregnancy requires the use of assessment, advocacy, and counselling skills. Assessment begins with the accurate measurement of the client's blood pressure at each encounter. In addition, nurses need to assess for

subjective complaints that may indicate progression of the disease—visual changes, severe headaches, unusual bleeding or bruising, right upper quadrant pain, sudden weight gain, or nausea and vomiting (Mistovich, Krost, & Limmer, 2008). The significant signs of gestational hypertension—proteinuria and hypertension—occur without the woman's awareness. Unfortunately, by the time symptoms are noticed, gestational hypertension can be severe.

> ▷ **Take** NOTE!
>
> *The absolute blood pressure (value that validates elevation) of 140/90 mm Hg should be obtained on two occasions 6 hours apart to be diagnostic of gestational hypertension. Proteinuria is defined as 0.3 g or more of urinary protein per 24 hours or more than 1+ protein by chemical reagent strip or dipstick of at least two random urine samples collected at least 6 hours apart with no evidence of urinary tract infection (Magee et al., 2008).*

Health History and Physical Examination

Take a thorough history during the first antepartal visit to identify whether the woman is at risk for pre-eclampsia. Risk factors include:

- Primigravida status
- Multifetal pregnancy
- History of pre-eclampsia in a previous pregnancy
- Family history of pre-eclampsia (mother or sister)
- Lower socioeconomic group
- History of diabetes, hypertension, or renal disease
- Black race
- Age extremes (younger than 20 or older than 35)
- Obesity (Magee et al., 2008; Mistovich et al., 2008)

In addition, complete a nutritional assessment that includes the woman's usual intake of protein, calcium, daily calories, and fluids.

Women at risk for pre-eclampsia require more frequent prenatal visits throughout their pregnancy, and they require teaching about problems so that they can report them promptly.

Blood pressure must be measured carefully and consistently. Obtain all measurements with the woman in the same position (blood pressure is highest in the sitting position and lowest in the side-lying position) and by using the same technique (automated versus manual). This standardization in position and technique will yield the most accurate readings (Magee et al., 2008).

Obtain the client's weight (noting gain since last visit), and assess for amount and location of edema. Asking questions such as "Do your rings still fit on your fingers?" or "Is your face puffy when you get up in the morning?"

will help to determine whether fluid retention is present or if the woman's status has changed since her last visit.

▶ *Take* NOTE!

Although edema is not a cardinal sign of pre-eclampsia, weight should be monitored frequently to identify sudden gains in a short time span. Current research relies less on the classic triad of symptoms (hypertension, proteinuria, and edema or weight gain) and more on decreased organ perfusion, endothelial dysfunction (capillary leaking and proteinuria), and elevated blood pressure as key indicators (Carson & Gibson, 2012).

If edema is present, assess the distribution, degree, and pitting. Document your findings and identify whether the edema is dependent or pitting. Dependent edema is present on the lower half of the body if the client is ambulatory, where hydrostatic pressure is greatest. It is usually observed in the feet and ankles or in the sacral area if the client is on bed rest.

Pitting edema is edema that leaves a small depression or pit after finger pressure is applied to a swollen area (Brodovicz, McNaughton, Uemura, et al., 2009). Record the depth of pitting demonstrated when pressure is applied. Although subjective, the following is used to record relative degrees:

- 1+ pitting edema = 2-mm depression into skin; disappears rapidly
- 2+ pitting edema = 4-mm skin depression; disappears in 10 to 15 seconds
- 3+ pitting edema = 6-mm depression into skin; lasts more than 1 minute
- 4+ pitting edema = 8-mm depression into skin; lasts 2 to 3 minutes

At every antepartal visit, assess the fetal heart rate with a Doppler device. Also check a clean-catch urine specimen for protein using a dipstick.

Laboratory and Diagnostic Testing

Various laboratory tests may be performed to evaluate the woman's status. Typically these include a CBC, serum electrolytes, BUN, creatinine, and hepatic enzyme levels. Urine specimens are checked for protein; if levels are 1+ to 2+ or greater, a 24-hour urine collection is completed.

Nursing Management

Nursing management of the woman with gestational hypertension focuses on close monitoring of blood pressure and ongoing assessment for evidence of disease progression. Throughout the client's pregnancy, fetal surveillance is key.

Intervening with Pre-Eclampsia

The woman with mild pre-eclampsia requires frequent monitoring to detect changes because pre-eclampsia can progress rapidly. Instruct all women about the signs and symptoms of pre-eclampsia and urge them to contact their health care professional for immediate evaluation should any occur.

Typically women with mild pre-eclampsia can be managed at home if they have a good understanding of the disease process, are stable, have no abnormal laboratory test results, and demonstrate good fetal movement (Teaching Guideline 19.2). The home care nurse makes frequent visits and follow-up phone calls to assess the woman's condition, to assist with scheduling periodic

TEACHING GUIDELINE 19.2

Teaching for the Woman with Mild Pre-Eclampsia

- Rest in a quiet environment to prevent cerebral disturbances.
- Drink 8 to 10 glasses of water daily.
- Consume a balanced, high-protein diet including high-fibre foods.
- Obtain intermittent bed rest to improve circulation to the heart and uterus.
- Limit your physical activity to promote urination and subsequent decrease in blood pressure.
- Enlist the aid of your family so that you can obtain appropriate rest time.
- Perform self-monitoring as instructed, including:
  - Taking your own blood pressure twice daily
  - Checking and recording weight daily
  - Performing urine dipstick twice daily
  - Recording the number of fetal kicks daily
- Contact the home health nurse if any of the following occurs:
  - Increase in blood pressure
  - Protein present in urine
  - Gain of more than 450 g (1 lb) in 1 week
  - Burning or frequency when urinating
  - Decrease in fetal activity or movement
  - Headache (forehead or posterior neck region)
  - Dizziness or visual disturbances
  - Increase in swelling in hands, feet, legs, and face
  - Stomach pain, excessive heartburn, or epigastric pain
  - Decreased or infrequent urination
  - Contractions or low back pain
  - Easy or excessive bruising
  - Sudden onset of abdominal pain
  - Nausea and vomiting

DRUG GUIDE 19.3 MEDICATIONS USED WITH PRE-ECLAMPSIA AND ECLAMPSIA

Medication	Action/Indications	Nursing Implications
Magnesium sulphate	Blocks neuromuscular transmission, vasodilation Prevents and treats eclamptic seizures	Administer IV loading dose of 4–6 g over 30 min; continue maintenance infusion of 2–4 g/h as ordered. Monitor serum magnesium levels closely. Assess DTRs and check for ankle clonus. Have calcium gluconate readily available in case of toxicity. Monitor for signs and symptoms of toxicity, such as flushing, sweating, hypotension, and cardiac and central nervous system depression.
Methyldopa (Aldomet)	Antihypertensive Stimulates alpha-adrenergic receptor sites, decreasing sympathetic stimulation to heart and blood vessels	250–500 mg PO bid-qid (max 2 g/day) Sedation is common; caution patient about driving or other hazardous activities until effect is known Monitor for possible adverse effects such as jaundice and hepatitis
Hydralazine hydrochloride (Apresoline)	Vascular smooth muscle relaxant, thus improving perfusion to renal, uterine, and cerebral areas Reduction in blood pressure	Administer 5–10 mg by slow IV bolus every 20 min as needed Use parenteral form immediately after opening ampule. Withdraw drug slowly to prevent possible rebound hypertension. Monitor for adverse effects such as palpitations, headache, tachycardia, anorexia, nausea, vomiting, and diarrhea.
Labetalol hydrochloride (Normodyne)	Alpha-1 and beta blocker Reduces blood pressure	Be aware that drug lowers blood pressure without decreasing maternal heart rate or cardiac output. Administer IV bolus dose of 10–20 mg and then administer IV infusion of 2 mg/min until desired blood pressure value is achieved. Monitor for possible adverse effects such as gastric pain, flatulence, constipation, dizziness, vertigo, and fatigue.
Nifedipine (Procardia)	Calcium-channel blocker Dilates coronary arteries, arterioles, and peripheral arterioles Reduces blood pressure Stops preterm labour	Administer 10 mg orally for three doses and then every 4–8 h. Monitor for possible adverse effects such as dizziness, peripheral edema, angina, diarrhea, nasal congestions, cough.
Sodium nitroprusside	Causes rapid vasodilation (arterial and venous) Used for severe hypertension requiring rapid reduction in blood pressure	Administer via continuous IV infusion with dose titrated according to blood pressure levels. Wrap IV infusion solution in foil or opaque material to protect from light. Monitor for possible adverse effects, such as apprehension, restlessness, retrosternal pressure, palpitations, diaphoresis, abdominal pain.

121

Medication	Action/Indications	Nursing Implications
Furosemide (Lasix)	Diuretic action, inhibiting the reabsorption of sodium and chloride from the ascending loop of Henle Pulmonary edema (used only if condition is present)	Administer via slow IV bolus at a dose of 10–40 mg over 1–2 min. Monitor urine output hourly. Assess for possible adverse effects such as dizziness, vertigo, orthostatic hypotension, anorexia, vomiting, electrolyte imbalances, muscle cramps, and muscle spasms.

Sources: Brophy, K., Scarlett-Fergusen, H., & Webber, K. (2008). *Clinical drug therapy for Canadian practice* (1st Canadian ed.). Philadelphia: Lippincott Williams & Wilkins; Gilbert, E. S. (2011). *Manual of high-risk pregnancy and delivery* (5th ed.). St. Louis, MO: Mosby Elsevier; Karch, A. M. (2011). *2011 Lippincott's nursing drug guide.* Philadelphia: Lippincott Williams & Wilkins; King, T. L., & Brucker, M. C. (2011) *Pharmacology for women's health.* Sudbury, MA: Jones and Bartlett Publishers; and Magee, L. A., Helewa, M., Moutquin, J.-M., & von Dadelszen, P. (2008). SOGC clinical practice guidelines: Diagnosis, evaluation and management of the hypertensive disorders of pregnancy. *Journal of Obstetrics and Gynaecology Canada, 30*(3 Suppl. 1), S1–S52. Retrieved March 9, 2012 from http://www.sogc.org/guidelines/documents/gui206CPG0803_001.pdf.

evaluations of the fetus (such as nonstress tests), and to evaluate any changes that might suggest a worsening of the woman's condition.

Early detection and management of mild pre-eclampsia is associated with the greatest success in reducing progression of this condition. As long as the client carries out the guidelines of care as outlined by the health care provider and she remains stable, home care can continue to maintain the pregnancy until the fetus is mature. If disease progression occurs, hospitalization is required.

Intervening with Severe Pre-Eclampsia

The woman with severe pre-eclampsia requires hospitalization. Maintain the client on complete bed rest in the left lateral lying position. Ensure that the room is dark and quiet to reduce stimulation. Give sedatives as ordered to encourage quiet bed rest. The client is at risk for seizures if the condition progresses. Therefore, institute and maintain seizure precautions, such as padding the side rails and having oxygen, suction equipment, and call light readily available to protect the client from injury.

> ▶ **Take** NOTE!
>
> *Pre-eclampsia increases the risk for placental abruption, preterm birth, IUGR, and fetal distress during childbirth. Be prepared!*

Closely monitor the client's blood pressure. Administer antihypertensives as ordered to reduce blood pressure (Drug Guide 19.3). Assess the client's vision and level of consciousness. Report any changes and any complaints of headache or visual disturbances. Offer a high-protein diet with eight to 10 glasses of water daily. Monitor the client's intake and output every hour and administer fluid and electrolyte replacements as ordered. Assess the woman for signs and symptoms of pulmonary edema, such as crackles and wheezing heard on auscultation, dyspnea, decreased oxygen saturation levels, cough, anxiety, confusion, and restlessness (Sovari, Kocheril, & Bass, 2012).

To achieve a safe outcome for the fetus, prepare the woman for possible testing to evaluate fetal status as pre-eclampsia progresses. These may include the nonstress test, serial ultrasounds to track fetal growth, amniocentesis to determine fetal lung maturity, Doppler velocimetry to screen for fetal compromise, and biophysical profile to evaluate ongoing fetal well-being (Carson & Gibson, 2012).

Other laboratory tests may be performed to monitor the disease process and to determine whether it is progressing into HELLP syndrome. These include liver enzymes such as lactic dehydrogenase (LDH), ALT, and AST; chemistry panel, such as creatinine, BUN, uric acid, and glucose; CBC, including platelet count; coagulation studies, such as PT, PTT, fibrinogen, and bleeding time; and a 24-hour urine collection for protein and creatinine clearance.

Administer parenteral magnesium sulphate as ordered to prevent seizures. Assess DTRs to evaluate the effectiveness of therapy. Clients with pre-eclampsia commonly present with hyperreflexia. Severe pre-eclampsia causes changes in the cortex, which disrupts the equilibrium of impulses between the cerebral cortex and the spinal cord. Brisk reflexes (hyperreflexia) are the result of an irritable cortex and indicate central nervous system involvement (Lim, Sayah, Steinberg, et al., 2011).

Diminished or absent reflexes occur when the client develops magnesium toxicity. Because magnesium is a potent neuromuscular blocker, the afferent and efferent nerve pathways do not relay messages properly and hyporeflexia develops. Common sites used to assess DTRs are the biceps, triceps, patella, Achilles, and heel.

Nursing Procedure 19.1

ASSESSING THE PATELLAR REFLEX

Purpose: To Evaluate for Nervous System Irritability Related to Pre-Eclampsia

1. Place the woman in the supine position (or sitting upright with the legs dangling freely over the side of the bed or examination table).
2. If lying supine, have the woman flex her knee slightly.
3. Place a hand under the knee to support the leg and locate the patellar tendon. It should be midline just below the knee cap.
4. Using a reflex hammer or the side of your hand, strike the area of the patellar tendon firmly and quickly.
5. Note the movement of the leg and foot. A patellar reflex occurs when the leg and foot move (documented as 2+).
6. Repeat the procedure on the opposite leg.

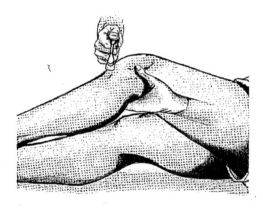

Nursing Procedure 19.1 highlights the steps for assessing the patellar reflex.

The National Institute of Neurological Disorders and Stroke (NINDS), a division of the US National Institutes of Health, published a scale in the early 1990s that, although subjective, remains widely in use today. It grades reflexes from 0 to 4+. Grades 2+ and 3+ are considered normal, whereas grades 0 and 4 may indicate pathology (Table 19.2). Because these are subjective assessments, to improve communication of reflex results, condensed descriptor categories such as absent, average, brisk, or clonus should be used rather than numeric codes (Gilbert, 2010).

Clonus is the presence of rhythmic involuntary contractions, most often at the foot or ankle. Sustained clonus confirms central nervous system involvement. Nursing Procedure 19.2 highlights the steps used to test for ankle clonus.

With magnesium sulphate administration, the client is at risk for magnesium toxicity. Closely assess the client

TABLE 19.2 GRADING DEEP TENDON REFLEXES

Description of Finding	Grade
Reflex absent, no response detected	0
Diminished, low normal	1
Average, normal	2
Brisker than average, may indicate disease	3
Hyperactive, brisk, clonus present	4

Source: Jarvis, C. (2009). *Physical examination & health assessment* (1st Canadian ed.). Toronto, Ontario: Saunders Elsevier.

for signs of toxicity, which include a respiratory rate of less than 12 breaths/minute, absence of DTRs, and a decrease in urinary output, below 30 mL per hour. Also monitor serum magnesium levels. Although exact levels may vary among agencies, serum magnesium levels ranging from 4 to 7 mEq/L are considered therapeutic, whereas levels higher than 8 mEq/dL are generally considered toxic. As levels increase, the woman is at risk for adverse effects:

- Respiratory paralysis
- Hypothermia

Nursing Procedure 19.2

TESTING FOR ANKLE CLONUS

Purpose: To Evaluate for Nervous System Irritability Related to Pre-Eclampsia

1. Place the woman in the supine position.
2. Have the client slightly bend her knee and place a hand under the knee to support it.
3. Dorsiflex the foot briskly and then quickly release it.
4. Watch for the foot to rebound smoothly against your hand. If the movement is smooth without any rapid contractions of the ankle or calf muscle, then clonus is not present; if the movement is jerky and rapid, clonus is present.
5. Repeat on the opposite side.

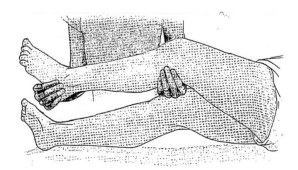

- Pulmonary edema
- Depressed reflexes
- Hypotension
- Flushing
- Drowsiness
- Depressed cardiac function
- Diaphoresis
- Hypocalcemia
- Hypophosphatemia
- Hyperkalemia
- Visual changes (Medscape Reference, 2011)

If signs and symptoms of magnesium toxicity develop, expect to administer calcium gluconate as the antidote.

Throughout the client's stay, closely monitor her for signs and symptoms of labour. Perform continuous electronic fetal monitoring to assess fetal well-being. Note trends in baseline rate and presence or absence of accelerations or decelerations. Also observe for signs of fetal distress and report them immediately. Administer glucocorticoid treatment as ordered to enhance fetal lung maturity and prepare for labour induction if the mother's condition warrants.

Keep the client and family informed of the woman's condition and educate them about the course of treatment. Provide emotional support for the client and family. Severe pre-eclampsia is very frightening for the client and her family, and most expectant mothers are very anxious about their own health as well as that of the fetus. To allay anxiety, use light touch to comfort and reassure her that the necessary actions are being taken. Actively listening to her concerns and fears and communicating them to the health care provider is important in keeping lines of communication open. Offering praise for small accomplishments can provide positive reinforcement for behaviours that should be continued.

Intervening with Eclampsia

The onset of seizure activity identifies eclampsia. Typically, eclamptic seizures are generalized and start with facial twitching. The body then becomes rigid, in a state of tonic muscular contraction. The clonic phase of the seizure involves alternating contraction and relaxation of all body muscles. Respirations stop during seizure activity and resume shortly after it ends. Client safety is the primary concern during eclamptic seizures. If possible, turn the client to her side and remain with her. Make sure that the side rails are up and padded. Dim the lights and keep the room quiet.

Document the time and sequence of events as soon as possible. After the seizure activity has ceased, suction the nasopharynx as necessary and administer oxygen. Continue the magnesium sulphate infusion to prevent further seizures. Ensure continuous electronic fetal monitoring, evaluating fetal status for changes. Also assess the client for uterine contractions. After the client is stabilized, prepare her for the birthing process as soon as possible to reduce the risk for perinatal mortality.

Providing Follow-Up Care

After delivery of the newborn, continue to monitor the client for signs and symptoms of pre-eclampsia/eclampsia for at least 48 hours. Expect to continue to administer magnesium sulphate infusion for 24 hours to prevent seizure activity, and monitor serum magnesium levels for toxicity.

Assess vital signs at least every 4 hours, along with routine postpartum assessments—fundus, lochia, breasts, bladder, bowels, and emotional state attention when performing the fundal assessment and assessing lochia. Monitor urine output closely. Diuresis is a positive sign that, along with a decrease in proteinuria, signals resolution of the disease.

HELLP

HELLP is an acronym for hemolysis, elevated liver enzymes, and low platelets. HELLP syndrome occurs in about 20% of pregnant women diagnosed with severe pre-eclampsia. Typically, HELLP develops in the third trimester, though it can develop either earlier in the pregnancy or up to 48 hours postpartum (Hagel-Fenton, 2008). HELLP syndrome leads to an increased maternal risk for liver hematoma or rupture, placental abruption, DIC, stroke, pulmonary edema, cerebral edema, renal damage, sepsis, and death as well as an increased fetal risk for respiratory distress, IUGR, and death (Haram, Svendsen, & Abildgaard, 2009).

Pathophysiology

The hemolysis that occurs is termed microangiopathic hemolytic anemia. It is thought to happen when red blood cells become fragmented as they pass through small, damaged blood vessels. Elevated liver enzymes are the result of reduced blood flow to the liver secondary to obstruction from fibrin deposits. Hyperbilirubinemia and jaundice result from liver impairment. Low platelet levels are caused by vascular damage, which results from vasospasm, and platelets aggregate at sites of damage, resulting in thrombocytopenia (Haram et al., 2009).

Therapeutic Management

The treatment for HELLP syndrome is based on the severity of the disease, the gestational age of the fetus, and the condition of the mother and the fetus. The client should be admitted or transferred to a tertiary centre with a neonatal intensive care unit. Additional treatments include magnesium sulphate, antihypertensives, and correction of the coagulopathies that accompany HELLP syndrome. After this syndrome is diagnosed and the woman's condition is stable, birth of the infant is indicated.

Magnesium sulphate is used prophylactically to prevent seizures. Antihypertensives such as hydralazine or labetalol are given to control blood pressure. Blood component therapy—such as fresh-frozen plasma, packed red cells, or platelets—is transfused to address the microangiopathic hemolytic anemia. Birth may be delayed up to 96 hours so that betamethasone or dexamethasone can be given to stimulate lung maturation in the preterm fetus.

Nursing Assessment

Nursing assessment of the woman with HELLP is similar to that for the woman with severe pre-eclampsia. Be alert for complaints of nausea (with or without vomiting), malaise, epigastric or right upper quadrant pain, and demonstrable edema. Perform systematic assessments frequently, as indicated by the woman's condition and response to therapy.

A diagnosis of HELLP syndrome is made based on laboratory test results, including:

- Low hematocrit that is not explained by any blood loss
- Elevated LDH (liver impairment)
- Elevated AST (liver impairment)
- Elevated ALT (liver impairment)
- Elevated BUN
- Elevated bilirubin level
- Elevated uric acid and creatinine levels (renal involvement)
- Low platelet count (less than $100,000 \times 10^9/L$)

Nursing Management

Nursing management of the woman diagnosed with HELLP syndrome is the same as that for the woman with severe pre-eclampsia. Closely monitor the client for changes and provide ongoing support throughout this experience.

Gestational Diabetes

Gestational diabetes is a condition involving glucose intolerance that occurs during pregnancy. It is discussed in greater detail in Chapter 20.

Blood Incompatibility

Blood incompatibility most commonly involves blood type or the Rh factor. Blood type incompatibility, also known as ABO incompatibility, is not as severe a condition as Rh incompatibility. ABO incompatibility rarely causes significant hemolysis, and antepartum treatment is not warranted. Rh sensitization occurs in approximately 0.4 in 1,000 births (Fung & Eason, 2003).

Dr. D. B. Chown, a Canadian physician living in Winnipeg, worked with Connaught Laboratories to manufacture the Rh immune serum, which was licensed in 1968. Approximately, 15% of white Canadian women are Rh negative (Beaulieu, 1993). About 35,000 Rh-negative women become pregnant every year and carry 24,500 Rh-positive fetuses who are at risk for Rh disease. Maternal alloimmunization occurs in 1% to 2% of Rh-negative women in Canada (Fung & Eason, 2003).

Pathophysiology

Hemolysis associated with ABO incompatibility is limited to mothers with type O blood whose fetuses have type A or B blood. In mothers with type A and B blood, naturally occurring antibodies are of the IgM class, which do not cross the placenta, whereas in type O mothers the antibodies are predominantly IgG in nature. Because A and B antigens are widely expressed in a variety of tissues besides red blood cells, only a small portion of antibodies crossing the placenta are available to bind to fetal red cells. In addition, fetal red cells appear to have less surface expression of A or B antigen, resulting in few reactive sites—hence the low incidence of significant hemolysis in affected neonates.

With ABO incompatibility, usually the mother is blood type O, with anti-A and anti-B antibodies in her serum; the infant is blood type A, B, or AB. The incompatibility arises as a result of the interaction of antibodies present in maternal serum and the antigen sites on the fetal red cells.

Rh incompatibility is a condition that develops when a woman with Rh-negative blood is exposed to Rh-positive blood cells and subsequently develops circulating titers of Rh antibodies. Individuals with an Rh-positive blood type have the D antigen present on their red cells, whereas individuals with an Rh-negative blood type do not. The presence or absence of the Rh antigen on the red blood cell membrane is genetically controlled. Fifteen percent to twenty percent of whites have Rh-negative blood (Salem, 2012).

Rh incompatibility most commonly arises with exposure of an Rh-negative mother to Rh-positive fetal blood during pregnancy or birth, during which time erythrocytes from the fetal circulation leak into the maternal circulation. After a significant exposure, alloimmunization or sensitization occurs. As a result, maternal antibodies are produced against the foreign Rh antigen.

Theoretically, fetal and maternal blood do not mix during pregnancy. In reality, however, small placental accidents (transplacental bleeds secondary to minor separation), abortions, ectopic pregnancy, abdominal trauma, trophoblastic disease, amniocentesis, placenta previa, and abruptio placentae allow fetal blood to enter the maternal circulation and initiate the production of antibodies to destroy Rh-positive blood. The amount of fetal blood necessary to produce Rh incompatibility varies. In one study, less than 1 mL of Rh-positive blood was shown to result in sensitization of women who are Rh negative (Salem, 2012).

Once sensitized, it takes approximately a month for Rh antibodies in the maternal circulation to cross over into the fetal circulation. In most cases, sensitization occurs during delivery (Salem, 2012). Thus, most firstborn infants with Rh-positive blood are not affected because the short period from first exposure of Rh-positive fetal erythrocytes to the birth of the infant is insufficient to produce a significant maternal IgG antibody response.

The risk and severity of alloimmune response increase with each subsequent pregnancy involving a fetus with Rh-positive blood. A second pregnancy with an Rh-positive fetus often produces a mildly anemic infant, whereas succeeding pregnancies produce infants with more serious hemolytic anemia.

Nursing Assessment

At the first prenatal visit, determine the woman's blood type and Rh status. Also obtain a thorough health history, noting any reports of previous events involving hemorrhage to delineate the risk for prior sensitization. When the client's history reveals an Rh-negative mother who may be pregnant with an Rh-positive fetus, prepare the client for an antibody screen (indirect Coombs test) to determine whether she has developed isoimmunity to the Rh antigen. This test detects unexpected circulating antibodies in a woman's serum that could be harmful to the fetus (Gilbert, 2010).

Nursing Management

If the indirect Coombs test is negative (meaning no antibodies are present), then the woman is a candidate for WinRho. If the test is positive, WinRho is of no value because isoimmunization has occurred. In this case, the fetus is monitored carefully for hemolytic disease.

The incidence of isoimmunization has declined dramatically as a result of prenatal and postnatal WinRho administration after any event in which blood transfer may occur. The standard dose is 300 μg, which is effective for 30 mL of fetal blood. Rh immunoglobulin helps to destroy any fetal cells in the maternal circulation before sensitization occurs, thus inhibiting maternal antibody production. This provides temporary passive immunity, thereby preventing maternal sensitization.

The current recommendation is that every Rh-negative nonimmunized woman receives WinRho at 28 weeks' gestation and again within 72 hours after giving birth. Other indications for WinRho include:

- Ectopic pregnancy
- Chorionic villus sampling
- Amniocentesis
- Prenatal hemorrhage
- Molar pregnancy
- Maternal trauma
- Percutaneous umbilical sampling
- Therapeutic or spontaneous abortion
- Fetal surgery (Fung & Eason, 2003; Koelewijn, de Haas, Vrijkotte, et al., 2009)

Despite the availability of WinRho and laboratory tests to identify women and newborns at risk, isoimmunization remains a serious clinical reality that continues to contribute to perinatal and neonatal mortality. Nurses, as client advocates, are in a unique position to make sure test results are brought to the health care provider's attention so appropriate interventions can be initiated. In addition, nurses must stay abreast of current literature and research regarding isoimmunization and its management. Stress to all women that early prenatal care can help identify and prevent this condition. Since Rh incompatibility is preventable with the use of WinRho, prevention remains the best treatment. Nurses can make a tremendous impact to ensure positive outcomes for the greatest possible number of pregnancies through education.

Amniotic Fluid Imbalances

Amniotic fluid develops from several maternal and fetal structures, including the amnion, chorion, maternal blood, fetal lungs, GI tract, kidneys, and skin. Any alteration in one or more of the various sources will alter the amount of amniotic fluid. Polyhydramnios and oligohydramnios are two imbalances associated with amniotic fluid.

Polyhydramnios

Polyhydramnios, also called hydramnios, is a condition in which there is too much amniotic fluid (more than 2,000 mL) surrounding the fetus between 32 and 36 weeks. It occurs in approximately 3% of all pregnancies and is associated with fetal anomalies of development (Rajiah, 2011). It is associated with poor fetal outcomes because of the increased incidence of preterm births, fetal malpresentation, and cord prolapse.

There are several causes of polyhydramnios. Generally, too much fluid is being produced, there is a problem with the fluid being taken up, or both. It can be associated with maternal disease and fetal anomalies, but it can also be idiopathic in nature.

Premature Rupture of Membranes

Premature rupture of membranes (PROM) is the rupture of the bag of waters before the onset of true labour. There are a number of associated conditions and complications, such as infection, prolapsed cord, abruptio placentae, and preterm labour. This is the single most common diagnosis associated with preterm births (Gilbert, 2010).

PROM occurs in approximately 6% to 19% of all births (Crane, 2001). If prolonged (greater than 24 hours), the woman's risk for infection (chorioamnionitis, endometritis, sepsis, and neonatal infections) increases, and this risk continues to increase as the duration of rupture time increases. The time interval from rupture of membranes to the onset of regular contractions is termed the latent period.

The terminology pertaining to PROM can be confusing. PROM is rupture of the membranes prior to the onset of labour and is used appropriately when referring to a woman who is beyond 37 weeks' gestation, has presented with spontaneous rupture of the membranes, and is not in labour. Related terms include **preterm premature rupture of membranes (PPROM)**, which is defined as rupture of membranes prior to the onset of labour in a woman who is *less* than 37 weeks of gestation. Perinatal risks associated with PPROM may stem from immaturity, including respiratory distress syndrome, intraventricular hemorrhage, patent ductus arteriosus, and necrotizing enterocolitis.

The exact cause of PROM is not known. In many cases, PROM occurs spontaneously.

Therapeutic Management

Treatment of PROM typically depends on the gestational age. Under no circumstances is an unsterile digital cervical examination done until the woman enters active labour, to minimize infection exposure. If the fetal lungs are mature, induction of labour is initiated. PROM is not a lone indicator for surgical birth. If the fetal lungs are immature, expectant management is carried out with adequate hydration, reduced physical activity, pelvic rest, and close observation for possible infection, such as with frequent monitoring of vital signs and laboratory test results (e.g., the white blood cell count). Corticosteroids may be given to enhance fetal lung maturity if lungs are immature, although this remains controversial. Recent studies have shown clear benefits of antibiotics to decrease neonatal morbidity associated with PPROM (Yudin, van Schalkwyk, & Van Eyk, 2009).

Nursing Assessment

Nursing assessment focuses on obtaining a complete health history and performing a physical examination to determine maternal and fetal status. An accurate assessment of the gestational age and knowledge of the maternal, fetal, and neonatal risks are essential to appropriate evaluation, counselling, and management of women with PROM and PPROM.

Health History and Physical Examination

Review the maternal history for risk factors such as infection, increased uterine size (hydramnios, macrosomia, multifetal gestation), uterine and fetal anomalies, lower socioeconomic status, STIs, cervical insufficiency, vaginal bleeding, and cigarette smoking during pregnancy. Ask about any history or current symptoms of urinary tract infection (frequency, urgency, dysuria, or flank pain) or pelvic or vaginal infection (pain or vaginal discharge).

Assess for signs and symptoms of labour, such as cramping, pelvic pressure, or back pain. Also assess her vital signs, noting any signs indicative of infection such as fever and tachycardia (Jazayeri, 2011).

Institute continuous electronic fetal heart rate monitoring to evaluate fetal well-being. Conduct a vaginal examination to ascertain the cervical status in PROM. If PPROM exists, a sterile speculum examination (where the examiner inspects the cervix but does not palpate it) is done rather than a digital cervical examination because digital examination may diminish latency (period of time from rupture of membranes to birth) and increase newborn morbidity (Cunningham, Leveno, Bloom, et al., 2010).

Observe the characteristics of the amniotic fluid. Note any evidence of meconium, or a foul odour. When meconium is present in the amniotic fluid, it typically indicates fetal distress related to hypoxia. Meconium stains the fluid yellow to greenish brown, depending on the amount present. A foul odour of amniotic fluid indicates infection. Also observe the amount of fluid. A decreased amount of amniotic fluid reduces the cushioning effect, thereby making cord compression a possibility. Key assessments are summarized in Box 19.4.

Laboratory and Diagnostic Testing

To diagnose PROM or PPROM, several procedures may be used: the Nitrazine test, fern test, or ultrasound.

BOX 19.4 Key Assessments with Premature Rupture of Membranes

For the woman with PROM, the following assessments are essential:

- Determine the date, time, and duration of membrane rupture by client interview.
- Ascertain the gestational age of the fetus based on date of mother's last menstrual period, fundal height, and ultrasound dating.
- Question the woman about possible history of or recent urinary tract infection or vaginal infection that might have contributed to PROM.
- Assess for any associated labour symptoms, such as back pain or pelvic pressure.
- Assist with or perform diagnostic tests to validate leakage of fluid, such as Nitrazine test, "ferning" on slide, and ultrasound.
- Continually assess for signs of infection, including:
  - Elevation of maternal temperature and pulse rate
  - Abdominal/uterine tenderness
  - Fetal tachycardia more than 160 bpm
  - Elevated white blood cell count and C-reactive protein
  - Cloudy, foul-smelling amniotic fluid

After the insertion of a sterile speculum, a sample of the fluid in the vaginal area is obtained. With a Nitrazine test, the pH of the fluid is tested; amniotic fluid is more basic (7.0) than normal vaginal secretions (4.5). Nitrazine paper turns blue in the presence of amniotic fluid. However, false-positive results can occur if blood, urine, semen, or antiseptic chemicals are also present; all will increase the pH.

For the fern test, a sample of vaginal fluid is place on a slide to be viewed directly under a microscope. Amniotic fluid will develop a fern-like pattern when it dries because of sodium chloride crystallization.

Other laboratory and diagnostic tests that may be used include:

- Urinalysis and urine culture for urinary tract infection or asymptomatic bacteriuria
- Cervical test or culture for chlamydia or gonorrhea
- Vaginal culture for bacterial vaginosis and trichomoniasis
- Vaginal introital/rectal culture for group B streptococcus

Nursing Management

Nursing management for the woman with PROM or PPROM focuses on preventing infection and identifying uterine contractions. The risk for infection is great because of the break in the amniotic fluid membrane and its close proximity to vaginal bacteria. Therefore, monitor maternal vital signs closely. Be alert for a temperature elevation or an increase in pulse, which could indicate infection. Also monitor the fetal heart rate continuously, reporting any fetal tachycardia (which could indicate a maternal infection) or variable decelerations (suggesting cord compression). If variable decelerations are present, anticipate amnioinfusion based on agency policy. Evaluate the results of laboratory tests such as a CBC. An elevation in white blood cells would suggest infection. Administer antibiotics if ordered.

Encourage the woman and her partner to verbalize their feelings and concerns. Educate them about the purpose of the protective membranes and the implications of early rupture. Keep them informed about planned interventions, including potential complications and required therapy. As appropriate, prepare the woman for induction or augmentation of labour as appropriate if she is near term.

If labour doesn't start within 48 hours, the woman with PPROM may be discharged home on expectant management, which may include:

- Antibiotics if cervicovaginal cultures are positive
- Activity restrictions
- Education about signs and symptoms of infection and when to call with problems or concerns (Teaching Guideline 19.3)

TEACHING GUIDELINE 19.3

Teaching for the Woman with PPROM

- Monitor your baby's activity by performing fetal kick counts daily.
- Check your temperature daily and report any temperature increases to your health care provider.
- Watch for signs related to the beginning of labour. Report any tightening of the abdomen or contractions.
- Avoid any touching or manipulating of your breasts, which could stimulate labour.
- Do not insert anything into your vagina or vaginal area.
- Maintain any specific activity restrictions as recommended.
- Wash your hands thoroughly after using the bathroom and make sure to wipe from front to back each time.
- Keep your perineal area clean and dry.
- Take your antibiotics as directed if your health care provider has prescribed them.
- Call your health care provider with changes in your condition, including fever, uterine tenderness, feeling like your heart is racing, and foul-smelling vaginal discharge.

- Frequent fetal testing for well-being
- Ultrasound every 3 to 4 weeks to assess amniotic fluid levels
- Possible corticosteroid treatment depending on gestational age
- Daily kick counts to assess fetal well-being

□▦■ Key Concepts

□ Identifying risk factors early on and throughout the pregnancy is important to ensure the best outcome for every pregnancy. Risk assessment should start with the first prenatal visit and continue with subsequent visits.

□ The three most common causes of hemorrhage early in pregnancy (first half of pregnancy) are spontaneous abortion, ectopic pregnancy, and GTD.

□ Ectopic pregnancies occur in about 1 in 50 pregnancies and have increased dramatically during the past few decades.

□ Having a molar pregnancy results in the loss of the pregnancy and the possibility of developing choriocarcinoma, a chronic malignancy from the trophoblastic tissue.

□ The classic clinical presentation for placenta previa is painless, bright-red vaginal bleeding occurring during the third trimester.

□ Treatment of abruptio placentae is designed to assess, control, and restore the amount of blood lost; to provide a positive outcome for both mother and infant; and to prevent coagulation disorders.

□ DIC can be described in simplest terms as a loss of balance between the clot-forming activity of thrombin and the clot-lysing activity of plasmin.

□ Hyperemesis gravidarum is a complication of pregnancy characterized by persistent, uncontrollable nausea and vomiting before the 20th week of gestation.

□ Gestational hypertension is the most common complication reported during pregnancy (Carson & Gibson, 2012).

□ HELLP is an acronym for hemolysis, elevated liver enzymes, and low platelets.

□ Rh incompatibility is a condition that develops when a woman of Rh-negative blood type is exposed to Rh-positive fetal blood cells and subsequently develops circulating titers of Rh antibodies.

□ Hydramnios occurs in approximately 3% to 4% of all pregnancies and is associated with fetal anomalies of development.

□ Nursing care related to the woman with oligohydramnios involves continuous monitoring of fetal well-being during nonstress testing or during labour and birth by identifying nonreassuring patterns on the fetal monitor.

□ The increasing number of multiple gestations is a concern because women who are expecting more than one infant are at high risk for preterm labour, hydramnios, hyperemesis gravidarum, anemia, pre-eclampsia, and antepartum hemorrhage.

□ Nursing care related to PROM centres on infection prevention and identification of preterm labour contractions.

□ Early identification of preterm labour would allow for appropriate interventions that may prolong the pregnancy, such as transferring the woman to a facility with a neonatal intensive care unit for prenatal care, administering glucocorticoids to the mother to promote fetal lung maturity, and giving appropriate antibiotics to treat infections to arrest the labour process.

□ It is essential that nurses teach all pregnant women how to detect the early symptoms of preterm labour and what to do if they experience contractions or cramping that does not go away.

REFERENCES

Arsenault, M. Y., & Lane, C. (2002). SOGC clinical practice guidelines: The management of nausea and vomiting in pregnancy. *Journal of Obstetrics and Gynaecology Canada, 24*(10), 817–823.

Bahar, A., Abusham, A., Eskandar, M., Sobande, A., & Alsunaidi, M. (2009). Risk factors and pregnancy outcome in different types of placenta previa. *Journal of Obstetrics and Gynaecology Canada, 31*(2), 126–131.

Beaulieu, M. D. (1993). *Screening for D (Rh) sensitization in pregnancy.* Retrieved March 9, 2012 from http://www.phac-aspc.gc.ca/publicat/clinic-clinique/pdf/s1c11e.pdf

Brodovicz, K. G., McNaughton, K., Uemura, N., Meininger, G., Girman, C. J., & Yale, S. H. (2009). Reliability and feasibility of methods to quantitatively assess peripheral edema. *Clinical Medicine and Research, 7*(1–2), 21–31.

Brophy, K., Scarlett-Fergusen, H., & Webber, K. (2008). *Clinical drug therapy for Canadian practice* (1st Canadian ed.). Philadelphia: Lippincott Williams & Wilkins.

Canadian Institute for Health Information. (2004). *Giving birth in Canada: Providers of maternity and infant care.* Retrieved March 9, 2012 from http://dsp-psd.pwgsc.gc.ca/Collection/H118-25-2004E.pdf

Carson, M. P., & Gibson, P. (2012). *Hypertension and pregnancy.* Retrieved March 9, 2012 from http://emedicine.medscape.com/article/261435-overview#showall

Carter, B. S., & Boyd, R. L. (2012). *Pediatric polyhydramnios and oligohydramnios medication.* Retrieved March 9, 2012 from http://emedicine.medscape.com/article/975821-medication#showall

Cole, L. (2010). Biological functions of hCG and hCG-related molecules. *Reproductive Biology and Endocrinology, 8*, 102. doi:10.1186/1477-7827-8-102

Crane, J. (2001). SOGC clinical practice guideline: Induction of labour at term. *Journal of Obstetrics and Gynaecology Canada, 23*(8), 717–728. Retrieved March 9, 2012 from http://www.sogc.org/guidelines/public/107E-CPG-August2001.pdf

Cunningham, F. G. N. F., Leveno, K. J., Bloom, S., Hauth, J. C., Rouse, D., & Sponc, C. (2010). *Williams' obstetrics* (23rd ed.). New York: McGraw-Hill.

Day, R., Paul, P., Williams, B., Smeltzer, S., & Bare, B. (2010). *Brunner & Suddarth's textbook of medical-surgical nursing* (2nd Canadian ed.). Philadelphia: Lippincott Williams & Wilkins.

Deering, S. (2011). *Abruptio placentae.* Retrieved March 9, 2012 from http://emedicine.medscape.com/article/252810-overview#showall

Deglin, J., Vallerand, A., Sanoski, C. (2011). *Davis's drug guide for nurses* (12th ed.). Philadelphia: FA Davis Company.

Einarson, A., Choi, J., Einarson, T. R., & Koren, G. (2009). Rates of spontaneous and therapeutic abortions following use of antidepressants in pregnancy: Results from a large prospective database. *Journal of Obstetrics and Gynaecology Canada, 31*(5), 452–456.

Einarson, A., Maltepe, C., Boskovic, R., & Koren, G. (2007). *Treatment of nausea and vomiting in pregnancy.* Retrieved March 9, 2012 from http://www.motherisk.org/women/updatesDetail.jsp?content_id=875

Fletcher, G., Zach, T., Pramanik, A. K., & Ford, S. P. (2009). *Multiple births.* Retrieved March 9, 2012 from http://emedicine.medscape.com/article/977234-overview#showall

Fox, N. S., & Chervenak, F. A. (2008). Cervical cerclage: A review of the evidence. *Obstetrical and Gynecological Survey, 63*(1), 58–65.

Fung, K., & Eason, E. (2003). SOGC clinical practice guidelines: Prevention of RH alloimmunization. *Journal of Obstetrics and Gynaecology Canada, 25*(9), 765–773. Retrieved March 9, 2012 from http://www.sogc.org/guidelines/public/133e-cpg-september2003.pdf

Gerulath, A. H. (2002). SOGC clinical practice guidelines: Gestational trophoblastic disease. *Journal of Obstetrics and Gynaecology Canada, 24*(5), 434–439. Retrieved March 9, 2012 from http://www.sogc.org/guidelines/public/114E-CPG-May2002.pdf

Gibbs, R. S., Danforth, D. N., Karlan, B. Y., & Haney, A. F. (2008). *Danforth's obstetrics and gynecology* (10th ed.). Philadelphia: Lippincott Williams & Wilkins.

Gilbert, E. (2010). *Manual of high-risk pregnancy and delivery* (5th ed.). St. Louis, MO: Mosby.

Hagel-Fenton, D. J. (2008). Beyond preeclampsia: HELLP syndrome. *RN, 71*(3), 22–26.

Hajenius, P. J., Mol, F., Mol, B. W. J., Bossuyt, P. M. M., Ankum, W. M., & van der Veen, F. (2009). Interventions for tubal ectopic pregnancy. *Cochrane Database of Systematic Reviews, 1*, CD000324. doi: 10.1002/14651858.CD000324.pub2

Han, C., & Norwitz, E. R. (2011). Expectant management of severe preeclampsia remote from term: Not for everyone. *Contemporary OB/GYN, 56*(2), 50–55.

Haram, K., Svendsen, E., & Abildgaard, U. (2009). The HELLP syndrome: Clinical issues and management. A review. *BMC Pregnancy and Childbirth, 9*, 8. Retrieved March 9, 2012 from http://www.ncbi.nlm.nih.gov/pmc/articles/PMC2654858/?tool=pubmed. doi:10.1186/1471-2393-9-8

Hernandez, E. (2012). Gestational trophoblastic neoplasia. Retrieved March 9, 2012 from http://emedicine.medscape.com/article/279116-overview#showall

Jarvis, C. (2009). *Physical examination & health assessment* (1st Canadian ed.). Toronto, Ontario: Saunders Elsevier.

Jazayeri, A. (2011). *Premature rupture of membranes.* Retrieved April 28, 2011 from http://emedicine.medscape.com/article/261137-overview#

Joy, S., Lyon, D., & Stone, R. A. (2010). *Placenta previa.* Retrieved March 9, 2012 from http://emedicine.medscape.com/article/262063-overview

Karch, A. M. (2011). *2011 Lippincott's nursing drug guide.* Philadelphia: Lippincott Williams & Wilkins.

Ko, P., & Yoon, Y. (2011). *Placenta previa in emergency medicine clinical presentation. eMedicine.* Retrieved March 9, 2012 from http://emedicine.medscape.com/article/796182-clinical#showall

Koelewijn, J. M., de Haas, M., Vrijkotte, T. G. M., van der Schoot, C. E., & Bonsel, G. E. (2009). Risk factors for RhD immunisation despite antenatal and postnatal anti-D prophylaxis. *British Journal of Obstetrics and Gynaecology, 116*(10), 1304–1314.

Lavanya, R., Deepika, K., & Patil, M. (2009). Successful pregnancy following medical management of heterotopic pregnancy. *Journal of Human Reproductive Science, 2*(1), 35–40.

Levi, M., & Schmaier, A. H. (2011). *Disseminated intravascular coagulation treatment & management.* Retrieved March 9, 2012 from http://emedicine.medscape.com/article/199627-treatment#a1127

Lim, K., Butt, K., & Crane, J. M. (2011). SOGC clinical practice guidelines: Ultrasonographic cervical length assessment in predicting preterm birth in singleton pregnancies. *Journal of Obstetrics and Gynaecology Canada, 25*(9), 765–773. Retrieved March 9, 2012 from http://www.sogc.org/guidelines/documents/gui257CPG1106E.pdf

Lim, K. H., Sayah, A. J., Steinberg, G., Semenovskaya, Z., Erogul, M., & Zwanger, M. (2011). *Preeclampsia.* Retrieved March 9, 2012 from http://www.emedicine.com/med/topic1905.htm

Lindheimer, M. D., Taler, S. J., & Cunningham, F. G. (2008). Hypertension in pregnancy. *Journal of the American Society of Hypertension, 2*(6), 484–494.

Lipscomb, G. H. (2011). Ectopic pregnancy. In E. T. Bope, R. Kellerman, & R. E. Rakel (Eds.), *Conn's current therapy 2011.* Philadelphia: Saunders Elsevier.

Liston, R., Sawchuk, D., & Young, D. (2007). Fetal health surveillance: Antepartum and intrapartum consensus guideline. *Journal of Obstetrics and Gynaecology Canada, 29*(9 Suppl. 4), S3–S56. Retrieved March 9, 2012 from http://www.sogc.org/guidelines/documents/gui197CPG0709.pdf

Madani, Y. (2008). The use of ultrasonography in the diagnosis of ectopic pregnancy: A case report and review of the literature. *The Medscape Journal of Medicine, 10*(2), 35.

Magee, L. A., Helewa, M., Moutquin, J.-M., & von Dadelszen, P. (2008). SOGC clinical practice guidelines: Diagnosis, evaluation and management of the hypertensive disorders of pregnancy. *Journal of Obstetrics and Gynaecology Canada, 30*(3 Suppl. 1), S1–S52. Retrieved March 9, 2012 from http://www.sogc.org/guidelines/documents/gui206CPG0803_001.pdf

Mancuso, M., & Owen, J. (2009). Prevention of preterm birth based on a short cervix: Cerclage. *Seminars in Perinatology, 33*(5), 325–333. doi:10.1053/j.semperi.2009.06.005

McParlin, C., Graham, R. H., & Robson, S. C. (2008). Caring for women with nausea and vomiting in pregnancy: New approaches. *British Journal of Midwifery, 16*(5), 280–285.

Medscape Reference. (2011). *Magnesium sulfate (Rx).* Retrieved March 9, 2012 from http://reference.medscape.com/drug/mgso4-magnesium-sulfate-344444#0

Mistovich, J. J., Krost, W. S., & Limmer, D. D. (2008). Beyond the basics: Preeclampsia and eclampsia. *EMS Magazine, 37*(11), 51–55.

Murray, H., Baakdah, H., Bardell, T., & Tulandi, T. (2005). Diagnosis and treatment of ectopic pregnancy. *Canadian Medical Association Journal, 173*(8), 905–912.

Norwitz, E. R., & Schorge, J. O. (2010). *Obstetrics and gynecology at a glance* (3rd ed.). Malden, MA: Blackwell Publishing Ltd.

Ogunyemi, D. A., Fong, A., & Chen Herrero, T. (2011). *Hyperemesis gravidarum.* Retrieved March 9, 2012 from http://emedicine.medscape.com/article/254751-overview

Oxlund, B., Ørtoft, G., Brüel, A., Danielsen, C., Oxlund, H., & Uldbjerg, N. (2010). Cervical collagen and biomechanical strength in non-pregnant women with a history of cervical insufficiency. *Reproductive Biology and Endocrinology, 8*, 92. doi:10.1186/1477-7827-8-92

Peel, A. (2009). Diagnosis of an interstitial ectopic pregnancy with two-dimensional transvaginal sonography. *Ultrasound, 17*(2), 93–95.

Public Health Agency of Canada. (2008). *Canadian perinatal health report, 2008 edition.* Retrieved March 9, 2012 from http://www.phac-aspc.gc.ca/publicat/2008/cphr-rspc/pdf/cphr-rspc08-eng.pdf

Rajiah, P. (2011). *Polyhydramnios.* Retrieved March 9, 2012 from http://emedicine.medscape.com/article/404856-overview

Reid, H., Power, M., & Cheshire, K. (2009). Factors influencing antenatal depression, anxiety and stress. *British Journal of Midwifery, 17*(8), 501–508.

Ross, M. (2011). *Eclampisa.* Retrieved March 9, 2012 from http://emedicine.medscape.com/article/253960-overview#aw2aab6c10

Salem, L. (2012). *Rh incompatibility.* Retrieved April 28, 2011 from http://emedicine.medscape.com/article/797150-overview#showall

Sepilian, V. (2011). *Ectopic pregnancy treatment and management.* Retrieved March 9, 2012 from http://emedicine.medscape.com/article/258768-treatment

Sepilian, V., & Wood, E. (2011). *Ectopic pregnancy.* Retrieved March 9, 2012 from http://emedicine.medscape.com/article/258768-overview#showall

Sierra-Bergua, B., Sánchez-Marteles, M., Cabrerizo-García, J. L., & Sanjoaquin-Conde, I. (2008). Choriocarcinoma with pulmonary and cerebral metastases. *Singapore Medical Journal, 49*(10), 286–288.

Silver, R. M. (2009). Evaluation of fetal death from nongenetic causes. *Contemporary OB/GYN, 54*(12), 35–43.

Society of Obstetrics and Gynaecologists of Canada. (2010). *Women's health information: Nausea and vomiting in pregnancy.* Retrieved March 9, 2012 from http://www.sogc.org/health/pregnancy-nausea_e.asp

Sovari, A. A., Kocheril, A. G., & Bass, A. S. (2012). *Cardiogenic pulmonary edema clinical presentation.* Retrieved March 9, 2012 from http://emedicine.medscape.com/article/157452-clinical#showall

Stan, C. M., Boulvian, M., Pfister, R., & Hirsbrunner-Almagbaly, P. (2009). Hydration for treatment of preterm labour. *Cochrane Database of Systematic Reviews, 2,* CD003096.

Statistics Canada. (2008). Live births and fetal deaths (stillbirths), by geography—Type of birth (single or multiple). Retrieved March 9, 2012 from http://www.statcan.gc.ca/pub/84f0210x/2008000/t025-eng.pdf

Statistics Canada. (2011). *Deaths, by cause—Chapter XV: Pregnancy, childbirth and the puerperium (O00 to O99), age group and sex, Canada.* Retrieved March 9, 2012 from http://www5.statcan.gc.ca/cansim/a05?lang=eng&id=1020535

Stephenson, M. (2008). Recurrent early pregnancy less: Is miscarriage evaluation the missing link? *Contemporary OB/GYN, 53*(10), 50–55.

Stokes, B. (2011). Hypertensive disease of pregnancy. In E. T. Bope, R. Kellerman, & R. E. Rakel (Eds.), *Conn's current therapy 2011.* Philadelphia: Saunders Elsevier.

Stucki, D., & Buss, J. (2008). The ectopic pregnancy, a diagnostic and therapeutic challenge. *Journal of Medicine and Life, 1*(1), 40–48.

Varma, R., & Gupta, J. (2009). Tubal ectopic pregnancy. *Clinical Evidence, 1406,* 1–15.

Wilcox, S. R. (2010). *Pregnancy, hyperemesis gravidarum.* Retrieved March 9, 2012 from http://emedicine.medscape.com/article/796564-overview

Yudin, M. H., van Schalkwyk, J., & Van Eyk, N. (2009). SOGC clinical practice guideline: Antibiotic therapy in preterm premature rupture of the membranes. *Journal of Obstetrics and Gynaecology Canada, 31*(9), 863–867. Retrieved March 9, 2012 from http://www.sogc.org/guidelines/documents/gui233CPG0909.pdf

Zeltzer, J. S. (2011). Vaginal bleeding in late pregnancy. In R. D. Kellerman & E. T. Bope (Eds.), *Conn's current therapy 2011.* Philadelphia: Saunders Elsevier.

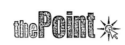

Most women describe pregnancy as an exciting time in their life, but the development of an unexpected problem can suddenly change this description dramatically. Consider the woman who has had a problem-free pregnancy and then suddenly develops a condition during labour, changing a routine situation into a possible crisis. Many complications occur with little or no warning and present challenges for the perinatal health care team as well as the family. The nurse plays a major role in identifying the problem quickly and coordinating immediate intervention, ultimately achieving a positive outcome.

This chapter addresses several conditions occurring during labour and birth that may increase the risk for an adverse outcome for the mother and the fetus. It also describes birth-related procedures that may be necessary for the woman who develops a condition that increases her risk or that may be needed to reduce the woman's risk for developing a condition, thus promoting optimal maternal and fetal outcomes. Nursing management of the woman and her family focuses on professional support and compassionate care.

Dystocia

Dystocia, defined as abnormal or difficult labour, can be influenced by a vast number of maternal and fetal factors. Dystocia is said to exist when the progress of active labour deviates from normal; it is characterized by a slow and abnormal progression of labour (Joy et al., 2011) and has been identified in approximately 10% of hospital deliveries in Canada. Dystocia is the leading indicator for cesarean section (Public Health Agency of Canada [PHAC], 2008).

To characterize a labour as abnormal, a basic understanding of normal labour is essential. Normal labour starts with regular uterine contractions that are strong enough to result in cervical effacement and dilation. Early in labour, uterine contractions are irregular and cervical effacement and dilation occur gradually. When cervical dilation reaches 4 cm and uterine contractions become more powerful, the active phase of labour begins. Because dystocia cannot be predicted or diagnosed with certainty, the term "failure to progress" is often used. This term includes lack of progressive cervical dilation (>4 hours with <0.5 cm per hour) and lack of descent of the fetal head (>1 hour of effective pushing with no descent of the head) (Cheng & Caughey, 2012). An adequate trial of labour is needed to declare with confidence that dystocia or "failure to progress" exists. Understanding normal labour patterns and early identification of factors associated with dystocia are essential to reducing the prevalence and risk related to dystocia.

According to the Society of Obstetricians and Gynaecologists of Canada (SOGC, 2008), dystocia can be prevented through prenatal education, allowing for spontaneous onset of labour, and providing continuous labour support, free movement in labour, no routine interventions, and appropriate non-pharmacologic and pharmacologic pain relief measures.

Early identification of and prompt interventions for dystocia are essential to minimize the risk to the woman and the fetus. Factors associated with an increased risk for dystocia include epidural analgesia, excessive analgesia, multiple gestation, hydramnios, maternal exhaustion, ineffective maternal pushing technique, occiput posterior position, unripe cervix with induction, longer first stage of labour, nulliparity, contracted pelvis, short maternal stature, fetal macrosomia, maternal obesity, fetal malpresentation, fetal anomalies (hydrocephalus), maternal age older than 35 years, gestational age more than 41 weeks, chorioamnionitis, ineffective uterine contractions, and high fetal station at complete cervical dilation (Joy et al., 2011).

Dystocia can result from problems or abnormalities involving the expulsive forces (known as the "powers"); presentation, position, and fetal development (the "passenger"); the maternal bony pelvis or birth canal (the "passageway"); and maternal stress (the "psyche"). Table 21.1 summarizes the diagnosis, therapeutic management, and nursing management of the common problems associated with dystocia (Joy et al., 2011).

Problems with the Powers

When the expulsive forces of the uterus become dysfunctional, the uterus may either never fully relax (hypertonic contractions), placing the fetus in jeopardy, or relax too much (hypotonic contractions), causing ineffective contractions. Still another dysfunction can occur when the uterus contracts so frequently and with such intensity that a very rapid birth will take place (precipitous labour).

Hypertonic uterine dysfunction occurs when the uterus never fully relaxes between contractions. Subsequently, contractions are erratic and poorly coordinated because more than one uterine pacemaker is sending signals for contraction. Placental perfusion becomes compromised, thereby reducing oxygen to the fetus. These hypertonic contractions exhaust the mother, who is experiencing frequent, intense, and painful contractions with little progression (Watts, 2010).

Hypotonic uterine dysfunction occurs during active labour (dilation more than 4 cm) when contractions become poor in quality and lack sufficient intensity to dilate and efface the cervix. Contributing factors to hypotonic uterine function are overdistention, malposition of the fetus, and excessive analgesia (Watts, 2010). The major risk with this complication is hemorrhage after giving birth because the uterus cannot contract effectively to compress blood vessels.

Precipitous labour is one that is completed in less than 3 hours. Women experiencing precipitous labour

(text continues on page 676)

TABLE 21.1 DIAGNOSIS AND MANAGEMENT OF COMMON PROBLEMS ASSOCIATED WITH DYSTOCIA

Problem	Description	Diagnosis	Therapeutic Management	Nursing Management
Problems with the powers				
Hypertonic uterine dysfunction	• Occurs in the latent phase of the first stage of labour (cervical dilation <4 cm), uncoordinated • Force of contraction typically in the midsection of the uterus at the junction of the active upper and passive lower segments of the uterus rather than in the fundus • Loss of downward pressure to push the presenting part against the cervix (Watts, 2010) • Woman commonly becomes discouraged due to lack of progress; also has increased pain secondary to uterine anoxia	Characteristic hypertonicity of the contractions and the lack of labour progress	• Therapeutic rest with the use of sedatives to promote relaxation and stop the abnormal activity of the uterus • Hydration to promote fluid and electrolyte balance • Identification of and intervention for any contributing factors • Ruling out placental abruption (also associated with high resting tone and persistent pain) • Onset of a normal labour pattern occurs in many women after a 4–6 h rest period (Watts, 2010).	• Institute bed rest and sedation to promote relaxation and reduce pain. • Assist with measures to rule out fetopelvic disproportion and fetal malpresentation. • Evaluate fetal tolerance to labour pattern, such as monitoring of FHR patterns. • Assess for signs of maternal infection. • Promote adequate hydration through IV therapy. • Provide pain management via epidural or IV analgesics. • Assist with amniotomy to augment labour. • Explain to woman and family about dysfunctional pattern. • Plan for operative birth if normal labour pattern is not achieved.
Hypotonic uterine dysfunction	• Often termed secondary uterine inertia because the labour begins normally and then the frequency and intensity of contractions decrease • Possible contributing factors: overdistended uterus (i.e., multifetal pregnancy, macrosomia, polyhydramnios), too much pain medicine given too early in labour, fetal malposition, and regional anesthesia (Watts, 2010)	Evaluation of the woman's labour to confirm that she is having hypotonic active labour rather than a long latent phase Evaluation of maternal pelvis and fetal presentation and position to ensure that they are not contributing to the prolonged labour without noticeable progress	• Identification of possible cause of inefficient uterine action (a malpositioned fetus, a too small maternal pelvis, overdistention of the uterus with fluid or a macrosomic fetus) • Rupture of amniotic sac (amniotomy) if all causes ruled out • Possible augmentation with oxytocin (Syntocin) to stimulate effective uterine contractions • Cesarean birth if amniotomy and augmentation ineffective	• Administer oxytocin as ordered once fetopelvic disproportion is ruled out. • Assist with amniotomy if membranes are intact. • Provide fetal surveillance as appropriate. • Monitor vital signs, contractions, and cervix continually. • Assess for signs of maternal and fetal infection. • Explain to woman and family about dysfunctional pattern. • Plan for surgical birth if normal labour pattern is not achieved or fetal distress occurs.

Precipitous labour	Abrupt onset of higher-intensity contractions occurring in a shorter period of time instead of the more gradual increase in frequency, duration, and intensity that typifies most spontaneous labours	Identification based on the rapidity of progress through the stages of labour	Vaginal delivery if maternal pelvis is adequate	Closely monitor woman with previous history. Anticipate use of scheduled induction to control labour rate. Stay in constant attendance to monitor progress. Be prepared for delivery in the absence of the primary care provider. Anticipate postpartum hemorrhage.
Problems with the passenger				
Persistent occiput posterior position	Engagement of fetal head in the left or right occipito-transverse position with the occiput rotating posteriorly rather than into the more favourable occiput anterior position (fetus born facing upward instead of the normal downward position) Labour usually much longer and more uncomfortable (causing increased back pain during labour) if fetus remains in this position Possible extensive caput succedaneum and moulding from the sustained occiput posterior position	Leopold manoeuvres and vaginal examination to determine position of fetal head in conjunction with the mother's complaints of severe back pain (back of fetal head pressing on mother's sacrum and coccyx)	Labour to proceed, preparing the woman for a long labour (spontaneous resolution possible) Comfort measures and maternal positioning to help promote fetal head rotation	Assess for complaints of back pain in first stage of labour. Perform fetal surveillance as appropriate. Encourage maternal position changes to promote fetal head rotation: hands and knees and rocking pelvis back and forth; side-lying position; side lunges during contractions; sitting, kneeling, or standing while leaning forward; squatting position to give birth and enlarge pelvic outlet (Simkin, 2010). Apply low back counter-pressure during contractions to ease the discomfort. Use other helpful measures to attempt to rotate the fetal head, including lateral abdominal stroking in the direction that the fetal head should rotate; assisting the client into a hands-and-knees position (all fours); and squatting, pelvic rocking, stair climbing, assuming a side-lying position toward the side that the fetus should rotate, and side lunges.

(continued)

669

TABLE 21.1 DIAGNOSIS AND MANAGEMENT OF COMMON PROBLEMS ASSOCIATED WITH DYSTOCIA (continued)

Problem	Description	Diagnosis	Therapeutic Management	Nursing Management
				Provide measures to reduce anxiety, including continuous support.
				Continuously reinforce the woman's progress.
				Teach the woman and support person(s) about measures to facilitate fetal head rotation.
				Administer agents as ordered for pain relief (effective pain relief is crucial to help the woman to tolerate the back discomfort).
				Assess for prolonged second stage of labour with arrest of descent (common with this malposition).
				Anticipate possible use of forceps to rotate to anterior position at birth or manual rotation to anterior position at end of second stage.
				Prepare for possible cesarean birth if rotation is not achieved.
Face and brow presentation	Face presentation with complete extension of the fetal head	Diagnosis via vaginal examination only once labour is well established; palpation of facial features as the presenting part rather than the fetal head	Vaginal birth possible with face presentation with an adequate maternal pelvis and fetal head rotation; cesarean birth if head rotates backward	Assist with evaluating for feto-pelvic disproportion.
	Brow presentation: fetal head between full extension and full flexion so that the largest fetal skull diameter presents to the pelvis		Cesarean birth for brow presentation unless head flexes	Anticipate cesarean birth if vertex position is not achieved.
				Explain fetal malposition to the woman and her partner.
				Provide close observation for any signs of fetal hypoxia, as evidenced by late decelerations on the *fetal monitor.*

Breech presentation			

Breech presentation

Fetal buttocks, or breech, presenting first rather than the head

1. Frank breech: buttock as the presenting part, with hips flexed and legs and knees extended upward
2. Complete breech (or full breech): buttock as presenting part, with hips flexed and knees flexed in a "cannonball" position
3. Footling or incomplete breech: One or two feet as the presenting part, with one or both hips extended

Vaginal examination to determine breech presentation. Ideally, ultrasound to confirm a clinically suspected presentation and to identify any fetal anomalies

The optimal method of birth is controversial and depends on a variety of factors: anticipated size of fetus, maternal pelvis, cord position, availability of early labour ultrasound assessment, comfort of care provider with breech delivery, and availability of cesarean birth

Regardless of the birth method selected, the risk for trauma is high. Breech vaginal births are recommended by SOGC only when early labour ultrasound is available, no contraindications to vaginal breech delivery exist, and the estimated fetal weight is between 2,500 and 4,000 g (Kotaska et al., 2009).

Vaginal delivery: fetus allowed to spontaneously deliver up to the umbilicus; then manoeuvres to assist in the delivery of the remainder of the body, arms, and head; fetal membranes left intact as long as possible to act as a dilating wedge and to prevent cord prolapse; anesthesiologist and pediatrician present

Caesarean birth: use of external cephalic version to reduce the chance of breech presentation at birth; attempted after the 36th week of gestation but before the start of labour (some fetuses spontaneously turn to a cephalic

Assess for associated conditions such as placenta previa, hydramnios, fetal anomalies, and multiple gestation.

Arrange for ultrasound to confirm fetal presentation.

Assist with external cephalic version possible after 36 weeks, and administer tocolytics to assist with external cephalic version.

Anticipate trial labour for 4–6 h to evaluate progress if version is unsuccessful.

Plan for cesarean birth if no progress is seen or fetal distress occurs.

After external cephalic version, administer RhoGAM to the Rh-negative woman to prevent a sensitization reaction if trauma has occurred and the potential for mixing of blood exists (Hofmeyr & Kulier, 2010).

(continued)

TABLE 21.1 DIAGNOSIS AND MANAGEMENT OF COMMON PROBLEMS ASSOCIATED WITH DYSTOCIA (continued)

Problem	Description	Diagnosis	Therapeutic Management	Nursing Management
			presentation on their own toward term, and some will return to the breech presentation if external cephalic version is attempted too early) (Hofmeyr & Kulier, 2010); variable success rates, with risk for fractured bones, ruptured viscera, abruptio placentae, fetomaternal hemorrhage, and umbilical cord entanglement; tocolytic drugs to relax the uterus, as well as other methods to facilitate external cephalic version at term; individual evaluation of each woman for all factors before any interventions are initiated (Fischer, 2011)	
Shoulder dystocia	Delivery of fetal head with neck not appearing; retraction of chin against the perineum; shoulders remaining wedged behind the mother's pubic bone, causing a difficult birth with potential for injury to both mother and baby If shoulders still above the brim at this stage, no advancement. Newborn's chest trapped within the vaginal vault; chest unable to expand with respiration (although nose and mouth are outside)	Emergency, often unexpected complication. Diagnosis made when newborn's head delivers without delivery of neck and remaining body structures; "turtle sign" Primary risk factors, including suspected infant macrosomia, maternal diabetes mellitus, excessive maternal weight gain, abnormal maternal pelvic anatomy, maternal obesity,	If anticipated, preparatory tasks instituted: alerting of key personnel; education of woman and family regarding steps to be taken in the event of a difficult birth; emptying of woman's bladder to allow additional room for possible manoeuvres needed for the birth McRobert's maneuvre or suprapubic pressure (not fundal) (see Fig. 21.1). Combination of manoeuvres effective in more than 100% of cases of shoulder dystocia (Allen & Gurewitsch, 2010)	Intervene immediately due to cord compression. Perform McRobert's manoeuvre (application of suprapubic pressure) and be prepared to assist in other manoeuvres. Assist with positioning the woman in squatting position, hands-and-knees position, or lateral recumbent position for birth to free shoulder. Clear room of unnecessary clutter to make room for additional personnel and equipment.

(continued)

	Risk for umbilical cord compression between the fetal body and the maternal pelvis	post-dates pregnancy, short stature, a history of previous shoulder dystocia, precipitous second stage, multiple pregnancy, induction of labour, prolonged labour, operative vaginal delivery, and use of epidural analgesia (Allen & Gurewitsch, 2010; Davies, Maxwell, & McLeod, 2010).	Newborn resuscitation team readily available	After the birth, assess newborn for crepitus, deformity, Erb's palsy, or bruising, which might suggest neurologic damage or a fracture of clavicle or humorous (Allen & Gurewitsch, 2010).
Multiple gestation	More than one fetus, leading to uterine overdistention and possibly resulting in hypotonic contractions and abnormal presentations of the fetuses Fetal hypoxia during labour a significant threat due to placenta providing oxygen and nutrients to more than one fetus	Nearly all multiples are now diagnosed early by ultrasound. Most women go into labour before 37 weeks.	Admission to facility with specialized care unit if woman goes into labour Spontaneous progression of labour if woman has no complicating factors and first fetus is in longitudinal lie Separate monitoring of each FHR during labour and birth After birth of first fetus, clamping of cord and lie of the second twin assessed. Possible external cephalic version necessary to assist in providing a longitudinal lie. Second and subsequent fetuses at greater risk for birth-related complications, such as umbilical cord prolapse, malpresentation, and placental abruption regardless of the method of delivery (Schmitz, Carnavalet, Azria, et al., 2008). Cesarean birth if risk factors high.	Assess for hypotonic labour pattern due to overdistention. Evaluate for fetal presentation, maternal pelvic size, and gestational age to determine mode of delivery. Ensure presence of neonatal team for birth of multiples. Anticipate need for cesarean birth.

673

TABLE 21.1 DIAGNOSIS AND MANAGEMENT OF COMMON PROBLEMS ASSOCIATED WITH DYSTOCIA (continued)

Problem	Description	Diagnosis	Therapeutic Management	Nursing Management
Excessive fetal size and abnormalities	Macrosomia leading to fetopelvic disproportion (fetus unable to fit through the maternal pelvis to be born vaginally) Reduced contraction strength due to overdistention by large fetus leading to a prolonged labour and the potential for birth injury and trauma Fetal abnormalities possibly interfering with fetal descent, leading to prolonged labour and difficult birth	A diagnosis of fetal macrosomia can be confirmed by measuring the birth weight after birth. Suspicion of macrosomia based on increased fundal height measurements or ultrasound examination before onset of labour (if suspected due to conditions such as maternal diabetes or obesity, estimation of fetal weight via ultrasound). Leopold's manoeuvres to estimate fetal weight and position on admission to labour and birth unit	Possible trial of labour to evaluate progress. Possible planned cesarean section	Assess for inability of fetus to descend. Plan for cesarean birth if maternal parameters are inadequate to give birth to large fetus.
Problems with the passageway	Contraction of one or more of the three planes of the pelvis Poorer prognosis for vaginal birth in women with android and platypelloid types of pelvis Contracted pelvis involving reduction in one or more of the pelvic diameters interfering with progress of labour: inlet, midpelvis, and outlet contracture Obstruction in the birth canal, such as placenta previa that partially or completely obstructs the internal os of the cervix, fibroids in the	Shortest AP diameter <10 cm or greatest transverse diameter <12 cm (approximation of AP diameter via measurement of diagonal conjugate, which in the contracted pelvis is <11.5 cm) Interischial tuberous diameter of ≤8 cm possibly compromising outlet contracture (outlet and midpelvic contractures frequently occur together)	Focus on allowing natural forces of labour contractions to push the largest diameter (biparietal) of the fetal head beyond the obstruction or narrow passage	Assess for poor contractions, slow dilation, and prolonged labour. Evaluate bowel and bladder status to reduce soft tissue obstruction and allow increased pelvic space. Anticipate trial of labour; if no labour progression after an adequate trial, plan for cesarean birth.

lower uterine segment, a full bladder or rectum, an edematous cervix caused by premature bearing-down efforts, and human papillomavirus (HPV) warts

Problems with the psyche

Release of stress-related hormones (catecholamines, cortisol, epinephrine, beta-endorphin), which act on smooth muscle (uterus) and reduce uterine contractility (Romano & Lothian, 2008). Excessive release of catecholamines and other stress-related hormones not therapeutic.

Release also results in decreased uteroplacental perfusion and increased risk for poor newborn adjustment (Romano & Lothian, 2008).

Ruling out of other possible causes of dystocia

Treatment dependent on woman's responses, such as anxiety, fear, anger, frustration, or denial (highly variable due to woman's understanding of the condition itself, past experiences, previous coping mechanisms, and the amount of family and nursing support received)

Appropriate medical or surgical interventions depending on the underlying condition

Provide comfortable environment—dim lighting, music.

Encourage partner to participate.

Provide pain management to reduce anxiety and stress.

Ensure continuous presence of staff to allay anxiety.

Provide frequent updates concerning fetal status and progress.

Provide ongoing encouragement to minimize the woman's stress and help her to cope with labour and to promote a positive, timely outcome (Romano & Lothian, 2008).

Assist in relaxation and comfort measures to help her body work more effectively with the forces of labour.

Engage the woman in conversation about her emotional well-being; offer anticipatory guidance and reassurance to increase her self-esteem and ability to cope, decrease frustration, and encourage cooperation.

675

141

typically have soft perineal tissues that stretch readily, permitting the fetus to pass through the pelvis quickly and easily. Maternal complications are rare if the maternal pelvis is adequate and the soft tissues yield to a fast fetal descent, although perineal lacerations and postpartum hemorrhage are possible. Potential fetal complications may include head trauma, such as intracranial hemorrhage or nerve damage, and hypoxia due to the rapid progression of labour (Cunningham, Leveno, Bloom, et al., 2010).

Problems with the Passenger

Any presentation other than occiput anterior or a slight variation of the fetal position or size increases the probability of dystocia. These variations can affect the contractions or fetal descent through the maternal pelvis. Common problems involving the fetus include occiput posterior position, breech presentation, multifetal pregnancy, excessive size (macrosomia) as it relates to cephalopelvic disproportion, and structural anomalies.

Persistent occiput posterior is one of the most common malpositions. The reasons for this malposition are often unclear. This position presents slightly larger diameters to the maternal pelvis, thus slowing fetal descent. A fetal head that is poorly flexed may be responsible. In addition, poor uterine contractions may not push the fetal head down into the pelvic floor to the extent that the fetal occiput sinks into it rather than being pushed to rotate in an anterior direction. Persistent occiput posterior may be associated with a more painful labour, prolonged labour, and dystocia (Hunter, Hofmeyr, & Kulier, 2007).

Face and brow presentations are rare and are associated with fetal malformations and polyhydramnios (Bashiri, Burstein, Bar-David, et al., 2008).

Breech presentation, which occurs in 3% to 4% of labours, is frequently associated with high parity with uterine relaxation, previous breech delivery, uterine anomalies, multifetal pregnancies, placenta previa, oligohydramnios, polyhydramnios, preterm births, and fetal anomalies such as hydrocephaly and anencephaly (Cunningham et al., 2010). Perinatal mortality is increased with a breech presentation, regardless of the mode of delivery (Hofmeyr & Hannah, 2010). Women with breech presentation at term may be offered external cephalic version, which is an attempt to turn the fetus to cephalic presentation and is performed under carefully controlled clinical conditions (Hofmeyr & Kulier, 2010).

Shoulder dystocia is defined as the obstruction of fetal descent and birth by the axis of the fetal shoulders after the fetal head has been delivered. It is one of the most anxiety-provoking emergencies encountered in labour. Failure of the shoulders to deliver spontaneously places both the woman and the fetus at risk for injury. Postpartum hemorrhage, secondary to uterine atony or vaginal lacerations, is the major complication to the mother. Transient Erb's or Duchenne's brachial plexus palsies and clavicular or humeral fractures are the most common fetal injuries encountered with shoulder dystocia. Failure to deliver the whole body within 6 minutes has been shown to increase the incidence of acidosis, asphyxia, permanent central nervous system impairment, and death (Allen & Gurewitsch, 2010). Risks for shoulder dystocia include a history of shoulder dystocia, macrosomia, maternal diabetes, excessive weight gain, maternal obesity, postterm pregnancy, precipitous second stage, operative delivery (forceps or vacuum), and prolonged second stage. Prompt recognition and appropriate management, such as with McRobert's manoeuvre or suprapubic pressure, can reduce the severity of injuries to the mother and the newborn (Fig. 21.1).

> ▶ **Take** NOTE!
>
> *Prompt recognition and appropriate management of shoulder dystocia can reduce the severity of injuries to the mother and the infant. Immediately assess the infant for signs of trauma such as a fractured clavicle, Erb's palsy, or neonatal asphyxia. Assess the mother for excessive vaginal bleeding and blood in the urine from bladder trauma.*

Multiple gestation refers to twins, triplets, or more infants within a single pregnancy (Box 21.1). The incidence of multiple gestation is increasing, primarily as a result of infertility treatment (medical and surgical) and an increased number of women giving birth at older ages. The incidence of multiple births in Canada is 3 in 100 births (PHAC, 2008). The most common maternal complication is postpartum hemorrhage resulting from uterine atony.

Excessive fetal size and abnormalities can also contribute to labour and birth dysfunctions. **Macrosomia**, in which a newborn weighs more than 4,000 g (8 pounds 13 oz) at birth, complicates approximately 10% of all pregnancies but has a higher incidence in Aboriginal women (PHAC, 2008). Fetal abnormalities may include hydrocephalus, ascites, or a large mass on the neck or head. Complications associated with dystocia related to excessive fetal size and anomalies include an increased risk for postpartum hemorrhage, dysfunctional labour, increased incidence of instrumental delivery and cesarean section, increased length of hospital stay, fetopelvic disproportion, soft tissue laceration during vaginal birth, fetal injuries or fractures, asphyxia, lower Apgar scores, and increased incidence of neonatal intensive care unit admission (Pundir & Sinha, 2009).

Problems with the Passageway

Problems with the passageway (pelvis and birth canal) are related to a contraction of one or more of the three

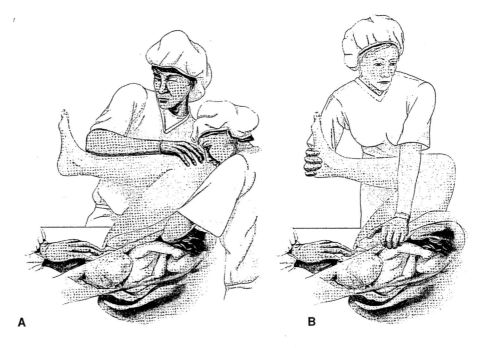

FIGURE 21.1 Manoeuvres to relieve shoulder dystocia. (**A**) McRobert's manoeuvre. The mother's thighs are flexed and abducted as much as possible to straighten the pelvic curve. (**B**) Suprapubic pressure. Pressure is applied just above the pubic bone, pushing the fetal anterior shoulder downward to displace it from above the mother's symphysis pubis. The newborn's head is depressed toward the mother's anus while suprapubic pressure is applied.

A   **B**

BOX 21.1   Multiple Gestation

As the name implies, multiple gestation involves more than one fetus. These fetuses can result from fertilization of a single ovum or multiple ova. Twin pregnancies that are single-ovum conceptions (monozygotic twins) share one chorion (membrane closest to the uterus), and each twin has his or her own amnion (membrane surrounding the amniotic fluid). One fertilized ovum splits into two separate individuals who are said to be natural clones. They have separate amniotic sacs and placentas, are identical in appearance, and are always the same gender. Twin pregnancies that are multiple-ova conceptions (dizygotic twins) result from two ova fertilized by two sperm. Genetically, dizygotic twins are as alike (or unlike) as any other pair or siblings (Fletcher, 2009).

The fetuses of a twin gestation, whether monozygotic or dizygotic, are slightly "squashed" because two fetuses develop in a space usually occupied by one. This compression is reflected in the slowing of weight gain in both twins compared with that for singletons.

Multiple births other than twins can be of the identical type, the fraternal type, or combinations of the two. Triplets can occur from the division of one zygote into two, with one dividing again, producing identical triplets, or they can come from two zygotes, one dividing into a set of identical twins, and the second zygote developing as a single fraternal sibling, or from three separate zygotes (Fletcher, 2009). In recent years, fertility drugs used to induce ovulation have resulted in a greater frequency of quadruplets, quintuplets, sextuplets, and even octuplets.

planes of the maternal pelvis: inlet, midpelvis, and outlet. The female pelvis can be classified into four types based on the shape of the pelvic inlet, which is bounded anteriorly by the posterior border of the symphysis pubis, posteriorly by the sacral promontory, and laterally by the linea terminalis. The four basic types are gynecoid, anthropoid, android, and platypelloid (see Chapter 12 for additional information). Contraction of the midpelvis is more common than inlet contraction and typically causes an arrest of fetal descent. Obstructions in the maternal birth canal, such as swelling of the soft maternal tissue and cervix, termed soft tissue dystocia, also can hamper fetal descent and impede labour progression outside the maternal bony pelvis.

Problems with the Psyche

Many women experience an array of emotions during labour, which may include fear, anxiety, helplessness, being alone, and weariness. These emotions can lead to psychological stress, which indirectly can cause dystocia.

Nursing Assessment

Begin the assessment by reviewing the client's history to look for risk factors for dystocia. Include in the assessment the mother's frame of mind to identify fear, anxiety, stress, lack of support, and pain, which can interfere with uterine contractions and impede labour progress. Helping the woman to relax will promote normal labour progress.

Assess the woman's vital signs. Note any elevation in temperature (might suggest an infection) or changes in heart rate or blood pressure (might signal hypovolemia). Evaluate the uterine contractions for frequency and intensity. Question the woman about any changes in her contraction pattern, such as a decrease or increase in frequency or intensity, and report these. Assess fetal heart rate (FHR) and pattern, reporting any abnormal patterns immediately.

Assess fetal position via Leopold's manoeuvres to identify any deviations in presentation or position, and report any deviations. Assist with or perform a vaginal examination to determine cervical dilation, effacement, and engagement of the fetal presenting part. Evaluate for evidence of membrane rupture. Report any malodorous fluid.

Nursing Management

Nursing management of the woman with dystocia, regardless of the etiology, requires patience. The nurse should provide physical and emotional support to the client and her family. The final outcome of any labour depends on the size and shape of the maternal pelvis, the quality of the uterine contractions, and the size, presentation, and position of the fetus. Thus, dystocia is diagnosed not at the start of labour but rather after labour has progressed for a time.

Promoting the Progress of Labour

The nurse plays a major role in determining the progress of labour. Continue to assess the woman, frequently monitoring cervical dilation and effacement, uterine contractions, and fetal descent, and document that all assessed parameters are progressing. Evaluate progress in active labour by using a partogram. When the woman's membranes rupture, if they have not already ruptured, observe for colour, odour, and visible cord prolapse. Continue to assess fetal well-being and document the FHR on the partogram.

> ▶ **Take** NOTE!
>
> *If a dysfunctional labour occurs, contractions will slow or fail to advance in frequency, duration, or intensity; the cervix will fail to respond to uterine contractions by dilating and effacing; and the fetus will fail to descend.*

Throughout labour, assess the woman's fluid balance status. Check skin turgor and mucous membranes. Monitor intake and output. Also monitor the client's bladder for distention at least every 2 hours and encourage her to empty her bladder often. In addition, monitor her bowel status. A full bladder or rectum can impede descent.

Continue to monitor fetal well-being. If the presenting part is high or the fetus is in the breech position, be especially observant for visible cord prolapse and note any variable decelerations in heart rate. If either occurs, report it immediately.

Be prepared to administer a labour stimulant such as oxytocin (Syntocin) if ordered to treat hypotonic labour contractions. Anticipate the need to assist with manipulations if shoulder dystocia is diagnosed. Prepare the woman and her family for the possibility of a cesarean birth if labour does not progress.

Providing Physical and Emotional Comfort

Employ physical comfort measures to promote relaxation and reduce stress. Offer blankets for warmth and a backrub, if the client wishes, to reduce muscle tension. Provide an environment conducive to rest so the woman can conserve her energy. Lower the lights and reduce external noise by closing the hallway door. Offer a warm shower or bath to promote relaxation (if not contraindicated). Use pillows to support the woman in a comfortable position, changing her position every 30 minutes to reduce tension and to enhance uterine activity and efficiency. Offer her fluids/food as appropriate to moisten her mouth and replenish her energy (Fig. 21.2).

Assist with providing counter-pressure along with backrubs if the fetus is in the occiput posterior position. Encourage the woman to ambulate or assume different positions to promote fetal rotation. Upright positions are helpful in facilitating fetal rotation and descent. Also encourage the woman to visualize the descent and birth of the fetus.

Assess the woman's level of pain and degree of distress. Administer analgesics as ordered or according to the facility's protocol.

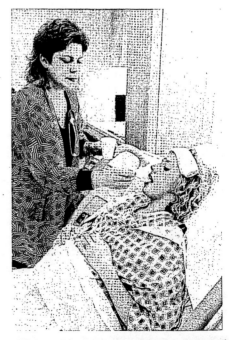

FIGURE 21.2 The nurse applies a cool, moist washcloth to the forehead and offers ice chips to combat thirst and provide comfort for the woman experiencing dystocia.

Evaluate the mother's level of fatigue throughout labour, such as verbal expressions of feeling exhausted, inability to cope in early labour, or inability to rest or calm down between contractions. Praise the woman and her partner for their efforts. Provide empathetic listening to increase the client's coping ability, and remain with the client to demonstrate caring (Romano & Lothian, 2008).

Promoting Empowerment

Educate the client and family about dysfunctional labour and its causes and therapies. Explain therapeutic interventions that may be needed to assist with the labour process. Encourage the client and her partner to participate in decision making about interventions.

Assist the woman and partner in expressing their fears and anxieties. Provide encouragement to help them to maintain control. Support the client and her partner in their coping efforts. Keep the woman and her partner informed of progress and advocate for them.

Preterm Labour

Preterm labour is defined as the occurrence of regular uterine contractions accompanied by cervical effacement and dilation before the end of the 37th week of gestation. If not halted, it leads to preterm birth. Contributing factors include infection, prior preterm birth, periodontal disease, genetic influence, working during pregnancy, lifestyle (e.g., cigarette smoking, illicit drug use, inadequate weight gain, psychological factors such as anxiety or chronic stress), and ethnicity (e.g., Aboriginal women and in the African background in the United States) (Cunningham et al., 2010; Women's Health Data Directory, 2011). The exact cause of preterm labour is not known. Currently, prevention is the goal.

Preterm births remain one of the biggest contributors to perinatal morbidity and mortality in the world. According to PHAC (2008), about 8.2% of births in Canada are preterm. One percent to 2% of deliveries occur before 34 weeks. Late preterm deliveries (between 34 and 37 weeks) occurring in a level III centre have a 99% to 100% survival rate, with the infant often appearing to be the "same" as a term baby; however, these infants require observation and interventions to maintain thermoregulation and glycemic control (Ishiguro, Namai, & Yoichi, 2009).

Preterm birth is one of the most common obstetric complications, and its sequelae have a profound effect on the survival and health of the newborn. The rate of preterm births in Canada has increased over the past 25 years. Preterm births prior to 32 weeks' gestation account for 50% of neurologic morbidity and 60% of perinatal mortality (PHAC, 2008). Infants born prematurely also are at risk for serious sequelae such as respiratory distress syndrome, respiratory failure, central nervous system hemorrhage, infections, thermoregulation problems that can lead to acidosis and weight loss, gastrointestinal complications including necrotizing enterocolitis and feeding difficulties, and long-term cognitive, visual, motor, hearing, growth, and behavioural problems (PHAC, 2008; Ross & Eden, 2011). Although great strides have been made in neonatal intensive care, prematurity remains the leading cause of infant death in Canada (PHAC, 2008).

Therapeutic Management

Predicting the risk for preterm labour is valuable only if there is an available intervention that is likely to improve the situation. Many factors influence the decision to intervene when women present with symptoms of preterm labour, including the probability of progressive labour, gestational age, and the risks of treatment. Accurate dating of the fetus is essential (Ross & Eden, 2011).

The treatment for preterm labour often includes tocolysis and varying degrees of activity restriction (Fig. 21.3). Antibiotics may be prescribed to treat presumed or confirmed infections. Steroids may be given to enhance fetal lung maturity between 24 weeks and 34 weeks' gestation.

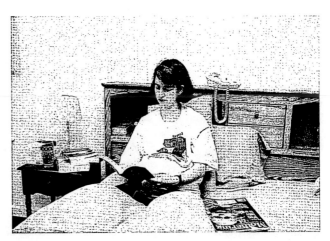

FIGURE 21.3 The mother with preterm labour resting in bed at home.

Nursing Assessment

Obtain a thorough history to determine the estimated date of birth. Many women are unsure of the date of their last menstrual period, so the date given may be unreliable. Despite numerous methods used to date pregnancies, many are still misdated. Accurate gestational dating via ultrasound is essential.

Antepartum assessment for a postterm pregnancy typically includes daily fetal movement counts done by the woman, nonstress tests done twice weekly, amniotic fluid assessments as part of the biophysical profile, and weekly cervical examinations to evaluate for ripening. In addition, assess the following:

- Client's understanding of the various fetal well-being tests
- Client's stress and anxiety concerning her lateness
- Client's coping ability and support network

Nursing Management

Once the dates are established and postdate status is confirmed, monitoring fetal well-being becomes critical. When determining the plan of care for a woman with a postterm pregnancy, the first decision is whether to deliver the baby or wait. If the decision is to wait, then fetal surveillance is the key. If the decision is to have the woman deliver, labour induction is initiated. Both decisions remain controversial, and there is no clear answer about which option is more appropriate. Therefore, the plan must be individualized.

*T*hink back to Jennifer, who is scheduled for labour induction. What ongoing nursing assessments would be important when providing care for her?

Providing Support

The intense surveillance is time-consuming and intrusive, adding to the anxiety and worry already being experienced by the woman about her overdue status. Be alert to the woman's anxiety and allow her to discuss her feelings. Provide reassurance about the expected time range for birth and the well-being of the fetus based on the assessment tests. Validating the woman's stressful state due to the prolonged pregnancy provides an opportunity for her to verbalize her feelings openly.

Educating the Woman and Her Partner

Teach the woman and her partner about the testing required and the reasons for each test. Also describe the methods that may be used for cervical ripening if indicated.

Explain about the possibility of induction if the woman's labour isn't spontaneous or if a dysfunctional labour pattern occurs. Also prepare the woman for the possibility of a surgical delivery if fetal distress occurs.

Providing Care During the Intrapartum Period

During the intrapartum period, continuously assess and monitor FHR to identify potential fetal compromise early (e.g., atypical or abnormal FHR) so that interventions can be initiated. Also monitor the woman's hydration status to ensure maximal placental perfusion. When the membranes rupture, assess amniotic fluid characteristics (colour, amount, and odour) to identify previous fetal hypoxia and prepare for prevention of meconium aspiration. Report meconium-stained amniotic fluid immediately when the membranes rupture. Anticipate the need for amnioinfusion to minimize the risk for meconium aspiration by diluting the meconium in the amniotic fluid expelled by the hypoxic fetus. In addition, monitor the woman's labour pattern closely because dysfunctional patterns are common.

Encourage the woman to verbalize her feelings and concerns, and answer all her questions. Provide support, presence, information, and encouragement throughout this time.

Women Requiring Labour Induction and Augmentation

Ideally, all pregnancies go to term, with labour beginning spontaneously. However, many women need help to initiate or sustain the labour process. **Labour induction** involves the stimulation of uterine contractions by medical or surgical means to produce delivery before the onset of spontaneous labour. The labour induction rate in Canada is approximately 20% (PHAC, 2008). Evidence is compelling that medical induction of labour increases the risk for cesarean birth (Wilson, Effken, & Butler, 2010).

Labour induction is not an isolated event: it brings about a cascade of other interventions that may or may not produce a favourable outcome. Labour induction also involves intravenous therapy, continuous electronic fetal monitoring, and significant discomfort from stimulating uterine contractions. It may also involve increased use of epidural analgesia/anesthesia and a prolonged stay on the labour unit.

Labour augmentation enhances ineffective contractions after labour has begun. Continuous electronic FHR monitoring is necessary.

There are multiple medical and obstetric reasons for inducing labour, the most common being postterm gestation. Other indications for inductions include prelabour rupture of membranes, hypertensive disorders, renal disease, chorioamnionitis, intrauterine fetal demise, and preexisting diabetes (PHAC, 2008). According to the SOGC, contraindications to labour induction are the same as contraindications to labour and vaginal delivery and may include complete placenta previa, transverse fetal lie, prolapsed umbilical cord, a prior classic uterine incision that entered the uterine cavity, previous myomectomy, previous uterine rupture, vasa previa, invasive cervical cancer, active genital herpes infection, and abnormal FHR patterns (Crane, 2001). In general, labour induction is indicated when the benefits of birth outweigh the risks to the mother or the fetus for continuing the pregnancy. However, the balance between risk and benefit remains controversial. See Evidence-based Practice 21.1.

> ### ▷ *Take NOTE!*
>
> *Before labour induction is started, fetal maturity (dating, ultrasound, amniotic fluid studies) and cervical readiness (vaginal examination, Bishop scoring) must be assessed. Both need to be favourable for a successful induction.*

Therapeutic Management

The decision to induce labour is based on a thorough evaluation of maternal and fetal status. Typically, this includes an assessment to evaluate fetal size, position, and gestational age; nonstress test to evaluate fetal well-being; Nitrazine paper and/or fern test to confirm ruptured membranes; complete blood count; and vaginal examination to evaluate the cervix for inducibility. Accurate dating of the pregnancy is also essential before cervical ripening and induction are initiated to prevent a preterm birth.

Cervical Ripening

There has been increasing awareness that if the cervix is unfavourable or unripe, a successful vaginal birth is less likely. Cervical ripeness is an important variable when labour induction is being considered. A ripe cervix is shortened, centred (anterior), softened, and partially dilated. An unripe cervix is long, closed, posterior, and firm. Cervical ripening usually begins prior to the onset of labour contractions and is necessary for cervical dilation and the passage of the fetus.

Various scoring systems to assess cervical ripeness have been introduced, but the Bishop score is most

---

EVIDENCE-BASED PRACTICE 21.1
Labour Induction and Outcomes for Women Beyond Term

● Study
Postterm pregnancies may adversely affect both the mother and the fetus or newborn. Placental perfusion decreases as the placenta ages and becomes less efficient at delivering oxygen and nutrients to the fetus. Amniotic fluid volume also begins to decline by 40 weeks of gestation, increasing the fetus's risk for oligohydramnios, meconium aspiration, and cord compression. However, questions arise: what is the best time for inducing labour in a postterm pregnancy? Does labour induction improve maternal and fetal outcomes, or would it be better to wait for spontaneous labour to begin?

A study was conducted to compare the effects of inducing labour in women between 41 and 42 weeks of gestation or waiting for spontaneous labour to begin. A search was conducted for randomized, controlled trials that compared labour induction with expectant management in women who were greater than 41 + 0 weeks of gestation. Two review authors collected the data and analyzed the trials. A total of 19 trials were evaluated.

▲ Findings
Based on the trials analyzed, fewer perinatal deaths occurred in women who were offered labour induction at 41 + 0 weeks of gestation. There was a statistically significant rate of cesarean sections performed in the group that was not induced. There were fewer instances of fetal distress and fewer newborns experienced meconium aspiration syndrome with induction at 41 weeks or more. Statistical analysis; however, showed that these differences were not significant.

▣ Nursing Implications
Nurses need to be aware of the potential benefits and limitations associated with labour induction so that they can provide women and their families with the most appropriate information about options for a postterm pregnancy. Nurses can integrate information from this study in their teaching about the risks associated with postterm pregnancy. They can also use this information to help answer the couple's questions about induction and its effectiveness as well as provide anticipatory guidance about the procedure. Doing so fosters empowerment of the woman and her family, promoting optimal informed decision making.

Source: Delaney, M., & Roggensack, A. (2008). SOGC clinical practice guideline: Guidelines for management of pregnancy at 41 + 0 to 42 + 0 weeks. *Journal of Obstetrics and Gynaecology Canada*, 30(9), 800–1810. Retrieved February 28, 2012 from http://www.sogc.org/guidelines/documents/gui214CPG0809.pdf.

TABLE 21.2 BISHOP SCORING SYSTEM

Score	Dilation (cm)	Effacement (%)	Station	Cervical Consistency	Position of Cervix
0	Closed	0%–30%	−3	Firm	Posterior
1	1–2	40%–50%	−2	Medium	Midposition
2	3–4	60%–70%	−1 or 0	Soft	Anterior
3	5–6	80%	+1 or +2	Very soft	Anterior

Modified from: Bishop, E. H. (1964). Pelvic scoring for elective induction. *Obstetrics & Gynecology*, 24(2), 267.

commonly used today. The Bishop score helps identify women who would be most likely to achieve a successful induction (Table 21.2). The duration of labour is inversely correlated with the Bishop score: a score over 8 indicates a successful vaginal birth. Bishop scores of less than 6 usually indicate that a cervical ripening method should be used prior to induction (Blickstein, 2009).

Non-Pharmacologic Methods

Non-pharmacologic methods for cervical ripening are less frequently used today, but nurses need to be aware of them and question clients about their use. Methods may include herbal agents such as evening primrose oil, black haw, black and blue cohosh, and red raspberry leaves. In addition, castor oil, hot baths, and enemas are used for cervical ripening and labour induction. The risks and benefits of these agents have not been adequately studied.

Other non-pharmacologic methods suggested for labour induction are sexual intercourse and breast stimulation. Both actions promote the release of oxytocin, which stimulates uterine contractions. In addition, human semen is a biological source of prostaglandins used for cervical ripening. Sexual intercourse with breast stimulation may be beneficial, but its effectiveness has not been fully compared with other induction methods; therefore, this method for labour induction is not validated by research (Blickstein, 2009).

Mechanical Methods

Mechanical methods are used to open the cervix and stimulate the progression of labour. All share a similar mechanism of action—application of local pressure stimulates the release of prostaglandins to ripen the cervix. Potential advantages of mechanical methods, compared with pharmacologic methods, may include simplicity or preservation of the cervical tissue or structure, lower cost, and fewer side effects. The risks associated with these methods include infection, bleeding, membrane rupture, and placental disruption (Delaney & Roggensack, 2008).

For example, an indwelling (Foley) catheter (e.g., 26 French) can be inserted into the endocervical canal to ripen and dilate the cervix. This direct pressure stimulates the release of prostaglandins (Caughey & Butler, 2011).

Hygroscopic dilators such as laminaria (a type of dried seaweed) absorb endocervical and local tissue fluids. As they enlarge, they expand the endocervix and provide controlled mechanical pressure. Absorption of water leads to expansion of the dilators and opening of the cervix (Caughey & Butler, 2011).

Surgical Methods

Surgical methods used to ripen the cervix and induce labour include stripping of the membranes and performing an amniotomy. Stripping of the membranes is accomplished by inserting a finger through the internal cervical os and moving it in a circular direction. This motion causes the membranes to detach. Manual separation of the amniotic membranes from the cervix is thought to induce cervical ripening and the onset of labour (Boulvain, Stan, & Irion, 2005).

An amniotomy involves inserting a cervical hook (Amniohook) through the cervical os to deliberately rupture the membranes. This promotes pressure of the presenting part on the cervix and stimulates an increase in the activity of prostaglandins locally. Risks associated with these procedures include umbilical cord prolapse or compression, maternal or neonatal infection, FHR deceleration, bleeding, and client discomfort (Joy et al., 2011).

When either of these techniques is used, amniotic fluid characteristics (such as whether it is clear, bloody, or meconium is present) and the FHR pattern must be monitored closely.

Pharmacologic Agents

The use of pharmacologic agents has revolutionized cervical ripening. The use of prostaglandins to attain cervical ripening has been found to be highly effective in producing cervical changes independent of uterine contractions (Blickstein, 2009). In some cases, women will go into labour, requiring no additional stimulants for induction. Induction of labour with prostaglandins offers the advantage of promoting both cervical ripening and uterine contractility. A drawback of prostaglandins is their ability to induce excessive uterine contractions, which can increase maternal and perinatal morbidity (Crane, 2001; Kho, Sadler, & McCowan, 2008). Prostaglandin analogues commonly used for cervical ripening include dinoprostone gel (Prepidil), dinoprostone inserts (Cervidil), and misoprostol (Cytotec). Misoprostol, a synthetic PGE1 analogue, is a gastric cytoprotective agent used in the treatment and prevention of peptic ulcers. It can be administered intravaginally or orally to ripen the cervix or induce labour. Since the best route and dose of misoprostal have not been established, it is not used in Canada for induction of labour with a live fetus (Crane, 2001) (Drug Guide 21.2). Furthermore, it is contraindicated for women with prior uterine scars and therefore should not be used for cervical ripening in women attempting a **vaginal birth after cesarean (VBAC)**.

Oxytocin

Oxytocin is a potent endogenous uterotonic agent used for both artificial **induction** and **augmentation** of labour and is the most common induction agent used worldwide (Blickstein, 2009). It is produced naturally by the posterior pituitary gland and stimulates contractions of the uterus. For women with low Bishop scores, cervical ripening is typically initiated before oxytocin is administered. Once the cervix is ripe, oxytocin is the most popular pharmacologic agent used for inducing or augmenting labour. A woman with an unfavourable cervix may be admitted the evening before induction to ripen her cervix with one of the prostaglandin agents. Then induction begins with oxytocin the next morning if she has not already gone into labour. Doing so markedly enhances the success of induction.

Response to oxytocin varies widely: some women are very sensitive to even small amounts. The most common adverse effect of oxytocin is uterine hyperstimulation, leading to fetal compromise and impaired oxygenation (Hayes & Weinstein, 2008). The response of the uterus to

---

DRUG GUIDE 21.2   DRUGS USED FOR CERVICAL RIPENING AND LABOUR INDUCTION

Drug	Action/Indications	Nursing Implications
Dinoprostone (Cervidil insert; Prepidil gel)	Directly softens and dilates the cervix/to ripen cervix and induce labour	Provide emotional support. Administer pain medications as needed. Frequently assess degree of effacement and dilation. Monitor uterine contractions for frequency, duration, and strength. Assess maternal vital signs and FHR pattern frequently. Monitor woman for possible adverse effects such as headache, nausea and vomiting, and diarrhea.
Misoprostol (Cytotec)	Ripens cervix/to induce labour with intrauterine fetal demise. Misoprostol is not recommended for use with induction for live births.	Instruct client about purpose and possible adverse effects of medication. Ensure informed consent is signed per hospital policy. Assess vital signs frequently. Monitor client's reaction to drug. Initiate oxytocin for labour induction at least 4 h after last dose was administered. Monitor for possible adverse effects such as nausea and vomiting, diarrhea, and uterine hyperstimulation.
Oxytocin (Syntocin)	Acts on uterine myofibrils to contract/to initiate or reinforce labour	Administer as an IV infusion via pump, increasing dose based on protocol until adequate labour progress is achieved. Assess baseline vital signs and FHR and then frequently after initiating oxytocin infusion. Determine frequency, duration, and strength of contractions frequently. Notify health care provider of any uterine hypertonicity or abnormal FHR patterns. Maintain careful intake and output, being alert for water intoxication. Keep client informed of labour progress. Monitor for possible adverse effects such as hyperstimulation of the uterus, impaired uterine blood flow leading to fetal hypoxia, rapid labour leading to cervical lacerations or uterine rupture, water intoxication (if oxytocin is given in electrolyte-free solution or at a rate exceeding 20 mU/min), and hypotension.

the drug is closely monitored throughout labour so that the oxytocin infusion can be titrated appropriately. In addition, oxytocin has an antidiuretic effect, resulting in decreased urine flow that may lead to water intoxication. Symptoms to watch for include headache and vomiting.

Oxytocin is administered via an intravenous infusion pump piggybacked into the main intravenous line at the port most proximal to the insertion site. Usually 10 units of oxytocin is added to 1 L of isotonic solution to achieve an infusion rate of 0.5 to 20 mU/minute (6 to 120 mL/hour) with consistent assessment (Crane, 2001). The dose is titrated according to protocol to achieve stable contractions every 2 to 3 minutes lasting 40 to 60 seconds (Hayes & Weinstein, 2008; Joy et al., 2011). The uterus should relax between contractions. If the resting uterine tone remains above 20 mm Hg, uteroplacental insufficiency and fetal hypoxia can result. This underscores the importance of continuous FHR monitoring.

Oxytocin has many advantages: it is potent and easy to titrate, it has a short half-life (3 to 10 minutes), and it is generally well tolerated. Induction using oxytocin has side effects (water intoxication, hypotension, and uterine hypertonicity), but because the drug does not cross the placental barrier, no direct fetal problems have been observed (Hayes & Weinstien, 2008) (Fig. 21.4).

*R*emember *Jennifer, the young woman described at the beginning of the chapter? After her cervix is ripened, an oxytocin infusion is started and her progress is slow. What encouragement can the nurse offer? After a few hours, her contractions begin to increase in intensity and frequency. What typical pain management measures can the nurse implement, and how would the nurse evaluate the effectiveness of these measures?*

Nursing Assessment

Nursing assessment of the woman who is undergoing labour induction or augmentation involves a thorough history and physical examination. Review the woman's history for relative indications for induction or augmentation, such as diabetes, hypertension, postterm status, dysfunctional labour pattern, prolonged ruptured membranes, and maternal or fetal infection, and for contraindications such as placenta previa, overdistended uterus, active genital herpes, fetopelvic disproportion, fetal malposition, or severe fetal distress.

Assist with determining the gestational age of the fetus to prevent a preterm birth. Assess fetal well-being to validate the client's and fetus's ability to withstand labour contractions. Evaluate the woman's cervical status, including cervical dilation and effacement, and station via vaginal examination as appropriate before cervical ripening or induction is started. Determine the Bishop score to determine the probable success of induction.

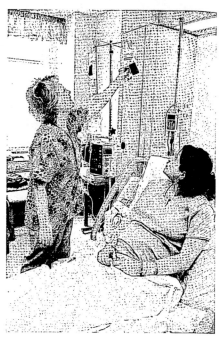

FIGURE 21.4 The nurse monitors an intravenous infusion of oxytocin being administered to a woman in labour.

▶ *Take* NOTE!

Nurses working with women in labour play an important role acting as the "eyes" and "ears" for the birth attendant because they remain at the client's bedside throughout the entire experience. Close, frequent assessment and follow-up interventions are essential to ensure the safety of the mother and her unborn child during cervical ripening and labour induction or augmentation.

Nursing Management

Explain to the woman and her partner about the induction or augmentation procedure clearly, using simple terms (Teaching Guideline 21.2). Ensure that an informed consent has been signed after the client and her partner have received complete information about the procedure, including its advantages, disadvantages, and potential risks. Ensure that the Bishop score has been determined before proceeding. Nursing Care Plan 21.1 presents an overview of the nursing care for a woman undergoing labour induction.

Administering Oxytocin

If not already done, prepare the oxytocin infusion by diluting 10 units of oxytocin in 1,000 mL of lactated Ringer's solution. Use an infusion pump on a secondary line connected to the primary infusion. Start the oxytocin infusion in mU/minute or mL/hour as ordered. Typically,

Teaching in Preparation for Labour Induction

- Your health care provider may recommend that you have your labour induced. This may be necessary for a variety of reasons, such as elevated blood pressure, a medical condition, prolonged pregnancy over 41 weeks, or problems with FHR patterns or fetal growth.
- Your health care provider may use one or more methods to induce labour, such as stripping the membranes, breaking the amniotic sac to release the fluid, administering medication close to or in the cervix to soften it, or administering a medication called oxytocin (Syntocin) to stimulate contractions.
- Labour induction is associated with some risks and disadvantages, such as overactivity of the uterus; nausea, vomiting, or diarrhea; and changes in FHR.
- Prior to inducing your labour, your health care provider may perform a procedure to ripen your cervix to help ensure a successful induction.
- Medication may be placed around your cervix the day before you are scheduled to be induced.
- During the induction, your contractions may feel stronger than normal. However, the length of your labour may be reduced with induction.
- Medications for pain relief and comfort measures will be readily available.
- Health care staff will be present throughout labour.

the initial dose is 1 to 2 mU/minute; anticipate increasing the rate in increments of 1 to 2 mU/minute every 30 minutes to a maximum of 20 mU/minute. Maintain the rate once the desired contraction frequency has been reached. To ensure adequate maternal and fetal surveillance during induction or augmentation, the SOGC recommends a nurse-to-client ratio that does not exceed 1:1 (Rowe, 2007).

During induction or augmentation, monitoring of the maternal and fetal status is essential. Apply an external electronic fetal monitor or assist with placement of an internal device. Obtain the mother's vital signs and the FHR every 15 minutes during the first stage. Evaluate and document the contractions (frequency, duration, and intensity) and resting tone, and adjust the oxytocin infusion rate accordingly. Monitor and document the FHR, including baseline rate, baseline variability, and decelerations, to determine whether the oxytocin rate needs adjustment. Discontinue the oxytocin and notify the birth attendant if uterine hyperstimulation or an abnormal

FHR pattern occurs. Perform or assist with periodic vaginal examinations to determine cervical dilation and fetal descent, and document labour progress on the partogram.

Continue to monitor the FHR continuously and document it every 15 minutes during the active phase of labour and every 5 minutes during the second stage. Assist with pushing efforts during the second stage.

Measure and record intake and output to prevent excess fluid volume. Encourage the client to empty her bladder every 2 hours to prevent soft tissue obstruction.

Providing Pain Relief and Support

Assess the woman's level of pain. Ask her frequently to rate her pain and provide pain management as needed. Offer position changes and other non-pharmacologic measures. Note her reaction to any medication given, and document its effect. Monitor her need for comfort measures as contractions increase.

Throughout induction and augmentation, frequently reassure the woman and her partner about the fetal status and labour progress. Provide them with frequent updates on the condition of the woman and the fetus. Assess the woman's ability to cope with stronger contractions. Provide support and encouragement as indicated.

After a very long day, Jennifer gives birth to a healthy baby boy with Apgar scores of 9 at 1 minute and 10 at 5 minutes. When transferring her to the postpartum unit, what information is essential to include for the accepting nurse? What specific nursing information should be given to the nursery nurse regarding the labouring experience? With such a lengthy labour, what assessments might the postpartum nurse be especially focused on for the first few hours after birth?

Intrauterine Fetal Demise

When an unborn life suddenly ends with fetal loss, the family members are profoundly affected. The sudden loss of an expected child is tragic and the family's grief can be very intense: it can leave families struggling with a variety of mental health challenges (Bennett, Litz, Maguen, et al., 2008).

Fetal death can be due to numerous conditions, such as infection, hypertension, advanced maternal age, maternal obesity, multiple pregnancy, diabetes, congenital anomalies, umbilical cord accident, placental abruption, hemorrhage, or coagulopathies; or it may go unexplained (PHAC, 2008). Early pregnancy loss (less than 20 weeks' gestation) may be through a spontaneous abortion (miscarriage), an induced abortion (therapeutic abortion), or a ruptured ectopic pregnancy. A wide spectrum of feelings

Nursing Care Plan 21.1

OVERVIEW OF THE WOMAN UNDERGOING LABOUR INDUCTION

Rose, a 29-year-old primipara, is admitted to the labour and birth suite at 40 weeks' gestation for induction of labour. Assessment reveals that her cervix is ripe and 80% effaced, and dilated to 2 cm. Rose says, "I'm a bit nervous about being induced. I've never been through labour before and I'm afraid that I'll have a lot of pain from the medicine used to start the contractions." She consents to being induced but wants reassurance that this procedure won't harm the baby. Upon examination, the fetus is engaged and in a cephalic presentation, with the vertex as the presenting part. Her partner is at her side. Induction is initiated with oxytocin. Rose reports that contractions have started and are beginning to get stronger.

NURSING DIAGNOSIS: Anxiety related to induction of labour and lack of experience with labour *as evidenced by statements about being nervous, not having gone through labour before, and fear of pain*

Outcome Identification and Evaluation
Client will experience decrease in anxiety as evidenced by ability to verbalize understanding of procedures involved and use of positive coping skills to reduce anxious state.

Interventions: Minimizing Anxiety
- Provide a clear explanation of the labour induction process *to provide client and partner with a knowledge base.*
- Maintain continuous physical presence *to provide physical and emotional support and demonstrate concern for maternal and fetal well-being.*
- Explain each procedure before carrying it out and answer questions *to promote understanding of procedure and rationale for use and decrease fears of the unknown.*
- Review with client measures used in the past to deal with stressful situations *to determine effectiveness;* encourage use of past effective coping strategies *to aid in controlling anxiety.*
- Instruct client's partner in helpful measures to assist client in coping and encourage their use *to foster joint participation in the process and feelings of being in control and to provide support to the client.*
- Offer frequent reassurance of fetal status and labour progress *to help alleviate client's concerns and foster continued participation in the labour process.*

NURSING DIAGNOSIS: Risk for injury (maternal or fetal) related to induction procedure *as evidenced by client's concerns about fetal well-being and possible adverse effects of oxytocin administration*

Outcome Identification and Evaluation
Client will remain free of complications associated with induction *as evidenced by progression of labour as expected, delivery of healthy newborn, and absence of signs and symptoms of maternal and fetal adverse effects.*

Interventions: Promoting Maternal and Fetal Safety
- Follow agency's protocol for medication use and infusion rate *to ensure accurate, safe drug administration.*
- Set up oxytocin IV infusion to piggyback into the primary IV infusion line *to allow for prompt discontinuation should adverse effects occur.*
- Use an infusion pump *to deliver accurate dose as ordered.*
- Gradually increase oxytocin dose in increments of 1 to 2 mU/minute every 30 to 60 minutes based on assessment findings and protocol *to promote effective uterine contractions.*
- Maintain oxytocin rate once desired frequency of contractions has been reached *to ensure continued progress in labour.*
- Accurately monitor contractions for frequency, duration, and intensity and resting tone *to prevent development of hypertonic contractions.*
- Monitor FHR via continuous electronic fetal monitoring to observe the FHR response to titrated medication rate *to ensure fetal well-being and identify adverse effects immediately.*
- Obtain maternal vital signs every 1 to 2 hours or as indicated by agency's protocol, reporting any deviations, *to promote maternal well-being and allow for prompt detection of problems.*
- Communicate with birth attendant frequently concerning progress *to ensure continuity of care.*
- Discontinue oxytocin infusion if tetanic contractions (>90 seconds), uterine hyperstimulation (<2 minutes apart), elevated uterine resting tone, or an atypical or abnormal FHR pattern occurs *to minimize the risk for adverse drug effects.*
- Provide client with frequent reassurance of maternal and fetal status *to minimize anxiety.*

Nursing Care Plan 21.1 (continued)

NURSING DIAGNOSIS: Pain related to uterine contractions as evidenced by client's statements about contractions increasing in intensity and expected effect of oxytocin administration

Outcome Identification and Evaluation

Client will report a decrease in pain as evidenced by statements of increased comfort and pain rating of 3 or less on numeric pain rating scale.

Interventions: Promoting Comfort and Pain Relief

- Explain to the client that she will experience discomfort sooner than with naturally occurring labour *to promote client's awareness of events and prepare client for the experience.*
- Frequently assess client's pain using a pain rating scale *to quantify client's level of pain and evaluate effectiveness of pain-relief measures.*
- Provide comfort measures, such as hygiene, backrubs, music, and distraction, and encourage the use of breathing and relaxation techniques *to help promote relaxation.*
- Provide support for her partner *to aid in alleviating stress and concerns.*
- Employ non-pharmacologic methods, such as position changes, birthing ball, hydrotherapy, visual imagery, and effleurage, *to help manage pain and foster feelings of control over situation.*
- Administer pharmacologic agents such as analgesia or anesthesia as appropriate and as ordered *to control pain.*
- Continuously reassess client's pain level *to evaluate effectiveness of pain management techniques used.*

---

may be expressed, from relief to sadness and despair. A stillbirth can occur at any gestational age (after 20 weeks' gestation), and typically there is little or no warning other than reduced fetal movement.

The period following a fetal death is extremely difficult for the family. For many women, emotional healing takes much longer than physical healing. The feelings of loss can be intense. The grief response in some women may be so great that their relationships become strained, and healing can become hampered unless appropriate interventions and support are provided.

Fetal death also affects the health care staff. Despite the trauma that the loss of a fetus causes, some staff members avoid dealing with the bereaved family, never talking about or acknowledging their grief. This seems to imply that not discussing the problem will allow the grief to dissolve and vanish. As a result, the family's needs go unrecognized. Failing to keep the lines of communication open with a bereaved client and her family closes off some of the channels to recovery and healing that may be desperately needed. Subsequently, the bereaved family members may feel isolated.

Nursing Assessment

History and physical examination are of limited value in the diagnosis of fetal death, since the only history tends to be recent absence of fetal movement. An inability to obtain fetal heart sounds on examination suggests fetal demise, but an ultrasound is necessary to confirm the absence of fetal cardiac activity. Once fetal demise is confirmed, induction of labour is indicated.

Nursing Management

The nurse can play a major role in assisting the grieving family. With skillful intervention, the bereaved family may be better prepared to resolve their grief and move forward. To assist families in the grieving process, include the following measures:

- Provide accurate, understandable information to the family.
- Encourage discussion of the loss and venting of feelings of grief and guilt.
- Provide the family with baby mementos and pictures to validate the reality of death.
- Allow unlimited time with the stillborn infant after birth to validate the death; provide time for the family members to be together and grieve; offer the family the opportunity to see, touch, and hold the infant.
- Use appropriate touch, such as holding a hand or touching a shoulder.
- Inform the chaplain or the religious leader of the family's denomination about the death and request his or her presence.
- Assist the parents with the funeral arrangements or disposition of the body.
- Provide the parents with brochures offering advice about how to talk to other siblings about the loss.
- Refer the family to a local support group designed for those who have lost an infant through abortion, miscarriage, fetal death, stillbirth, or other tragic circumstances.
- Make community referrals to promote a continuum of care after discharge.

Women Experiencing an Obstetric Emergency

Obstetric emergencies are challenging to all labour and birth personnel because of the increased risk for adverse outcomes for the mother and fetus. Quick clinical judgment and good critical decision making will increase the odds of a positive outcome for both mother and fetus. This chapter discusses a few of these emergencies: umbilical cord prolapse, placental abruption, uterine rupture, and amniotic fluid embolism.

Umbilical Cord Prolapse

An **umbilical cord prolapse** is the protrusion of the umbilical cord alongside (occult) or ahead of the presenting part of the fetus (Fig. 21.5). This condition occurs in 0.6% of deliveries and requires prompt recognition and intervention for a positive outcome (Beall & Ross, 2012). The risk is increased further when the presenting part does not fill the lower uterine segment, as is the case with incomplete breech presentations (5% to 10%), premature infants, and multiparous women (Beall & Ross, 2012). With a 50% perinatal mortality rate, cord prolapse is one of the most catastrophic events in the intrapartum period (Rodgers & Schiavone, 2008).

Pathophysiology

Prolapse usually leads to total or partial occlusion of the cord. Since this is the fetus's only lifeline, fetal perfusion deteriorates rapidly. Complete occlusion renders the fetus helpless and oxygen-deprived. The fetus will die if the cord compression is not relieved.

Nursing Assessment

Prevention is the key to managing cord prolapse by identifying clients at risk for this condition. Carefully assess each client to help predict her risk status. Be aware that cord prolapse is more common in pregnancies involving mal-presentation, prematurity, ruptured membranes with a fetus at a high station, polyhydramnios, grand multiparity, and multifetal gestation (Beall & Ross, 2012). Continuously assess the client and fetus to detect changes and to evaluate the effectiveness of any interventions performed.

▶ **Take** NOTE!

When the presenting part does not fully occupy the pelvic inlet, prolapse is more likely to occur.

Nursing Management

Prompt recognition of a prolapsed cord is essential to reduce the risk for fetal hypoxia resulting from prolonged cord compression. When membranes are artificially ruptured, assist with verifying that the presenting part is well applied to the cervix and engaged into the pelvis. If pressure or compression of the cord occurs, assist with measures to relieve the compression. Typically, the examiner places a sterile gloved hand into the vagina and holds the presenting part of the umbilical cord until delivery. Changing the woman's position to a modified Sims, Trendelenburg, or knee–chest position also helps relieve cord pressure. Monitor FHR, maintain bed rest, and administer oxygen if ordered. Provide emotional support and explanations as to what is going on to allay the woman's fears and anxiety. If the mother's cervix is not fully dilated, prepare the woman for an emergency cesarean birth to save the fetus's life.

Placental Abruption

Placental abruption refers to premature separation of a normally implanted placenta from the maternal myometrium. Placental abruption occurs in about 1% of all

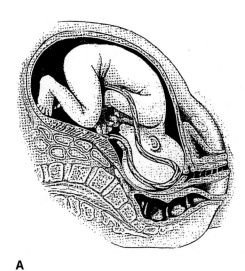

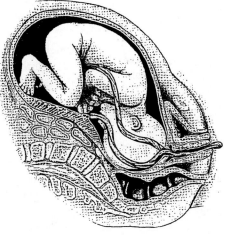

A   B

FIGURE 21.5 Prolapsed cord.
(**A**) Prolapse within the uterus.
(**B**) Prolapse with the cord visible at the vulva.

pregnancies throughout the world. Risk factors include hypertensive disorders, intrauterine growth restriction, prolonged rupture of membranes, chorioamnionitis, advanced maternal age, seizure activity, uterine rupture, trauma, smoking, cocaine use, coagulation defects, previous history of abruption, trauma (including domestic violence), and placental pathology. These conditions may force blood into the underlayer of the placenta and cause it to detach (Neilson, 2003).

Management of placental abruption depends on the gestational age, the extent of the hemorrhage, and maternal–fetal oxygenation perfusion/reserve status (see Chapter 19 for additional information on abruptio placenta). Treatment is based on the circumstances. Typically once the diagnosis is established, the focus is on maintaining the cardiovascular status of the mother and developing a plan to deliver the fetus quickly. A cesarean birth takes place if the fetus is still alive. A vaginal birth may take place if there is fetal demise.

Uterine Rupture

Uterine rupture is a catastrophic tearing of the uterine wall into the abdominal cavity. Its onset is often marked only by sudden fetal bradycardia, and treatment requires rapid surgery for good outcomes. From the time of diagnosis to delivery, only 10 to 37 minutes are available before clinically significant fetal morbidity occurs. Fetal morbidity occurs secondary to catastrophic hemorrhage, fetal anoxia, or both (Nahum & Pham, 2010).

Nursing Assessment

Review the mother's history for risk conditions such as previous uterine surgery (including cesarean section), prior rupture, trauma, prior invasive molar pregnancy, history of placenta percreta or increta, malpresentation, labour induction with excessive uterine stimulation, dystocia, overdistended uterus (multiple gestation or polyhydramnios), and crack cocaine use (Nahum & Pham, 2010). Reviewing a client's history for risk factors might prove to be life-saving for both mother and fetus.

Generally, the first and most reliable symptom of uterine rupture is sudden fetal distress. Other signs may include decreased baseline uterine pressure, loss of uterine contractility, abdominal pain with or without an epidural, hemorrhage, irregular abdominal wall contour, loss of station in the fetal presenting part, and hypovolemic shock in the woman, fetus, or both (Nahum & Pham, 2010).

Timely management of uterine rupture depends on prompt detection. Because many women desire a trial of labour after a previous cesarean birth, the nurse must be familiar with the signs and symptoms of uterine rupture. It is difficult to prevent uterine rupture or to predict which women will experience rupture, so constant preparedness is necessary.

Screening all women with previous uterine surgical scars is important, and continuous electronic fetal monitoring should be used during labour because this may provide the only indication of an impending rupture.

Nursing Management

Because the presenting signs may be nonspecific, the initial management will be the same as that for any other cause of acute fetal distress. Urgent delivery by cesarean birth is usually indicated. Monitor maternal vital signs and observe for hypotension and tachycardia, which might indicate hypovolemic shock. Assist in preparing for an emergency cesarean birth by alerting the operating room staff, anesthesia provider, and neonatal team. Insert an indwelling urinary (Foley) catheter if one is not in place already. Inform the woman of the seriousness of this event and remind her that the health care staff will be working quickly to ensure her health and that of her fetus. Remain calm and provide reassurance that everything is being done to ensure a safe outcome for both.

The life-threatening nature of uterine rupture is underscored by the fact that the maternal circulatory system delivers approximately 500 mL of blood to the term uterus every minute. Maternal death is a real possibility without rapid intervention. Newborn outcome after rupture depends largely on the speed with which surgical rescue is carried out.

▶ **Take** NOTE!

When excessive bleeding occurs during the childbirth process and it persists or signs such as bruising or petechiae appear, disseminated intravascular coagulation (DIC) should be suspected.

Amniotic Fluid Embolism

Amniotic fluid embolism is a rare and often fatal event characterized by the sudden onset of hypotension, hypoxia, and coagulopathy. Amniotic fluid containing particles of debris (e.g., hair, skin, vernix, or meconium) enters the maternal circulation and obstructs the pulmonary vessels, causing respiratory distress and circulatory collapse (Spiliopoulos, Puri, Neetu, et al., 2009). The incidence is approximately 1 case per 8,000 to 80,000 pregnancies. Due to improvements in early recognition and treatment, the maternal mortality rate has decreased to 61% (Toy, 2009).

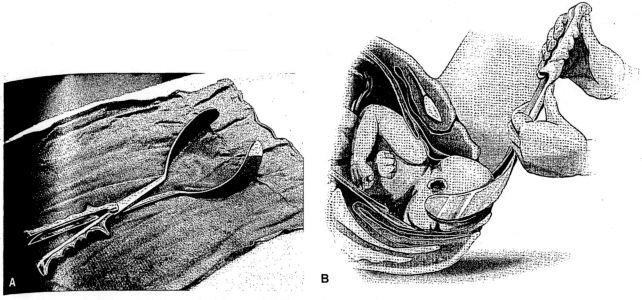

FIGURE 21.6 Forceps delivery. (**A**) Example of forceps. (**B**) Forceps being applied to the fetus.

When caring for the woman who is receiving an amnioinfusion, include the following:

- Explain the need for the procedure, what it involves, and how it may solve the problem.
- Inform the mother that she will need to remain on bed rest during the procedure.
- Assess the mother's vital signs and associated discomfort level.
- Maintain intake and output records.
- Assess the duration and intensity of uterine contractions frequently to identify overdistention or increased uterine tone.
- Monitor the FHR pattern to determine whether the amnioinfusion is improving the fetal status.
- Prepare the mother for a possible cesarean birth if the FHR does not improve after the amnioinfusion.

Forceps- or Vacuum-Assisted Birth

Forceps or a vacuum extractor may be used to apply traction to the fetal head or to provide a method of rotating the fetal head during birth. **Forceps** are stainless-steel instruments, similar to tongs, with rounded edges that fit around the fetus's head. Some forceps have open blades and some have solid blades. Outlet forceps are used when the fetal head is crowning and low forceps are used when the fetal head is at a +2 station or lower but not yet crowning. The forceps are applied to the sides of the fetal head. The type of forceps used is determined by the birth attendant. All forceps have a locking mechanism that prevents the blades from compressing the fetal skull (Fig. 21.6).

A **vacuum extractor** is a cup-shaped instrument attached to a suction pump used for extraction of the fetal head (Fig. 21.7). The suction cup is placed against

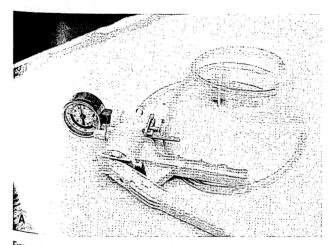
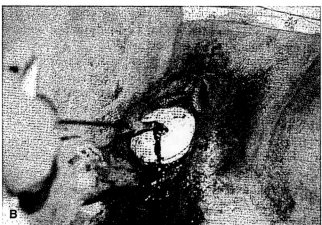

FIGURE 21.7 Vacuum extractor for delivery. (**A**) Example of a vacuum extractor. (**B**) Vacuum extractor applied to the fetal head to assist in delivery.

the occiput of the fetal head. The pump is used to create negative pressure (suction) of approximately 50 to 60 mm Hg. The birth attendant then applies traction until the fetal head emerges from the vagina.

According to the SOGC, the indications for the use of either method are similar and include a prolonged second stage of labour, abnormal FHR pattern, failure of the presenting part to fully rotate to the occiput anterior position, presumed fetal jeopardy or fetal compromise, maternal heart disease, maternal cerebrovascular malformations, and maternal fatigue (Cargill & MacKinnon, 2004).

The use of forceps or a vacuum extractor poses the risk for tissue trauma to the mother and the newborn. Maternal trauma may include lacerations of the cervix, vagina, or perineum; hematoma; extension of the episiotomy incision into the anus; hemorrhage; and infection. Potential newborn trauma includes ecchymosis, facial and scalp lacerations, facial nerve injury, cephalhematoma, intracranial hemorrhage, and caput succedaneum (Cargill & MacKinnon, 2004).

Prevention is the key to reducing the use of these techniques. Preventive measures include frequently changing the client's position, encouraging upright posture and ambulation if permitted, frequently reminding the client to empty her bladder to allow maximum space for birth, and providing adequate hydration throughout labour. Additional measures include assessing maternal vital signs, the contraction pattern, the fetal status, and the maternal response to the procedure. Provide a thorough explanation of the procedure and the rationale for its use. Reassure the mother that any marks or swelling on the newborn's head or face will disappear without treatment within 2 to 3 days. Alert the postpartum nursing staff about the use of the technique so that they can observe for any bleeding or infection related to genital lacerations.

Cesarean Birth

A **cesarean birth** is the delivery of the fetus through an incision in the abdomen and uterus. A classic (vertical) or low transverse incision may be used; today, the low transverse incision is more common (Fig. 21.8).

The number of cesarean births has risen steadily in Canada; approximately 26% of infants are delivered via this method today compared with approximately 17% in 1996 (PHAC, 2008). Several factors may explain the increased incidence of cesarean deliveries, including the widespread use of continuous electronic fetal monitoring, which identifies fetal distress early; the reduced number of forceps-assisted births; maternal obesity; older maternal age and reduced parity, with more nulliparous women having infants; convenience to the client and doctor; elective repeat cesarean sections; elective cesarean section for breech presentation as a result of the Term Breech Trial; and attitudes of clients, nurses, and physicians about birth

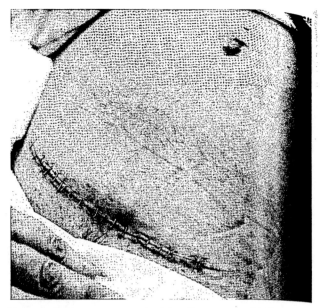

FIGURE 21.8 Low transverse incision for cesarean birth.

(Hewer, Boschma, & Hall, 2009; Kotaska, Menticoglou, & Gagnon, 2009; PHAC, 2008).

High cesarean birth rates are an international concern. Cesarean birth is a major surgical procedure with a fourfold increase in mortality compared with a vaginal birth. The client is at risk for complications such as infection, hemorrhage, aspiration, venous thromboembolus, and bowel and urinary tract trauma. Fetal injury and respiratory difficulty for the newborn also may occur (Cargill & MacKinnon, 2004).

Spinal, epidural, or general anesthesia is used for cesarean births. Epidural anesthesia is most commonly used today because it is associated with less risk and most women wish to be awake and aware of the birth experience.

Nursing Assessment

Review the woman's history for indications associated with cesarean birth and complete a physical examination. Any condition that obstructs or prevents the safe passage of the fetus through the birth canal or that seriously compromises maternal or fetal well-being may be an indication for a cesarean birth. Examples include active genital herpes, suspected fetopelvic disproportion after a trial of labour, prolapsed umbilical cord, placental abnormality (placenta previa or abruptio placentae), previous classic uterine incision or scar, HIV in women who have not received optimal anti-retroviral therapy or who choose an elective cesarean section, and dystocia. Fetal indications include malpresentation, congenital anomalies (neural tube defects, hydrocephalus), and fetal compromise (Joy & Contag, 2011).

Nursing Management

Once the decision has been made to proceed with a cesarean birth, assess the woman's knowledge of the procedure and necessary preparation. Assist with obtaining diagnostic tests as ordered. These tests are usually ordered to ensure the well-being of both parties and may include a complete blood count; blood type and cross-match so that blood is available for transfusion if needed; and an ultrasound to determine fetal position and placental location.

Although the nurse's role in a cesarean birth can be very technical and skill-oriented at times, the focus must remain on the woman, not the equipment surrounding the bed. Care should be centred on the family, not the surgery. Provide education and minimize separation of the mother, father, and newborn. Remember that the client is anxious and concerned about her welfare as well as that of her child. Use touch, eye contact, therapeutic communication, and genuine caring to provide couples with a positive birth experience, regardless of the type of delivery.

Providing Preoperative Care

Client preparation varies depending on whether the cesarean birth is planned or unplanned. The major difference is the time allotted for preparation and teaching. In an unplanned cesarean birth, institute measures quickly to ensure the best outcomes for the mother and the fetus. Ensure that the woman has signed an informed consent, and allow for discussion of fears and expectations. Provide essential teaching and explanations to reduce the woman's fears and anxieties.

Ascertain the client's and family's understanding of the surgical procedure. Reinforce the reasons for surgery given by the surgeon. Outline the procedure and expectations of the surgical experience. Ensure that all diagnostic tests ordered have been completed, and evaluate the results. Explain to the woman and her family about what to expect postoperatively. Reassure the woman that pain management will be provided throughout the procedure and afterward. Encourage the woman to report any pain.

Ask the woman about the time she last had anything to eat or drink. Document the time and what was consumed. Throughout the preparations, assess maternal and fetal status frequently.

Provide preoperative teaching to reduce the risk for postoperative complications. Demonstrate the use of the incentive spirometer and deep-breathing and leg exercises. Instruct the woman on how to splint her incision.

Complete the preoperative procedures, which may include:

• Preparing the surgical site as ordered
• Starting an intravenous infusion for fluid replacement therapy as ordered
• Inserting an indwelling (Foley) catheter and informing the client about how long it will remain in place (usually 24 hours)
• Administering any preoperative medications as ordered; documenting the time administered and the client's reaction

Maintain a calm, confident manner in all interactions with the client and the family. Help transport the client and her partner to the operative area.

Providing Postoperative Care

Postoperative care for the mother who has had a cesarean delivery is similar to that for one who has had a vaginal birth, with a few additional measures. Assess vital signs and lochia flow every 15 minutes for the first hour, then every 30 minutes for the next hour, and then every 4 hours if stable. Assist with perineal care and instruct the client in the same. Inspect the abdominal dressing and document the description, including any evidence of drainage. Assess uterine tone to determine fundal firmness. Check the patency of the intravenous line, making sure the infusion is flowing at the correct rate. Inspect the infusion site frequently for redness.

Assess the woman's level of consciousness if sedative drugs were administered. Institute safety precautions until the woman is fully alert and responsive. If a regional anesthetic was used, monitor for the return of sensation to the legs.

Assess for evidence of abdominal distention and auscultate bowel sounds. Assist with early ambulation to prevent respiratory and cardiovascular problems and to promote peristalsis. Monitor intake and output at least every 4 hours initially and then every 8 hours as indicated.

Encourage the woman to cough, perform deep-breathing exercises, and use the incentive spirometer every 2 hours. Administer analgesics as ordered and provide comfort measures, such as splinting the incision and pillows for positioning. Assist the client to move in bed and turn side to side to improve circulation. Also encourage the woman to ambulate to promote venous return from the extremities.

Encourage early touching and holding of the newborn to promote bonding. Assist with breastfeeding initiation and offer continued support. Suggest alternate positioning techniques to reduce incisional discomfort while breastfeeding.

Review with the couple their perception of the surgical birth experience. Allow them to verbalize their feelings and assist them in positive coping measures. Prior to discharge, teach the woman about the need for adequate rest, activity restrictions such as lifting, and signs and symptoms of infection.

Vaginal Birth After Cesarean

Vaginal birth after cesarean describes a woman who gives birth vaginally after having at least one previous cesarean birth. SOGC guidelines suggest that most women who have had a cesarean birth are candidates for vaginal birth and should be offered a trial of labour for subsequent pregnancies (Martel & MacKinnon, 2005).

The choice of a vaginal or a repeat cesarean birth can be offered to women who had a lower abdominal incision. However, controversy remains. The argument against VBAC focuses on the risk for uterine rupture and hemorrhage. Although the risk for uterine rupture is relatively low, 1 in 200, the rate of fetal mortality in the event of a uterine rupture is extremely high (Nahum & Pham, 2010).

Contraindications to VBAC include a prior classic uterine incision, prior hysterotomy or myomectomy, previous uterine rupture, or the presence of a contraindication to labour (Martel & MacKinnon, 2005). Most women go through a trial of labour to see how they progress, but this must be performed in an environment capable of providing continuous electronic fetal monitoring and cesarean section if needed. The use of prostaglandin E2 and misoprostol (Cytotec) increases the risk for uterine rupture and thus is not recommended in VBAC clients. The woman considering induction of labour after a previous cesarean birth needs to be informed of the increased risk for uterine scar dehiscence with an induction than with spontaneous labour (Martel & MacKinnon, 2005).

Women are the primary decision makers about the choice of birth method, but they need education about VBAC during their prenatal course. Management is similar for any women experiencing labour, but certain areas require special focus:

- Consent: fully informed consent is essential for the woman who wants to have a trial of labour after cesarean birth. The client must be advised about the risks as well as the benefits. She must understand the ramifications of uterine rupture, even though the risk is small.
- Documentation: recordkeeping is an important component of safe client care. If an emergency occurs, it is imperative not only to take care of the client but also to keep track of the plan of care, interventions and their timing, and the client's response. Events and activities can be written right on the fetal monitoring tracing to correlate with the change in fetal status.
- Surveillance: an abnormal fetal monitor tracing in a woman undergoing a trial of labour after a cesarean birth should alert the nurse to the possibility of uterine rupture. Terminal bradycardia must be considered an emergency situation, and the nurse should prepare the team for an emergency delivery.
- Readiness for emergency: according to SOGC criteria for a safe trial of labour for a woman who has had a previous cesarean birth, the physician, anesthesia provider, and operating room team must be available. Anything less would place the women and fetus at risk (Martel & MacKinnon, 2005).

Nurses must act as advocates, giving input on the appropriate selection of women who wish to undergo VBAC. Nurses also need to become experts at reading fetal monitoring tracings to identify an atypical or abnormal pattern and set in motion an emergency delivery. Including all these nursing strategies will make VBAC safer for all.

☐▨■ Key Concepts

- ▨ Risk factors for dystocia include epidural analgesia, excessive analgesia, multiple gestation, maternal exhaustion, hydramnios, ineffective pushing, unripe cervix with induction, maternal obesity, malpresentation, fetal anomalies, occiput posterior position, longer first stage of labour, nulliparity, short maternal stature, maternal age older than 35 years, gestational age more than 41 weeks, chorioamnionitis, pelvic contractions, macrosomia, and high station at complete cervical dilation.
- ▨ Dystocia may result from problems in the powers, passenger, passageway, or psyche.
- ▨ Problems involving the powers that lead to dystocia include hypertonic uterine dysfunction, hypotonic uterine dysfunction, and precipitous labour.
- ▨ Management of hypertonic labour pattern involves therapeutic rest with the use of sedatives to promote relaxation and stop the abnormal activity of the uterus.
- ▨ Any presentation other than occiput or a slight variation of the fetal position or size increases the probability of dystocia.
- ▨ Multiple gestation may result in dysfunctional labour due to uterine overdistention, which may lead to hypotonic dystocia, and abnormal presentations of the fetuses.
- ▨ During labour, evaluation of fetal descent, cervical effacement and dilation, and characteristics of uterine contractions are paramount to determine progress or lack thereof.
- ▨ Antepartum assessment for a postterm pregnancy typically includes daily fetal movement counts done by the woman, nonstress tests done twice weekly, amniotic fluid assessments as part of the biophysical profile, and weekly cervical examinations to check for ripening for induction.
- ▨ Once the cervix is ripe, oxytocin is the most popular pharmacologic agent used for inducing or augmenting labour.
- ▨ Generally, the first and most reliable symptom of uterine rupture is fetal distress.
- ▨ Amniotic fluid embolism is a rare but often fatal event characterized by the sudden onset of hypotension, hypoxia, and coagulopathy.
- ▨ Cesarean births have steadily risen in Canada; today, approximately one in four births occurs this way. Cesarean birth is a major surgical procedure and has increased risks over vaginal birth.

REFERENCES

Allen, R. H., & Gurewitsch, E. D. (2010). *Shoulder dystocia.* Retrieved February 28, 2012 from http://emedicine.medscape.com/article/1602970-overview

Bashiri, A., Burstein, E., Bar-David, J., Levy, A., & Mazor, M. (2008). Face and brow presentation: Independent risk factors. *The Journal of Maternal-Fetal and Neonatal Medicine, 21*(6), 357–360. doi:10.1080/14767050802037647

Beall, M. H., & Ross, M. G. (2012). *Umbilical cord complications.* Retrieved February 28, 2012 from http://emedicine.medscape.com/article/262470-overview

Bennett, S. M., Litz, B. T., Maguen, S., & Ehrenreich, J. T. (2008). An exploratory study of the psychological impact and clinical care of perinatal loss. *Journal of Loss and Trauma, 13*(6), 485–510. doi:10.1080/15325020802171268

Bishop, E. H. (1964). Pelvic scoring for elective induction. *Obstetrics and Gynecology, 24*(2), 267.

Blickstein, I. (2009). Induction of labour. *Journal of Maternal-Fetal and Neonatal Medicine, 22*(S2), 31–37.

Boulvain, M., Stan, C. M., & Irion, O. (2005). Membrane sweeping for induction of labour. *Cochrane Database of Systematic Reviews, 1,* CD000451. doi:10.1002/14651858.CD000451.pub2

Brownfoot, F. C., Crowther, C. A., & Middleton, P. (2008). Different corticosteroids and regimens for accelerating fetal lung maturity for women at risk for preterm birth. *Cochrane Database of Systematic Reviews, 4.* doi:10.1002/14651858.CD0006764.pub2

Cargill, Y. M., & MacKinnon, C. J. (2004). Guidelines for operative vaginal birth. *Journal of Obstetrics and Gynaecology Canada, 26*(8), 747–753.

Carter, B. S., & Boyd, R. L. (2012). *Pediatric polyhydramnios and oligohydramnios.* Retrieved February 28, 2012 from http://www.emedicine.com/ped/topic1854.htm

Caughey, A. B., & Butler, J. R. (2011). *Postterm pregnancy.* Retrieved February 28, 2012 from http://www.emedicine.medscape.com/article/261369-overview

Cheng, Y., & Caughey, A. B. (2012). Normal labor and delivery. Retrieved February 28, 2012 from http://emedicine.medscape.com/article/260036-overview

Clark, M. B., & Clark, D. A. (2010). Meconium aspiration syndrome. Retrieved February 28, 2012 from http://emedicine.medscape.com/article/974110-overview

Crane, J. M. (2001). SOGC clinical practice guideline: Induction of labour at term. *Journal of Obstetrics and Gynaecology Canada, 23*(8), 717–728. Retrieved February 28, 2012 from http://www.sogc.org/guidelines/public/107E-CPG-August2001.pdf

Cunningham, F., Leveno, K., Bloom, S., Hauth, J., Rouse, D., & Spong, C. (2010). *Williams obstetrics.* New York: McGraw-Hill.

Currell, R., Urquhart, C, Harlow, F., & Callow, L. (2009). Home uterine monitoring for detecting preterm labour. *Cochrane Database of Systematic Reviews, 4,* CD006172. doi:10.1002/14651858.CD006172

Davies, G. A. L., Maxwell, C., & McLeod, L. (2010). SOGC clinical practice guideline: Obesity in pregnancy. *Journal of Obstetrics and Gynaecology Canada, 32*(2), 165–173. Retrieved February 28, 2012 from http://www.sogc.org/guidelines/documents/gui239ECPG1002.pdf

Delaney, M., & Roggensack, A. (2008). SOGC clinical practice guideline: Guidelines for management of pregnancy at 41 + 0 to 42 + 0 weeks. *Journal of Obstetrics and Gynaecology Canada, 30*(9), 800–1810. Retrieved February 28, 2012 from http://www.sogc.org/guidelines/documents/gui214CPG0809.pdf

Fischer, R. (2011). *Breech presentation.* Retrieved February 28, 2012 from http://emedicine.medscape.com/article/262159-overview

Fletcher, G. E. (2009). *Multiple birth.* Retrieved February 28, 2012 from http://emedicine.medscape.com/article/977234-overview

Hayes, E. J., & Weinstein, L. (2008). Improving patient safety and uniformity of care by a standardized regimen for the use of oxytocin. *American Journal of Obstetrics and Gynecology, 198,* 622.e1–622.e7.

Health Canada. (2011). *Drugs and health products.* Retrieved September 1, 2011 from http://www.hc-sc.gc.ca/dhp-mps/prodpharma/index-eng.php

Hewer, N., Boschma, G., & Hall, W. A. (2009). Elective cesarean section as a transformative technological process: Players, power, and context. *Journal of Advanced Nursing, 65*(8), 1762–1771. doi:10.1111/j.1365-2648.2009.05021.x

Hofmeyr, G. J., & Hannah, M. (2010). Planned cesarean section for term breech delivery. *Cochrane Database of Systematic Reviews, 8,* CD 000166. doi:10.1002.14651858.CD000166

Hofmeyr, G. J., & Kulier, R. (2010). External cephalic version for breech presentation at term. *Cochrane Database of Systematic Reviews, 1,* CD000083. doi:10.1002/14651858.Cd000083

Hofmeyr, G. J., & Xu, H. (2010). Amnioinfusion for meconium-stained liquor in labour. *Cochrane Database of Systematic Reviews, 1,* CD000014. doi:10.1002/14651888.CD000014.pub3

Hunter, S., Hofmeyr, G. J., & Kulier, R. (2007). Hands and knees posture in late pregnancy or labour for fetal malposition (lateral or posterior). *Cochrane Database of Systematic Reviews, 4,* CD 001063. doi:10.1002/14651858.CD001063.pub3

Ishiguro, A., Namai, Y., & Yoichi, M. I. (2009). Managing "healthy" late preterm infants. *Pediatrics International, 51*(5), 720–725. doi:10.1111/j.1442-200X.2009.02837.x

Joy, S., & Contag, S. A. (2011). *Cesarean delivery.* Retrieved February 28, 2012 from http://emedicine.medscape.com/article/263424-overview#Indications

Joy, S., Scott, P. L., & Lyon, D. (2011). *Abnormal labour.* Retrieved February 28, 2012 from http://www.emedicine.medscape.com/article/273053-overview

Kho, E. M., Sadler, L., & McCowan, L. (2008). Induction of labour: A comparison between controlled-release dinoprostone vaginal pessary (Cervadil®) and dinoprostone intravaginal gel (Prostin E2®). *Australian and New Zealand Journal of Obstetrics and Gynecology, 48,* 473–477. doi:10.1111/j.1479-828X.2008.00901.x

Kiefer, D. G., & Vintzileous, A. M. (2008). The utility of fetal fibronectin in the prediction and prevention of spontaneous preterm birth. *Reviews in Obstetrics and Gynecology, 1*(3), 106–112.

Kotaska, A., Menticoglou, S., & Gagnon, R. (2009). SOGC clinical practice guideline: Vaginal delivery of breech presentation. *Journal of Obstetrics and Gynaecology Canada, 31*(6), 557–566. Retrieved February 28, 2012 from http://www.sogc.org/guidelines/documents/gui226CPG0906.pdf

Martel, M., & MacKinnon, C. J. (2005). SOGC clinical practice guideline: Guidelines for a vaginal birth after previous Caesarean birth. *Journal of Obstetrics and Gynaecology Canada, 27*(2), 164–174. Retrieved February 28, 2012 from http://www.sogc.org/guidelines/public/155E-CPG-February2005.pdf

Menon, R. (2008). Spontaneous preterm birth, a clinical dilemma: Etiologic, pathophysiologic and genetic heterogeneities and racial disparity. *Acta Obstetricia et Gynecologica Scandinavica, 87*(6), 590–600. doi:10.1080/00016340802005126

Moore, L. E. (2012). *Amniotic fluid embolism.* Retrieved February 28, 2012 from http://emedicine.medscape.com/article/253068-zoverview

Nahum, G. G., & Pham, K. Q. (2010). Uterine rupture in pregnancy. Retrieved February 28, 2012 from http://emedicine.medscape.com/article/275854-overview

Neilson, J. P. (2003). Interventions for treating placental abruption. *Cochrane Database of Systematic Reviews, 1,* CD003247. doi:10.1002/14651858.CD003247

Prieto, A. P., Badillo, M. P. C., Galán, S. M., & Ventoso, F. M. (2008). Prophylactic intrapartum transcervical amnioinfusion. *Current Women's Health Reviews, 4*(2), 133–140.

Public Health Agency of Canada. (2008). *Canadian perinatal health report, 2008 edition.* Retrieved February 28, 2012 from http://www.phac-aspc.gc.ca/publicat/2008/cphr-rspc/index-eng.php

Pundir, J., & Sinha, P. (2009). Non-diabetic macrosomia: An obstetrical dilemma. *Journal of Obstetrics and Gynecology, 29*(3), 200–205. doi:10.1080/01443610902735140

Rodgers, C., & Schiavone, N. (2008). Cord prolapse audit: Recognition, management and outcome. *British Journal of Midwifery, 16*(5), 315–318.

Romano, A. M., & Lothian, J. A. (2008). Promoting, protecting, and supporting normal birth: A look at the evidence. *Journal of Obstetric, Gynecologic, & Neonatal Nursing, 37*(1), 94–105. doi:10.1111/j.1552-6909.2007.00210.x

Ross, M. G., & Eden, R. D. (2011). *Preterm labour.* Retrieved February 28, 2012 from http://emedicine.medscape.com/article/260998-overview

Rowe, T. (2007). Fetal health surveillance: Antepartum and intrapartum consensus guideline. *Journal of Obstetrics and Gynaecology Canada, 29*(9 Suppl. 4), S1–S56.

Schmitz, T., Carnavalet, C. C., Azria, E., Lopez, E., Carbrol, D., & Goffinet, F. (2008). Neonatal outcomes of twin pregnancy according to the planned mode of delivery. *Obstetrics and Gynecology, 111*(3), 695–703. doi:10.1097/AOG.0b013e318163c435

Simkin, P. (2010). The fetal occiput posterior position: State of science and a new perspective. *BIRTH, 37*(1), 61–71.

Society of Obstetricians and Gynaecologists of Canada. (2006). *Preterm labour.* Retrieved February 28, 2012 from http://www.sogc.org/health/pdf/preterme.pdf

Society of Obstetricians and Gynaecologists of Canada. (2008). Joint policy statement on normal childbirth. *Journal of Obstetrics and Gynaecology Canada, 30*(12), 1163–1165.

Spiliopoulos, M., Puri, I., Neetu, J., Kruse, L., Mastrogiannis, D., & Dandolu, V. (2009). Amniotic fluid embolism-risk factors, maternal and neonatal outcomes. *Journal of Maternal-Fetal and Neonatal Medicine, 22*(5), 439–444. doi:10.1080/14767050902787216

Toy, H. (2009). Amniotic fluid embolism. *European Journal of General Medicine, 6*(2), 108–115.

Watts, N. (2010). High-risk labour and childbirth. In R. J. Evans, M. K. Evans, Y. M. Brown, & S. Orshan (Eds.), *Canadian maternity, newborn, & women's health.* Philadelphia: Lippincott Williams & Wilkins.

Wilson, B. L., Effken, J., & Butler, R. J. (2010). The relationship between cesarean section and labour induction. *Journal of Nursing Scholarship, 64*(4), 371–377.

Women's Health Data Directory. (2011). Premature/preterm birth. Retrieved March 6, 2012 from http://www.womenshealthdata.ca/category.aspx?catid=95&rt=1

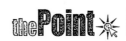

Emotional Status

Assess the woman's emotional status by observing how she interacts with her family, her level of independence, energy levels, eye contact with her infant (within a cultural context), posture and comfort level while holding the newborn, and sleep and rest patterns. Be alert for mood swings, irritability, or crying episodes.

Remember Raina and her "quiet" husband, the Muslim couple? The postpartum nurse informs Raina that her doctor, Nancy Schultz, has been called away for emergency surgery and won't be available the rest of the day. The nurse explains that Dr. Robert Nappo will be making rounds for her. Raina and her husband become upset. Why? Is culturally competent care being provided to this couple?

Bonding and Attachment

Nurses can be instrumental in promoting attachment by assessing attachment behaviours (positive and negative) and intervening appropriately if needed. Nurses must be able to identify any family discord that might interfere with the attachment process. Remember, however, that mothers from different cultures may behave differently from what is expected in your own culture. Use of herbal remedies after childbirth, for example, may be common among women of Aboriginal or Chinese descent (London et al., 2011). Don't assume that different behaviour is wrong. Engaging in conversation with the woman regarding different practices can be helpful for both the nurse and the patient in order to deepen cultural awareness.

Meeting their newborn for the first time after birth can be an exhilarating experience for parents. Although the mother has spent many hours dreaming of her unborn child and how he or she will look, it is not until after birth that they meet face to face. They both need to get to know one another and to develop feelings for one another.

Bonding is the close emotional attraction to a newborn by the parents that optimally develops during the first 30 to 60 minutes after birth. It is unidirectional, from parent to infant. It is thought that optimal bonding of the parents to a newborn requires a period of close contact within the first few minutes to a few hours after birth (Society of Obstetricians and Gynaecologists of Canada [SOGC], 2010). The mother initiates bonding when she caresses her infant and exhibits certain behaviours typical of a mother tending her child. Skin-to-skin contact, wherein the unclothed baby is next to the mother's skin, is encouraged as soon after the birth as is feasible (BCC, 2011). The infant's responses to the initial contact with the mother, including body and eye movements, are thought to be a necessary part of the process. During this initial period, the infant is in a quiet, alert state, looking directly at the holder.

▷ **Take** NOTE!

The length of time necessary for bonding depends on the health of the infant and mother as well as the circumstances surrounding the labour and birth (London et al., 2011).

Attachment is the development of strong affection between an infant and a significant other (mother, father, sibling, or caretaker) (McKinney, James, Murray, et al., 2009). The process of attachment follows a progressive or developmental course that changes over time. Attachment is an individualized and multifactorial process that differs based on the health of the infant, the mother, and environmental circumstances such as the need to care for other children (McKinney et al., 2009). It occurs through mutually satisfying experiences. Maternal attachment begins during pregnancy as the result of fetal movement and maternal fantasies about the infant and continues through the birth and postpartum periods. Attachment behaviours include seeking, staying close to, and exchanging gratifying experiences with the infant. In a high-risk pregnancy, the attachment process may be complicated by premature birth (lack of time to develop a relationship with the unborn baby) and by parental stress due to the fetal and/ or maternal vulnerability (McKinney et al., 2009).

Bonding is a vital component of the attachment process and is necessary in establishing parent–infant attachment and a healthy, loving relationship. During this early period of acquaintance, mothers touch their infants in a very characteristic manner. Mothers visually and physically "explore" their infants, initially using their fingertips on the infant's face and extremities and progressing to massaging and stroking the infant with their fingers. This is followed by palm contact on the trunk. Eventually, mothers draw their infant toward them and hold the infant. Mothers also interact with their infants through eye-to-eye contact in the *en face* position (Fig. 16.5) (McKinney et al., 2009).

Generally, research on attachment has found that the process is similar for fathers as for mothers. Fathers develop an emotional tie with their infants in a variety of ways. They seek and maintain closeness with the infant

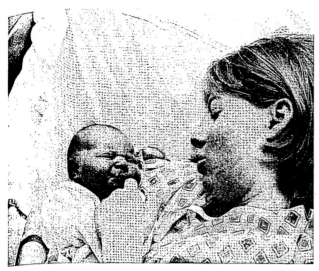

FIGURE 16.5 *En face* position.

and can recognize characteristics of the infant. Initially, the father (like the mother) will spend time inspecting the new infant and experience the euphoria that can be a part of the birth experience. For the father, attachment increases as the baby responds to him. It is important for the father to be included in the teaching and care of the infant so that his involvement will be as complete as possible (McKinney et al., 2009). Attachment is a process; it does not occur instantaneously, even though many parents believe in a romanticized version of attachment, which happens right after birth. A delay in the attachment process can occur if a mother's physical and emotional states are adversely affected by exhaustion, pain, the absence of a support system, anesthesia, or an unwanted outcome (London et al., 2011).

> ▷ **Take** *NOTE!*
>
> *Many midwives teach fathers to massage their partners, which has been proven to have a positive effect on the pregnancy, labour, bonding and attachment, and perhaps on family dynamics (Whitehouse, 2006).*

The developmental task for the infant is learning to differentiate between trust and mistrust. If the mother or caretaker is consistently responsive to the infant's care, meeting the baby's physical and psychological needs, the infant will likely learn to trust the caretaker, view the world as a safe place, and grow up to be secure, self-reliant, trusting, cooperative, and helpful. However, if the infant's needs are not met, the child is more likely to face developmental delays, neglect, and child abuse (Logsdon, Wisner, Pinto-Foltz, 2006).

"Becoming" a parent may take 4 to 6 months. The transition to parenthood involves four stages:

1. Commitment, attachment, and preparation for an infant during pregnancy, including the choice of care provider for the birth, acquiring prenatal instruction, and seeking out mentors and role models to learn about mothering behaviours.
2. Acquaintance with, and increasing attachment to, the infant, learning how to care for the infant, and physical restoration during the first weeks after birth. This phase often requires many supports from family, friends, and care providers. Women are intent on learning how to interpret their baby's cues.
3. Moving toward a new normal routine in the first 4 months after birth. Mothers gain confidence about their abilities to mother the infant based on their individual situation, as opposed to relying on textbooks or following other's instructions without question.
4. Achievement of a parenthood role around 4 months, wherein mothers have integrated the role of parent into their lives.

The stages overlap, and the timing of each is affected by variables such as the environment, family dynamics, and the partners (McKinney et al., 2009).

Factors Affecting Attachment

Attachment behaviours are influenced by three major factors:

1. Parents' background (includes the care that the parents received when growing up, cultural practices, relationship within the family, experience with previous pregnancies and planning and course of events during pregnancy, postpartum depression)
2. Infant (includes the infant's temperament and health at birth)
3. Care practices (the behaviours of physicians, midwives, nurses, and hospital personnel; care and support during labour; first day of life in separation of mother and infant; and rules of the hospital or birthing centre) (Grossman, Grossman, Waters, 2006)

Attachment occurs more readily with the infant whose temperament, health, appearance, and gender fit the parent's expectations. If the infant does not meet these expectations, parents may grieve the loss of the fantasy that they held about the infant during the pregnancy (McKinney et al., 2009).

Factors associated with the health care facility or birthing unit can also hinder attachment. These include:

- Separation of infant and parents immediately after birth and for long periods during the day
- Policies that discourage unwrapping and exploring the infant

- Intensive care environment, restrictive visiting policies
- Staff indifference or lack of support for parent's care-taking attempts and abilities

Critical Attributes of Attachment

The terms "bonding" and "attachment" are often used interchangeably, even though they involve different time frames and interactions. Bonding refers to the initial connection toward the infant that is felt by the parents during pregnancy and the initial contact 30 to 60 minutes following the birth. Attachment is a reciprocal process that continues to develop as mutually satisfying interactions occur between the parents and the child. Parents who are sensitive and responsive to their infant's cues will promote the infant's development and growth. Parents who become skilled at recognizing the ways their infant communicates will respond appropriately by smiling, vocalizing, and touching.

Maternal behaviours that facilitate attachment include:

- "Fingertipping," in which the mother explores the baby's face, fingers, and toes with her fingertips only
- Stroking the baby's chest with her palm, beginning to enfold the child, and engaging in consoling behaviours
- Beginning to identify specific features of the infant, including resemblance to family members
- Speaking to the infant in a high-pitched and soothing voice, and referring to the infant according to the child's gender rather than as "it" (McKinney et al., 2009)

In centrality, parents place the infant at the centre of their lives. They acknowledge and accept their responsibility to promote the infant's safety, growth, and development. Parent role exploration is the parents' ability to find their own way and integrate the parental identity into themselves (McKinney et al., 2009).

Positive and Negative Attachment Behaviours

Positive bonding behaviours include maintaining close physical contact, making eye-to-eye contact, speaking in soft, high-pitched tones, and touching and exploring the infant. Table 16.1 highlights typical positive and negative behaviours of attachment.

Nursing Interventions

In terms of postpartum hospital stays today, "less is more." If the woman had a vaginal delivery, she may be discharged in 24 hours or less, depending on her condition and her preferences. If she had a cesarean birth, she may remain hospitalized for 72 hours. This shortened stay leaves little time for nurses to prepare the woman and her family for the many changes that will occur when she returns home. Nurses need to use this limited time to address the following topics: pain and discomfort, immunizations, nutrition, activity and exercise, lactation, discharge teaching, sexuality and contraception, and follow-up (Nursing Care Plan 16.1).

TABLE 16.1 POSITIVE AND NEGATIVE ATTACHMENT BEHAVIOURS

	Positive Behaviours	Negative Behaviours
Infant	Smiles; is alert; demonstrates strong grasp reflex to hold parent's finger; sucks well, feeds easily; enjoys being held close; makes eye-to-eye contact; follows parent's face; appears facially appealing; is consolable when crying	Feeds poorly, regurgitates often; cries for long periods, colicky and inconsolable; shows flat affect, rarely smiles even when prompted; resists holding and closeness; sleeps with eyes closed most of the time; stiffens body when held; is unresponsive to parents; doesn't pay attention to parents' faces
Parent	Makes direct eye contact; assumes *en face* position when holding infant; claims infant as family member, pointing out common features; expresses pride in infant; assigns meaning to infant's actions; smiles and gazes at infant; touches infant, progressing from fingertips to holding; names infant; requests to be close to infant as much as allowed; speaks positively about infant	Expresses disappointment or displeasure in infant; fails to "explore" infant visually or physically; fails to claim infant as part of family; avoids caring for infant; finds excuses not to hold infant close; has negative self-concept; appears uninterested in having infant in room; frequently asks to have infant taken back to nursery to be cared for; assigns negative attributes to infant and calls infant inappropriate, negative names (e.g., frog, monkey, tadpole)

Sources: Grossman, K. E., Grossman, K., & Waters, E. (2006). *Attachment from infancy to adulthood.* New York: Guilford Publications, Inc; Nash, L. R. (2007). Postpartum care. In R. E. Rakel & E. T. Bope (Eds.), *Conn's current therapy 2007.* Philadelphia: Saunders Elsevier; & Oppenheim, D., & Goldsmith, D. F. (2007). *Attachment theory in clinical work with children: Bridging the gap between research and practice.* New York: Guilford Publications, Inc.

Nursing Care Plan 16.1

OVERVIEW OF THE POSTPARTUM WOMAN

Belinda, a 26-year-old G2P2, is a patient on the mother–baby unit after giving birth to a term 3.7 kg (8 lb, 2 oz) baby boy yesterday. The night nurse reports that she has an episiotomy, complains of a pain rating of 7 points on a scale of 1 to 10, is having difficulty breastfeeding, and had heavy lochia most of the night. The nurse also reports that the patient seems focused on her own needs and not on her infant. Assessment this morning reveals the following:

B: Breasts are soft with colostrum leaking; nipples cracked
U: Uterus is one fingerbreadth below the umbilicus; deviated to right
B: Bladder is palpable; patient states she hasn't been up to void yet
B: Bowels have not moved; bowel sounds present; passing flatus
L: Lochia is moderate; perineal pad soaked from night accumulation
E: Episiotomy site intact; swollen, bruised; hemorrhoids present

E: Extremities; no edema over tibia, no warmth or tenderness in calf
E: Emotional status is "distressed" as a result of discomfort and fatigue

NURSING DIAGNOSIS: Impaired tissue integrity related to episiotomy

Outcome Identification and Evaluation

The woman remains free of infection, without any signs and symptoms of infection, and exhibits evidence of progressive healing as demonstrated by a clean, dry, intact episiotomy site.

Interventions: Promoting Tissue Integrity

- Monitor episiotomy site *to check for redness, edema, and signs of infection.*
- Assess vital signs at least every 4 hours *to identify changes suggesting infection.*
- Apply ice pack to episiotomy site *to reduce swelling.*
- Instruct patient on use of sitz bath *to promote healing, hygiene, and comfort.*
- Encourage frequent perineal care and perineal pad changes *to prevent infection.*
- Recommend ambulation *to improve circulation and promote healing.*
- Instruct patient on positioning *to relieve pressure on perineal area.*
- Demonstrate use of anesthetic sprays *to numb perineal area.*

NURSING DIAGNOSIS: Pain related to episiotomy, sore nipples, and hemorrhoids

Outcome Identification and Evaluation

The woman experiences a decrease in pain, reporting that her pain has diminished to a tolerable level, rating it as 2 points or less.

Interventions: Providing Pain Relief

- Thoroughly inspect perineum *to rule out hematoma as cause of pain.*
- Administer analgesic medication as ordered *to promote comfort.*
- Carry out comfort measures to episiotomy as outlined earlier *to reduce pain.*
- Explain discomforts and reassure the client that they are time-limited to assist in coping with pain.
- Apply Tucks pads to swollen hemorrhoids *to induce shrinkage and reduce pain.*
- Suggest frequent use of sitz bath *to reduce hemorrhoid pain.*
- Administer stool softener and laxative *to prevent straining with first bowel movement.*
- Observe positioning and latching-on technique during breastfeeding. Offer suggestions based on observations to correct positioning/latching-on *to minimize trauma to the breast.*
- Suggest air-drying of nipples after breastfeeding and use of plain water *to prevent nipple cracking.*
- Teach relaxation techniques when breastfeeding *to reduce anxiety and discomfort.*

(continued)

Nursing Care Plan 16.1 (continued)

NURSING DIAGNOSIS: Risk for ineffective coping related to mood alteration and pain

Outcome Identification and Evaluation

The woman copes with mood alterations, as evidenced by positive statements about newborn and participation in newborn care.

Interventions: Promoting Effective Coping

- Provide a supportive, nurturing environment and encourage the mother to vent her feelings and frustrations to relieve anxiety.
- Provide opportunities for the mother to rest and sleep *to combat fatigue.*
- Encourage the mother to eat a well-balanced diet *to increase her energy level.*
- Provide reassurance and explanations that mood alterations are common after birth secondary to waning hormones after pregnancy *to increase the mother's knowledge.*
- Allow the mother relief from newborn care *to afford opportunity for self-care.*
- Discuss with partner expected behaviour from mother and how additional support and help are needed during this stressful time *to promote partner's participation in care.*
- Make appropriate community referrals for mother–infant support *to ensure continuity of care.*
- Encourage frequent skin-to-skin contact and closeness between mother and infant *to facilitate bonding and attachment behaviours.*
- Encourage client to participate in infant care and provide instructions as needed *to foster a sense of independence and self-esteem.*
- Offer praise and reinforcement of positive mother–infant interactions *to enhance self-confidence in care.*

▷ *Take NOTE!*

Always adhere to standard precautions when providing direct care to reduce the risk of disease transmission.

Providing Optimal Cultural Care

As Canadian culture becomes more diverse, nurses must be prepared to care for childbearing families from various cultures. In many cultures, women and their families are cared for and nurtured by their community for weeks and even months after the birth of a new family member. Box 16.3 highlights some of the major cultural variants during the postpartum period.

Many Aboriginal women from remote areas are encouraged to relocate to major centres to await the birth of a child, since their home communities are not seen as having the appropriate resources to deliver babies. These women may experience a sense of social and cultural isolation from family and loved ones and may be separated from their other children or partners. The SOGC (2010) recommends a new model of care for women whose pregnancies are considered low risk so that they can stay in their home communities and be attended by local health care providers such as midwives or physicians. Resource development in remote communities (in the form of trained care providers) would be necessary before the current model of care could be changed (SOGC, 2010). Nurses need to remember that childbearing practices and beliefs vary across cultures. To provide appropriate nursing care, the nurse should determine the patient's preferences before intervening. Cultural practices may include dietary restrictions, certain clothes, taboos, activities for maintaining mental health, and the use of silence, prayer, or meditation.

Raina and her husband are upset at the thought of having a male doctor care for her because Muslim women are very modest and prefer having a same-sex care provider. What should the nurse do in this situation?

Promoting Comfort

The postpartum woman may have discomfort and pain from a variety of sources, such as an episiotomy, perineal lacerations, an edematous perineum, inflamed hemorrhoids, engorged breasts, afterbirth pains secondary to uterine contractions in breastfeeding and multiparous mothers, and sore nipples if breastfeeding. Non-pharmacologic and pharmacologic measures can be used to decrease pain and discomfort. See Evidence-based Practice 16.1.

Applications of Cold and Heat

Commonly, an ice pack is the first measure used after a vaginal birth to relieve perineal discomfort from edema,

French Canadian

Traditional French Canadian culture is comprised of people of European and Aboriginal heritage. Historically, contraceptive practices in French Canada were closely tied with the Roman Catholic religion. However, that is no longer the case and women today exercise conscious health and lifestyle decision making. In recent years, "francophones" of other origins who are French speaking (such as people from French-speaking African countries) also comprise French Canadian culture. If the nurse has the ability, speaking French with the family is a helpful way to include the extended family and connect with community resources (Evans et al., 2010).

- The practice of "la culbute" is when a parent holds the baby above the crib and rotates him or her in hopes that the infant will sleep during the night and be awake during the day.

First Nations

Aboriginal women comprise a diverse population in which unique cultural practices may be passed down using the oral tradition. Cultural practices may therefore be communicated among specific groups and may differ from one another. Because these cultural practices are communicated orally, it is important for the nurse to gain understanding by direct communication with the mother and her family (L. Barney, personal communication, January 20, 2011).

The importance of extended family is deeply embedded in the traditions and beliefs of Aboriginal people. Therefore, the nurse should consider individual accommodations such as encouraging the elder woman to be present when needed. The person who will be the infant's primary caregiver (which may not be the mother) should be included in all teaching. Health care services, in general, attempt to accommodate traditional native healing practices whenever possible, as those practices attempt to foster harmony with the environment and with the family (Evans et al., 2010).

Asian

The term "Asian" refers to people from Korea, China, Japan, the Philippines, and Southeast Asia. The importance of family is a core value, as are honour and harmony. In general, mothers of Asian descent tend to exhibit more protective behaviour of their children compared with Western approaches. The authority of the elders is unquestioned (Evans et al., 2010).

Japanese

- Cleanliness and protection from cold are essential components of newborn care. Nurses should give the daily bath to the infant.
- Newborns routinely are not taken outside the home because it is believed that they should not be exposed to outside or cold air. Infants should be kept in a quiet, clean, warm place for the first month of life.
- Breastfeeding is the primary method of feeding.
- Many women stay in their parents' home for 1 to 2 months after birth.
- Bathing the infant can be the centre of family activity at home (Bowers, 2007).

Filipino

- Grandparents often assist in the care of their grandchildren.
- Breastfeeding is encouraged, and some mothers breastfeed their children for up to 2 years.
- Women have difficulty discussing birth control and sexual matters.
- Strong religious beliefs prevail, and bedside prayer is common.
- Families are very close-knit, and numerous visitors can be expected at the hospital after childbirth (Srivastava, 2007).

Hispanic

People from Latin America, Central America, and South America are represented by the term "Hispanic." The Hispanic culture is primarily patriarchal, but in matters of health the woman usually makes the decisions, as her role is to care for the women and children. Often the extended family members are consulted before the medical community in case of illness. Home remedies and folk remedies may be valued (Evans et al., 2010).

Mexican

- The newborn's grandmother lives with the mother for several weeks after birth to help with housekeeping and child care.
- Most women will breastfeed more than 1 year. The infant is carried in a *rebozo* (shawl) that allows easy access for breastfeeding.
- Women may avoid eye contact and may not feel comfortable being touched by a stranger. Nurses need to respect this feeling.
- Some women may bring religious icons to the hospital and may want to display them in their room (Srivastava, 2007).

Muslim

Muslim families are patriarchal, but within the marriage the woman may have considerable influence over decision making. Culturally, the birth of a child is welcomed, as it promotes family status. Because Muslim women are concerned with modesty, they may have a preference for female birth attendants only (Evans et al., 2010).

- Modesty is a primary concern; nurses need to protect the client's modesty.
- Muslims are not permitted to eat pork; check all food items before serving.
- Male–female touching is prohibited except in an emergency situation.
- A Muslim woman stays in the house for 40 days after birth, being cared for by the female members of her family.
- Most Muslim women will breastfeed, but religious events call for periods of fasting, which may increase the risk of dehydration or malnutrition.
- Women are exempt from obligatory five-times-daily prayers as long as lochia is present.
- Extended family is likely to be present throughout much of the woman's hospital stay. They will need an empty room to perform their prayers without having to leave the hospital (Cassar, 2006).

EVIDENCE-BASED PRACTICE 16.1
Administration of Paracetamol (Acetaminophen) to Relieve Postpartum Perineal Pain

The perineum often incurs trauma following a vaginal delivery because of the stretching and/or tearing of tissue that occurs during the birth, especially if forceps or vacuum extraction is used or an episiotomy has been performed. Perineal pain and swelling can interfere with mobilization, breastfeeding positioning, and general well-being of new mothers.

● Study

Because the discomfort in the sensitive perineal area has the potential to diminish the quality of experience in the important first few days of the postpartum period, a meta-analysis of studies was conducted to ascertain whether administration of acetaminophen (at a dose of 500 to 1,000 mg) would alleviate discomfort in the perineal region.

It is important to note that this medication is generally assumed to be safe with breastfeeding.

▲ Findings

The use of acetaminophen was more effective than the placebo for treating perineal pain.

▦ Nursing Implications

This study concluded that women should be offered pain relief for perineal pain, even though some women may choose to decline it. It appears that a dose of either 500 or 1,000 mg of acetaminophen is effective, and there does not appear to be any rise in adverse effects if the medication is used according to instructions. Women can also be reassured that the medication does not pose a heightened risk to their breastfeeding newborn.

Source: Chou, D., Abalos, E., Gyte, G. M. L., Gülmezoglu, A. M. (2010). Paracetamol/acetaminophen (single administration) for perineal pain in the early postpartum period [review]. *The Cochrane Library,* 3:CD008407

an episiotomy, or laceration. It is applied during the fourth stage of labour and can be used for the first 24 hours to reduce perineal edema and prevent hematoma formation, thus reducing pain and promoting healing. Ice packs are wrapped in a disposable covering or clean washcloth and are applied to the perineal area. Usually the ice pack is applied for 20 minutes and removed for 10 minutes. Many commercially prepared ice packs are available, but a latex glove filled with crushed ice and covered can also be used if the mother is not allergic to latex. Ensure that the ice pack is changed frequently to promote good hygiene and to allow for periodic assessments.

The **peri bottle** is a plastic squeeze bottle filled with warm tap water that is sprayed over the perineal area after each voiding and before applying a new perineal pad. Usually the peri bottle is introduced to the woman when she is assisted to the bathroom to freshen up and void for the first time—in most instances, once vital signs are stable after the first hour. Provide the woman with instructions on how and when to use the peri bottle. Reinforce this practice each time she changes her pad, voids, or defecates, making sure that she understands to direct the flow of water from front to back. The woman can take the peri bottle home and use it over the next several weeks until her lochia discharge stops. The peri bottle can be used by women who had either vaginal or cesarean births to provide comfort and hygiene to the perineal area.

After the first 24 hours, a **sitz bath** with warm water may be prescribed and substituted for the ice pack to reduce local swelling and promote comfort for

an episiotomy, perineal trauma, or inflamed hemorrhoids. The change from cold to warm therapy enhances vascular circulation and healing (London et al., 2011). Before using a sitz bath, the woman should cleanse the perineum with a peri bottle or take a shower using mild soap.

Most health care agencies use plastic disposable sitz baths that women can take home. The plastic sitz bath

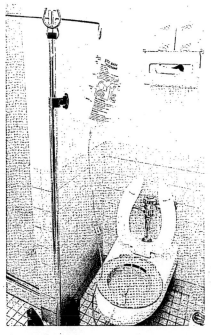

FIGURE 16.6 Sitz bath setup.

consists of a basin that fits on the commode; a bag filled with warm water is hung on a hook and connected via a tube onto the front of the basin (Fig. 16.6). Teaching Guideline 16.1 highlights the steps in using a sitz bath.

Advise the woman to use the sitz bath several times daily to provide hygiene and comfort to the perineal area. Encourage her to continue this measure after discharge.

Keep in mind that tremendous hemodynamic changes are taking place within the mother during this early postpartum period, and her safety must be a priority. Fatigue, blood loss, the effects of medications, and lack of food may cause her to feel weak when she stands up. Assisting the woman to the bathroom to instruct her on how to use the peri bottle and sitz bath is necessary to ensure her safety. Many women become lightheaded or dizzy when they get out of bed and need direct physical assistance. Staying in the woman's room, ensuring that the emergency call light is readily available, and being available if needed during this early period will ensure safety and prevent accidents and falls.

Topical Preparations

Several treatments may be applied topically for temporary relief of pain and discomfort. One such treatment is a

local anesthetic spray such as Dermoplast or Americaine. These agents numb the perineal area and are used after cleansing the area with water via the peri bottle and/or a sitz bath.

For hemorrhoid discomfort, cool witch hazel pads, such as Tucks Medicated Pads, can be used. The pads are placed at the rectal area, between the hemorrhoids and the perineal pad. These pads cool the area, help relieve swelling, and minimize itching.

Analgesics

Analgesics such as acetaminophen (Tylenol) and oral nonsteroidal anti-inflammatory drugs (NSAIDs) such as ibuprofen (Motrin) are prescribed to relieve mild postpartum discomfort. For moderate to severe pain, a narcotic analgesic such as codeine or oxycodone in conjunction with aspirin or acetaminophen may be prescribed. Instruct the woman about the possible adverse effects of any medication prescribed. Common adverse effects of oral opioid analgesics include dizziness, lightheadedness, nausea and vomiting, constipation, urinary retention, myoclonus, and sedation (Potter & Perry, 2010).

Also inform the woman that the drugs are secreted in breast milk. Nearly all medications that the mother takes are passed into her breast milk; however, mild analgesics (e.g., acetaminophen or ibuprofen) are considered relatively safe for breastfeeding mothers (Moretti, Lee, Ito, 2000). Administering a mild analgesic approximately an hour before breastfeeding will usually relieve afterpains and/or perineal discomfort.

Assisting with Elimination

The bladder is edematous, hypotonic, and congested immediately postpartum. Consequently, bladder distention, incomplete emptying, and inability to void are common. A full bladder interferes with uterine contraction and may lead to hemorrhage because it will displace the uterus out of the midline. Encourage the woman to void. Often, assisting her to assume the normal voiding position on the commode facilitates this. If the woman has difficulty voiding, pouring warm water over the perineal area, listening to the sound of running tap water, blowing bubbles through a straw, taking a warm shower, drinking fluids, or placing her hand in a basin of warm water may stimulate the urge to void. If these actions do not stimulate urination within 4 to 6 hours after giving birth, catheterization may be needed. Palpate the bladder for distention and ask the woman if she is voiding in small amounts (less than 100 mL) frequently (retention with overflow). If catheterization is necessary, use sterile technique to reduce the risk of infection.

Decreased bowel motility during labour, high iron content in prenatal vitamins, postpartum fluid loss, and the adverse effects of pain medications and/or anesthesia may predispose the postpartum woman to constipation.

TEACHING GUIDELINE 16.1

Using a Sitz Bath

1. Close clamp on tubing before filling bag with water to prevent leakage.
2. Fill sitz bath basin and plastic bag with warm water (comfortable to touch).
3. Place the filled basin on the toilet with the seat raised and the overflow opening facing toward the back of the toilet.
4. Hang the filled plastic bag on a hook close to the toilet or on an IV pole.
5. Attach the tubing to the opening on the basin.
6. Position the basin on the toilet seat and release the clamp to allow warm water to irrigate the perineum.
7. Remain seated on the basin for approximately 15 to 20 minutes.
8. Stand up and pat the perineum area dry. Apply a clean perineal pad.
9. Tip the basin to remove any remaining water and flush the toilet.
10. Wash the basin with warm water and soap and dry it in the sink.
11. Store basin and tubing in a clean, dry area until the next use.
12. Wash hands with soap and water.

In addition, the woman may fear that bowel movements will cause pain or injury, especially if she had an episiotomy or a laceration that was repaired with sutures.

Usually a stool softener, such as docusate (Colace), with or without a laxative might be helpful if the client has difficulty with bowel elimination. Other measures, such as ambulating and increasing fluid and fibre intake, may also help. Nutritional instruction might include increasing fruits and vegetables in the diet; drinking plenty of fluids (8 to 12 cups daily) to keep the stool soft; drinking small amounts of prune juice and/or hot liquids to stimulate peristalsis; eating high-fibre foods such as bran cereals, whole grains, dried fruits, fresh fruits, and raw vegetables; and walking daily.

Promoting Activity, Rest, and Exercise

The postpartum period is an ideal time for nurses to promote the importance of physical fitness, help women incorporate exercise into their lifestyle, and encourage them to overcome barriers to exercise. The lifestyle changes that occur postpartum may affect a woman's health for decades. Early ambulation is encouraged to reduce the risk of thromboembolism and to improve strength.

Many changes occur postpartum, and caring for a newborn alters the woman's eating and sleeping habits, work schedules, and time allocation. Postpartum fatigue is common during the early days after childbirth, and it may continue for weeks or months. Fatigue should be assessed as a symptom of postpartum depression or a thyroid condition (London et al., 2011). Fatigue affects the mother's relationships with significant others and her ability to fulfill household and child care responsibilities. Be sure that the mother recognizes her need for rest and sleep and is realistic about her expectations. Some suggestions for new mothers include the following:

- Nap when the infant is sleeping, because getting uninterrupted sleep at night is difficult.
- Reduce participation in outside activities and limit the number of visitors.
- Determine the infant's sleep–wake cycles and attempt to increase wakeful periods during the day so the baby sleeps for longer periods at night.
- Eat a balanced diet to promote healing and to increase energy levels.
- Share household tasks to conserve your energy.
- Ask the father or other family members to provide infant care during the night periodically so that you can get an uninterrupted night of sleep.
- Review your family's daily routine and see if you can "cluster" activities to conserve energy and promote rest.

The demands of parenthood may reduce or prevent exercise in even the most committed person, but walking at a brisk pace or pushing the baby in a stroller are excellent ways for new mothers to maintain healthy exercise. In some communities, fitness classes for postnatal women can provide exercise and an important supportive social outlet. Women are encouraged to take a few months to lose the pregnancy weight while ensuring they are attending to important nutritional needs (SOGC, 2009). Emphasize the following benefits of a regular exercise program:

- Helps the woman to lose pregnancy weight
- Increases energy level so the woman can cope with her new responsibilities
- Speeds the return to pre-pregnant size and shape
- Provides an outlet for stress

Breastfeeding and exercise may help to control weight in the long term (SOGC, 2009).

> ▷ **Take** NOTE!
>
> *Women with a body mass index greater than 29 have both the least weight gain during pregnancy and the least weight loss after birth. From 6 to 18 months after giving birth, women weigh an average of 3.6 kg more than their pre-pregnancy weight (Evans et al., 2010).*

The postpartum woman may face some obstacles to exercising, including physical changes (ligament laxity), competing demands (newborn care), lack of information about weight retention (inactivity equates to weight gain), and stress incontinence (leaking of urine during activity).

A healthy woman with an uncomplicated vaginal birth can resume exercise in the immediate postpartum period. Women who experience cesarean birth should follow the advice of their physician about when to safely resume exercise. Encourage the woman to start slowly and increase the level of exercise over a period of several weeks as tolerated. Jogging strollers may be an option for some women, allowing them to exercise with their newborns. Also, exercise videos and DVDs, television programs, and home exercise equipment allow mothers to work out while the newborn naps.

Exercising after giving birth promotes feelings of well-being and restores muscle tone lost during pregnancy. Routine exercise should be resumed gradually, beginning with Kegel exercises on the first postpartum day and progressing as appropriate for the type of delivery. Walking is an excellent form of early exercise as long as the woman avoids jarring and bouncing movements, because joints do not stabilize until 6 to 8 weeks postpartum. Exercising too much too soon can cause the woman to bleed more, and her lochia may return to bright red.

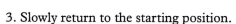

TEACHING GUIDELINE 16.2

Exercising During the Postpartum Period

Abdominal Breathing

1. While lying on a flat surface (floor or bed), take a deep breath through your nose and expand your abdominal muscles (they will rise up from your midsection).
2. Slowly exhale and tighten your abdominal muscles for 3 to 5 seconds.
3. Repeat this several times.

Head Lift

1. Lie on a flat surface with the knees flexed and feet flat on the surface.
2. Lift your head off the flat surface, tuck it onto your chest, and hold for 3 to 5 seconds.
3. Relax your head and return to the starting position.
4. Repeat this several times.

Modified Sit-Ups

1. Lie on a flat surface and raise your head and shoulders 14 to 18 cm (6 to 8 inches) so that your outstretched hands reach your knees.
2. Keep your waist on the flat surface.

3. Slowly return to the starting position.
4. Repeat, increasing in frequency as your comfort level allows.

Double Knee Roll

1. Lie on a flat surface with your knees bent.
2. While keeping your shoulders flat, slowly roll your knees to your right side to touch the flat surface (floor or bed).
3. Roll your knees back over your body to the left side until they touch the opposite side of the flat surface.
4. Return to the starting position on your back and rest.
5. Repeat this exercise several times.

Pelvic Tilt

1. Lie on your back on a flat surface with your knees bent and your arms at your side.
2. Slowly contract your abdominal muscles while lifting your pelvis up toward the ceiling.
3. Hold for 3 to 5 seconds and slowly return to your starting position.
4. Repeat several times.

Should that occur, women can take it as a sign that they need to decrease their activity level (London et al., 2011).

Recommended exercises for the first few weeks postpartum include abdominal breathing, head lifts, modified sit-ups, double knee roll, and pelvic tilt (Teaching Guideline 16.2). The number of exercises and their duration are gradually increased as the woman gains strength.

Remember that cultures may have different attitudes toward exercise. Some cultures expect new mothers to observe a specific period of bed rest or activity restriction. It would be inappropriate to recommend active exercise during the early postpartum period, since that recommendation may indicate a lapse in attention to cultural competence in nursing, which is of the utmost importance in the maternal/child setting (Evans et al., 2010).

Preventing Stress Incontinence

Stress incontinence refers to urine loss associated with coughing, sneezing, laughing, or lifting. Weak pelvic floor muscles and supportive tissue often account for the condition (Potter & Perry, 2010). Therefore, the more vaginal deliveries a woman has had, the more likely she is to have stress incontinence, as each pregnancy and delivery challenges the tone of the pelvic

floor. Postpartum women might consider low-impact activities such as walking, biking, swimming, or low-impact aerobics so they can resume physical activity while strengthening the pelvic floor.

Suggestions to prevent stress incontinence include:

- Start a regular program of Kegel exercises after childbirth.
- Lose weight if necessary; obesity is associated with stress incontinence.
- Avoid smoking; limit intake of alcohol and caffeinated beverages, which irritate the bladder.

Kegel exercises help to strengthen the pelvic floor muscles if done properly and regularly, since they facilitate structural support and maintain the bladder neck in position so as not to leak during increases in intra-abdominal pressure (Potter & Perry, 2010). Kegel exercises were originally developed by Dr. Arnold Kegel as a method of controlling incontinence in women after childbirth. While providing postpartum care, instruct women on primary prevention of stress incontinence by discussing the value and purpose of Kegel exercises. Approach the subject sensitively, avoiding the term "incontinent." The terms "leakage," "loss of urine," or "bladder control issues" are more acceptable to most women.

Women can perform Kegel exercises, doing ten 5-second contractions, whenever they change diapers,

TEACHING GUIDELINE 16.3

Performing Kegel Exercises

1. Identify the correct pelvic floor muscles by contracting them to stop the flow of urine while sitting on the toilet.
2. Repeat this contraction several times to become familiar with it.
3. Start the exercises by emptying the bladder.
4. Tighten the pelvic floor muscles and hold for 10 seconds.
5. Relax the muscle completely for 10 seconds.
6. Perform 10 exercises at least three times daily. Progressively increase the number that you perform.
7. Perform the exercises in different positions, such as standing, lying, and sitting.
8. Keep breathing during the exercises.
9. Don't contract your abdominal, thigh, leg, or buttocks muscles during these exercises.
10. Relax while doing Kegel exercises and concentrate on isolating the right muscles.
11. Attempt to tighten your pelvic muscles before sneezing, jumping, or laughing.
12. Remember that you can perform Kegel exercises anywhere without anyone noticing.

talk on the phone, or watch TV. Teach the woman to perform Kegel exercises properly; help her to identify the correct muscles by trying to stop and start the flow of urine when sitting on the toilet (Teaching Guideline 16.3). Kegel exercises can be done without anyone knowing.

Assisting with Self-Care Measures

Demonstrate and discuss with the woman ways to prevent infection during the postpartum period. Because she may experience lochia drainage for as long as a month after childbirth, describe practices to promote well-being and healing. These measures include:

• Frequently change perineal pads (at least four times daily) by applying and removing them from front to back to prevent spreading contamination from the rectal area to the genital area.
• Avoid using tampons after giving birth to decrease the risk of infection.
• Shower once or twice daily using a mild soap. Avoid using soap on the nipples.
• Use a sitz bath after every bowel movement to cleanse the rectal area and relieve enlarged hemorrhoids.

• Use the peri bottle filled with warm water after urinating and before applying a new perineal pad
• Wash your hands before changing perineal pads, after disposing of soiled pads, and after voiding (London et al., 2011).

To reduce the risk for infection at the episiotomy site, reinforce proper perineal care with the client, showing her how to rinse her perineum with the peri bottle after she voids or defecates. Stress the importance of always patting gently from front to back and washing her hands thoroughly before and after perineal care. For hemorrhoids, have the client apply witch hazel-soaked pads (Tucks Medicated Pads), ice packs to relieve swelling, or hemorrhoidal cream or ointment if ordered.

Ensuring Safety

One of the safety concerns during the postpartum period is orthostatic hypotension. When the woman moves rapidly from a lying or sitting position to a standing one, her blood pressure can drop suddenly, causing her pulse rate to increase. She may become dizzy and faint. Be aware of this problem and initiate the following safeguards:

• Check blood pressure first before ambulating the client.
• Elevate the head of the bed for a few minutes before ambulating the client.
• Have the client sit on the side of the bed for a few moments before getting up.
• Help the client to stand up, and stay with her.
• Ambulate alongside the client and provide support if needed.
• Frequently ask the client how her head feels.
• Stay close by to assist if she feels lightheaded.

Additional topics to address concern infant safety. Instruct the woman to place the newborn back in the crib on his or her back if she is feeling sleepy. If the woman falls asleep while holding the infant, she might drop him or her. Also, instruct mothers to keep the door to their room closed when their infant is in their room with them. They should check the identification of anyone who enters their room or who wants to take the infant out of the room. Many hospitals emphasize safety strategies to parents and have added security measures to protect families from infant abduction.

Counselling About Sexuality and Contraception

Sexuality is an important part of every woman's life. Women want to get back to "normal" as soon as possible after giving birth, but the couple's sexual relationship cannot be isolated from the psychological and psychosocial adjustments that both partners are going through.

Most couples wait to have sexual intercourse for about 4 to 6 weeks after the delivery (SOGC, 2009). Fatigue, the physical demands made by the infant, and the stress of new roles and responsibilities may stress the emotional reserves of couples. To promote comfort, the body needs time to recover from the delivery and for the organs to return to their pre-pregnant state. Body image issues may also be a factor for women whose bodies are still changed. New parents may not get much privacy or rest, both of which are necessary for sexual pleasure (SOGC, 2009).

Men may feel they now have a secondary role within the family, and they may not understand their partner's daily routine. These issues, combined with the woman's increased investment in the mothering role, can strain the couple's sexual relationship.

Although couples are reluctant to ask, they often want to know when they can safely resume sexual intercourse after childbirth. Typically, sexual intercourse can be resumed once bright-red bleeding has stopped and the perineum is healed from an episiotomy or lacerations. This is usually by the third to the sixth week postpartum. However, there is not a set, prescribed time to resume sexual intercourse after childbirth. Each couple must set their own time frame when they feel it is appropriate to resume sexual intercourse (SOGC, 2009).

When counselling the couple about sexuality, determine what knowledge and concerns the couple have about their sexual relationship. Inform them that fluctuations in sexual interest are normal. Also inform the couple about what to expect when resuming sexual intercourse and how to prevent discomfort. Precoital vaginal lubrication may be impaired during the postpartum period, especially in women who are breastfeeding. Use of water-based gel lubricants (K-Y jelly, Astroglide) can help, as can position changes during intercourse (SOGC, 2009). Pelvic floor exercises, in addition to preventing stress incontinence, can also enhance sensation.

Contraceptive options should be included in the discussions with the couple so that they can make an informed decision before resuming sexual activity. Many couples are overwhelmed with the amount of new information given to them during their brief hospitalization, so many are not ready for a lengthy discussion about contraceptives. Presenting a brief overview of the options, along with literature, may be appropriate. It may be suitable to ask them to think about contraceptive needs and preferences and advise them to use a barrier method (condom with spermicidal gel or foam) until they choose another form of contraceptive. This advice is especially important if the follow-up appointment will not occur for 4 to 6 weeks after childbirth, as many couples will resume sexual activity before this time. Some postpartum women ovulate before their menstrual period returns and thus need contraceptive

protection to prevent another pregnancy. It is important to emphasize that there is a chance to become pregnant, even if women are breastfeeding and experiencing amenorrhea. Contraception is therefore an important consideration.

Open and effective communication is necessary for effective contraceptive counselling so that information is clearly understood. Provide clear, consistent information appropriate to the woman and her partner's language, culture, and educational level. Recommending resources such as *Healthy Beginnings* (SOGC, 2009) or other pamphlets about contraception that have been developed in the local community could also be helpful.

Promoting Nutrition

The postpartum period can be a stressful one for myriad reasons, such as fatigue, the physical stress of pregnancy and birth, and the nonstop work required to take care of the newborn and to meet the needs of other family members. As a result, the new mother may ignore her own nutrition needs. Whether she is breastfeeding or bottle-feeding, encourage the new mother to take good care of herself and eat a healthy diet so that the nutrients lost during pregnancy can be replaced and she can return to a healthy weight. In general, nutrition recommendations for the postpartum woman include the following:

- Eat a wide variety of foods with high nutrient density.
- Eat meals that require little or no preparation.
- Avoid high-fat fast foods.
- Drink plenty of fluids daily—at least 2,500 mL (approximately 84 oz).
- Avoid fad weight-reduction diets and harmful substances such as alcohol, tobacco, and drugs.
- Avoid excessive intake of fat, salt, sugar, and caffeine.
- Eat the recommended daily servings from each food group.

The following summary outlines Canada's Food Guide daily nutrition requirements for postpartum women (Health Canada, 2011):

- Seven to eight servings of vegetables and fruits
- Six or seven servings of grain products
- Two servings of milk or milk alternatives
- Two servings of meat or meat alternatives
- 30 to 45 mL (2 to 3 tbsp) of unsaturated oils and fats

The breastfeeding mother's nutritional needs are higher than they were during pregnancy. The mother's diet and nutritional status influence the quantity and quality of breast milk. To meet the needs for milk production, breastfeeding women require an extra two or three Food Guide servings per day. These servings can be included as additions to regular meals or as extra snacks.

Following are some examples of dietary additions to achieve these additional requirements:

- One piece of fruit and 175 g (¾ cup) of yogurt
- An extra piece of toast at breakfast and an extra 250 mL (1 cup) of milk at supper
- Half a bagel (45 g) with 50 g (1½ oz) of cheese
- 30 g of cereal with 250 mL (1 cup) of milk
- Spinach salad made with 250 mL (1 cup) of spinach, one hard-boiled egg, and 30 mL (2 tbsp) of walnuts (Health Canada, 2011)

According to Food Guide recommendations (Health Canada, 2011), breastfeeding mothers should take a daily multivitamin that contains 400 µg (0.4 mg) of folic acid. When combined with foods rich in folic acid, daily requirements will be met.

Certain foods (usually gaseous or strong-flavoured ones) eaten by the mother may affect the flavour of the breast milk or cause gastrointestinal problems for the infant. Not all infants are affected by the same foods. If the particular food item seems to cause a problem, urge the mother to eliminate that food for a few days to see if the problem disappears.

> ▶ *Take* NOTE!
>
> *During the woman's brief stay in the health care facility, she may demonstrate a healthy appetite and eat well. Nutritional problems usually start at home when the mother needs to make her own food selections and prepare her own meals. This is a crucial area to address during follow-up.*

Supporting the Woman's Choice of Feeding Method

While there is considerable evidence that breastfeeding has numerous health benefits, many mothers choose to feed their infants formula for the first year of life. Nurses must be able to deliver sound, evidence-based information to help the new mother choose the best way to feed her infant and must support her in her decision (London et al., 2011).

Many factors affect a woman's choice of feeding method, such as culture, employment demands, support from significant others and family, and knowledge base. Although breastfeeding is encouraged, be sure that couples have the information they need to make an informed decision. Whether a couple chooses to breast-feed or bottle-feed their newborn, support and respect their choice.

Certain women should not breastfeed. Drugs such as antithyroid drugs, antineoplastic drugs, alcohol, or street drugs (amphetamines, cocaine, PCP, marijuana) enter the breast milk and will harm the infant, so women taking these substances should not breastfeed. Women with mental health challenges face decision making concerning the safety of breastfeeding while taking anti-depressant or antipsychotic medication. Many medications are considered safe in the context of breastfeeding, but not all, so women will need information about the safety of their particular medication in the context of breastfeeding. Despite reassurances about the safety of a given medication, some women may choose not to breastfeed because they are uncomfortable with the knowledge that the medications will be transferred to the infant through the breast milk. To prevent HIV transmission to the newborn, women who are HIV positive should not breastfeed. Other contraindications to breastfeeding include a newborn with an inborn error of metabolism such as galactosemia or phenylketonuria, a current pregnancy, or a serious mental health disorder that would prevent the mother from remembering to feed the infant consistently.

Providing Assistance with Breastfeeding and Bottle-Feeding

First-time mothers often have many questions about feed-ing, and even women who have had experience with feed-ing a newborn may have questions. Regardless of whether the postpartum woman is breastfeeding or bottle-feeding her newborn, she can benefit from instruction.

Providing Assistance with Breastfeeding
WATCH & LEARN

The World Health Organization (WHO) and UNICEF (2009) and the Breastfeeding Committee for Canada (BCC, 2011) recommend breastfeeding for all full-term newborns. Exclusive breastfeeding is sufficient to support optimal growth and development for approximately the first 6 months of life. Breastfeeding for the first 6 months of life and up to 2 years of age or older is optimal (SOGC, 2009). Education and support for a mother regarding breastfeeding choice will increase the likelihood of a suc-cessful breastfeeding experience.

At birth, all newborns should be quickly dried, assessed and, if stable, placed immediately in uninter-rupted skin-to-skin contact with their mother. This is good practice whether the mother is going to breastfeed or bottle-feed her infant. Skin-to-skin care provides the newborn with optimal physiologic stability, warmth, and opportunities for the first feed (BCC, 2011; WHO, UNICEF, 2009). The benefits of breastfeeding are clear (see Chapter 18). To promote breastfeeding, the Baby-Friendly Hospital Initiative, an international program of the World Health Organization and the United Nations Children's Fund, was started in 1991 (UNICEF, n.d.). As part of this program, the hospital or birth centre should take the following 10 steps to provide "an optimal environment for the promotion, protection, and support of breastfeeding":

1. Have a written breastfeeding policy that is communicated to all staff.
2. Educate all staff to implement this written policy.
3. Inform all women about the benefits and management of breastfeeding.
4. Show all mothers how to initiate breastfeeding within 30 minutes of birth.
5. Give no food or drink other than breast milk to all newborns.
6. Demonstrate to all mothers how to initiate and maintain breastfeeding.
7. Encourage breastfeeding on demand.
8. Allow no pacifiers to be given to breastfeeding infants.
9. Establish breastfeeding support groups and refer mothers to them.
10. Practice rooming-in 24 hours daily (BCC, 2011; WHO, UNICEF, 2009)

The nurse is responsible for encouraging breastfeeding when appropriate. For the woman who chooses to breastfeed her infant, the nurse or lactation consultant will need to spend time instructing her how to do so successfully. Many women have the impression that breastfeeding is simple. Although it is a natural process, women may experience some difficulty in breastfeeding their newborns. Nurses can assist mothers with this transition. Assist and provide one-to-one support for breastfeeding mothers, especially first-time breastfeeding mothers, to encourage appropriate technique. Suggestions are highlighted in Teaching Guideline 16.4.

> ▶ *Take* NOTE!
>
> *Some newborns "latch on and catch on" right away, while others take more time and patience. Inform new mothers about this to reduce their frustration and uncertainty about their ability to breastfeed.*

Encourage mothers to believe in themselves and their ability to accomplish successful breastfeeding. They should not panic if breastfeeding does not go smoothly at first; it takes time and practice. Additional suggestions to help mothers relax and feel more comfortable while breastfeeding, especially when they return home, include the following:

- Select a quiet corner or room where you won't be disturbed.
- Use a rocking chair to soothe both you and your infant.
- Take long, slow deep breaths to relax before nursing.
- Drink while breastfeeding to replenish body fluids.
- Listen to soothing music while breastfeeding.
- Cuddle and caress the infant while feeding.
- Set out extra cloth diapers within reach to use as burping cloths.
- Allow sufficient time to enjoy each other in an unhurried atmosphere.
- Involve other family members in all aspects of the infant's care from the start.

Providing Assistance with Bottle-Feeding

If the mother or couple has chosen to bottle-feed their newborn, the nurse should respect and support their decision. Some women experience feelings of guilt and stigmatization as a result of the decision to feed their infant with formula. That potential needs to be understood and addressed by nurses. Discuss with the parents what type of formula they will use. Commercial formulas are classified as cow's milk-based (Enfamil, Similac), soy protein-based (Isomil, Prosobee, Nursoy), or specialized or therapeutic formulas for infants with protein allergies (Nutramigen, Pregestimil, Alimentum). The Canadian Pediatric Society (2009) advises caution regarding the use of soy formula in cases in which there is neither a cultural reason to avoid cow's milk nor an allergy to cow's milk. Some studies indicate that there can be short- or long-term consequences for the infant (such as hormonal disturbances or thyroid malfunction) as a result of exposure to soy products.

Because of the emphasis on breastfeeding promotion in maternal/child care settings, nurses can overlook the need for education around formula preparation. There are many considerations for new parents around formula use, including the methods of maintaining asepsis, sterility, the importance of the concentration of formula, and other issues associated with safe feeding practice, and these should be addressed with the new parents (London et al., 2011).

Commercial formulas can be purchased in various forms: powdered (must be mixed with water), condensed liquid (must be diluted with equal amounts of water), ready to use (poured directly into bottles), and prepackaged (ready to use in disposable bottles). One way to calculate the amount of formula an infant will require per day is to give 150 to 200 mL (5 to 6 oz) of formula milk per kilogram of body weight each day. The amount required also depends on the baby's age, however, and guidelines change as the baby ages. For example, a newborn only needs 30 to 60 mL per feed for the first week of life. This amount will increase to 90 to 120 mL per feed by 1 month of age and 120 to 180 mL per feed from 2 to 6 months. After that, the infant will take 180 to 220 mL at

TEACHING GUIDELINE 16.4

Breastfeeding Suggestions

- Explain that breastfeeding is a learned skill for both parties.
- Offer a thorough explanation about the procedure.
- Instruct the mother to wash her hands before starting.
- Inform the mother that her afterpains will increase during breastfeeding.
- Make sure the mother is comfortable (pain-free) and not hungry.
- Tell the mother to start the feeding with an awake and alert infant showing hunger signs.
- Assist the mother to position herself correctly for comfort.
- Urge the mother to relax to encourage the let-down reflex.
- Guide the mother's hand to form a "C" to access the nipple.
- Have the mother lightly tickle the infant's upper lip with her nipple to stimulate the infant to open the mouth wide.
- Help her to latch on by bringing the infant rapidly to the breast with a wide-open mouth.
- Show her how to check that the newborn's mouth position is correct, and tell her to listen for a sucking noise.
- Demonstrate correct removal from the breast, using her finger to break the suction.
- Instruct the mother on how to burp the infant between breasts.
- Show her different positions, such as cradle and football holds and side-lying positions (see Chapter 18).
- Reinforce and praise the mother for her efforts.
- Allow ample time to answer questions and address concerns.
- Refer the mother to support groups and community resources.

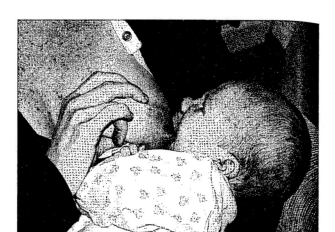

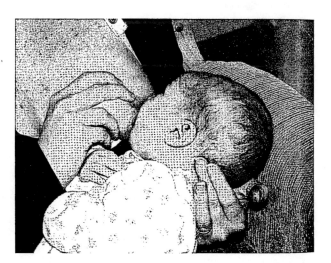

each feeding. The baby's cues will be the guide for how much to feed (rooting, crying) and when to discontinue the feeding (Babycenter, 2011). After 6 months of age, the number of feedings declines to accommodate other foods in the baby's diet, such as fruits, cereals, and vegetables (Babycenter, 2012). For more information on newborn nutrition and bottle-feeding, see Chapter 18.

When teaching parents and other caretakers about bottle-feeding, provide the following guidelines:

- Make feeding a relaxing time, a time to provide both food and comfort to your newborn.

- Use the feeding period to promote bonding by smiling, singing, making eye contact, and talking to the infant.
- Always hold the newborn when feeding. Never prop the bottle as this can cause choking and/or dental carries. Cuddle the baby close and ensure that the baby's head is higher than his or her body. Support the head to make swallowing easier.
- Use a comfortable position when feeding the newborn. Place the newborn in your dominant arm, which is supported by a pillow. Alternatively, have the newborn in a semi-upright position supported in the

crook of your arm (this position reduces choking and the flow of milk into the middle ear).

• Tilt the bottle so that the nipple and the neck of the bottle are always filled with formula. This prevents the infant from taking in too much air. Let the baby set the pace.

• Stimulate the sucking reflex by touching the nipple to the infant's lips.

• Observe expiry dates on formula containers. When purchasing formula, avoid cans with bumps or indents.

• Refrigerate any powdered formula that has been combined with tap water after constitution.

• Discard any formula not taken; do not save it for future feedings.

• Follow the baby's cues for hunger before feeding, and stop feeding when the baby shows signs of feeling full (such as turning away).

• Burp the infant frequently, and place the baby on his or her back for sleeping.

• Do not let the baby hold the bottle until after 1 year of age.

• Use only iron-fortified infant formula for first year (HealthLink, 2010).

Teaching About Breast Care

Regardless of whether or not the mother is breastfeeding her newborn, urge her to wear a very supportive, snug bra 24 hours a day to support enlarged breasts and promote comfort. A woman who is breastfeeding should wear a supportive bra throughout the lactation period. A woman who is not nursing should wear a supportive bra until engorgement ceases and then should wear a less restrictive one. The bra should fit snugly while still allowing the mother to breathe without restriction. All new mothers should use plain water to clean their breasts, especially the nipple area; soap is drying and should be avoided.

Assessing the Breasts

Instruct the mother how on to examine her breasts daily. Daily assessment includes the milk supply (breasts will feel full as they are filling), the condition of the nipples (red, bruised, fissured, or bleeding), and the success of breastfeeding. The fullness of the breasts may progress to engorgement in the breastfeeding mother if feedings are delayed or breastfeeding is ineffective. Palpating both breasts will help identify whether the breasts are soft, filling, or engorged. A similar assessment of the breasts should be completed on the nonlactating mother to identify any problems, such as engorgement or mastitis.

Alleviating Breast Engorgement

Breast engorgement usually occurs during the first week postpartum. It is a common response of the breasts to the sudden change in hormones and the presence of an increased amount of milk. Reassure the woman that this condition is temporary and usually resolves within 72 hours.

Alleviating Breast Engorgement in the Breastfeeding Woman

If the mother is breastfeeding, encourage frequent feedings, at least every 2 to 3 hours, using manual expression just before feeding to soften the breast so the newborn can latch on more effectively. Advise the mother to allow the newborn to feed on the first breast until it softens before switching to the other side. See Chapter 18 for more information on alleviating breast engorgement and other common breastfeeding concerns.

Alleviating Breast Engorgement and Suppressing Lactation in the Bottle-Feeding Woman

If the woman is bottle-feeding, explain that breast engorgement is a self-limiting phenomenon that disappears as increasing estrogen levels suppress milk formation (i.e., lactation suppression). Encourage the woman to use ice packs, to wear a snug, supportive bra 24 hours a day, and to take mild analgesics such as acetaminophen. Encourage her to avoid any stimulation to the breasts that might foster milk production, such as warm showers or pumping or massaging the breasts. Medication is no longer given to hasten lactation suppression. Teaching Guideline 16.5 provides tips on lactation suppression.

TEACHING GUIDELINE 16.5

Suppressing Lactation

1. Wear a supportive, snugly fitting bra starting at approximately 6 hours post-delivery. Remove the bra only when taking showers.
2. Milk suppression may take 5 to 7 days to accomplish.
3. Take mild analgesics to reduce breast discomfort.
4. Let shower water flow over your back rather than your breasts so that the heat of the water does not stimulate milk production and delay the suppression process.
5. Avoid any breast stimulation in the form of sucking or massage.
6. Ice packs may be applied over axillary area of each breast for 20 minutes at a time four times daily.
7. Medications to suppress lactation are no longer recommended. (London et al., 2011).

Promoting Family Adjustment and Well-Being

The postpartum period involves extraordinary physiologic, psychological, and sociocultural changes in the life of a woman and her family. Adapting to the role of a parent is not an easy process. The postpartum period is a "getting-to-know-you" time when parents begin to integrate the newborn into their lives as they reconcile the fantasy child with the real one. This can be a very challenging period for families. Nurses play a major role in assisting families to adapt to the changes, promoting a smooth transition into parenthood. Appropriate and timely interventions can help parents adjust to the role changes and promote attachment to the newborn.

For couples who already have children, the addition of a new member may bring role conflict and challenges. The nurse should provide anticipatory guidance about siblings' responses to the new baby, increased emotional tension, child development, and meeting the multiple needs of the expanding family. Although the multiparous woman has had experience with newborns, do not assume that her knowledge is current and accurate, especially if some time has elapsed since her previous child was born. Reinforcing information is important for all families.

Promoting Parental Roles

Parents' roles develop and grow when they interact with their newborn (see Chapter 15 for information on maternal and paternal adaptation). The pleasure they derive from this interaction stimulates and reinforces this behaviour. With repeated, continued contact with the newborn, parents learn to recognize cues and understand the newborn's behaviour. This positive interaction contributes to family harmony.

Nurses need to know the stages parents go through as they make their new parenting roles fit into their life experience. Assess the parents for attachment behaviours (normal and deviant), adjustment to the new parental role, family member adjustment, social support system, and educational needs. To promote parental role adaptation and parent–newborn attachment, include the following nursing interventions:

- Provide as much opportunity as possible for parents to interact with their newborn. Encourage exploration, holding, and providing care.
- Model behaviours by holding the newborn close and speaking positively.
- Always refer to the newborn by name in front of the parents.
- Speak directly to the newborn in a calm voice.
- Encourage both parents to pick up and hold the newborn.
- Point out the newborn's response to parental stimulation.
- Point out the positive physical features of the newborn.
- Involve both parents in the newborn's care and praise them for their efforts.
- Evaluate the family's strengths and weaknesses and readiness for parenting.
- Assess for risk factors such as lack of social support and the presence of stressors.
- Observe the effect of culture on the family interaction to determine whether it is appropriate.
- Monitor parental attachment behaviours to determine whether alterations require referral. Positive behaviours include holding the newborn closely or in an *en face* position, talking to or admiring the newborn, or demonstrating closeness. Negative behaviours include avoiding contact with the newborn, calling the baby derogatory names, or showing a lack of interest in caring for the newborn (see Table 16.1).
- Monitor the parents' coping behaviours to determine alterations that need intervention. Positive coping behaviours include positive conversations between the partners, both parents wanting to be involved with newborn care, and lack of arguments between the parents. Negative behaviours include not visiting, limited conversations or periods of silence, and heated arguments or conflict.
- Identify the support systems available to the new family and encourage them to ask for help. Ask direct questions about home or community support. Make referrals to community resources to meet the family's needs.
- Arrange for community home visits in high-risk families to provide positive reinforcement of parenting skills and nurturing behaviours with the newborn.
- To reduce the new parents' frustration, provide anticipatory guidance about the following before discharge:
  - Newborn sleep–wake cycles (they may be reversed)
  - Variations in newborn appearance
  - Infant developmental milestones (growth spurts)
  - How to interpret crying cues (hunger, wet, discomfort)
  - Techniques to quiet a crying infant (e.g., car ride)
  - Sensory enrichment/stimulation (e.g., colourful mobile)
  - Signs and symptoms of illness and how to assess for fever
  - Important phone numbers, follow-up care, and needed immunizations
  - Physical and emotional changes associated with the postpartum period

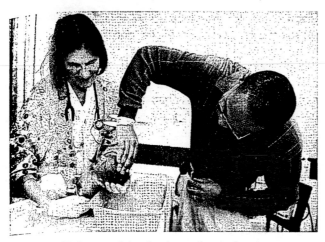

FIGURE 16.7 Father participating in newborn care.

- Need to integrate siblings into care of the newborn; stress that sibling rivalry is normal and offer ways to reduce it
- Ways for the couple to make time together
- Appropriate community referral resources

In addition, nurses can help fathers to feel more competent in assuming their parental role by teaching and providing information (Fig. 16.7). Education can dispel any unrealistic expectations they may have, helping them to cope more successfully with the demands of fatherhood and thereby fostering a nurturing family relationship.

Explaining Sibling Roles

It can be overwhelming to a young child to have another family member introduced into his or her small, stable world. Although most parents try to prepare siblings for the arrival of their new little brother or sister, many young children experience stress. They may view the new infant as competition or fear that they will be replaced in the parents' affection. All siblings need extra attention from their parents and reassurance that they are loved and important.

Many parents need reassurance that sibling rivalry is normal. Suggest the following to help parents minimize sibling rivalry:

- Expect and tolerate some regression (thumb-sucking, bedwetting).
- Explain childbirth in an appropriate way for the child's age.
- Encourage discussion about the new infant during relaxed family times.
- Encourage the sibling(s) to participate in decisions, such as the baby's name and toys to buy.
- Take the sibling on the tour of the maternity suite.

► **Consider** *THIS!*

Katie and Molly have been excited about having a new baby sister since they were told about their mother's pregnancy. The 6-year-old twins are eagerly looking out the front window, waiting for their parents to bring their new sister, Jessica, home. The girls are big enough to help their mother care for their new sibling, and for the past few months they have been fixing up the new nursery and selecting baby clothes. They practiced diapering their dolls—their mother was specific about not using any powder or lotion on Jessica's bottom—and holding them correctly to feed them bottles. Finally, their mother arrives home from the hospital with Jessica in her arms!

The girls notice that their mother is very protective of Jessica and watches them carefully when they care for her. They fight over the opportunity to hold her or feed her. What is special to both of them is the time they spend alone with their parents. Although a new family member has been added, the twins still feel special and loved by their parents.

Thoughts: Bringing a new baby into an established family can cause conflict and jealousy. What preparation did the older siblings have before Jessica arrived? Why is it important for parents to spend time with each sibling separately?

- Buy a T-shirt that says "I'm the [big brother or big sister]."
- Spend "special time" with the child.
- Read with the child. Some suggested title include *Things to Do with A New Baby* (Ormerod, 1984); *Betsy's Baby Brother* (Wolde, 1975); *The Berenstain Bears' New Baby* (Berenstain, 1974); and *Mommy's Lap* (Horowitz & Sorensen, 1993).
- Plan time for each child throughout the day.
- Role-play safe handling of a newborn, using a doll. Give the preschooler or school-age child a doll to care for.
- Encourage older children to verbalize emotions about the newborn.
- Purchase a gift that the child can give to the newborn.
- Purchase a gift that can be given to the child by the newborn.
- Arrange for the child to come to the hospital to see the newborn (Fig. 16.8).
- Move the sibling from his or her crib to a youth bed months in advance of the birth of the newborn.
- Encourage grandparents to pay attention to the older child when visiting (Rector, 2007).

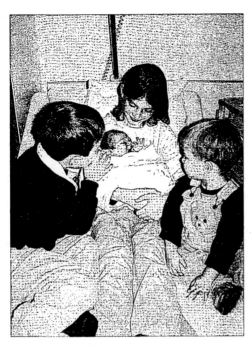

FIGURE 16.8 Sibling visitation.

Discussing Grandparents' Role

Grandparents can be a source of support and comfort to the postpartum family if effective communication skills are used and roles are defined. The grandparents' role and involvement will depend on how close they live to the family, their willingness to become involved, and cultural expectations of their role. Just as parents and siblings go through developmental changes, so too do grandparents. These changes can have a positive or negative effect on the relationship.

Newborn care, feeding, and childrearing practices have changed since the grandparents raised the parents. New parents may lack parenting skills but nonetheless want their parents' support without criticism. A grandparent's "take-charge approach" may not be welcome by new parents who are testing their own parenting roles, and family conflict may ensue. However, many grandparents respect their adult children's wishes for autonomy and remain "resource people" for them when requested.

▷ *Take* NOTE!

Grandparents' involvement can enrich the lives of the entire family if accepted in the right context and dose by the family.

Nurses can assist in the grandparents' role transition by assessing their communication skills, role expectations, and support skills during the prenatal period. Find out whether the grandparents are included in the couple's social support network and whether their support is wanted or helpful. If they are, and it is, then encourage the grandparents to learn about the parenting, feeding, and childrearing skills their children have learned in childbirth classes. This information is commonly found in "grandparenting" classes, which introduce new parenting concepts and bring the grandparents up to date on current childbirth practices.

Teaching About Postpartum Blues

Issues such as sleep deprivation and exhaustion are important for the nurse to assess during the early postpartum period. Not only is a woman adjusting to the needs of her infant over a 24-hour period but she may also be coping with interruptions and visitors while in the hospital. In general, it is difficult for women to achieve the societal expectations of motherhood, which include high levels of coping and capability (Evans et al., 2010). The postpartum period is typically a happy yet stressful time because the birth of an infant is accompanied by enormous physical, social, and emotional changes.

The postpartum woman may report feelings of emotional lability, such as crying one minute and laughing the next. **Postpartum blues** are transient emotional disturbances beginning in the first week after childbirth and are characterized by a wide range of labile emotions such as uneven energy capacities, insomnia, difficulty with decision making, emotional insecurity, and grieving for a former sense of self and body image. These symptoms typically begin 3 to 4 days after childbirth and resolve by day 10 (SOGC, 2009). These mood swings may be confusing to new mothers but are usually self-limiting.

Postpartum blues are thought to affect up to 70% of all new mothers (Evans et al., 2010). In mothers who maintain contact with reality and enjoy a firm support system, the symptoms tend to resolve spontaneously without therapy within 1 to 2 weeks.

▷ *Take* NOTE!

If the baby blues do not resolve but become more severe and last longer than 2 weeks, it is possible that postpartum depression is developing. Typical manifestations of postpartum depression include feelings of hopelessness, isolation, and despair. Thoughts of harming oneself or one's baby may persist. Immediate medical attention is warranted (SOGC, 2009)

Postpartum blues requires no formal treatment other than support and reassurance because it does not usually interfere with the woman's ability to function and care for her infant. Further evaluation is necessary, however, if symptoms persist more than 2 weeks (SOGC, 2009). Nurses can ease a mother's distress by encouraging her to vent her feelings and by demonstrating patience and understanding with her and her family. Suggest that getting outside help with housework and infant care might help her to feel less overwhelmed until the blues ease. Provide telephone numbers she can call when she feels down during the day. Making women aware of postpartum blues while they are pregnant will increase their knowledge about this mood disturbance, which may lessen their embarrassment and increase their willingness to ask for and accept help if it does occur.

The postpartum woman also is at risk for postpartum depression and postpartum psychosis; these conditions are discussed in Chapter 22.

Preparing for Discharge

The length of stay in the health care facility should be individualized for each mother and baby, but in Canada the average hospital stay is 2.1 days following a vaginal birth and 3.8 days following a cesarean birth (Public Health Agency of Canada [PHAC], 2009). A shortened hospital stay may be indicated if the following criteria are met:

• Mother is afebrile and vital signs are within normal range.
• Lochia is appropriate in amount and colour for stage of recovery.
• Hemoglobin and hematocrit values are within normal range.
• Uterine fundus is firm; urinary output is adequate.
• ABO blood groups and RhD status are known and, if indicated, anti-D immunoglobulin has been administered.
• Surgical wounds are healing and no signs of infection are present.
• Mother is able to ambulate without difficulty.
• Food and fluids are taken without difficulty.
• Self-care and infant care are understood and demonstrated.
• Family or other support system is available to care for both mother and baby.
• Mother is aware of possible complications

Teaching About Safe Sleeping

PHAC (2011a) recently issued the following recommendations about infant safe sleeping:

1. Provide a smoke-free environment before and after birth.
2. Always place the baby on his or her back to sleep.
3. Place the baby to sleep in a crib next to the adult's bed for the first 6 months.
4. Use a safe crib environment that has no toys or loose bedding.

Bed-sharing (referring to adults sharing any sleep surface with infants) is not recommended as it is associated with a higher risk of sudden infant death syndrome (SIDS) and suffocation.

Providing Immunizations

Prior to discharge, check the immunity status for rubella for all mothers and give a subcutaneous injection of rubella vaccine if the mother is not serologically immune (titer less than 1:10). Be sure that the client signs a consent form to receive the vaccine. Nursing mothers can be vaccinated because the live, attenuated rubella virus is not communicable. Inform all mothers receiving immunization about adverse effects (rash, joint symptoms, and a low-grade fever 5 to 21 days later) and the need to avoid pregnancy for at least 3 months after being vaccinated because of the risk of teratogenic effects (PHAC, 2011b).

If the client is Rh negative, check the Rh status of the newborn. Verify that the woman is Rh negative and has not been sensitized, that the Coombs' test is negative, and that the newborn is Rh positive. Mothers who are Rh negative and have given birth to an infant who is Rh positive should receive an injection of Rh immunoglobulin within 72 hours after birth to prevent a sensitization reaction in the Rh-negative woman who received Rh-positive blood cells during the birthing process. The usual protocol for the Rh-negative woman is to receive two doses of Rh immunoglobulin (RhoGAM), one dose at 28 weeks' gestation and the second within 72 hours after childbirth. A signed consent form is needed after a thorough explanation about the procedure is provided, including its purpose, possible adverse effects, and effect on future pregnancies.

Ensuring Follow-Up Care

New mothers and their families need to be attended to over an extended period of time by nurses knowledgeable about mother care, infant feeding (breastfeeding and bottle-feeding), infant care, and nutrition. Although continuous nursing care stops on discharge from the hospital or birthing centre, extended episodic nursing care needs to be provided at home. Some of the challenges faced by families after discharge are described in Box 16.4.

Many new mothers are reluctant to "cut the cord" after their brief stay in the health care facility and need expanded community services. Women who are discharged too early from the hospital run the risk of uterine subinvolution, discomfort at an episiotomy or cesarean site, infection, fatigue, and maladjustment to their new role. Postpartum nursing care should include a range of family-focused care, including telephone calls, out-patient

BOX 16.4 Challenges Facing Families After Discharge

- Lack of role models for breastfeeding and infant care
- Lack of support from the new mother's own mother if she did not breastfeed
- Increased mobility of society, which means that extended family may live far away and cannot help care for the newborn and support the new family
- Feelings of isolation and limited community ties for women who work full-time
- Shortened hospital stays: parents may be overwhelmed by all the information they are given during the brief hospital stay
- Prenatal classes usually focus on the birth itself rather than on skills parents need to care for themselves and the newborn during the postpartum period
- Limited access to education and support systems for families from diverse cultures

Source: Nash, L. R. (2007). Postpartum care. In R. E. Rakel & E. T. Bope (Eds.), *Conn's current therapy 2007.* Philadelphia: Saunders Elsevier.

clinics, and home visits. Typically, public health nurses or community nurses will provide postpartum care after hospital discharge. Ideally, a postpartum home visit or a telephone call from a public health nurse will occur within a week of discharge (PHAC, 2009). It is important for the postpartum nurse to document any concerns that may require follow-up in the community.

Providing Telephone Follow-Up

Telephone follow-up typically occurs during the first week after discharge to check on how things are going at home. Calls can be made by perinatal nurses within the agency as part of follow-up care or by the local public health nurses. A disadvantage to a phone call assessment is that the nurse cannot see the client and thus must rely on the mother's or family's observations. The experienced nurse needs to be able to recognize distress and give appropriate advice and referral information if needed.

Providing Out-Patient Follow-Up

For mothers with established health care providers, such as midwives, family physicians, pediatricians, and obstetricians, visits to the office are arranged soon after discharge. For the woman with an uncomplicated vaginal birth, an office visit is usually scheduled for 4 to 6 weeks after childbirth. A woman who has had a cesarean birth frequently is seen within 2 weeks after hospital discharge. Hospital discharge orders will specify when these visits

should be made. Newborn examinations and further diagnostic laboratory studies are scheduled within the first week.

▶ Take NOTE!

In Canada, women may deliver at home under the care of a registered midwife. Women may also choose midwifery care but deliver in hospital and leave within hours of delivery. In both cases, women and babies are followed at home daily for several days by the midwife. Guidelines for follow-up with mothers and infants vary according to the nature of the professional providing maternal/child care.

Out-patient clinics are available in many communities. If family members run into a problem, the local clinic is available to provide assessment and treatment. Clinic visits can replace or supplement home visits. Although these clinics are open during daytime hours only and the staff members are unfamiliar with the family, they can be a valuable resource for the new family with a problem or concern.

Providing Home Visit Follow-Up

Depending on the part of the country, home visits are usually made within the first week after discharge to assess the mother and newborn. During the home visit, the nurse assesses for and manages common physical and psychosocial problems. In addition, the home nurse can help the new parents adjust to the change in their lives. The postpartum home visit usually includes the following:

- Maternal assessment: general well-being, vital signs, breast health and care, abdominal and musculoskeletal status, voiding status, fundus and lochia status, psychological and coping status, family relationships, proper feeding technique, environmental safety check, newborn care knowledge and health teaching needed (Fig. 16.9 shows sample assessment forms)
- Infant assessment: physical examination, general appearance, vital signs, home safety check, child development status, any education needed to improve parents' skills
- The homecare nurse must be prepared to support and educate the woman and her family in the following areas:
- Breastfeeding or bottle-feeding technique and procedures
- Appropriate parenting behaviour and problem solving
- Maternal/newborn physical, psychosocial, and culture-environmental needs

(text continues on page 498)

Maternal Assessment

Maternal/Newborn Record System

Page 1 of 2

PATIENT IDENTIFICATION

Record No. _____

Name _____

Home
address _____
STREET

CITY   STATE   ZIP

Date MO / DAY / YR   Time begin: _____   Date of delivery MO / DAY / YR
Time end: _____

Medication allergy ☐ None   Identify_____
Significant health history ☐ None   Identify_____

PHYSICAL

TEMP.	PULSE	RESP.	BP /

Breasts ☐ Nursing ☐ Non-nursing
Color ☐ Normal ☐ Reddened
Condition ☐ Soft ☐ Firm ☐ Engorged ☐ Blocked ducts
Secretion ☐ Colostrum ☐ Milk ☐ Other
Support bra ☐ No ☐ Yes, fit ☐ Appropriate
☐ Inappropriate

Nipples (If nursing) ☐ Erect ☐ Flat ☐ Inverted
Condition ☐ Intact ☐ Bruised ☐ Blistered
☐ Fissured ☐ Bleeding ☐ Scabbed
Care ☐ Water only ☐ Soap ☐ Air dry
☐ Topical agent (type/frequency) _____

☐ Other _____
Self-exam ☐ Accurate ☐ Inaccurate/instructed

Abdomen
Diastasis recti ☐ Absent ☐ Present_____cm
☐ Exercise taught
Incision ☐ None
Type ☐ Transverse ☐ Vertical ☐ Umbilical
Closure ☐ Staples ☐ Sutures ☐ Steri-strips
Condition ☐ Approximated ☐ Open_____cm
☐ Redness _____
☐ Swelling _____
☐ Discharge _____
☐ Other_____

Reproductive Tract
Uterus ☐ Firm ☐ Firm with massage ☐ Boggy
Height _____ ☐ Midline ☐ Displaced L R
☐ Non tender ☐ Tender ☐ With touch ☐ Constant
Lochia ☐ Rubra ☐ Serosa ☐ Alba
☐ Clots (describe)_____
☐ Fleshy odor ☐ Foul odor
Pads Type _____ Number/day _____
Saturation %_____
0   25   50   75   100

Perineum ☐ Intact ☐ Laceration
☐ Episiotomy Type _____ Extension _____
Condition ☐ Redness _____
☐ Edema _____
☐ Ecchymoses _____
☐ Discharge _____
☐ Approximation _____
Care ☐ Front-to-back cleansing ☐ Peri-bottle
☐ Soap/water
☐ Ice ☐ Sitz bath ☐ Warm ☐ Cool
☐ Topical agent (type/frequency) _____

☐ Other _____

Elimination
Urinary tract
Voiding pattern ☐ Normal ☐ Incontinence
☐ Bladder distention ☐ Catheter (type) _____
Signs of infection ☐ None/reviewed ☐ Urgency ☐ Frequency
☐ Dysuria ☐ CVA tenderness L R
Gastrointestinal tract
Bowel pattern ☐ Normal ☐ No BM
☐ Constipation ☐ Diarrhea
☐ Meds/treatments (type, frequency, effect) _____

Hemorrhoids ☐ No ☐ Yes (describe) _____
☐ Meds/treatments (type, frequency, effect) _____

Lower Extremities
Edema ☐ None ☐ Pedal ☐ Ankle ☐ Pretibial ☐ Thigh
☐ Pitting (describe)
Signs of thrombophlebitis ☐ None

	L	R		L	R
Homan's sign	☐	☐	Redness	☐	☐
Pain	☐	☐	Warmth	☐	☐
Swelling	☐	☐			

Pain	**No**	**Yes**	
		Managed	Problematic
Abdominal incision	☐	☐	☐
Back	☐	☐	☐
Breasts	☐	☐	☐
Headache	☐	☐	☐
Hemorrhoid	☐	☐	☐
Nipple	☐	☐	☐
Perineum	☐	☐	☐
Uterine cramping	☐	☐	☐
Other _____	☐	☐	☐

Analgesic ☐ No
☐ Yes (type/dose/frequency) _____

Reportable danger signs ☐ Aware ☐ Unaware/instructed

TESTS ☐ None
☐ Urinalysis
☐ CBC
☐ _____

IDENTIFIED NEEDS
_____
_____
_____
_____
_____
_____
_____
_____

Signature _____

A

FIGURE 16.9 Sample postpartum home visit assessment form. (A) Maternal
assessment. (continued)

Maternal Assessment
Maternal/Newborn Record System

Page 2 of 2

PATIENT IDENTIFICATION

Record No. _____

Name _____

Home address _____
STREET

CITY _____ STATE _____ ZIP

ACTIVITIES OF DAILY LIVING - 24 HOUR HISTORY

Date MO / DAY / YR

Nutrition

Appetite	☐ Good	☐ Fair	☐ Poor
Usual pattern	☐ Yes	☐ No	_____
Special diet	☐ No	☐ Yes	_____
Food intolerance/allergy	☐ No	☐ Yes	_____
Vitamin/mineral supplement	☐ No	☐ Yes	_____

Fluid intake (type/amount) _____

BREAKFAST	LUNCH	DINNER	SNACKS

General Hygiene ☐ Adequate ☐ Inadequate (describe)

Sleep/Activity

Amount of Activity

Night, uninterrupted _____ hrs

Naps ☐ No ☐ Yes _____ hrs

Fatigue ☐ None ☐ Minimal ☐ Moderate ☐ Exhausted

Activities

Limitations ☐ None Identify _____

	Appropriate	Inappropriate/instructed
☐ Self-care	☐ Infant care	
Stair climbing	☐	☐
Lifting	☐	☐
Household tasks	☐	☐
Outside home	☐	☐
Other _____		

Exercise

☐ None

	Accurate	Inaccurate/instructed
Kegel	☐	☐
Postpartum	☐	☐
Other		

PSYCHOLOGICAL

Review of Labor and Birth

Missing pieces	☐ No	☐ Yes
Unmet expectations	☐ No	☐ Yes
Unresolved feelings	☐ No	☐ Yes

Pertinent data _____

Emotional Status ☐ Happy ☐ Ambivalent ☐ Anxious

☐ Sad ☐ Other _____

Postpartum-depression (Key on reverse side)

☐ 0 ☐ 1 ☐ 2 ☐ 3 ☐ 4

☐ Signs/Symptoms Reviewed

General Comments (body image, role changes, concerns) _____

Postpartum Timetable (Key on reverse side)

☐ Taking in ☐ Taking hold ☐ Letting go

SEXUALITY

	Aware	Unaware/instructed
Relationship with partner		
Adjustment	☐	☐
Expressions of affection	☐	☐
Resuming Intercourse		
Timing (lack of lochia, comfort)	☐	☐
Vaginal dryness	☐	☐
Milk ejection (if lactating)	☐	☐
Position variation	☐	☐
Libidinal changes	☐	☐
Return of Menses	☐	☐

Contraceptive Method

☐ None ☐ Undecided/aware of options

☐ Natural family planning

☐ Cervical cap

☐ Condom

☐ Diaphragm

☐ Hormones ☐ Pill ☐ Injection ☐ Implant

☐ IUD

☐ Spermicide

☐ Sterilization ☐ Female ☐ Male

☐ Other _____

Accurate use ☐ Yes ☐ No/instructed

IDENTIFIED NEEDS

_____

_____

_____

Signature _____

FIGURE 16.9 (continued)

Newborn Assessment
Maternal/Newborn Record System

PATIENT IDENTIFICATION

Record No. _____

Name _____

Home
address _____
STREET

CITY   STATE   ZIP

Date MO / DAY / YR   Time begin: _____ Date of Birth MO / DAY / YR
                      Time end: _____
Significant history ☐ None   Identify _____

PHYSICAL

Temp _____ Pulse (rate/rhythm) _____ Resp _____
Weight _____ Birth weight _____ % Change _____
Length _____ Head _____ Chest _____

HEAD/NECK

	Level	Bulging	Depressed
1. Fontanels			
Anterior	☐	☐	☐
Posterior	☐	☐	☐

Sutures   ☐ Open   ☐ Closed   ☐ Overriding
2. Variations ☐ Molding ☐ Caput ☐ Cephalhematoma

	NORMAL	ABNORMAL	DETAIL VARIATIONS/ABNORMAL FINDINGS
3. Face (symmetry)	☐	☐	
4. Eyes (symmetry, conjunctiva, sciera, eyelids, PERL)	☐	☐	
5. Ears (shape, position, auditory response)	☐	☐	
6. Nose (patency)	☐	☐	
7. Mouth (lip, mucous membranes, tongue, palate)	☐	☐	
8. Neck (ROM, symmetry)	☐	☐	
Chest			
9. Appearance (shape, breasts, nipples)	☐	☐	
10. Breath sounds	☐	☐	
11. Clavicles	☐	☐	
Cardiovascular			
12. Heart sounds	☐	☐	
13. Brachial/femoral pulses (compare strength, equality)	☐	☐	
Abdomen			
14. Appearance (shape, size)	☐	☐	
15. Cord (condition)	☐	☐	
16. Liver (less than or equal to 3 cm ↓ ®costal margin)	☐	☐	
Genitalia			
17. Female (labia, introitus, discharge	☐	☐	
18. Male (meatus, scrotum, testes)	☐	☐	
19. Circumcision ☐ No ☐ Yes	☐	☐	
Musculoskeletal			
20. Muscle tone	☐	☐	
21. Extremities (symmetry, digits, ROM)	☐	☐	
22. Hips (symmetry, ROM)	☐	☐	
23. Spine (alignment, integrity)	☐	☐	
Neurologic			
24. Reflexes (presence, symmetry)			
Moro	☐	☐	
Grasp	☐	☐	
Babinski	☐	☐	
25. Cry (presence, quality)	☐	☐	

PHYSICAL (CONT'D)
Skin
Turgor   ☐ Good   ☐ Poor
Condition ☐ Smooth ☐ Dry, cracked ☐ Peeling
Color   ☐ Pink ☐ Ruddy ☐ Cyanotic ☐ Pale
          ☐ Jaundice (note levels)
            ☐ Head (3 mg/dl)
            ☐ Head and upper chest (6 mg/dl)
            ☐ Head and entire chest (9 mg/dl)
            ☐ Head, chest and abdomen to umbilicus (12 mg/dl)
            ☐ Head, chest and entire abdomen (15 mg/dl)
            ☐ Head, chest, abdomen, legs and feet (18 mg/dl)
Variations (Rashes, lesions, birthmarks). _____

NUTRITION
Feeding
Reflexes ☐ Root ☐ Suck ☐ Swallow
Hunger cues identified ☐ Yes ☐ No/instructed

BREAST	FORMULA
Frequency _____ times in _____ hours	Type _____
Time per breast _____ min _____ min	Amount _____ oz.
Positioning ☐ Correct	Frequency _____
☐ Incorrect _____	Preparation ☐ Correct
Latch ☐ Correct	☐ Incorrect _____
☐ Incorrect _____	
Appropriate audible swallows	☐ Correct
☐ Yes ☐ No	☐

Satiation demonstrated ☐ Yes
  ☐ No (describe) _____
Regurgitation ☐ No ☐ Yes (describe) _____
Pacifier use ☐ No ☐ Yes (type/pattern) _____

Stool (number/day, color, consistency) _____
Urine (number/day, color) _____

BEHAVIOR
Sleep/Activity Pattern (24 hours)
Sleep (16–20 hrs)   ☐ Yes ☐ No (describe) _____

Awake-alert (2–3 hrs)   ☐ Yes ☐ No (describe) _____

Awake-crying (2–4 hrs)   ☐ Yes ☐ No (describe) _____

Consolability (Key on reverse) ☐ 0 ☐ 1 ☐ 2 ☐ 3 ☐ 4

TESTS ☐ None   Time
☐ Metabolic screen kit no. _____   _____
☐ Bilirubin   _____
☐ Hematocrit   _____
☐ _____   _____
☐ _____

IDENTIFIED NEEDS _____

Signature _____

B

FIGURE 16.9 (continued) (**B**) Newborn assessment. (Used with permission: Copyright Briggs Corporation. Professional Nurse Associates.)

- Emotional needs of the new family
- Warning signs of problems and how to prevent or eliminate them
- Sexuality issues, including contraceptive use
- Immunization needs for both mother and infant
- Family dynamics for smooth transition
- Links to health care providers and community resources

□■■ Key Concepts

- ⊡ The transitional adjustment period between birth and parenthood includes education about baby care basics, the role of the new family, emotional support, breastfeeding or bottle-feeding support, and maternal mentoring.
- ⊡ Sensitivity to how childbearing practices and beliefs vary for multicultural families and knowledge about how best to provide appropriate nursing care to meet their needs are important during the postpartum period.
- ⊡ A thorough postpartum assessment is the key to preventing complications, as is frequent handwashing by the nurse, especially between handling mothers and infants.
- ⊡ The postpartum assessment using the acronym BUBBLE-EE (breasts, uterus, bowel, bladder, lochia, episiotomy/perineum, extremities, and emotions) is a helpful guide in performing a systematic head-to-toe postpartum assessment.
- ⊡ Lochia is assessed according to its amount, colour, and change with activity and time. It proceeds from lochia rubra to serosa to alba.
- ⊡ Because of shortened agency stays, nurses must use this brief time with the client to address areas of comfort, elimination, activity, rest and exercise, self-care, sexuality and contraception, nutrition, family adaptation, discharge, and follow-up.
- ⊡ The BCC (2011) and the SOGC (2009) advocate breastfeeding for all full-term newborns, maintaining that, ideally, breast milk should be the sole nutrient for infants for the first 6 months, followed by breastfeeding along with foods until 12 months of age or longer.
- ⊡ Successful parenting is a continuous and complex interactive process that requires the acquisition of new skills and the integration of the new member into the existing family unit.
- ⊡ Bonding is a vital component of the attachment process and is necessary in establishing parent–infant attachment and a healthy, loving relationship; attachment behaviours include seeking and maintaining close proximity to, and exchanging gratifying experiences with, the infant.
- ⊡ Nurses can be instrumental in facilitating attachment by first understanding attachment behaviours

(positive and negative) of newborns and parents, and intervening appropriately to promote and enhance attachment.

- ⊞ New mothers and their families need to be attended to over an extended period of time by nurses knowledgeable about mother care, newborn feeding (breastfeeding and bottle-feeding), newborn care, and nutrition.

REFERENCES

Babycenter. (2011). *How do I know if my baby is getting enough formula?* Retrieved February 28, 2012 from http://www.babycenter.ca/baby/formula/gettingenoughexpert/

Babycenter. (2012). *How much formula milk does my baby need?* Retrieved February 28, 2012 from http://www.babycenter.ca/baby/formula/howmuchmilk/

Bowers, P. (2007). *Cultural perspectives in childbearing.* Retrieved February 28, 2012 from http://www.nurse.com/ce/course.html?CCID=3245

Breastfeeding Committee for Canada. (2011). *Summary 1: Integrated 10 steps practice indicators for hospitals and community health services.* Retrieved March 10, 2012 from http://breastfeedingcanada.ca/documents/2011-03-30_BCC_BFI_Integrated_10_Steps_summary.pdf

Canadian Paediatric Society. (2009). Concerns for the use of soy-based formulas in infant nutrition. *Paediatrics and Child Health, 14*(3):109–113.

Cassar, L. (2006). Cultural expectations of Muslims and Orthodox Jews in regard to pregnancy and the postpartum period: A study in comparison and contrast. *International Journal of Childbirth Education, 21*(2), 27–30.

Evans, R. J., Evans, M. K., Brown, Y. M. R., & Orshan, S. A. (2010). *Canadian maternity, newborn & women's health nursing.* Philadelphia: Lippincott Williams & Wilkins.

Grossman, K. E., Grossman, K., & Waters, E. (2006). *Attachment from infancy to adulthood.* New York: Guilford Publications, Inc.

Health Canada. (2011). *Canada's Food Guide: Pregnancy and breastfeeding.* Retrieved August 30, 2011 from http://hc-sc.gc.ca/fn-an/food-guide-aliment/choose-choix/advice-conseil/women-femmes-eng.php

HealthLink, B. C. (2010). *Formula feeding your baby; getting started.* Retrieved February 28, 2012 from http://www.hc-sc.gc.ca/fn-an/food-guide-aliment/choose-choix/advice-conseil/women-femmes-eng.php

Logsdon, M. C., Wisner, K. L., & Pinto-Foltz, M. D. (2006). The impact of postpartum depression on mothering. *Journal of Obstetric, Gynecologic, and Neonatal Nursing, 35*(5), 652–658.

London, M. L., Ladewig, P. W., Ball, J. W., Bindler, R. C., & Cowen, K. J. (2011). In M. Connor (Ed.), *Maternal and child nursing care* (3rd ed.). Upper Saddle River, NJ: Pearson.

McKinney, E. S., James, S. R., Murray, S. S., & Ashwill, J. W. (Eds.). (2009). *Maternal-child nursing* (3rd ed.). Canada: Saunders Elsevier.

Moretti, M. E., Lee, A., Ito, S. (2000). *Cancer in pregnancy: Which drugs are contraindicated during breastfeeding?* Retrieved February 28, 2012 from http://www.motherisk.org/prof/commonDetail.jsp?content_id=232

Nash, L. R. (2007). Postpartum care. In R. E. Rakel & E. T. Bope (Eds.), *Conn's current therapy 2007.* Philadelphia: Saunders Elsevier.

Oppenheim, D., & Goldsmith, D. F. (2007). *Attachment theory in clinical work with children: Bridging the gap between research and practice.* New York: Guilford Publications, Inc.

Potter, P. A., & Perry, A. G. (2010). Urinary elimination. In P. A. Potter, A. G. Perry, M. J. Wood & J. C. Ross-Kerr (Eds.), *Canadian fundamentals of nursing* (4th ed.). Toronto, ON: Mosby Elsevier.

Public Health Agency of Canada. (2009). *What mothers say: The Canadian maternity experiences survey.* Retrieved February 28, 2012 from http://www.phac-aspc.gc.ca/rhs-ssg/pdf/survey-eng.pdf

Public Health Agency of Canada. (2011a). *Sleep safe for your baby.* Retrieved February 28, 2012 from http://www.phac-aspc.gc.ca/hp-ps/dca-dea/stages-etapes/childhood-enfance_0–2/sids/index-eng.php

Typically, recovery from childbirth proceeds normally in both physiologic and psychological aspects. It is a time filled with many changes and wide-ranging emotions, and the new mother commonly experiences a great sense of accomplishment. However, the woman can experience deviations from the norm, developing a postpartum condition that places her at risk. The development of a high-risk condition or complication can become a life-threatening event. This chapter addresses the nursing management of the most common conditions that place the postpartum woman at risk: hemorrhage, infection, thromboembolic disease, and postpartum emotional disorders.

Postpartum Hemorrhage

Postpartum hemorrhage (PPH) is a potentially life-threatening complication of both vaginal and cesarean births. It occurs in 5% of deliveries and is the leading cause of maternal death worldwide, with an estimated mortality rate of 140,000 per year or one maternal death every 4 minutes (Leduc, Senikas, & Lalonde, 2009). In Canada, the incidence of direct maternal mortality from hemorrhage is 2.5 per 1,000,000 live births (Public Health Agency of Canada [PHAC], 2008).

Primary or early PPH is defined as excessive bleeding that occurs in the first 24 hours after delivery (Leduc et al., 2009). Blood loss that occurs 24 hours to 6 weeks after birth is termed secondary or late PPH. Traditionally, the definition of PPH has been blood loss greater than 500 mL after vaginal birth and more than 1,000 mL after abdominal birth (Leduc et al., 2009). However, this definition is arbitrary because estimates of blood loss at birth are subjective and generally inaccurate. Studies have suggested that health care providers consistently underestimate actual blood loss (Leduc et al., 2009; Maslovitz, Barkai, Lessing, et al., 2008; Tebruegge, Misra, Pantazidou, et al., 2009). A more objective definition of PPH would be any amount of bleeding that places the mother in hemodynamic instability (Leduc et al., 2009).

Factors that place a woman at risk for PPH are listed in Box 22.1.

Etiology

Excessive bleeding can occur at any time between the separation of the placenta and its expulsion or removal. The most common cause of PPH is **uterine atony**, failure of the uterus to contract and retract after birth. The uterus must remain contracted after birth to control bleeding from the placental site. Any factor that causes the uterus to relax after birth will cause bleeding—even a full bladder that displaces the uterus.

Over the course of a pregnancy, maternal blood volume increases by approximately 50% (4 to 6 L). The

BOX 22.1 Factors Placing A Woman at Risk for Postpartum Hemorrhage

- Prolonged first, second, or third stage of labour
- Previous history of postpartum hemorrhage
- Multiple gestation
- Uterine infection
- Manual extraction of placenta
- Arrest of descent
- Maternal exhaustion, malnutrition, or anemia
- Mediolateral episiotomy
- Pre-eclampsia
- Precipitous birth
- Maternal hypotension
- Previous placenta previa
- Coagulation abnormalities
- Birth canal lacerations
- Operative birth (forceps or vacuum)
- Augmented labour with medication
- Coagulation abnormalities
- Grand multiparity
- Hydramnios

Sources: Gilbert, E. S. (2011). *Manual of high risk pregnancy & delivery* (5th ed.). St. Louis, MO: Mosby Elsevier; & Leduc, D., Senikas, V., & Lalonde, A. B. (2009). SOGC clinical practice guideline: Active management of the third stage of labour: Prevention and treatment of postpartum hemorrhage. *Journal of Obstetrics and Gynaecology Canada, 31*(10), 980–993. Retrieved March 12, 2012 from http://www.sogc.org/guidelines/documents/gui235CPG0910.pdf.

plasma volume increases somewhat more than the total red blood cell volume, leading to a fall in the hemoglobin and hematocrit levels. The increase in blood volume meets the perfusion demands of the low-resistance uteroplacental unit and provides a reserve for the blood loss that occurs at delivery (Blackburn, 2008). Given this increase, the typical signs of hemorrhage (i.e., falling blood pressure, increasing pulse rate, and decreasing urinary output) do not appear until as much as 1,800 to 2,100 mL has been lost (Gilbert, 2011). In addition, accurate determination of actual blood loss is difficult because of pooling inside the uterus and on peripads, mattresses, and the floor. Because no universal clinical standard exists, nurses must be vigilant of risk factors, checking clients carefully before letting the primary care provider leave.

Other causes of PPH include lacerations of the genital tract, episiotomy, retained placental fragments, uterine inversion, coagulation disorders, and hematomas of the vulva, vagina, or subperitoneal areas (Cabero Roura & Keith, 2009). A helpful way to remember the causes of PPH is the "4T's": tone, tissue, trauma, and thrombosis (Leduc et al., 2009).

Tone

Altered uterine muscle tone most commonly results from overdistention of the uterus. Overdistention can be caused by multifetal gestation, fetal macrosomia, hydramnios, fetal abnormality, or placental fragments. Other causes might include prolonged or rapid, forceful labour, especially if stimulated; bacterial toxins (e.g., chorioamnionitis, endomyometritis, septicemia); use of anesthesia, especially halothane; and magnesium sulfate used in the treatment of pre-eclampsia (Leduc et al., 2009). Overdistention of the uterus is a major risk factor for uterine atony, the most common cause of early PPH, which can lead to hypovolemic shock.

Tissue

Uterine contraction and retraction lead to detachment and expulsion of the placenta after birth. Complete detachment and expulsion of the placenta permit continued contraction and optimal occlusion of blood vessels. Failure of complete separation of the placenta and expulsion does not allow the uterus to contract fully, since retained fragments occupy space and prevent the uterus from contracting fully to clamp down on blood vessels; this can lead to hemorrhage. After the placenta is expelled, a thorough inspection is necessary to confirm its intactness; tears or fragments left inside may indicate an accessory lobe or placenta accreta. Placenta accreta is an uncommon condition in which the chorionic villi adhere to the myometrium. This causes the placenta to adhere abnormally to the uterus and not separate and deliver spontaneously. Profuse hemorrhage results because the uterus cannot contract fully.

A prolapse of the uterine fundus to or through the cervix so that the uterus is turned inside out after birth is called **uterine inversion**. This condition is associated with abnormal adherence of the placenta, excessive traction on the umbilical cord, vigorous fundal pressure, precipitous labour, or vigorous manual removal of the placenta. Acute postpartum uterine inversion is rare, with an estimated incidence of 1 per 2,500 births (Mirza & Gaddipati, 2009). Prompt recognition and rapid treatment to replace the inverted uterus will avoid morbidity and mortality for this serious complication (Majd, Nawaz, Ismail, et al., 2009).

Subinvolution refers to the incomplete involution of the uterus or failure to return to its normal size and condition after birth (Al-Mehaisen, Al-Kuran, Amarin, et al., 2008). Complications of subinvolution include hemorrhage, pelvic peritonitis, salpingitis, and abscess formation (Leduc et al., 2009). Causes of subinvolution include retained placental fragments, distended bladder, uterine myoma, and infection. The clinical picture includes a postpartum fundal height that is higher than expected, with a boggy uterus; the lochia fails to change colour from red to serosa to alba within a few weeks. This condition is usually identified at the woman's postpartum examination 4 to 6 weeks after birth via a bimanual vaginal examination or ultrasound. Treatment is directed toward stimulating the uterus to expel fragments with a

uterine stimulant, and antibiotics are given to prevent infection.

Trauma

Damage to the genital tract may occur spontaneously or through the manipulations used during birth. For example, a cesarean birth results in more blood loss than a vaginal birth. The amount of blood loss depends on suturing, vasospasm, and clotting for hemostasis. Uterine rupture more common in women with previous cesarean scars or those who have undergone any procedure resulting in disruption of the uterine wall, including myomectomy, uteroplasty for a congenital anomaly, perforation of the uterus during a dilation and curettage (D&C), biopsy, or intrauterine device (IUD) insertion (Cabero Roura & Keith, 2009).

Trauma can also occur after prolonged or vigorous labour, especially if the uterus has been stimulated with oxytocin or prostaglandins. Trauma can also occur after extrauterine or intrauterine manipulation of the fetus.

Cervical lacerations commonly occur during a forceps delivery or in mothers who have not been able to resist bearing down before the cervix is fully dilated. Vaginal sidewall lacerations are associated with operative vaginal births but may occur spontaneously, especially if the fetal hand presents with the head. Lacerations can arise during manipulations to resolve shoulder dystocia. Lacerations should always be suspected in the face of a contracted uterus with bright-red blood continuing to trickle out of the vagina.

Thrombosis

Thrombosis (blood clots) helps to prevent PPH immediately after birth by providing a homeostasis in the woman's circulatory system. As long as there is a normal clotting mechanism that is activated, postpartum bleeding will not be exacerbated. Disorders of the coagulation system do not always appear in the immediate postpartum period due to the efficiency of stimulating uterine contractions through medications to prevent hemorrhage. Fibrin deposits and clots in supplying vessels play a significant role in the hours and days after birth. Coagulopathies should be suspected when postpartum bleeding persists without any identifiable cause (Peyvandi, Menegatti, & Siboni, 2011).

Ideally, the client's coagulation status is determined during pregnancy. However, if she received no prenatal care, coagulation studies should be ordered immediately to determine her status. Abnormal results typically include decreased platelet and fibrinogen levels; increased prothrombin time, partial thromboplastin time, and fibrin degradation products; and a prolonged bleeding time (Kadir, Chi, & Bolton-Maggs, 2009). Conditions associated with coagulopathies in the postpartum client include idiopathic thrombocytopenic purpura (ITP), von

Willebrand disease (vWD), and disseminated intravascular coagulation (DIC).

Idiopathic Thrombocytopenia Purpura

ITP is a disorder of increased platelet destruction caused by the development of autoantibodies to platelet-membrane antigens. The incidence of ITP in young women is approximately 1 to 2 per 1,000 pregnancies (Belkin, Levy, & Sheiner, 2009). Thrombocytopenia, capillary fragility, and increased bleeding time define the disorder. Clinical manifestations include easy bruising, bleeding from mucous membranes, menorrhagia, epistaxis, bleeding gums, hematomas, and severe hemorrhage after a cesarean birth or lacerations (Fujita, Sakai, Matsuura, et al., 2010). Glucocorticoids and immune globulin are the mainstays of medical therapy.

von Willebrand Disease

vWD is a congenital bleeding disorder, inherited as an autosomal dominant trait, that is characterized by a prolonged bleeding time, a deficiency of von Willebrand factor, and impairment of platelet adhesion (Peyvandi et al., 2011). It is estimated to affect 1 in 1,000 or 30,000 Canadians (Canadian Hemophilia Society, 2007). Most cases remain undiagnosed from lack of awareness, difficulty in diagnosis, a tendency to attribute bleeding to other causes, and variable symptoms (Castaman, Tosetto, & Rodeghiero, 2010). Symptoms include excessive bruising, prolonged nosebleeds, and prolonged oozing from wounds after surgery and after childbirth. The goal of therapy is to correct the defect in platelet adhesiveness by raising the level of von Willebrand factor with medications (Castaman et al., 2010).

Disseminated Intravascular Coagulation

DIC is a life-threatening, acquired pathologic process in which the clotting system is abnormally activated, resulting in widespread clot formation in the small vessels throughout the body (Peyvandi et al., 2011). It can cause PPH by altering the blood clotting mechanism. DIC is always a secondary diagnosis that occurs as a complication of abruptio placentae, amniotic fluid embolism, intrauterine fetal death with prolonged retention of the fetus, severe pre-eclampsia, septicemia, and hemorrhage. Clinical features include petechiae, ecchymoses, bleeding gums, tachycardia, uncontrolled bleeding during birth, and acute renal failure (Thachil & Toh, 2009). The treatment goal is to maintain tissue perfusion through aggressive administration of fluid therapy, oxygen, and blood products.

Nursing Management

Pregnancy and childbirth involve significant health risks, even for women with no preexisting health problems. There are approximately 50 cases of pregnancy-related hemorrhage per 1,000 pregnancies every year in Canada, with some of these women bleeding to death (PHAC, 2008). Most of these deaths occur within 4 hours of giving birth and are a result of problems during the third stage of labour (Leduc et al., 2009). The period after the birth and the first hours of postpartum are crucial times for the prevention, assessment, and management of bleeding. Compared with other maternal risks such as infection, bleeding can rapidly become life-threatening, and nurses, along with other health care providers, need to identify this condition quickly and intervene appropriately.

Nursing Assessment

Since the most common cause of immediate severe PPH is uterine atony (failure of the uterus to properly contract after birth), assessing uterine tone after birth by palpating the fundus for firmness and location is essential. A soft, boggy fundus indicates uterine atony.

> ▶ **Take** NOTE!
>
> *A soft, boggy uterus that deviates from the midline suggests a full bladder interfering with uterine involution. If the uterus is not in correct position (midline), it will not be able to contract to control bleeding.*

Assess the amount of bleeding. If bleeding continues even though there are no lacerations, suspect retained placental fragments. The uterus remains large with painless dark-red blood mixed with clots. This cause of hemorrhage can be prevented by carefully inspecting the placenta for intactness.

If trauma is suspected, attempt to identify the source and document it. Typically, the uterus will be firm with a steady stream or trickle of unclotted bright-red blood noted in the perineum. Most deaths from PPH are not due to gross bleeding, but rather to inadequate management of slow, steady blood loss (Cabero Roura & Keith, 2009).

Assessment for a suspected hematoma would reveal a firm uterus with bright-red bleeding. Observe for a localized bluish bulging area just under the skin surface in the perineal area (Fig. 22.1). Often, the woman will report severe perineal or pelvic pain and will have difficulty voiding. In addition, she will have hypotension, tachycardia, and anemia (Gilbert, 2011).

Assessment for coagulopathies as a cause of PPH would reveal prolonged bleeding from the gums and venipuncture sites, petechiae on the skin, and ecchymotic areas. The amount of lochia would be much greater also. Urinary output would be diminished, with signs of acute renal failure. Vital signs would show an increase in pulse rate and a decrease in level of consciousness. Signs of

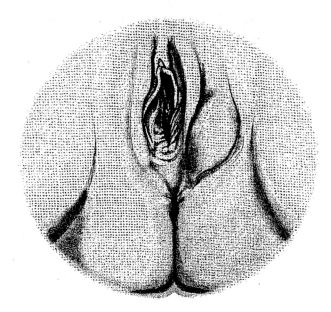

FIGURE 22.1 Perineal hematoma. Note the bulging, swollen mass.

shock do not appear until hemorrhage is far advanced due to the increased fluid and blood volume of pregnancy.

Nursing Management

Massage the uterus if uterine atony is noted. The uterine muscles are sensitive to touch; massage aids in stimulating the muscle fibers to contract. Massage the boggy uterus while supporting the lower uterine segment to stimlate contractions and expression of any accumulat blood clots. As blood pools in the vagina, stasis of blo causes clots to form; they need to be expelled as pressu is placed on the fundus. Overly forceful massage can ti the uterine muscles, resulting in further uterine atony a increased pain. See Nursing Procedure 22.1 for the ste in massaging the fundus.

If repeated fundal massage and expression of clc fail, medication is probably needed to contract the uter to control bleeding from the placental site. The injecti of a uterotonic drug immediately after birth is an impo tant intervention used to prevent PPH. Oxytocin (Pitoc Syntocinon); methylergonovine maleate (Methergin ergonovine maleate (Ergotrate); a synthetic analogue prostaglandin E1 misoprostol (Cytotec); and prostagla din F2-alpha (PGF2-alpha, carboprost [Hemabate]) a drugs used to manage PPH (Drug Guide 22.1). T choice of which uterotonic drug to use for management bleeding depends on the clinical judgment of the heal care provider, the availability of drugs, and the risks a benefits of the drug.

Remember Joan, the woman described at the beginning c the chapter? The nurse assesses her and finds that her uteru is boggy. What would the nurse do next? What additional nursing measures might be used if Joan's fundus remains boggy? When should the health care provider be notified?

Nursing Procedure 22.1

MASSAGING THE FUNDUS

Purpose: To Promote Uterine Contraction

1. After explaining the procedure to the woman, place one gloved hand (usually the dominant hand) on the fundus.
2. Place the other gloved hand on the area above the symphysis pubis (this helps to support the lower uterine segment).
3. With the hand on the fundus, gently massage the fundus in a circular manner. Be careful not to over massage the fundus, which could lead to muscle fatigue and uterine relaxation.
4. Assess for uterine firmness (uterine tissue responds quickly to touch).
5. If firm, apply gentle yet firm pressure in a downward motion toward the vagina to express any clots that may have accumulated.
6. Do not attempt to express clots until the fundus is firm because the application of firm pressure on an uncontracted uterus could cause uterine inversion, leading to massive hemorrhage.

7. Assist the woman with perineal care and applying a new perineal pad.
8. Remove gloves and wash hands.

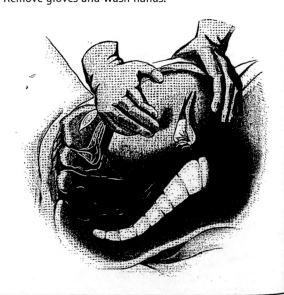

DRUG GUIDE 22.1   DRUGS USED TO CONTROL POSTPARTUM HEMORRHAGE

Drug	Action/Indication	Nursing Implications
Oxytocin (Pitocin, Syntocinon)	Stimulates the uterus to contract to control bleeding from the placental site	Assess fundus for evidence of contraction and compare amount of bleeding every 15 minutes or according to orders. Monitor vital signs every 15 minutes. Monitor uterine tone to prevent hyperstimulation. Reassure client about the need for uterine contraction and administer analgesics for comfort. Offer explanation to client and family about what is happening and the purpose of the medication. Provide non-pharmacologic comfort measures to assist with pain management. Set up the IV infusion to be piggybacked into a primary IV line. This ensures that the medication can be discontinued readily if hyperstimulation or adverse effects occur while maintaining the IV site and primary infusion.
Misoprostol (Cytotec)	Stimulates the uterus to contract to reduce bleeding; a prostaglandin analogue	As above. Very effective drug therapy for acute postpartum hemorrhage Contraindications: allergy, active CVD, pulmonary or hepatic disease; use with caution in women with asthma
Ergonovine maleate (Ergotrate)	Stimulates the uterus/to prevent and treat postpartum hemorrhage due to atony or subinvolution	Assess baseline bleeding, uterine tone, and vital signs every 15 minutes or according to protocol. Offer explanation to client and family about what is happening and the purpose of the medication. Monitor for possible adverse effects, such as nausea, vomiting, weakness, muscular pain, headache, or dizziness.
Prostaglandin (PGF2-alpha, carboprost [Hemabate])	Stimulates uterine contractions/to treat postpartum hemorrhage due to uterine atony when not controlled by other methods	Assess vital signs, uterine contractions, client's comfort level, and bleeding status as per protocol. Offer explanation to client and family about what is happening and the purpose of the medication. Monitor for possible adverse effects, such as fever, chills, headache, nausea, vomiting, diarrhea, flushing, and bronchospasm.

Sources: King, T.L., and Brucker, M.C. (2011). *Pharmacology for women's health.* Sudbury, MA: Jones and Bartlett Publishers; Lilley, L., Collins, S.R., Harrington, S., and Snyder, J. (2011). *Pharmacology and the nursing process.* St. Louis, MO: Mosby Elsevier; Skidmore-Roth, L. (2012). *Mosby's 2012 nursing drug reference.* (25th edition), St. Louis, MO: Mosby Elsevier; and Society of Obstetrics and Gynaecologists of Canada. (2009). Active management of the third stage of labour: Prevention and treatment of postpartum hemorrhage. *Clinical practice guideline.* Retrieved April 4, 2012 from http://www.sogc.org/guidelines/documents/gui235CPG0910.pdf.

Maintain the primary IV infusion and be prepared to start a second infusion at another site in case blood transfusions are necessary. Draw blood for type and cross-match and send it to the laboratory. Administer oxytocics as ordered, correlating and titrating the IV medication infusion rate to assessment findings of uterine firmness and lochia. Assess for visible vaginal bleeding, and count or weigh perineal pads.

▶ ***Take*** *NOTE!*

When weighing perineal pads to determine blood loss, remember that 1 g of pad weight is equivalent to 1 mL of blood loss (Gilbert, 2011; Leduc et al., 2009).

Check vital signs every 15 to 30 minutes, depending on the acuity of the mother's health status. Monitor her complete blood count to identify any deficit or assess the adequacy of replacement. In addition, assess the woman's level of consciousness to determine changes that may result from inadequate cerebral perfusion.

If a full bladder is present, assist the woman to empty her bladder to reduce displacement of the uterus. If the woman cannot void, anticipate the need to catheterize her to relieve bladder distention.

Retained placental fragments usually are manually separated and removed by the birth attendant. Be sure that the birth attendant remains long enough after birth to assess the bleeding status of the woman and determine the etiology. Assist the birth attendant with suturing any lacerations immediately to control hemorrhage and repair the tissue.

For the woman who develops ITP, glucocorticoids, intravenous immunoglobulin, intravenous anti-Rho D, and platelet transfusions may be administered. A splenectomy may be needed if the bleeding tissues do not respond to medical management.

In vWD, there is a decrease in von Willebrand factor, which is necessary for platelet adhesion and aggregation. It binds to and stabilizes factor VIII of the coagulation cascade (Peyvandi et al., 2011). Desmopressin, a synthetic form of vasopressin (antidiuretic hormone), may be used to treat vWD. This drug stimulates the release of stored factor VIII and von Willebrand factor from the lining of blood vessels, which increases platelet adhesiveness and shortens bleeding time. Other treatments that may be ordered include clotting factor concentrates, replacement of von Willebrand factor and factor VIII (Alphanate, Humate-P), antifibrinolytics (Amicar), and nonsteroidal anti-inflammatory drugs (NSAIDs) that do not cause platelet dysfunction (Bextra) (Castaman et al., 2010).

Be alert for women with abnormal bleeding tendencies, ensuring that they receive proper diagnosis and treatment. Teach them how to prevent severe hemorrhage by learning how to feel for and massage their fundus when boggy, assisting the nurse to keep track of the number of and amount of bleeding on perineal pads, and avoiding any medications with antiplatelet activity such as aspirin, antihistamines, or NSAIDS.

If the woman develops DIC, institute emergency measures to control bleeding and impending shock and prepare to transfer her to the intensive care unit. Identification of the underlying condition and elimination of the causative factor are essential to correct the coagulation problem. Be ready to replace fluid volume, administer blood component therapy, and optimize the mother's oxygenation and perfusion status to ensure adequate cardiac output and end-organ perfusion. Continually reassess the woman's coagulation status via laboratory studies.

Monitor vital signs closely, being alert for changes that signal an increase in bleeding or impending shock.

Observe for signs of bleeding, including spontaneous bleeding from gums or nose, petechiae, excessive bleeding from the cesarean incision site, hematuria, and blood in the stool. These findings correlate with decreased blood volume, decreased organ and peripheral tissue perfusion, and clots in the microcirculation (Pacheco, Costantine, Saade, et al., 2010).

> ▶ *Take* NOTE!
>
> *Always remember the four causes of PPH and the appropriate intervention for each: 1. Uterine atony—massage and oxytocics; 2. Retained placental tissue—evacuation and oxytocics; 3. Lacerations or hematoma—surgical repair; 4. Thrombosis (bleeding disorders)—blood products.*

Institute measures to avoid tissue trauma or injury, such as giving injections and drawing blood. Also provide emotional support to the client and her family throughout this critical time by being readily available and providing explanations and reassurance.

An IV oxytocin infusion is started for Joan. What assessments will need to be done frequently to make sure Joan is not losing too much blood? What discharge instructions need to be reinforced with Joan?

Thromboembolic Conditions

A thrombosis (blood clot within a blood vessel) can cause an inflammation of the blood vessel lining (**thrombophlebitis**), which in turn can lead to a possible thromboembolism (obstruction of a blood vessel by a blood clot carried by the circulation from the site of origin). Thrombi can involve the superficial or deep veins in the legs or pelvis. Superficial venous thrombosis usually involves the saphenous venous system and is confined to the lower leg. In some women, superficial thrombophlebitis may be caused by the use of the lithotomy position during birth. Deep venous thrombosis can involve deep veins from the foot to the calf, thighs, or pelvis. In both locations, thrombi can dislodge and migrate to the lungs, causing pulmonary embolism (PE) (James, 2009).

PE is a potentially fatal thromboembolic condition that occurs when the pulmonary artery is obstructed by a blood clot that has travelled from another vein into the lungs, causing an obstruction and infarction. When the clot is large enough to block one or more of the pulmonary vessels that supply the lungs, it can result in sudden death. PE is one of the leading causes of pregnancy-related deaths worldwide (Liu, Rouleau, Joseph, et al., 2009).

The incidence of PE in Canada is 5 in 1,000,000 live births (PHAC, 2008).

Pathophysiology

The major causes of a thrombus formation (blood clot) are venous stasis, injury to the innermost layer of the blood vessel, and hypercoagulation. Venous stasis and hypercoagulation are both common in the postpartum period. Other factors that place women at risk for thrombosis include prolonged bed rest, diabetes, obesity, cesarean birth, smoking, progesterone-induced distensibility of the veins of the lower legs during pregnancy, severe anemia, history of previous thrombosis, varicose veins, diabetes mellitus, advanced maternal age (older than 35 years), multiparity, and use of oral contraceptives before pregnancy (Jacobsen, Skjeldestad, & Sandset, 2008; Liu et al., 2009).

Nursing Assessment

Assess the woman closely for risk factors and signs and symptoms of thrombophlebitis. Look for risk factors in the woman's history such as use of oral contraceptives before the pregnancy, employment that necessitates prolonged standing, history of thrombophlebitis or endometritis, or evidence of current varicosities. Suspect superficial venous thrombosis in a woman with varicose veins who reports tenderness and discomfort over the site of the thrombosis, most commonly in the calf area. The area appears reddened along the vein and is warm to the touch. The woman will report increased pain in the affected leg when she ambulates and bears weight.

Manifestations of deep venous thrombosis are often absent and diffuse. If they are present, they are caused by an inflammatory process and obstruction of venous return. Calf swelling, erythema, warmth, tenderness, and pedal edema may be noted. A positive Homans sign (pain in the calf upon dorsiflexion) is not a definitive diagnostic sign because pain can also be caused by a strained muscle or contusion (Lindqvist, Torsson, Almqvist, et al., 2008; Liu et al., 2009).

Assess for signs and symptoms of PE, including unexplained sudden onset of shortness of breath, tachypnea, sudden chest pain, tachycardia, cardiac arrhythmias, apprehension, profuse sweating, hemoptysis, and sudden change in mental status as a result of hypoxemia (Liu et al., 2009). Expect a lung scan to be done to confirm the diagnosis.

Nursing Management

The three most common thromboembolic conditions occurring during the postpartum period are superficial venous thrombosis, deep venous thrombosis, and PE.

Preventing Thrombotic Conditions

Prevention of thrombotic conditions is an essential aspect of nursing management. Many deaths related to these conditions can be prevented by the routine use of simple measures:

- Developing public awareness about risk factors, symptoms, and preventive measures
- Preventing venous stasis by encouraging activity that causes leg muscles to contract and promotes venous return (leg exercises and walking)
- Using intermittent sequential compression devices to produce passive leg muscle contractions until the woman is ambulatory
- Elevating the woman's legs above her heart level to promote venous return
- Stopping smoking to reduce or prevent vascular vasoconstriction
- Applying compression stockings and removing them daily for inspection of legs
- Performing passive range-of-motion exercises while in bed
- Using postoperative deep-breathing exercises to improve venous return by relieving the negative thoracic pressure on leg veins
- Reducing hypercoagulability with the use of warfarin, aspirin, and heparin
- Preventing venous pooling by avoiding pillows under the knees, not crossing the legs for long periods, and not leaving the legs up in stirrups for long periods
- Padding stirrups to reduce pressure against the popliteal angle
- Avoiding sitting or standing in one position for prolonged periods
- Using a bed cradle to keep linens and blankets off extremities
- Avoiding trauma to legs to prevent injury to the vein wall
- Increasing fluid intake to prevent dehydration
- Avoiding the use of oral contraceptives

In women at risk, early ambulation is the easiest and most cost-effective method of prevention. Use of elastic compression stockings (TED hose or Jobst stockings) decreases distal calf vein thrombosis by decreasing venous stasis and augmenting venous return (Liu et al., 2009). Women who are at a high risk for thromboembolic disease based on risk factors or previous history of deep vein thrombosis or PE may be placed on prophylactic heparin therapy during pregnancy. Standard heparin or a low-molecular-weight heparin such as enoxaparin (Lovenox) can be given, since neither of these crosses the placenta. It is typically discontinued during labour and birth and then restarted during the postpartum period.

Treating Thromboembolic Disorders

Although thromboembolic disorders occur in less than 1% of all postpartum women, pulmonary embolus can be fatal if a clot obstructs the lung circulation; thus, early identification and treatment are paramount. For the woman with superficial venous thrombosis, care includes administering NSAIDs for analgesia, providing for rest and elevation of the affected leg, applying warm compresses to the affected area to promote healing, and using antiembolism stockings to promote circulation to the extremities.

Nursing interventions for a woman with deep vein thrombosis include bed rest and elevation of the affected extremity to decrease interstitial swelling and promote venous return from that leg. Apply antiembolism stockings to both extremities as ordered. Fit the stockings correctly and urge the woman to wear them at all times. Sequential compression devices can also be used for women with varicose veins, a history of thrombophlebitis, or a surgical birth. Anticoagulant therapy using a continuous IV infusion of heparin is started to prolong clotting time and prevent extension of the thrombosis. Monitor the woman's coagulation studies closely; these might include activated partial thromboplastin time (APTT), whole blood partial thromboplastin time, and platelet levels. Therapeutic APTT values typically range from 35 to 45 seconds, depending on which standard values are used (Liu et al., 2009). Also apply warm, moist compresses to the affected leg and administer analgesics as ordered to decrease the discomfort.

After several days of IV heparin therapy, expect to begin oral anticoagulant therapy with warfarin (Coumadin) as ordered. In most cases, the woman will continue to take this medication for several months after discharge.

For the woman who develops a PE, institute emergency measures immediately. The objectives of treatment are to prevent further growth or multiplication of thrombi in the lower extremities, prevent further thrombi from travelling to the pulmonary vascular system, and provide cardiopulmonary support if needed. Interventions include administering oxygen via mask or cannula and continuous IV heparin titrated according to the laboratory results, maintaining the client on bed rest, and administering analgesics for pain relief. Thrombolytic agents, such as tissue plasminogen activator (t-PA), might be used to dissolve pulmonary emboli and the source of the thrombus in the pelvis or deep leg veins, thus reducing the potential for a recurrence.

Educating the Client

Provide teaching about the use of anticoagulant therapy and possible danger signs (Teaching Guideline 22.1). Additional interventions include providing anticipatory guidance, support, and education about anticoagulants and associated signs of complications and risks. Focus discharge teaching on the importance of the following:

- Eliminating modifiable risk factors for deep vein thrombosis (smoking, use of oral contraceptives, a sedentary lifestyle, and obesity)
- Using compression stockings

TEACHING GUIDELINE 22.1

Teaching to Prevent Bleeding Related to Anticoagulant Therapy

- Watch for possible signs of bleeding and notify your health care provider if any occur:
  - Nosebleeds
  - Bleeding from the gums or mouth
  - Black, tarry stools
  - Brown "coffee ground" vomitus
  - Red to brown speckled mucus from a cough
  - Oozing at incision, episiotomy site, cut, or scrape
  - Pink-, red-, or brown-tinged urine
  - Bruises, "black and blue marks"
  - Increased lochia discharge (from present level)
- Practice measures to reduce your risk for bleeding:
  - Brush your teeth gently using a soft toothbrush.
  - Use an electric razor for shaving.
  - Avoid activities that could lead to injury, scrapes, bruising, or cuts.
  - Do not use any over-the-counter products containing aspirin or aspirin-like derivatives.
  - Avoid consuming alcohol.
  - Inform other health care providers about the use of anticoagulants, especially dentists.
  - If you accidentally cut or scrape yourself, apply firm direct pressure to the site for 5 to 10 minutes. Do the same after receiving any injections or having blood specimens drawn.
  - Avoid constrictive clothing and prolonged standing or sitting in a motionless, leg-dependent position.

- Making sure to comply with follow-up laboratory testing as scheduled
- Wearing an identification bracelet or band that indicates that you are taking an anticoagulant
- Knowing the danger signs and symptoms (sudden onset of chest pain, dyspnea, and tachypnea) to report to the health care provider

Postpartum Infection

Infection during the postpartum period is a common cause of maternal morbidity and mortality. Overall, postpartum infection is estimated to occur in up to 8% of all births. There is a higher occurrence in cesarean birth than in vaginal births (Belfort, Clark, Saade, et al., 2010; Clark, Belfort, Dildy, et al., 2008). The incidence of postpartum infections is expected to increase because of the earlier discharge of postpartum women from the hospital (Wong & Rosh, 2010).

Postpartum infection is defined as a fever of 38°C or higher after the first 24 hours after childbirth, occurring on at least 2 of the first 10 days after birth, exclusive of the first 24 hours (Gilbert, 2011; Wong & Rosh, 2010). Infections can easily enter the female genital tract externally and ascend through the internal genital structures. In addition, the normal physiologic changes of childbirth increase the risk for infection by decreasing the vaginal acidity due to the presence of amniotic fluid, blood, and lochia, all of which are alkaline. An alkaline environment encourages the growth of bacteria. Because today women are commonly discharged 24 to 48 hours after giving birth, nurses must assess new mothers for risk factors and identify early subtle signs and symptoms of an infectious process.

The common bacterial etiology of postpartum infections involves organisms that constitute the normal vaginal flora, typically a mix of aerobic and anaerobic species. Postpartum infections generally are polymicrobial and involve the following microorganisms: *Staphylococcus aureus, Escherichia coli, Klebsiella, Gardnerella vaginalis,* gonococci, coliform bacteria, group A or B hemolytic streptococci, *Chlamydia trachomatis,* and the anaerobes that are common to bacterial vaginosis (Arianpour, Safari, & Hatami, 2009; Paruk, 2008). Common postpartum infections include metritis, wound infections, urinary tract infections, and mastitis. Signs and symptoms of these postpartum infections are listed in Table 22.1.

Metritis

Although usually referred to clinically as endometritis, postpartum uterine infections typically involve more than just the endometrial lining. Metritis is an infectious condition that involves the endometrium, decidua, and adjacent myometrium of the uterus. Extension of metritis can result in parametritis, which involves the broad ligament and possibly the ovaries and fallopian tubes, or septic pelvic thrombophlebitis, which results when the infection spreads along venous routes into the pelvis (Wong & Rosh, 2010).

The uterine cavity is sterile until rupture of the amniotic sac. As a consequence of labour, birth, and associated manipulations, anaerobic and aerobic bacteria can contaminate the uterus. In most cases, the bacteria responsible for pelvic infections are those that normally reside in the bowel, vagina, perineum, and cervix, such as *E. coli, Klebsiella pneumoniae,* or *G. vaginalis.*

The risk for metritis increases dramatically after a cesarean birth; it complicates 10% to 20% of cesarean births. This is typically an extension of chorioamnionitis that was present before birth (indeed, that may have been why the cesarean birth was performed). In addition, trauma to the tissues and a break in the skin (incision) provide portals for bacteria to enter the body and multiply (Belfort et al., 2010).

Primary prevention of metritis is key and focuses on reducing the risk factors and incidence of cesarean

TABLE 22.1 SIGNS AND SYMPTOMS OF POSTPARTUM INFECTIONS

Postpartum Infection	Signs and Symptoms
Metritis	Lower abdominal tenderness or pain on one or both sides Temperature elevation (>38°C) Foul-smelling lochia Anorexia Nausea Fatigue and lethargy Leukocytosis and elevated sedimentation rate
Wound infection	Weeping serosanguineous or purulent drainage Separation of or unapproximated wound edges Edema Erythema Tenderness Discomfort at the site Maternal fever Elevated white blood cell count
Urinary tract infection	Urgency Frequency Dysuria Flank pain Low-grade fever Urinary retention Hematuria Urine positive for nitrates Cloudy urine with strong odour
Mastitis	Flu-like symptoms, including malaise, fever, and chills Tender, hot, red, painful area on one breast Inflammation of breast area Breast tenderness Cracking of skin or around nipple or areola Breast distention with milk

births. When metritis occurs, broad-spectrum antibiotics are used to treat the infection. Management also includes measures to restore and promote fluid and electrolyte balance, provide analgesia, and offer emotional support. In most treated women, reduction of fever and elimination of symptoms will occur within 48 to 72 hours after the start of antibiotic therapy.

Wound Infections

Any break in the skin or mucous membranes provides a portal for bacteria. In the postpartum woman, sites of wound infection include cesarean surgical incisions, the

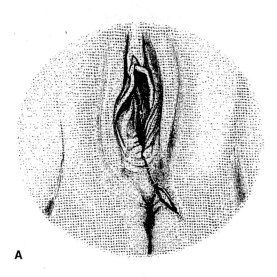

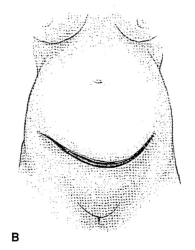

A

B

FIGURE 22.2 Postpartum wound infections. (**A**) Infected episiotomy site. (**B**) Infected cesarean birth incision.

episiotomy site in the perineum, and the genital tract as a result of laceration (Fig. 22.2). Wound infections are usually not identified until the woman has been discharged from the hospital because symptoms may not manifest until 24 to 48 hours after birth. Therefore, instructions about signs and symptoms to look for should be included in all discharge teaching. When a low-grade fever (<38°C), poor appetite, and a low energy level persist for a few days, a wound infection should be suspected.

Management of wound infections involves recognition of the infection followed by opening of the wound to allow drainage. Aseptic wound management with sterile gloves and frequent dressing changes if applicable, good handwashing, frequent perineal pad changes, hydration, and ambulation to prevent venous stasis and improve circulation are initiated to prevent development of a more serious infection or spread of the infection to adjacent structures. Parenteral antibiotics are the mainstay of treatment. Analgesics are also important because women often experience discomfort at the wound site.

Urinary Tract Infections

Urinary tract infections are most commonly caused by bacteria often found in bowel flora, including *E. coli, Klebsiella, Proteus,* and *Enterobacter* species. Any form of invasive manipulation of the urethra, such as urinary catheterization, frequent vaginal examinations, and genital trauma increase the likelihood of a urinary tract infection. Treatment consists of administering fluids if dehydration exists and antibiotics if appropriate.

Mastitis

Mastitis is an inflammation of the breast tissue caused by milk stasis and bacterial invasion that can develop in the first several postpartum weeks (Lowdermilk, Perry, Cashion, et al., 2011; Wilson-Clay & Hoover, 2008). Signs and symptoms of mastitis are the appearance of a

painful, hot and reddened area on the breast, fatigue, fever, flu-like symptoms, tachycardia, and headache (see Table 22.1). The infection is usually unilateral and located in the outer breast quadrants (Fig. 22.3) (Riordan & Wambach, 2010).

A number of risk factors predispose a woman to mastitis, including stress and fatigue, cracked nipples, plugged or blocked ducts, ample milk supply and/or decrease in number of feedings, and engorgement and stasis (Riordan & Wambach, 2010). Mastitis can be caused by a missed infant feeding, constriction from a bra that is too tight, breast trauma, poor drainage of duct and alveolus, poor maternal nutrition, vigorous exercise, or an infection.

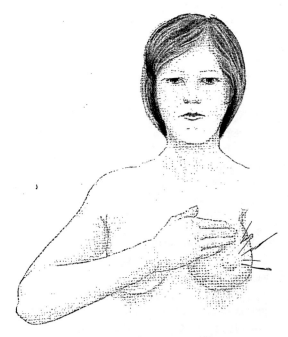

FIGURE 22.3 With mastitis, an area on one breast is tender, hot, red, and painful.

BOX 22.2   Factors Placing A Woman at Risk for Postpartum Infection

- Prolonged (>6 hours) premature rupture of membranes (removes the protective barrier to fetus and amniotic fluid so bacteria can ascend)
- Insertion of fetal scalp electrode or intrauterine pressure catheter for internal fetal monitoring during labour (provides entry into uterine cavity)
- Cesarean birth (allows bacterial entry due to break in protective skin barrier)
- Instrument-assisted childbirth, such as forceps or vacuum extraction (increases risk for trauma to genital tract, which provides bacteria access to grow)
- Urinary catheterization (could allow entry of bacteria into bladder due to break in aseptic technique)
- Regional anesthesia that decreases perception to void (causes urinary stasis and increases risk for urinary tract infection)
- Unwell staff attending to woman (promotes droplet infection from personnel)
- Compromised health status, such as anemia, obesity, smoking, drug abuse (reduces the body's immune system and decreases ability to fight infection)

- Preexisting colonization of lower genital tract with bacterial vaginosis, *C. trachomatis,* group B streptococci, *S. aureus,* and *E. coli* (allows microbes to ascend)
- Retained placental fragments (provides medium for bacterial growth)
- Manual removal of a retained placenta (causes trauma to the lining of the uterus and thus opens up sites for bacterial invasion)
- Trauma to the genital tract, such as episiotomy or lacerations (provides a portal of entry for bacteria)
- Prolonged labour with frequent vaginal examinations to check progress (allows time for bacteria to multiply and increases potential exposure to microorganisms or trauma)
- Poor nutritional status (reduces body's ability to repair tissue)
- Gestational diabetes (decreases body's healing ability and provides higher glucose levels on skin and in urine, which encourages bacterial growth)
- Break in aseptic technique during surgery or birthing process by the birth attendant or nurses (allows entry of bacteria)

The most common infecting organism is *S. aureus,* which comes from the breastfeeding infant's mouth or throat (Wong & Rosh, 2010). Infection can be transmitted from the lactiferous ducts to a secreting lobule, from a nipple fissure to periductal lymphatics, or by circulation (Riordan & Wambach, 2010).

The diagnosis is usually made without a culture being taken. Unless mastitis is treated adequately, it may progress to a breast abscess. Treatment of mastitis focuses on two areas: emptying the breasts and controlling the infection. The breast can be emptied either by the infant sucking or by manual expression. Increasing the frequency of nursing is advised. Lactation need not be suppressed. Control of infection is achieved with antibiotics. In addition, ice or warm packs and analgesics may be needed.

> ▶ **Take** NOTE!
>
> *Regardless of the etiology of mastitis, the focus is on reversing milk stasis, maintaining milk supply, and continuing breastfeeding, along with providing maternal comfort and preventing recurrence.*

Nursing Assessment

Perinatal nurses are primary caregivers for postpartum women and have the unique opportunity to identify subtle changes that place women at risk for infection. Because women today are commonly discharged 24 to 48 hours after giving birth, nurses must assess new mothers for

risk factors (Box 22.2) and identify early signs and symptoms of an infectious process, which may be subtle or specific depending on the type and location of the infection (see Table 22.1).

Review the client's history and physical examination and labour and birth record for factors that might increase her risk for developing an infection. Then complete the assessment (using the "BUBBLE-EE" parameters discussed in Chapter 16), paying particular attention to areas such as the abdomen and fundus, breasts, urinary tract, episiotomy, lacerations, or incisions, being alert for signs and symptoms of infection (see Table 22.1).

> ▶ **Take** NOTE!
>
> *A postpartum infection is commonly associated with an elevated temperature. Other generalized signs and symptoms may include chills, foul-smelling vaginal discharge, headache, malaise, restlessness, anxiety, and tachycardia. In addition, the woman may have specific signs and symptoms based on the type and location of the infection.*

When assessing the episiotomy site, use the acronym "REEDA" (redness, erythema or ecchymosis, edema, drainage or discharge, and approximation of wound edges) to ensure complete evaluation of the site (Gilbert, 2011; Wong & Rosh, 2010). Monitor the woman's vital signs, especially her temperature, for changes that may signal an infection.

Nursing Management

Nursing care focuses on preventing postpartum infections. Use the following guidelines to help reduce the incidence of postpartum infections:

- Maintain aseptic technique when performing invasive procedures such as urinary catheterization, when changing dressings, and during all surgical procedures.
- Use good handwashing technique before, after, and in between each patient care activity.
- Reinforce measures for maintaining good perineal hygiene.
- Use adequate lighting and turn the client to a side-lying position to assess the episiotomy site.
- Screen all visitors for any signs of active infections to reduce the client's risk for exposure.
- Review the client's history for preexisting infections or chronic conditions.
- Monitor vital signs and laboratory results for any abnormal values.
- Monitor the frequency of vaginal examinations and length of labour.
- Assess frequently for early signs of infection, especially fever and the appearance of lochia.
- Inspect wounds frequently for inflammation and drainage.
- Encourage rest, adequate hydration, and healthy eating habits.
- Reinforce preventive measures during any interaction with the client.

Client teaching is essential. Review the signs and symptoms of infection, emphasizing the danger signs and symptoms that need to be reported to the health care provider. Most importantly, stress proper handwashing, especially after perineal care and before and after breastfeeding. Also reinforce measures to promote breastfeeding, including proper breast care (see Chapter 16).

If the woman develops an infection, also review treatment measures, such as antibiotic therapy if ordered, and any special care measures, such as dressing changes (Nursing Care Plan 22.1). Teaching Guideline 22.2 highlights the major teaching points for a woman with a postpartum infection.

Postpartum Emotional Disorders

The postpartum period involves extraordinary physiologic, psychological, and social and cultural changes in the life of a woman and her family. Women have varied reactions to their childbearing experiences, exhibiting a wide range of emotions. The norm of some cultures is that birth is a happy time for all new mothers and is associated with positive feelings such as joy and gratitude for a healthy infant. But for others, it may not be a happy event. New mothers may also feel weepy, overwhelmed,

TEACHING GUIDELINE 22.2

Teaching for the Woman with a Postpartum Infection

- Continue your antibiotic therapy as prescribed:
  - Take the medication exactly as ordered and continue with the medication until it is finished.
  - Do not stop taking the medication even when you are feeling better.
  - Check your temperature every day and call your health care provider if it is above 38°C.
  - Watch for other signs and symptoms of infection, such as chills, increased abdominal pain, change in the colour or odour of your lochia, or increased redness, warmth, swelling, or drainage from a wound site such as your cesarean incision or episiotomy. Report any of these to your health care provider immediately
- Practice good infection prevention:
  - Always wash your hands thoroughly before and after eating, using the bathroom, touching your perineal area, or providing care for your newborn.
  - Wipe from front to back after using the bathroom.
  - Remove your perineal pad using a front-to-back motion. Fold the pad in half so that the inner sides of the pad that were touching your body are against each other. Wrap in toilet tissue or place in a plastic bag and discard.
  - Wash your hands before applying a new pad.
  - Apply a new perineal pad using a front-to-back motion. Handle the pad by the edges (top and bottom or sides) and avoid touching the inner aspect of the pad that will be against your body.
  - When performing perineal care with the peri bottle, angle the spray of water to that it flows from front to back.
  - Drink plenty of fluids each day and eat a variety of foods that are high in vitamins, iron, and protein.
  - Be sure to get adequate rest at night and periodically throughout the day.

or unsure of what is happening to them. They may experience fear about loss of control; they may feel scared, alone, or guilty, or as if they have somehow failed. Although the exact cause is unknown, a lower incidence of postpartum emotional disorders occurs in cultures that promote open expression of emotions and woman-centred care (Lowdermilk et al., 2011).

Postpartum emotional disorders have been documented for years, but only recently have they received medical attention. Plummeting levels of estrogen and progesterone immediately after birth can contribute to postpartum mood disorders. It is believed that the greater the change in these hormone levels between pregnancy and

Nursing Care Plan 22.1

OVERVIEW OF THE WOMAN WITH A POSTPARTUM COMPLICATION

Jennifer, a 16-year-old G1P1, gave birth to a boy by cesarean 3 days ago due to cephalopelvic disproportion following 25 hours of labour with ruptured membranes. Her temperature is 39.2°C. She is complaining of chills and malaise and severe pain at the incision site. The site is red and warm to the touch with purulent drainage. Jennifer's lochia is scant and dark red, with a strong odour. She tells the nurse to take her baby back to the nursery because she doesn't feel well enough to care for him.

NURSING DIAGNOSIS: Ineffective thermoregulation related to bacterial invasion *as evidenced by fever, complaints of chills and malaise, and statement of not feeling well.*

Outcome Identification and Evaluation
Jennifer will exhibit a return to normothermia *as evidenced by a body temperature being maintained around 37°C, reports of a decrease in chills and malaise, and statements of feeling better.*

Interventions: Promoting Fever Reduction
- Assess vital signs every 2 to 4 hours and record results *to monitor progress of infection.*
- Offer cool bed bath or shower *to reduce temperature.*
- Place cool cloth on forehead and/or back of neck *for comfort.*
- Change bed linen and gown when damp from diaphoresis *to provide comfort and hygiene.*
- Administer antipyretics as ordered *to reduce temperature.*
- Administer antibiotic therapy and wound care as ordered *to treat infection.*
- Use aseptic technique *to prevent spread of infection.*
- Force fluids to 2,000 mL per shift to hydrate patient; document intake and output *to assess hydration status.*

NURSING DIAGNOSIS: Impaired skin integrity related to wound infection as *evidenced by purulent drainage, redness, swelling, and separation of wound edges*

Outcome Identification and Evaluation
Jennifer will experience a resolution of wound infection as *evidenced by a reduction in redness, swelling, and drainage from wound, absence of purulent drainage, and beginning signs and symptoms of wound healing.*

Interventions: Promoting Wound Healing
- Administer antibiotic therapy as ordered *to treat infection.*
- Perform frequent dressing changes and wound care as ordered *to promote wound healing;* monitor dressing for drainage, including amount, colour, and characteristics, *to evaluate for resolution of infection.*
- Use aseptic technique *to prevent spread of infection.*
- Encourage fluid intake *to maintain fluid balance;* encourage adequate dietary intake, including protein, *to promote healing.*

NURSING DIAGNOSIS: Acute pain related to infectious process

Outcome Identification and Evaluation
Patient reports decreased pain *as evidenced by a rating of 0 or 1 on pain scale, verbalization of relief with pain management, and statements of feeling better and ability to rest comfortably.*

Interventions: Relieving Pain
- Place client in semi-Fowler's position to facilitate drainage and relieve pressure.
- Assess pain level on pain scale of 0 to 10 to quantify pain; reassess pain level after intervening to determine effectiveness of intervention.
- Assess fundus gently to ensure appropriate involution.
- Administer analgesics as needed and on time as ordered to maintain pain relief.
- Provide for rest periods to allow for the healing process.
- Encourage good dietary intake to promote healing.
- Assist with positioning in bed with pillows to promote comfort. Offer a backrub or other non-pharmacologic pain relief measure to ease aches and discomfort if desired.

(continued)

Nursing Care Plan 22.1 (continued)

NURSING DIAGNOSIS: Risk for impaired parental/infant attachment related to effects of postpartum infection *as evidenced by mother's request to take baby back to the nursery.*

Outcome Identification and Evaluation
Client begins to bond with newborn appropriately with each exposure *as evidenced by desire to spend time with newborn, expression of positive feelings toward newborn when holding him or her, increasing participation in care of newborn as client's condition improves, and statements about help and support at home to care for self and newborn.*

Interventions: Promoting Mother–Newborn Interaction
- Promote adequate rest and sleep *to promote healing.*
- Bring newborn to mother after she is rested and had an analgesic *to allow mother to focus her energies on the child.*
- Progressively allow the client to care for or comfort her infant as her energy level and pain level improve *to promote self-confidence in caring for the newborn.*
- Offer praise and positive reinforcement for caretaking tasks; stress positive attributes of newborn to mother while caring for him or her *to facilitate bonding and attachment.*
- Contact family members to participate in care of the newborn *to allow mother to rest and recover from infection.*
- Encourage mother to care for herself first and then the newborn *to ensure adequate energy for newborn's care.*
- Arrange for assistance and support after discharge from hospital *to aid in providing necessary backup.*
- Refer to community health nurse for follow-up care of mother and newborn at home *to foster continued development of maternal–infant relationship.*

---

postpartum, the greater the chance is for developing a mood disorder (Joy, Contag, & Templeton, et al., 2012).

Many types of emotional disorders occur in the postpartum period. Although their description and classification may be controversial, the disorders are commonly classified on the basis of their severity as postpartum or baby blues, postpartum depression, and postpartum psychosis.

Postpartum or Baby Blues

Many postpartum women (approximately 50% to 85%) experience the "baby blues." The woman exhibits mild depressive symptoms of anxiety, irritability, mood swings, tearfulness, increased sensitivity, and fatigue (Joy et al., 2012). The "blues" typically peak on postpartum days 4 and 5 and usually resolve by postpartum day 10. Although the woman's symptoms may be distressing, they do not reflect psychopathology and usually do not affect the mother's ability to function and care for her infant. Baby blues are usually self-limiting and require no formal treatment other than reassurance and validation of the woman's experience, as well as assistance in caring for herself and the newborn. However, follow-up of women with postpartum blues is important, as up to 20% go on to develop postpartum depression (Doucet, Dennis, Letourneau, et al., 2009).

Postpartum Depression

Depression is more prevalent in women than in men, which may be related to biological, hormonal, and psy-

chosocial factors. If the symptoms of postpartum blues last beyond 6 weeks and seem to get worse, the mother may be experiencing **postpartum depression**, a major depressive episode associated with childbirth (Joy et al., 2012). In Canada, as many as 8% to 23% of mothers develop postpartum depression in the first year following childbirth (Sharma & Penava, 2010). Unlike the postpartum blues, women with postpartum depression feel worse over time, and changes in mood and behaviour do not go away on their own.

The exact etiology is unknown but it appears to be a multi-factorial disorder and several factors can increase a mother's risk for developing postpartum depression:

- History of previous depression
- History of postpartum depression
- Evidence of depressive symptoms during pregnancy
- Family history of depression
- Life stress
- Childcare stress
- Prenatal anxiety
- Lack of social support
- Relationship stress
- Difficult or complicated pregnancy
- Traumatic birth experience
- Birth of a high-risk or special-needs infant (Doucet et al., 2009; Sharma & Penava, 2010)

Postpartum depression affects not only the woman but also the entire family. Identifying depression early can substantially improve the client and family outcomes. Postpartum depression usually has a more gradual onset

As an assertive practicing attorney in her thirties, my first pregnancy was filled with nagging feelings of doubt about this upcoming event in my life. Throughout my pregnancy I was so busy with trial work that I never had time to really evaluate my feelings. I was always reading about the bodily changes that were taking place, and on one level I was feeling excited, but on another level I was emotionally drained. Shortly after the birth of my daughter, those suppressed nagging feelings of doubt surfaced big time and practically immobilized me. I felt exhausted all the time and was only too glad to have someone else care for my daughter. I didn't breastfeed because I thought it would tie me down too much. Although at the time I thought this "low mood" was normal for all new mothers, I have since found out it was postpartum depression. How could any woman be depressed about this wondrous event?

Thoughts: Now that postpartum depression has been recognized as a real emotional disorder, it can be treated. This woman showed tendencies during her pregnancy but was able to suppress the feelings and go forward. Her description of her depression is very typical of many women who suffer in silence, hoping to get over these feelings in time. What can nurses do to promote awareness of this disorder? Can it be prevented?

and becomes evident within the first 6 weeks postpartum. Some of the common manifestations are listed in Box 22.3.

Postpartum depression lends itself to prophylactic intervention because its onset is predictable, the risk

BOX 22.3 Common Manifestations of Postpartum Depression

- Loss of pleasure or interest in life
- Low mood, sadness, tearfulness
- Exhaustion that is not relieved by sleep
- Feelings of guilt
- Irritability
- Inability to concentrate
- Anxiety
- Despair
- Compulsive thoughts
- Loss of libido
- Loss of confidence
- Sleep difficulties (insomnia)
- Loss of appetite
- Feelings of failure as a mother (Gilbert, 2011)

period for illness is well defined, and women at high risk can be identified using a screening tool. Prophylaxis starts with a prenatal risk assessment and education. Based on the woman's history of prior depression, prophylactic antidepressant therapy may be needed during the third trimester or immediately after giving birth. See Evidence-based Practice 22.1.

Management of postpartum depression mirrors that of any major depression—a combination of antidepressant medication, antianxiety medication, and psychotherapy in an out-patient or in-patient setting (Gilbert, 2011). Marital counselling may be necessary when marital problems may be contributing to the woman's depressive symptoms.

Postpartum Psychosis

At the severe end of the continuum of postpartum emotional disorders is postpartum psychosis, which occurs in 1 woman per 1,000 births (Sharma & Penava, 2010). It generally surfaces within 3 weeks of giving birth. Symptoms of postpartum psychosis include sleep disturbances, fatigue, depression, and hypomania. The mother will be tearful, confused, and preoccupied with feelings of guilt and worthlessness. Early symptoms resemble those of depression, but they may escalate to delirium, hallucinations, anger toward herself and her infant, bizarre behaviour, manifestations of mania, and thoughts of hurting herself and the infant. The mother frequently loses touch with reality and experiences a severe regressive breakdown, associated with a high risk for suicide or infanticide (Doucet et al., 2009).

Most women with postpartum psychosis are hospitalized for up to several months. Psychotropic drugs are almost always part of treatment, along with individual psychotherapy and support group therapy.

► *Take* NOTE!

The greatest hazard of postpartum psychosis is suicide. Infanticide and child abuse are also risks if the woman is left alone with her infant. Early recognition and prompt treatment of this disorder is imperative (Pacagnella, Cecatti, Camargo, et al., 2010).

Nursing Assessment
Postpartum emotional disorders are often overlooked and go unrecognized despite the large percentage of women who experience them (Pacagnella et al., 2010). The postpartum period is a time of increased vulnerability, but few women receive education about the possibility of depression after birth. In addition, many women

EVIDENCE-BASED PRACTICE 22.1
Psychosocial and Psychological Interventions to Prevent Postpartum Depression

● Study

Postpartum depression is a devastating condition that affects approximately 13% of new mothers. The negative maternal and newborn outcomes associated with postpartum depression are well documented in the literature. There is a lack of knowledge about its cause and mortality, and it often remains undetected, as women are reluctant to disclose symptoms of depression or seek treatment. The two clinical questions guided the study toward preventing postpartum depression: how can nurses confirm depressive symptoms in postpartum women, and what effective prevention interventions can nurses implement in practice?

Reviewers searched multiple databases to identify 106 peer-reviewed research articles and two guidelines published in English. A panel of experts and 46 stakeholders representing diverse perspectives, including women who experienced postpartum depression, reviewed the articles and guidelines. In total, 10 specific recommendations were developed, including two prevention recommendations.

▲ Findings

Women who received preventive psychosocial or psychological interventions for reducing the risk for developing postpartum depression suggest that intensive, professionally based support may prevent women from developing postpartum depression. The first practice recommendation is for individualized and flexible nursing preventive interventions based on the self-identification or diagnosis of depressive symptoms of at-risk families. Preventive interventions included antenatal and postnatal education, lay home visits, and early postpartum follow-up. The second recommendation is for nurses to initiate prevention strategies in the early postpartum period.

▦ Nursing Implications

The study provided some useful information for nurses to incorporate when providing care to pregnant women throughout the perinatal period. Nurses need to remain alert for risk factors associated with postpartum depression so they can initiate appropriate interventions for these vulnerable women and their families. Nurses can implement flexible and individually based psychosocial and psychological interventions during the prenatal period, keeping in mind that these interventions need to be continued throughout the postpartum period. They can also advocate for their clients upon discharge to ensure appropriate follow-up and support in the community and minimize impact on the family.

Source: McQueen, K., Montgomery, P., Lappan-Gracon, S., Evans, M., & Hunter, J. (2008). Evidence-based recommendations for depressive symptoms in postpartum women. *Journal of Obstetric, Gynecologic and Neonatal Nursing, 37,* 127–136. doi:10.1111/j.1552-6909.2008.00215.x

may feel ashamed of having negative emotions at a time when they "should" be happy; thus, they don't seek professional help. Nurses can play a major role in providing guidance about postpartum emotional disorders, detecting manifestations, and assisting women to obtain appropriate care.

Assessment should begin by reviewing the woman's history to identify risk factors that could predispose her to depression:

- Poor coping skills
- Low self-esteem
- Numerous life stressors
- Mood swings and emotional stress
- Previous psychological problems or a family history of psychiatric disorders
- Substance abuse
- Limited social support networks

Be alert for possible physical findings. Assess the woman's activity level, including her level of fatigue. Ask about her sleeping habits, noting any problems with insomnia. When interacting with the woman, observe for verbal and nonverbal indicators of anxiety as well as her ability to concentrate during the interaction. Difficulty concentrating and anxious behaviours suggest a problem. Also assess her nutritional intake: weight loss due to poor food intake may be seen. Assessment can identify women with a high-risk profile for depression, and the nurse can educate them and make referrals for individual or family counselling if needed.

Nursing Management

Nursing interventions that are appropriate to assist any postpartum woman to cope with the changes of this period include the following:

- Encourage the client to verbalize her feelings of what she is going through.
- Recommend that the woman seek help for household chores and child care.
- Stress the importance of good nutrition and adequate exercise and sleep.
- Encourage the client to develop a support system with other mothers.

- Assist the woman to structure her day to regain a sense of control.
- Emphasize the importance of keeping her expectations realistic.
- Discuss postponing major life changes, such as moving or changing jobs.
- Provide information about bodily changes (Canadian Mental Health Association, 2011).

The nurse can play an important role in assisting women and their partners with postpartum adjustment. Providing facts about the enormous changes that can occur during the postpartum period is critical. Review the signs and symptoms of all three emotional disorders. This information is typically included as part of prenatal visits and childbirth education classes. Know the risk factors associated with these disorders and review the history of clients and their families. Use specific, non-threatening questions to aid in early detection.

Discuss factors that may increase a woman's vulnerability to stress during the postpartum period, such as sleep deprivation and unrealistic expectations, so couples can understand and respond to those problems if they occur. Stress that many women need help after childbirth and that help is available from many sources, including people they already know. Assisting women to learn how to ask for help is important so they can gain the support they need. Also provide educational materials about postpartum emotional disorders. Have available referral sources for psychotherapy and support groups appropriate for women experiencing postpartum adjustment difficulties.

■■■ Key Concepts

- PPH is a potentially life-threatening complication of both vaginal and cesarean births. It is the leading cause of maternal mortality in Canada.
- A good way to remember the causes of PPH is the "4 T's": tone, tissue, trauma, and thrombosis.
- Uterine atony is the most common cause of early PPH, which can lead to hypovolemic shock.
- Oxytocin (Pitocin, Syntocinon), methylergonovine maleate (Methergine), ergonovine maleate (Ergotrate), and prostaglandin (PGF2-alpha, carboprost [Hemabate]) are drugs used to manage PPH.
- Failure of the placenta to separate completely and be expelled interferes with the ability of the uterus to contract fully, thereby leading to hemorrhage.
- Causes of subinvolution are retained placental fragments, distended bladder, uterine myoma, and infection.
- Lacerations should always be suspected when the uterus is contracted and bright-red blood continues to trickle out of the vagina.
- Conditions that cause coagulopathies may include ITP, vWD, and DIC.

- Pulmonary embolism is a potentially fatal condition that occurs when the pulmonary artery is obstructed by a blood clot that has travelled from another vein into the lungs, causing obstruction and infarction.
- The major causes of a thrombus formation (blood clot) are venous stasis and hypercoagulation, both of which are common in the postpartum period.
- Postpartum infection is defined as a fever of 38°C or higher after the first 24 hours after childbirth, occurring on at least 2 of the first 10 days exclusive of the first 24 hours.
- Common postpartum infections include metritis, wound infections, urinary tract infections, and mastitis.
- Postpartum emotional disorders are commonly classified on the basis of their severity: "baby blues," postpartum depression, and postpartum psychosis.
- Management of postpartum depression mirrors the treatment of any major depression—a combination of antidepressant medication, antianxiety medication, and psychotherapy in an out-patient or in-patient setting.

and may be treated as healthy newborns. Despite their appearance as term infants, late preterm infants (born at 34 to 36-6/7 weeks of gestation) are at increased risk for respiratory distress, temperature instability, hypoglycemia, apnea, feeding difficulties, and hyperbilirubinemia (Cooper, Holditch-Davis, Verklan, et al., 2012). Nurses working with healthy term infants must be cognizant of the risk factors for late preterm infants and watch for the development of problems related to the infant's immaturity. In an effort to identify these infants, a gestational-age assessment should be performed on all newborns soon after birth (Cooper et al., 2012).

The late preterm infant's care is further addressed in Chapter 28.

Common Newborn Concerns

Birth Injuries

Birth trauma includes any physical injury sustained by a newborn during labour and birth. Although most injuries are minor and resolve during the newborn period without treatment, some types of trauma require intervention; a few are serious enough to be fatal. See Chapter 29 for more information on birth injuries.

Soft-tissue injuries. Retinal and subconjunctival hemorrhages result from rupture of capillaries caused by increased pressure during birth. The hemorrhages clear within 5 days after birth and usually present no further problems. Parents need explanation about them and reassurance that these injuries are harmless.

Erythema, ecchymoses, petechiae, abrasions, lacerations, or edema of buttocks and extremities may be present. Localized discolouration can appear over a presenting part as a result of forceps or vacuum-assisted birth. Ecchymoses and edema can appear anywhere on the body. *Petechiae*, or pinpoint hemorrhagic areas, acquired during birth may extend over the upper trunk and face. These lesions are benign if they disappear within 2 or 3 days of birth and no new lesions appear. Ecchymoses and petechiae may be signs of a more serious disorder, such as thrombocytopenic purpura. To differentiate hemorrhagic areas from a skin rash or discolouration, the nurse can apply pressure to the skin with two fingers. Petechiae and ecchymoses do not blanch because extravasated blood remains within the tissues, whereas skin rashes and discolourations do blanch.

Trauma can occur during labour and birth to the presenting part. Caput succedaneum and cephalhematoma are normal and are discussed in Chapter 25 (see Fig. 25-10). Forceps injury and bruising from the vacuum cup occur at the site of application of the instruments. A forceps injury commonly produces a linear mark across both sides of the face in the shape of the blades of the forceps, with rarely skin integrity being compromised. These injuries usually resolve spontaneously within several days with no specific therapy. If small abrasions are evident the area should be kept clean to minimize the risk of infection. A topical ointment may be ordered by the primary health care provider to optimize healing. With increased use of the vacuum extractor, the incidence of these lesions has been significantly reduced.

Bruises over the face may be the result of face presentation (Fig. 26-5). In a breech presentation, bruising and swelling may

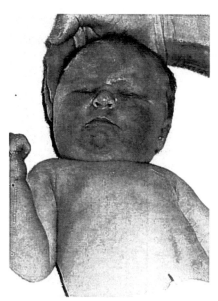

FIGURE 26-5 Marked bruising on the entire face of an infant born vaginally after face presentation. Less severe ecchymoses were present on the extremities. Phototherapy was required for treatment of jaundice resulting from the breakdown of accumulated blood. (From O'Doherty, N. [1986]. *Neonatology: Micro atlas of the newborn.* Nutley, NJ: Hoffmann–La Roche. Used with permission of F. Hoffmann–La Roche Ltd.)

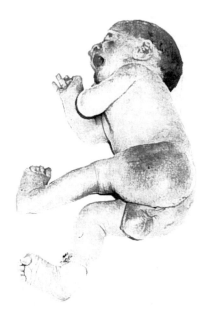

FIGURE 26-6 Swelling of genitalia and bruising of the buttocks after a breech birth. (From O'Doherty, N. [1986]. *Neonatology: Micro atlas of the newborn.* Nutley, NJ: Hoffmann–La Roche. Used with permission of F. Hoffmann–La Roche Ltd.)

be seen over the buttocks or genitalia (Fig. 26-6). The skin over the entire head may be ecchymotic and covered with petechiae caused by a tight nuchal cord or a precipitous delivery. If the hemorrhagic areas do not disappear spontaneously in 2 days or if the infant's condition changes, the primary health care provider should be notified.

Accidental lacerations can be inflicted with a scalpel during a Caesarean birth. These cuts may occur on any part of the body but are most often found on the scalp, buttocks, and thighs. Usually they are superficial and only need to be kept clean. If skin closure is needed, an adhesive substance or strips may be applied. Rarely are sutures needed.

Physiological Problems

Jaundice. Approximately 60% of all full-term newborns are visibly jaundiced (yellow) by the second through fifth day of life (Barrington, Sankaran, & CPS, 2007/2016). In most cases it is *physiological jaundice,* caused by increased levels of unconjugated bilirubin; physiological jaundice is usually self-limiting, requires no treatment, and resolves in a few days. Physiological jaundice or neonatal hyperbilirubinemia occurs in 80% of preterm newborns. The incidence of physiological jaundice is increased in Asian and Indigenous infants. It must be differentiated from pathological jaundice, or hyperbilirubinemia, which is associated with higher levels of unconjugated bilirubin. This type of jaundice can appear in the first 24 hours and often requires phototherapy to resolve. (See Chapter 25, pp. 653–655 for further discussion on pathophysiology of jaundice.)

Every newborn should be assessed for jaundice; this can be easily done when vital signs are assessed. Jaundice is generally first noticed in the head, especially the sclera and mucous membranes, and then progresses gradually to the thorax, abdomen, and extremities. Visual assessment of jaundice alone does not provide an accurate assessment of the level of serum bilirubin, especially in dark-skinned newborns; only 50% of babies with a total serum bilirubin (TSB) concentration greater than 128 mcmol/L appear jaundiced (Barrington et al., 2007/2016). To differentiate cutaneous jaundice from normal skin colour, the nurse applies pressure with a finger over a bony area (e.g., the nose, forehead, sternum) for several seconds to empty all the capillaries in that spot. If jaundice is present, the blanched area will look yellow before the capillaries refill. The conjunctival sacs and buccal mucosa are also assessed, especially in darker-skinned infants. Assessing for jaundice in natural light is recommended because artificial lighting and the reflection from walls can distort the actual skin colour.

Noninvasive monitoring of bilirubin via cutaneous reflectance measurements (transcutaneous bilirubinometry [TcB]) allows for repetitive estimations of bilirubin; however, there are limitations to the use of TcB monitors (Fig. 26-7). They are more accurate at lower TSB levels, are not accurate once phototherapy is initiated, and may be unreliable with changes in skin colour and thickness. TcB monitors may be used to screen clinically significant jaundice and decrease the need for serum bilirubin measurements (Barrington et al., 2007/2016). The CPS recommends monitoring healthy newborns at 35 weeks of gestation or greater before discharge from the hospital using hour-specific serum bilirubin levels to determine the infant's risk for development of hyperbilirubinemia requiring medical treatment or closer screening (Barrington et al., 2007/2016). Use of a nomogram (see Fig. 26-8) with three levels (high, intermediate, or low risk) of rising TSB values assists in the determination of newborns that might need further evaluation after discharge. Universal bilirubin screening based on

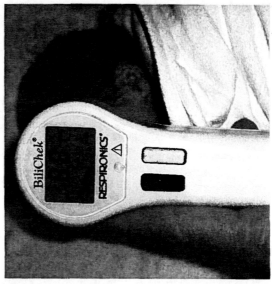

FIGURE 26-7 Transcutaneous monitoring of bilirubin with a transcutaneous bilirubinometry (TcB) monitor. (Courtesy Cheryl Briggs, BSN, RNC-NIC.)

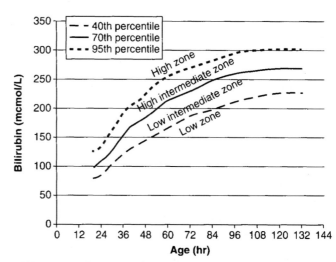

FIGURE 26-8 Nomogram for evaluation of screening total serum bilirubin (TSB) concentration in term and late preterm infants, according to the TSB concentration obtained at a known postnatal age in hours. (From Barrington, K. J., Sankaran, K., & Canadian Paediatric Society. [2007/2016]. Guidelines for detection, management and prevention of hyperbilirubinemia in term and late term newborn infants [35 or more weeks gestation]. *Paediatric Child Health, 12*[Suppl B], 1B–12B. Figure reproduced and adapted with permission from *Pediatrics, 114,* 297–316. Copyright © 2004 by the AAP.)

hour-specific TSB may be done at the same time as the routine newborn profile (phenylketonuria [PKU], galactosemia, and others) (Barrington et al., 2007/2016).

Risk factors that place infants in the high-risk category include gestational age 35 to 38 weeks, exclusive breastfeeding not well established and excessive weight loss, a sibling who had neonatal jaundice, visible bruising, cephalohematoma, DAT+ or other known hemolytic disease, G6PD deficiency (diagnosed at birth), ethnic background (East Asian), asphyxia (Apgar 0–3 beyond 5 minutes and cord PH less than 7), acidosis (ph less than 7 beyond initial cord sample), albumin less than 30 g/L, sepsis currently treated, temperature instability, and significant lethargy/poor feeding (Barrington et al., 2007/2016; Provincial Council for Maternal & Child Health [PCMCH] & Ministry of Health and Long-term Care, 2013). It is recommended that healthy infants (35 weeks or greater) receive assessment of bilirubin between 24 and 72 hours of life. If intervention is not required, further follow-up will depend on individual risk factors. If an infant is discharged before 24 hours of age, the infant needs further review within 24 hours by someone experienced in newborn care and with access to testing (Barrington et al., 2007/2016). Close follow-up of infants at risk for severe hyperbilirubinemia is essential; parents should be educated about the symptoms and encouraged to follow postdischarge recommendations.

If an infant is jaundiced in the first 24 hours of life, a TcB or TSB level should be measured and results interpreted on the basis of the newborn's age in hours according to the hour-specific nomogram for infants born at 35 weeks of gestation or later. Repeat testing is based on the risk level (low, intermediate, or high), the age of the newborn, and the progression of jaundice.

Pathological jaundice is that level of serum bilirubin which, if left untreated, can result in sensorineural hearing loss, mild cognitive delays, and kernicterus, which is the deposition of bilirubin in the brain. Kernicterus describes the yellow staining of the brain cells that may result in bilirubin encephalopathy. The damage occurs when the serum concentration reaches toxic levels, regardless of cause.

> **!) NURSING ALERT**
>
> Breastfeeding is essential in preventing hyperbilirubinemia. Newborns should breastfeed early (within the first hour after birth) and often (at least 8–12 times/24 hr). Colostrum acts as a laxative to promote stooling, which helps rid the body of bilirubin.

***Therapy for** hyperbilirubinemia.* The best therapy for hyperbilirubinemia is prevention. Because bilirubin is excreted in meconium, prevention can be facilitated by early and frequent feeding, which stimulates passage of meconium. However, despite early passage of meconium, some term infants may have trouble conjugating the increased amount of bilirubin derived from disintegrating fetal red blood cells (RBCs). As a result, the serum levels of unconjugated bilirubin may rise beyond normal limits, causing hyperbilirubinemia. The goal of treatment of hyperbilirubinemia is to help reduce the newborn's serum levels of unconjugated bilirubin. There are two ways to reduce unconjugated bilirubin levels: phototherapy and exchange blood transfusion.

Phototherapy. The purpose of phototherapy is to reduce the level of circulating unconjugated bilirubin or to keep it from increasing. Phototherapy uses light energy to change the shape and structure of unconjugated bilirubin and convert it to molecules that can be excreted. The dose and effectiveness of phototherapy are affected by the source of light. Phototherapy units vary in the spectrum of light they deliver and in the filters that are used. The most effective therapy is achieved with special blue fluorescent tubes or a specially designed light-emitting diode (LED). Phototherapy lights do not emit significant ultraviolet radiation; the small amount that is emitted does not cause erythema. Most of the ultraviolet light is absorbed by the glass wall of the fluorescent tube and by the plastic cover of the light (Kamath, Thilo, & Hernandez, 2011). Phototherapy is usually effective for treatment of hyperbilirubinemia that has not reached levels associated with acute bilirubin encephalopathy or kernicterus.

The effectiveness of phototherapy is related to the distance between the light and the newborn and on the area of skin that is exposed. During phototherapy, the unclothed infant is placed under a bank of lights approximately 45 to 50 cm from the light source. Research suggests that the newborn be placed supine for maximum exposure to the light source (Bhethanabhotia, Thurak, Sankar, et al., 2013). Phototherapy can be used for the infant in an isolette (Fig. 26-9) or in an open crib. The distance varies according to unit protocol and type of light used. The lamp's energy output should be monitored routinely with a photometer during treatment to ensure efficacy of therapy. Phototherapy is used until the infant's serum bilirubin level decreases to within an acceptable range. The decision to discontinue therapy is based on the observation of a definite downward trend in bilirubin values.

The infant's eyes must be protected by an opaque mask to prevent overexposure to the light. The eye shield should cover the eyes completely but not occlude the nares. Before the mask is applied, the infant's eyes should be closed gently to prevent excoriation of the corneas. The mask should be removed periodically and during infant feedings so that the eyes can be

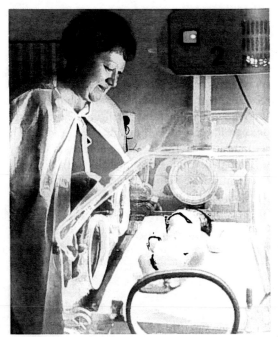

FIGURE 26-9 Infant under phototherapy lights while in isolette. (Olesia Bilkei/Shutterstock.com.)

209

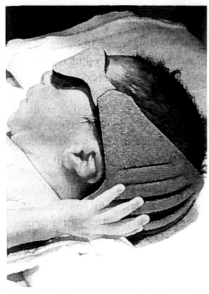

FIGURE 26-10 Infant with eyes covered while receiving phototherapy. (Courtesy Cheryl Briggs, BSN, RNC-NIC.)

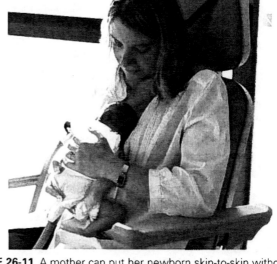

FIGURE 26-11 A mother can put her newborn skin-to-skin without interrupting phototherapy when a fibre-optic blanket is used. (Courtesy Mother and Childcare, Phillips Healthcare.)

FAMILY-CENTRED CARE

Phototherapy and Parent–Infant Interaction

The traditional use of phototherapy has evoked concerns regarding a number of psychobehavioural issues, including parent–infant separation, potential social isolation, decreased sensorineural stimulation, altered biological rhythms, altered feeding patterns, and activity changes. Parental anxiety is greatly increased, particularly at the sight of the newborn blindfolded and under special lights. The interruption of breastfeeding for phototherapy is a potential deterrent to successful maternal–infant attachment and interaction. Because research has demonstrated that bilirubin catabolism occurs primarily within the first few hours of the initiation of phototherapy, there is increased support for the removal of the infant from treatment for feeding and holding. Intermittent phototherapy may be just as effective as continuous therapy when used correctly.

checked and cleansed with water and the parents can have visual contact with the infant (see Family-Centred Care box and Fig. 26-10).

Phototherapy may cause changes in the infant's temperature, depending partially on the bed used: bassinet, isolette, or radiant warmer. When under a phototherapy light, infants are usually clothed only with a diaper. The infant's temperature should be closely monitored at least every 2 hours. Phototherapy lights can increase the rate of insensible water loss, which contributes to fluid loss and dehydration. Therefore, it is important that the infant be adequately hydrated. The healthy newborn is kept hydrated with human milk or infant formula; there is no advantage or benefit to administering oral glucose or plain water because these do not promote excretion of bilirubin in stools and may in fact perpetuate enterohepatic circulation, thus delaying bilirubin excretion.

It is important to closely monitor urinary output as an indicator of hydration status while the infant is receiving phototherapy. Urine output can be decreased or unaltered; the urine can have a dark gold or brown appearance.

The number and consistency of stools should also be monitored. Bilirubin breakdown increases gastric motility, which results in loose stools that can cause skin excoriation and breakdown. The infant's buttocks must be cleaned after each stool to maintain skin integrity. A fine maculopapular rash may appear during phototherapy, but this is transient.

Additional systems used for phototherapy include a bassinet system that provides special blue light above and beneath the infant. Another phototherapy device is a fibre-optic blanket that is connected to a light source (see Fig. 26-11). The blanket is flexible and can be placed around the infant's torso or underneath the infant in the bassinet. There are also bilirubin beds with LED lights in a pad that covers the surface of the bassinet. The LED lights do not produce heat and can be used with radiant warmers. These devices are usually less effective when used alone than with conventional phototherapy lights. They can be very useful in combination with overhead phototherapy lights. In certain instances, the infant's bilirubin levels increase rapidly and intensive phototherapy is required; this situation involves the use of a combination of conventional lights and fibre-optic blankets to maximize bilirubin reduction. Although fibre-optic lights do not produce heat as conventional lights do, staff should ensure that a covering pad is placed between the infant's skin and the fibre-optic device to prevent skin burns, especially in preterm infants. The newborn can remain in the mother's room in an open crib or in her arms during treatment. The use of eye patches depends on whether the devices are used alone or in combination with phototherapy lights.

Home phototherapy. The use of home phototherapy should be reserved for healthy term infants with bilirubin levels in the "optional phototherapy" range according to the nomogram. The concern is that home phototherapy units do not provide the same level of irradiance or body surface coverage as phototherapy devices used in the hospital.

Follow-up. Serum levels of bilirubin in the newborn continue to rise until the fifth day of life. Many parents leave the hospital within 24 hours of birth, and some as early as 6 hours after birth. Therefore, parents must receive education regarding jaundice and its treatment. They should have written instructions for assessing the infant's condition and the name of a contact person to whom they should report their findings and concerns.

Close follow-up is needed for infants who have been treated for hyperbilirubinemia. Repeat testing of serum bilirubin levels and follow-up visits with the pediatric health care provider are expected. When follow-up serum bilirubin levels are needed after discharge from the hospital, a health care technician or nurse may draw the blood for the specimen or the parents may take the baby to a laboratory to have blood drawn for a serum bilirubin. In some cases, parents take the newborn to an outpatient clinic or to the physician's office to be evaluated.

Exchange transfusion. When phototherapy is not effective in reducing serum bilirubin levels or in treating severe hyperbilirubinemia such as in hemolytic disease, exchange transfusion may be needed. This procedure is done in an intensive care setting. The infant's blood is replaced with a combination of blood products such as RBCs mixed with 5% albumin or fresh frozen plasma (Kaplan, Wong, Sibley, et al., 2011). This invasive procedure is rarely done and can be minimized by early management and treatment (see discussion in Chapter 29).

Hypoglycemia. Hypoglycemia during the early newborn period of a term infant is defined as a blood glucose concentration less than that needed to support adequate neurological, organ, and tissue function; however, there is a lack of consensus regarding the precise level at which this concentration occurs.

At birth, the maternal source of glucose is cut off with the clamping of the umbilical cord. Most healthy term newborns experience a transient decrease in glucose levels to as low as 1.7 mmol/L during the first 1 to 2 hours after birth, with a subsequent mobilization of free fatty acids and ketones to help maintain adequate glucose levels (Blackburn, 2013). Infants who are asphyxiated or have other physiological stress may experience hypoglycemia as a result of a decreased glycogen supply, inadequate gluconeogenesis, or overutilization of glycogen stored during fetal life. There is concern about neurological injury as a result of severe or prolonged hypoglycemia, especially in combination with ischemia (Kalhan & Devaskar, 2011).

There is no need to routinely assess glucose levels of healthy term infants (Aziz, Dancey, & CPS, 2004/2014). Breastfeeding early and often helps these newborns maintain adequate glucose levels.

Glucose levels should be measured in newborns at 34 weeks of gestation or more if risk factors or clinical manifestations of hypoglycemia are present. In infants who are at risk for altered metabolism as a result of maternal illness factors (diabetes, gestational hypertension) or newborn factors (perinatal hypoxia, infection, hypothermia, polycythemia, congenital malformations, hyperinsulinism, SGA, LGA, fetal hydrops), close observation and monitoring of blood glucose levels within 2 hours of birth, after an initial feeding, are recommended. The frequency of glucose testing is determined by the risk factors for each individual newborn. Infants of diabetic mothers should undergo glucose screening before feedings for at least

the first 12 hours after birth; further testing is done if glucose levels are less than 2.6 mmol/L. However, preterm and SGA infants may be vulnerable up to 36 hours of age so should be screened until 36 hour of age if feeding is established and blood glucose is maintained at 2.6 mmol/L or higher (Aziz et al., 2004/2014).

The CPS recommendations state that asymptomatic, at-risk babies should receive at least one effective feeding before a blood glucose check at 2 hours of age and should be encouraged to feed regularly thereafter. At-risk babies who have a blood glucose of less than 1.8 mmol/L at 2 hours of age despite one feeding (breastfeeding or approximately 5 mL/kg to 10 mL/kg of formula or glucose water) or less than 2.0 mmol/L after subsequent feeding should receive an intravenous (IV) dextrose infusion. At-risk babies who repeatedly have blood glucose levels of less than 2.6 mmol/L despite subsequent feeding should also be considered for IV therapy (Aziz et al., 2004/2014).

Glucose testing should be done in any infant with clinical signs of hypoglycemia. The clinical signs can be transient or recurrent and include jitteriness, lethargy, poor feeding, abnormal cry, hypotonia, temperature instability (hypothermia), respiratory distress, apnea, and seizures (Kalhan & Devaskar, 2011). It is important to remember that hypoglycemia can be present in the absence of clinical manifestations.

Hypoglycemia in the low-risk term infant is usually eliminated by feeding the infant a source of carbohydrate (i.e., preferably human milk) and putting the newborn skin-to-skin with a parent. Occasionally, the IV administration of glucose is required for infants with persistently high insulin levels or in those with depleted stores of glycogen.

> **! NURSING ALERT**
>
> Late preterm infants are at increased risk for hypoglycemia. They have decreased glycogen stores and lack hepatic enzymes for gluconeogenesis and glycogenolysis. Their hormonal regulation and insulin secretion are immature. The increased risk of cold stress and feeding difficulties adds to the risk for hypoglycemia (Cooper, Holditch-Davis, Verklan, et al., 2012).

Hypocalcemia. Hypocalcemia in infants is defined as serum calcium levels less than 2 mmol/L in the term infant and slightly lower (1.75 mmol/L) in the preterm infant. Hypocalcemia is common in critically ill newborns but also can occur in infants of mothers with diabetes or in those who experienced perinatal asphyxia or trauma and in low-birth-weight and preterm infants. Infants born to mothers treated with anticonvulsants during pregnancy are also at risk (Rigo, Mohamed, & De Curtis, 2011). Early-onset hypocalcemia usually occurs within the first 24 to 48 hours after birth. Signs of hypocalcemia include jitteriness, tremors, twitching, high-pitched cry, irritability, apnea, and laryngospasm, although some infants may be asymptomatic. Jitteriness is a symptom of both hypoglycemia and hypocalcemia; therefore, hypocalcemia must be considered if the therapy for hypoglycemia proves ineffective.

In most instances, early-onset hypocalcemia is self-limiting and resolves within 1 to 3 days. Treatment usually includes early

The activities of daily care during the newborn period are the best times for infant and family interactions. While caring for their newborn, the mother and father or partner (or other family member) can talk to the infant, play baby games, caress and cuddle the baby, and perhaps use infant massage. Feeding is an optimal time for interaction because the infant is usually awake and alert, at least at the beginning of the feeding. Too much stimulation should be avoided after feeding and before a sleep period. In Fig. 26-20 a great-grandmother and infant are shown engaging in arousal, imitation of facial expression, and smiling. Older children's contact with a newborn is encouraged and should be supervised according to the developmental level of the child (Fig. 26-21). Parents often keep memento books that record the birth, the hospital stay, and their infant's progress.

Discharge Planning and Teaching

Providing infant care can cause much anxiety for the new parent. Support from nursing staff can be an important factor in determining whether new mothers seek and accept help in the future. The nurse should try to avoid covering all the content at one time because the parents can be overwhelmed by too much information and become anxious. However, because new mothers go home quickly from the hospital, it is difficult for nurses to teach all the content that is necessary. It is important to start teaching on admission to the hospital. Community health nurses may visit families after birth and provide teaching, but this is not a standard practice across the country.

To set priorities for teaching, the nurse should follow parental cues. Learning needs should be identified before beginning to teach. Normal growth and development and the changing needs of the infant (e.g., for personal interaction and stimulation, growth milestones, exercise, injury prevention, and social contacts), as well as the topics that follow, should be included during discharge planning with parents. Safety issues should also be addressed (see Home Care box).

Temperature

Parents need to understand practical information related to thermoregulation. The nurse should discuss the following topics in parent teaching:

- The causes of elevation in body temperature (e.g., overwrapping, cold stress with resultant vasoconstriction, or response to infection) and the body's response to extremes in environmental temperature
- Ways to promote normal body temperature, such as dressing the infant appropriately for the environmental air temperature and protecting the infant from exposure to direct sunlight, and how to assess whether the infant is hot or cold by feeling the back of the neck
- Use of warm wraps or extra blankets in cold weather
- Technique for taking the newborn's axillary temperature, and normal values for axillary temperature
- Signs to be reported to the primary health care provider, such as high or low temperatures with accompanying fussiness, lethargy, irritability, poor feeding, and excessive crying

Respirations

The nurse can provide information to parents regarding the normal characteristics of newborn respirations, emergency

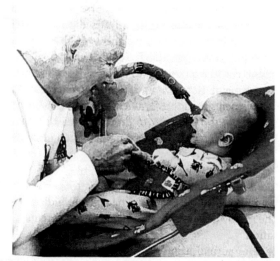

FIGURE 26-20 Great-grandmother and infant enjoying social interaction. (Courtesy Freida Belding.)

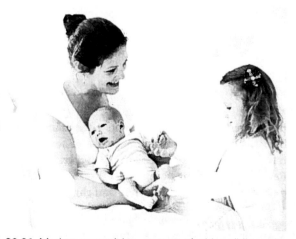

FIGURE 26-21 Mother supervising contact of older sibling with newborn. (FamVeld/Shutterstock.com.)

HOME CARE

Infant Safety

- Never leave your baby alone on a bed, couch, or table. Even newborns can move enough to eventually reach the edge and fall off.
- Never put your baby on a cushion, pillow, beanbag, or waterbed to sleep. Your baby may suffocate. Also, do not keep pillows, large floppy toys, or loose plastic sheeting in the crib.
- Always lay the baby flat in bed on his or her back for sleep. Do not place your infant on the abdomen or side for sleep.
- When using an infant carrier, place the carrier on the floor in a place where you can see the baby. It should never be on a high place, such as a table, couch, or store counter.
- Infant carriers do not keep your baby safe in a car. Always place your baby in an approved car safety seat when travelling in a motor vehicle (car, truck, bus, or van). Car safety seats are recommended for travel on trains and airplanes as well. Use the car safety seat for *every* ride. Your baby should be in a rear-facing infant car safety seat from birth until at minimum 1 year or until exceeding the car seat's limits for height and weight. Do not be in a rush to turn the car safety seat to the forward-facing position. The car safety seat should be in the back seat of the car (see Fig. 26-23). This precaution is especially important in vehicles with front passenger air bags because when air bags inflate, they can be fatal for infants and toddlers. If an infant must ride in the front seat, disable the air bag.
- When bathing your baby, never leave him or her alone. Newborns and infants can drown in 2 to 5 cm of water.
- Be sure that your hot water heater is set at 49°C (120°F) or less. Always check bath-water temperature with your elbow before putting your baby in the bath.
- Do not tie anything around your baby's neck. Pacifiers, for example, tied around the neck with a ribbon or string can strangle your baby.
- Check your baby's crib for safety. Slats should be no more than 5.7 cm apart. The space between the mattress and sides should be less than two fingerwidths. The bedposts should have no decorative knobs.
- There should be no bumper pads, blankets, stuffed toys, or other items in the baby's crib because of the risk for suffocation.
- Keep the crib or playpen away from window blind and drapery cords; your baby could strangle on them.
- Keep the crib and playpen well away from radiators, heat vents, and portable heaters. Linens in the crib or playpen can catch fire if they come into contact with these heat sources.
- Install smoke detectors on every floor of your home. Check them once a month to be sure they are working properly. Change batteries twice a year.
- Avoid exposing your baby to cigarette or cigar smoke in your home or other places. Passive exposure to tobacco smoke greatly increases the likelihood that your infant will have respiratory symptoms and illnesses.
- Be gentle with your baby. Do not pick your baby up or swing your baby by the arms or throw him or her up in the air. Never shake the baby.

procedures, and measures to protect the infant. It is helpful to discuss signs of the common cold and to offer suggestions related to care of the infant who experiences this type of illness. Review the following points:

- Normal variations in the rate and rhythm
- Reflexes such as sneezing to clear the airway (this is normal and does not mean the newborn has a cold)
- Steps to take if the infant appears to be choking
- The need to protect the infant from the following:

- Exposure to people with upper respiratory tract infections and respiratory syncytial virus
- Exposure to second-hand and third-hand tobacco smoke
- Suffocation from loose bedding, water beds, and beanbag chairs; drowning (in bath water); entrapment under excessive bedding or in soft bedding; anything tied around the infant's neck; blind cords near cribs; poorly constructed playpens, bassinets, or cribs
- Sleep position—on back when put to sleep
- Avoid the use of baby powder, which is a commonly aspirated substance. Whenever a powder is used, it should be placed in the caregiver's hand and then applied to the skin. It is kept away from the infant's face.
- Notify the health care provider if the infant develops symptoms such as difficulty breathing or swallowing, nasal congestion, excess drainage of mucus, coughing, sneezing, decreased interest in feeding, or fever.
- If the infant has a respiratory illness such as the "common cold," the following suggestions can be helpful:
  - Feed smaller amounts more often to prevent overtiring the infant.
  - Hold the baby in an upright position to feed.
  - For sleeping, raise the infant's head and chest by raising the mattress 30 degrees. (Do not use a pillow.)
  - Avoid drafts; do not overdress the baby.
  - Use only medications prescribed by a physician. Do not use over-the-counter medications without health care provider approval.
  - Use nasal saline drops in each nostril and suction well with bulb syringe to decrease and relieve secretions.

Feeding Patterns

Nurses instruct parents about infant feeding and provide assistance based on whether they have chosen breastfeeding or formula feeding. The infant should be put to breast ideally within the first hour after birth. Newborns should be allowed to feed when they awaken and demonstrate typical hunger cues, regardless of the amount of time since the previous feeding. This concept is commonly referred to as "cue-based" or "on-demand" feeding. Breastfed babies nurse more often than bottle-fed babies because breast milk is digested faster than formulas made from cow's milk and the stomach empties sooner as a result. Exclusively formula feeding newborns will typically awaken and cue to feed every 3 to 4 hours. Breastfed newborns feed an average of 10 to 12 times per day. Water and dextrose water supplements are not recommended in the newborn period since these have the tendency to decrease breastfeeding. For a thorough discussion of infant feeding, see Chapter 27.

Elimination

Awareness of the normal elimination patterns of newborns helps parents recognize problems related to voiding or stooling. The following points are included in teaching about elimination:

- Colour of normal urine and number of voidings to expect each day; one wet diaper for each day of life until fifth to sixth day; then 6 to 10 per day (see Fig. 27-9)

- Changes to be expected in the colour of the stool (i.e., meconium to transitional to soft yellow or golden yellow) and the number of bowel evacuations, plus the odour of stools for breastfed or formula-fed infants (see Box 25-1 and Fig. 25-5)
- Formula-fed infants may have as few as one stool every other day after the first few weeks of life; stools are pasty to semiformed.
- Breastfed infants should have at least three stools every 24 hours for the first few weeks. The stools are looser and resemble mustard mixed with cottage cheese.

Prevention of Sudden Infant Death Syndrome (SIDS)

By definition, sudden infant death syndrome (SIDS) is the sudden death of an infant under the age of 1 year. Current evidence explains SIDS as a disorder arising from a combination of environmental, genetic, and metabolic factors (PHAC et al., 2012). The rate of SIDS in Canada is 1 in every 3000 babies; the rate is higher among Indigenous infants (PHAC et al., 2012). The PHAC guideline recommends placing the infant to sleep in the supine position to prevent SIDS. The prone position has been associated with an increased incidence of SIDS (see Critical Thinking Case Study). Other recommendations for preventing SIDS include ensuring a smoke-free environment (before and after birth), providing a safe crib environment (no toys or loose bedding), room sharing for 6 months, avoiding instances of the infant being overheated, and no sleeping in waterbeds or on sofas (PHAC et al., 2012). Breastfeeding and pacifier use may also decrease the rate of SIDS (Leduc, Côté, Woods, et al., 2004/2014). In addition, co-bedding practices may contribute to unintentional suffocation caused by entrapment or overlaying, often occurring when the infant is sharing a sleep surface with an adult or another child (PHAC et al., 2012).

Anatomically, the infant's shape—a barrel chest and flat, curve-less spine—makes it easy for the infant to roll from the side to the prone position; thus, the side-lying position for sleep is not recommended. When the infant is awake, "tummy time" can be provided under parental supervision so that the infant may begin to develop appropriate muscle tone for eventual crawling; this tummy time is also effective in the prevention of a misshaped head (positional plagiocephaly). Newborns should be placed on their stomach several times per day for increasing lengths of time but always when they are awake and supervised by an adult (Cummings & CPS, 2011/2014).

Care must also be taken to prevent the infant from rolling off flat, unguarded surfaces. When an infant is on such a surface, the parent or nurse who must turn away from the infant even for a moment should always keep one hand placed securely on the infant. The infant should always be held securely with his or her head supported because newborns are unable to maintain an erect head posture for more than a few moments. Fig. 26-22 illustrates holding an infant with adequate support.

Rashes

Diaper rash. Most infants develop a diaper rash at some time. This dermatitis or skin inflammation appears as redness, scaling, blisters, or papules. Various factors contribute to diaper

Late Preterm Infant, Sudden Infant Death Syndrome, and Infant Sleep Position

Mary gave birth to a 35-week, 2250-g female infant whom she named Delilah. This is her third baby; the other children are 18 and 20 years old. Mary and Delilah are being discharged today.

The nurse has given her instructions about placing Delilah on her back for sleep. Mary says that she remembers her other two children slept best when they were on their "tummies" for sleep. When Mary was in college, she worked as a unit secretary in a newborn nursery and she recalls that when babies were on their backs, they tended to "spit up" and turn blue. Recently, her sister had a baby who had to be under bilirubin lights and the nurses turned the baby on her abdomen sometimes for sleep. Mary voices concerns to the nurse about putting Delilah down to sleep on her back at home. How should the nurse respond to Mary's concerns?

QUESTIONS

1. Evidence—Is there sufficient evidence to draw conclusions about the safety and efficacy of the supine position for sleep for the late preterm infant in reducing the incidence of sudden infant death syndrome (SIDS)?
2. Assumptions—What assumptions can be made about the following factors related to infant positioning?
   a. Risk for aspiration
   b. Sleep position in the hospital versus sleep position at home
   c. Sleep position for late preterm versus term infants
3. What implications and priorities for nursing care can be drawn at this time?
4. Does the evidence objectively support your conclusion?

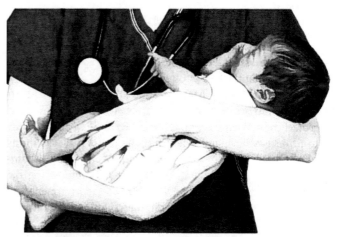

FIGURE 26-22 Holding baby securely with support for the head. (Duplass/Shutterstock.com.)

rash, including infrequent diaper changes, diarrhea, use of plastic pants to cover the diaper, or a change in the infant's diet, such as when solid foods are added.

Parents are instructed in measures to help prevent and treat diaper rash. Diapers should be checked often and changed as soon as the infant voids or stools. Plain water with mild soap is used to cleanse the diaper area; if baby wipes are used, they should be unscented and contain no alcohol. The infant's skin should be allowed to dry completely before applying another diaper. Because bacteria thrive in moist, dark areas, exposing the skin to dry air decreases bacterial proliferation. Zinc oxide ointments can be used to protect the infant's skin from moisture and further excoriation if a rash develops.

Although diaper rash can be alarming to parents and annoying to babies, most cases resolve within a few days with simple home treatments. There are instances when diaper rash is more serious and requires medical treatment.

The warm, moist atmosphere in the diaper area provides an optimal environment for *Candida albicans* growth; dermatitis appears in the perianal area, inguinal folds, and lower abdomen. The affected area is intensely erythematous with a sharply demarcated, scalloped edge, often with numerous satellite lesions that extend beyond the larger lesion. The usual source of infection is from handling by persons who do not practise adequate hand hygiene. It may also appear 2 to 3 days after an oral infection (thrush). Therapy consists of applications of an anticandidal ointment, such as clotrimazole or miconazole, with each diaper change. Sometimes the infant also is given an oral antifungal preparation such as nystatin or fluconazole to eliminate any gastrointestinal source of infection.

Other rashes. A rash on the cheeks may result from the infant's scratching with long unclipped fingernails or from rubbing the face against the crib sheets, particularly if regurgitated stomach contents are not washed off promptly. The newborn's skin begins a natural process of peeling and sloughing after birth. Dry skin may be treated with a neutral-pH lotion, but this should be used sparingly. Newborn rash, erythema toxicum, is a common finding and needs no treatment.

Clothing

Parents commonly ask how warmly they should dress their infant. A simple rule of thumb is to dress the child as they would dress themselves, adding or subtracting clothes and wraps for the child as necessary. Feeling the temperature of the skin at the back of the infant's neck is often an indicator of whether the child is too hot or cold. A cotton shirt and diaper may be sufficient clothing for the young infant. A hat or bonnet is needed to protect the scalp and minimize heat loss if the weather is cool, or to protect against sunburn and shade the eyes if it is sunny and hot. Overdressing in warm temperatures can cause discomfort, as can underdressing in cold weather. Overdressing the infant has also been associated with SIDS. Parents are encouraged to dress the infant in flame-retardant clothing. Infant sunglasses are available to protect the eyes when outdoors.

Safety: Use of Car Seat

Infants should travel only in federally approved, rear-facing safety seats secured in the rear seat (Fig. 26-23). The safest area of the car is in the middle of the back seat. A car seat that faces the rear gives the best protection for the infant's disproportionately weak neck and heavy head. In this position, the force of a frontal crash is spread over the head, neck, and back; the back of the car seat supports the spine. Car seats have expiration dates on them as well as Canadian Standards Association stickers, and parents need to ensure the car seat they are using is safe. A car seat that has been in a previous car accident should not be used. See Additional Resources for more information on car seat installation.

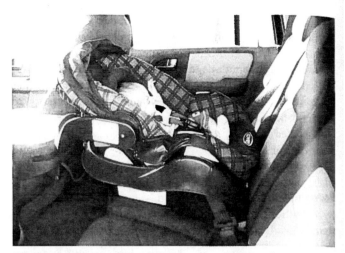

FIGURE 26-23 Rear-facing infant seat in rear seat of car. Infant is placed in seat when going home from the hospital. (Courtesy Brian and Mayannyn Sallee.)

> **! NURSING ALERT**
>
> Infants should use a rear-facing car seat from birth to 10 kg (22 lb), and the child must be able to walk unassisted. If the child meets these criteria and is under 1 year of age, they should remain in a rear-facing car seat. It is advisable to keep a child in a rear-facing car seat even after these criteria have been met.

To secure the infant in the rear-facing car safety seat, shoulder harnesses are placed in the slots at or below the level of the infant's shoulders. The harness is snug, and the retainer clip is placed at the level of the infant's armpits as opposed to on the abdomen or neck area. The car seat is secured by using the vehicle seat belts.

> **! NURSING ALERT**
>
> In cars equipped with air bags, rear-facing infant seats should not be placed in the front seat unless the air bag has been deactivated. Serious injury can occur if the air bag inflates because these types of infant seats fit closer to the dashboard than a passenger does.

Non-Nutritive Sucking

Sucking is the infant's chief pleasure. However, sucking needs may not be satisfied by breastfeeding or bottle-feeding alone. In fact, sucking is such a strong need that infants who are deprived of sucking, such as those with a cleft lip, will suck on their tongues. Some newborns are born with sucking pads on their fingers or lips that developed during in utero sucking. Several benefits of non-nutritive sucking have been demonstrated, such as an increased weight gain in preterm infants, greater ability to maintain an organized state, and less crying.

Problems arise when parents are concerned about the sucking of fingers, thumbs, or pacifiers and try to restrain this natural tendency. Before giving advice, nurses should investigate the parents' feelings and base the guidance they give on the information solicited. For example, some parents may see no problem with the use of a finger but may find the use of a pacifier objectionable. In general, there is no need to restrain either practice, unless thumb sucking persists past 4 years of age or past the time when the permanent teeth erupt. Parents are advised to consult with their health care provider on this topic.

There is compelling evidence that pacifiers help prevent SIDS. It is suggested that parents consider offering a pacifier for naps and bedtime (AAP Task Force on Sudden Death Syndrome, 2011; Ponti & CPS, 2003/2014). The pacifier should be used when the infant is placed supine for sleep, and it should not be reinserted once the infant falls asleep. No infant should be forced to take a pacifier. Pacifiers should be cleaned often and replaced regularly and should not be coated with any type of sweet solution. Pacifier use for breastfeeding infants should be delayed for 3 to 4 weeks to ensure that breastfeeding is well established.

A parent's excessive use of the pacifier to calm the child should also be explored, however. It is not unusual for parents to place a pacifier in the infant's mouth as soon as he or she begins to cry, thus reinforcing a pattern of distress-relief.

If parents choose to let their child use a pacifier, they need to be aware of certain safety considerations before purchasing one. Homemade, improvised, or poorly designed pacifiers can be dangerous because the entire object may be aspirated if it is small, or a portion may become lodged in the pharynx. Safe pacifiers are made of one piece that includes a shield or flange large enough to prevent entry into the mouth and a handle that can be grasped (Fig. 26-24).

Bathing and Umbilical Cord Care

Bathing. Bathing serves a number of purposes. It provides opportunities for (1) completely cleansing the infant, (2) observing the infant's condition, (3) promoting comfort, and (4) parent–child–family interaction.

An important consideration in skin cleansing is preservation of the skin's acid mantle, which is formed from the uppermost horny layer of the epidermis, sweat, superficial fat, metabolic products, and external substances such as amniotic fluid and microorganisms. To protect the newborn's skin, a cleanser with a neutral pH should be used.

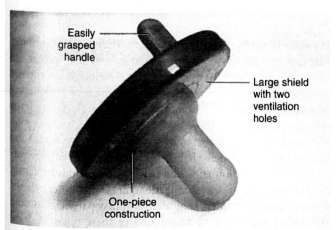

Easily grasped handle

Large shield with two ventilation holes

One-piece construction

FIGURE 26-24 Design of a safe pacifier. (Courtesy Julie Perry Nelson.)

Although the sponging technique may be used, bathing the newborn by immersion results in less heat loss and less crying and is thus recommended even with the umbilical cord still intact. It is recommended that the water is deep enough to cover the newborn's shoulders to ease discomfort from being cold (Association of Women's Health, Obstetrical and Neonatal Nurses [AWHONN], 2013). Immersion bathing is considered a safe alternative to sponge bathing provided the infant's condition is stable (no temperature instability or respiratory or cardiac illness) and he or she is dried off immediately afterward and kept warm (AWHONN, 2013). A daily bath is not necessary for achieving cleanliness and may do more harm by disrupting the integrity of the newborn's skin; cleansing the perineum after a soiled diaper and daily cleansing of the face may suffice. Until the initial bath is completed, hospital personnel must wear gloves to handle the newborn.

The infant bath time provides a wonderful opportunity for parent–infant social interaction. While bathing the baby, parents can talk to the infant, caress and cuddle the infant, and engage in arousal and imitation of facial expressions and smiling. Parents can pick a time for the bath that is easy for them and when the baby is awake, usually before a feeding.

Umbilical cord care. The goal of care is to prevent or decrease the risk for hemorrhage or infection. The umbilical cord stump is an excellent medium for bacterial growth and can become infected. Hospital protocol determines the technique for routine cord care. The current recommendations for cord care by the Association of Women's Health, Obstetric and Neonatal Nurses (AWHONN, 2013) include cleaning the cord with water (and cleanser if needed to remove debris) during the initial bath and subsequently cleaning with plain water if the umbilical stump is soiled with urine or stool. Evidence does not support the routine use of antiseptic or antimicrobial preparations for cord care (Lund & Durand, 2011).

The stump and base of the cord should be assessed for edema, erythema, and drainage with each diaper change. The area should be kept clean and dry and open to air or loosely covered with clothing. If soiled, the area is cleansed with plain water and dried with clean absorbent gauze. The diaper is folded down and away from the stump (AWHONN, 2013). The umbilical cord begins to dry, shrivel, and blacken by the second or third day of life. The stump deteriorates through the process of dry gangrene; thus, odour alone is not a positive indicator of *omphalitis* (infection of the umbilical stump).

The umbilicus should be inspected often for signs of infection (e.g., foul odour, redness, and purulent discharge), granuloma (i.e., small, red, raw-appearing polyp where the umbilical cord separates), bleeding, and discharge. The cord clamp may be removed when the cord is dry, in about 24 to 36 hours, although this is not routine practice in all hospitals (Fig. 26-25). Some institutions send the newborn home with the clamp still in place and it will fall off when the cord falls off. It is important to ensure that if a cord clamp remover is used, it is disinfected between uses.

Cord separation time is influenced by several factors, including type of cord care, type of birth, and other perinatal events. The average cord separation time is 10 to 14 days, although it can take up to 3 weeks for this to occur. Some dried blood may

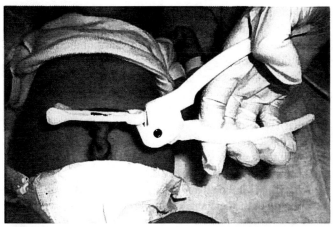

FIGURE 26-25 Using special scissors, remove clamp after cord begins drying (about 24 hours). (Courtesy Cheryl Briggs, BSN, RNC-NIC.)

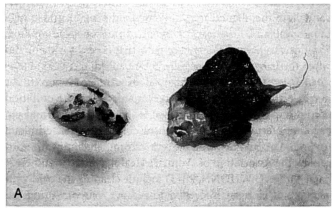

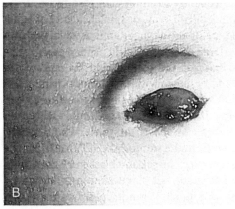

FIGURE 26-26 Cord separation. **A:** Cord separated with some dried blood still in the umbilicus. **B:** Umbilicus cleansed and beginning to heal. (Courtesy Cheryl Briggs, BSN, RNC-NIC.)

be seen in the umbilicus at separation (Fig. 26-26). Parents should be instructed in appropriate home cord care and the expected time of cord separation.

See the Home Care box for information regarding tub and sponge bathing, skin care, cord care, trimming nails, and dressing the infant.

Infant Follow-Up Care

With shorter hospital stays, the focus and site of infant care are changing. Across the country varying methods of early follow-up

health care visits have been implemented, including follow-up by a visiting nurse or community health team, and home visits by midwives and community health nurses to assess and support breastfeeding and wellness.

Parents should plan for their child's routine follow-up health care at the following ages: within 2 or 3 days to check for status of jaundice, feeding, and elimination; at 2 to 4 weeks of age; then every 2 months until 6 to 7 months of age; then every 3 months until 18 months; at 2 years; at 3 years; at preschool; and every 2 years thereafter.

Cardiopulmonary Resuscitation

All personnel working with infants must have current neonatal resuscitation (NRP). Parents should be encouraged to receive instruction in relieving airway obstruction and in CPR. Classes are often offered in hospitals and clinics during the prenatal period or to parents of newborns. Such instruction is especially important for parents whose infants were preterm or had cardiac or respiratory problems.

Practical Suggestions for the First Weeks at Home

Numerous changes occur during the first weeks of parenthood. Nursing care should be directed toward helping parents cope with infant care, role changes, altered lifestyle, and changes in family structure resulting from the addition of a new baby. Developing skill and confidence in caring for an infant can be especially challenging. The nurse's anticipatory guidance can help ease the transition home and decrease stress that might otherwise negate the parents' joy or cause them undue stress. For example, the nurse can teach parents several strategies that help quiet a fussy baby, prevent crying, and induce quiet attention or sleep. This is especially important for first-time parents. Even the simplest strategies can provide enormous support. Printed materials reinforcing education topics are helpful, as is a list of available community resources, both local and national, and websites that provide reliable information about child care. Classes in the prenatal period or during the postpartum stay are helpful. Instructions for the first days at home include relevant topics such as activities of daily living, dealing with visitors, and activity and rest.

Interpretation of Crying

Crying is an infant's first social communication. Some babies cry more than others, but all babies cry. They cry to communicate that they are hungry, uncomfortable, wet, ill, or bored and sometimes for no apparent reason at all. The longer parents are around their infants, the easier the task becomes of interpreting what a cry means. Many infants have a fussy period during the day, often in the late afternoon or early evening when everyone is naturally tired. Environmental tension adds to the length and intensity of crying spells. Babies also have periods of vigorous crying when no comforting can help. These periods of crying can last for long stretches until the infants seem to cry themselves to sleep. The nurse should inform new parents that time and infant maturation will take care of these types of cries. Many hospitals distribute a DVD on infant crying to new parents. *The Period of PURPLE Crying* is an example (see

HOME CARE

Newborn Bath

Timing
- Newborns do not need a bath every day. Every 2 to 3 days is often enough.
- Fit bath time into the family's schedule.
- Give a bath at any time convenient to you but not immediately after a feeding period because the increased handling can cause regurgitation.

Prevent Heat Loss
- The temperature of the room should be no cooler than 24°C (75°F), and the bathing area should be free of drafts.
- Control heat loss during the bath to conserve the infant's energy. Bathing the infant quickly, exposing only what is being washed, and thoroughly drying the infant are all important parts of the bathing technique.

Gather Supplies and Clothing Before Starting
- Clothing suitable for wearing indoors: diaper, shirt; sleeper or nightgown optional
- Towels for drying infant and a clean washcloth
- Receiving blanket
- Tub or sink for water
- Unscented, mild soap; with a neutral pH
- Diaper

Bathe the Baby
- Bring infant to the bathing area when all supplies are ready.
- Never leave the infant alone on the bath table or in bath water, not even for a second! If you have to leave, take the infant with you or put the infant back into the crib.
- Fill the tub to try to cover as much of the infant's body as you feel comfortable. Infants like to have as much of their body under water as possible (preferably to cover shoulders).
- Test temperature of the water. It should feel pleasantly warm to the elbow 38.0° to 40.0°C (100° to 104°F).
- Do not hold infant under running water—water temperature may change, and the infant may be scalded or chilled rapidly.
- If sponge bathing is to be performed (usually only necessary if circumcision is healing), undress the baby and wrap in a towel with the head exposed. Uncover the parts of the body you are washing, taking care to keep the rest of the baby covered as much as possible to prevent heat loss.
- Always work from clean to dirty. Start with the face, neck, and ears first. Do not use soap on the face. Cleanse the eyes from the inner canthus outward, using separate parts of a clean washcloth for each eye. For the first 2 or 3 days, there may be a discharge resulting from the reaction of the conjunctiva to the ointment used as a prophylactic measure against infection. Any discharge should be considered abnormal and reported to the health care provider.
- Cleanse ears and nose with twists of moistened cotton or a corner of the washcloth. Do not use cotton-tipped swabs because they may cause injury.
- Creases under the chin and arms and in the groin may need daily cleansing. The crease under the chin may be exposed by elevating the infant's shoulders 5 cm and letting the head drop back.
- When washing the infant's hair, hold the baby in a football hold. Wash infant's hair before or after body to prevent heat loss from prolonged

exposure to cold (scalp loses heat rapidly because of size). Wash the scalp with warm water and mild soap; dry thoroughly. Scalp desquamation, called *cradle cap*, often can be prevented by removing any scales with a fine-toothed comb or brush after washing. If the condition persists, notify the health care provider.
- Wash the body with mild soap (pH neutral); rinse and dry to decrease heat loss. Place your hand under the baby's shoulders and lift gently to expose the neck, lift the chin, and wash the neck, taking care to cleanse between the skin folds. Wash between the fingers and toes, and then rinse and dry thoroughly. Wash the genital area last. Pat dry gently.

Skin Care
- The skin of a newborn is sensitive and should be cleaned only with water between baths. Soap has drying properties, and its use is limited to bathing. Creams, lotions, ointments, or powders are not recommended. If the skin seems excessively dry during the first 2 to 3 weeks after birth, an unscented, non–alcohol-based lotion may be used; checking with the pediatric health care provider for suggestions on skin care products is best. Experts advise that baby clothes be laundered using a mild laundry detergent.
- The fragile skin can be injured by too vigorous cleansing. If stool or other debris has dried and caked on the skin, soak the area to remove it. Do not attempt to rub it off because abrasion may result. Gentleness, patting dry rather than rubbing, and using a mild soap without perfumes or colouring are recommended. Chemicals in the colouring and perfume can cause rashes on sensitive skin.
- Babies are very prone to sunburn and should be kept out of direct sunlight. Use of sunscreens should be discussed with the health care provider but are not recommended for the first 6 months of life.
- Babies often develop rashes that are normal. Neonatal acne resembles pimples and can appear at 2 to 4 weeks of age, resolving without treatment by 6 to 8 months. Heat rash is common in warm weather, which appears as a fine red rash around creases or folds where the baby sweats.

Cord Care
- Cleanse with plain water around base of the cord where it joins the skin. Notify the health care provider of any odour, discharge, or skin inflammation (redness) around the cord. The clamp may be removed when the cord is dry (approximately 24 to 48 hours after birth). The diaper should not cover the cord because a wet or soiled diaper will slow or prevent drying of the cord and foster infection. When the cord drops off after 10 to 14 days, a few small drops of blood may be seen. If there is active bleeding, notify the pediatric health care provider.

Nail Care
- Use caution cutting the nails—use blunt scissors, or a nail file. The nails have to grow out far enough from the skin so that the skin is not cut by mistake. Nails should be kept short so infants do not scratch themselves. Covering hands with mitts may frustrate infants who wants to suck on them, so it is better to keep nails short. The ideal time to trim the nails is when the infant is sleeping. Soft emery boards may be used to file the nails.

Continued

HOME CARE

Newborn Bath—cont'd

Genital Care

- Cleanse the infant's genitalia daily and after voiding or defecating.
- For girls, the genitalia may be cleansed by separating the labia slightly and gently washing from the pubic area to the anus.
- For uncircumcised boys, wash and rinse the penis with soap and warm water. Do not attempt to retract the foreskin. In most newborns, the inner layer of the foreskin adheres to the glans and the foreskin cannot be retracted. By age 3 years in 90% of boys, the foreskin can be retracted easily without causing pain or trauma. For others, the foreskin is not retractable until adolescence. As soon as the foreskin is partly retractable and the child is old enough, he can be taught self-care. Once healed, the circumcised penis does not require any special care other than cleansing with diaper changes.
- The infant's skin should be allowed to dry completely before applying another diaper. Exposing the buttocks to air can help dry up diaper rash. Zinc oxide ointments can be used to protect the infant's skin from moisture and further excoriation.

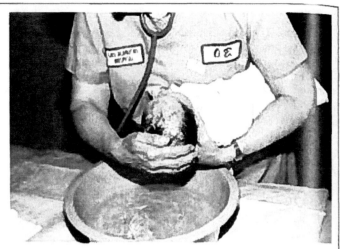

Wash hair with baby wrapped to prevent heat loss from wet scalp using the football hold. (Courtesy Marjorie Pyle, RNC, Lifecircle.)

FAMILY-CENTRED TEACHING

The Period of PURPLE Crying®

The Period of PURPLE Crying is a program to educate new parents about infant crying and the dangers of shaking a baby. Each letter in the acronym "PURPLE" represents key concepts:

P = Peak of crying. Your baby may cry more each week—the most at 2 months, then less at 3 to 5 months.

U = Unexpected. Crying can come and go and you don't know why.

R = Resists soothing. Your baby may not stop crying, no matter what you try.

P = Pain-like face. Crying babies may look like they are in pain, even when they are not.

L = Long lasting. Crying can last as much as 5 hours a day, or more.

E = Evening. Your baby may cry more in the later afternoon and evening.

From National Center on Shaken Baby Syndrome, PURPLEcrying.info.

Family-Centred Teaching box). It is intended to help parents understand that crying is normal and help them cope with infant crying. If parents have greater understanding of infant crying, they may be less likely to inflict harm such as occurs with "shaken-baby" syndrome.

Recognizing signs of illness

In addition to explaining the need for well-baby follow-up visits, the nurse should discuss with parents the signs of illness in newborns (see Patient Teaching box). Of particular importance is the parents' assessment of jaundice in newborns discharged early. Parents should be advised to call their pediatric care provider immediately if they notice increasing jaundice or signs of illness and to ask about over-the-counter medications, such as acetaminophen for infants, to keep at home.

PATIENT TEACHING

Signs of Illness

Notify the pediatric health care provider if any of these signs occur:

- Fever: temperature above 38°C (100.4°F) axillary; also a continual rise in temperature (**Note:** Tympanic [ear] thermometers are not recommended for infants younger than 3 months.)
- Hypothermia: temperature below 36.5°C (97.7°F) axillary and not able to increase temperature by putting on an extra layer of clothing or putting skin-to-skin
- Poor feeding or little interest in food: refusal to eat for two feedings in a row
- Vomiting: more than one episode of forceful vomiting or frequent vomiting (over a 6-hr period)
- Diarrhea: two consecutive green, watery stools (**Note:** Stools of breastfed infants are normally looser than stools of formula-fed infants. Diarrhea will leave a water ring around the stool, whereas breastfed stools will not.)
- Decreased bowel movement: in a breastfed infant, fewer than three stools per day; in a formula-fed infant, fewer than one stool every other day
- Decreased urination: fewer than six to eight wet diapers per day after 5 days of age
- Breathing difficulties: laboured breathing with flared nostrils or absence of breathing for more than 20 seconds (**Note:** A newborn's breathing is normally irregular and between 30 and 60 breaths/min. Count the breaths for a full minute but only if concerned.)
- Cyanosis (bluish skin colour) whether accompanying a feeding or not
- Lethargy: sleepiness, difficulty waking, or periods of sleep longer than 6 hours (most newborns sleep for short periods, usually from 1 to 4 hours, and wake to be fed)
- Inconsolable crying (attempts to quiet not effective) or continuous high-pitched cry
- Bleeding or purulent (yellowish) drainage from umbilical cord or circumcision; foul odour or redness at the site
- Drainage from the eyes

KEY POINTS

- Assessment of the newborn requires data from the prenatal, intrapartum, and postnatal periods.
- The immediate assessment of the newborn includes Apgar scoring and a general evaluation of physical status.
- Knowledge of biological and behavioural characteristics is essential for guiding assessment and interpreting data.
- Gestational-age assessment provides important information for predicting risks and guiding care management.
- Nursing care immediately after birth includes maintaining an open airway, preventing heat loss, and promoting parent–infant interaction.
- Providing a protective environment is a key responsibility of the nurse and includes such measures as careful

- identification procedures, support of physiological functions, and ways to prevent infection.
- The newborn has social and physical needs.
- Newborns require careful assessment for physiological and behavioural manifestations of pain.
- Nonpharmacological and pharmacological measures are used to reduce infant pain.
- Before hospital discharge, nurses provide anticipatory guidance for parents regarding feeding and elimination patterns; positioning and holding; comfort measures; car seat safety; bathing, skin care, cord care, and nail care; and signs of illness.

⊖volve WEBSITE

Visit the Evolve website for additional resources related to the content in this chapter such as Case Studies, Critical Thinking Case Study Answers, Nursing Care Plans, Nursing Processes, Nursing Skills, and Review Questions for Exam Preparation at: http://evolve.elsevier.com/Canada/Perry/maternal/

REFERENCES

American Academy of Pediatrics (AAP) Committee on Infectious Diseases. (2012). *Red book: 2012 report of the Committee on Infectious Diseases* (29th ed.). Elk Grove Village, IL: Author.

American Academy of Pediatrics (AAP) Task Force on Sudden Infant Death Syndrome. (2011). SIDS and other sleep-related infant deaths: Expansion of recommendations for a safe infant sleeping environment. *Pediatrics, 128*(5), e1341–e1367.

American College of Obstetricians and Gynecologists (ACOG) Committee on Obstetric Practice. (2006). Committee opinion no. 333: The Apgar score. *Obstetrics & Gynecology, 107*, 1209–1212. Reaffirmed 2010.

Araia, M. H., Wilson, B. J., Chakraborty, P., et al. (2012). Factors associated with knowledge of and satisfaction with newborn screening education: A survey of mothers. *Genetics in Medicine, 14*(12), 963–970.

Association of Women's Health, Obstetric and Neonatal Nurses (AWHONN). (2013). *Neonatal skin care: Evidence-based clinical practice guideline* (3rd ed.). Washington, DC: Author.

Aziz, K., Dancey, P., & Canadian Paediatric Society. (2004). Screening guidelines for newborns at risk for low blood glucose. *Paediatrics & Child Health, 9*(10), 723–729. Reaffirmed February 1, 2014.

Barrington, K. J., Batton, D. G., Finley, G. A., et al. (2007). Prevention and management of pain in the neonate: An update. A joint statement with the American Academy of Pediatrics. *Paediatrics & Child Health, 12*(2), 137–138. Reaffirmed 2015.

Barrington, K. J., Sankaran, K., & Canadian Paediatric Society. (2007). Guidelines for detection, management and prevention of hyperbilirubinemia in term and late term newborn infants [35 or more weeks gestation]. *Paediatrics & Child Health, 12*(Suppl. B), 1B–12B. Reaffirmed 2016.

Bates, E., Rouse, D., Chapman, V., et al. (2010). Fetal lung maturity testing before 39 weeks and neonatal outcomes. *Obstetrics & Gynecology, 116*(6), 1288–1295.

Bergomi, P., Chieppi, M., Maini, A., et al. (2014). Nonpharmacological techniques to reduce pain in preterm infants who receive heel-lance procedure: A randomized controlled trial. *Research and Theory for Nursing Practice, 28*(4), 335–348.

Bhethanabhotia, S., Thurak, A., Sankar, M., & Paul, V. (2013). Effect of position of infant during phototherapy in management of

hyperbilirubinemia in late preterm and term neonates: A randomized control trial. *Journal of Perinatology, 33*(10), 795–799.

Blackburn, S. T. (2013). *Maternal, fetal, and neonatal physiology: A clinical perspective* (4th ed.). St. Louis: Saunders.

Bramson, L., Lee, J. W., Moore, E., et al. (2010). Effect of early skin-to-skin mother-infant contact during the first 3 hours following birth on exclusive breastfeeding during the maternity hospital stay. *Journal of Human Lactation, 26*(2), 130–137.

Brown, V. D., & Landers, S. (2011). Heat balance. In S. L. Gardner, B. S. Carter, M. Enzman-Hines, et al. (Eds.), *Merenstein & Gardner's handbook of neonatal intensive care* (7th ed.). St. Louis: Mosby.

Bueno, M., Yamada, J., Harrison, D., et al. (2013). A systematic review and meta-analyses of non-sucrose sweet solutions for pain relief in neonates. *Pain Research & Management, 18*(3), 153–161.

Canadian Paediatric Society & College of Family Physicians of Canada. (1997). Routine administration of vitamin K to newborns. *Paediatrics & Child Health, 2*(6), 429–431. Reaffirmed 2014.

Chermont, A., Falcão, L., de Souza Silva, E., et al. (2009). Skin-to-skin contact and/or oral 25% sucrose for procedural pain relief for term newborn infants. *Pediatrics, 124*(6), e1102–e1107.

Cignacco, E. L., Sellam, G., Stoffel, L., et al. (2012). Oral sucrose with facilitated tucking is effective pain control for preterm infants: A randomized control trial. *Pediatrics, 129*(2), 299–308.

Cong, X., Ludington-Hoe, S., Vazquez, V., et al. (2013). *Neonatal Network, 32*(5), 353–357.

Cooper, B. M., Holditch-Davis, D., Verklan, M. T., et al. (2012). Newborn clinical outcomes of the AWHONN late preterm infant research-based practice project. *Journal of Obstetric, Gynecologic, & Neonatal Nursing, 41*(6), 774–785.

Craighead, D. V. (2012). Early term birth: Understanding the health risks to infants. *Nursing for Women's Health, 16*(2), 136–145.

Cummings, C., & Canadian Paediatric Society. (2011). Positional plagiocephaly. *Paediatrics & Child Health, 16*(8), 493–494. Reaffirmed February 1, 2014.

Finan, E., Aylward, D., Aziz, K., & Canadian Paediatric Society. (2011). Neonatal resuscitation guidelines update: A case-based review. *Paediatrics*

CHAPTER 27

Newborn Nutrition and Feeding

Maureen White

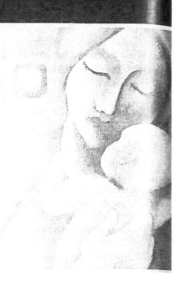

⊖volve WEBSITE

Visit the Evolve website for additional resources related to the content in this chapter such as Case Studies, Critical Thinking Case Study Answers, Nursing Care Plans, Nursing Processes, Nursing Skills, and Review Questions for Exam Preparation at: http://evolve.elsevier.com/Canada/Perry/maternal/

OBJECTIVES

On completion of this chapter the reader will be able to:
- Describe current recommendations for infant feeding.
- Explain the nurse's role in helping families choose an infant feeding method.
- Discuss the importance of breastfeeding for infants, mothers, families, and society.
- Describe the nutritional needs of newborns.
- Describe the anatomy and physiology of breastfeeding.
- Recognize newborn feeding-readiness cues.

- Explain maternal and infant indicators of effective breastfeeding.
- Examine nursing interventions to facilitate and promote successful breastfeeding.
- Analyze common problems associated with breastfeeding and interventions to help resolve them.
- Compare powdered, concentrated, and ready-to-use forms of commercial infant formula.
- Discuss patient teaching for the family who is formula-feeding their newborn.

Good nutrition in infancy fosters optimal growth and development. Infant feeding is more than the provision of nutrition; it represents an opportunity for social and psychological interaction between parent and infant. It can also establish a basis for developing good eating habits and influence lifelong health habits.

Through preconception and prenatal education and counselling, nurses play an instrumental role in helping parents make an informed decision about infant feeding. Scientific evidence is clear that human milk provides the best nutrition for infants, and parents should be strongly encouraged to choose breastfeeding. Although many consider commercial infant formula to be equivalent to breast milk, this belief is erroneous. Human milk is the gold standard for infant nutrition. It is species specific, uniquely designed to meet the needs of human infants. The composition of human milk changes to meet the nutritional needs of growing infants. It is highly complex, with anti-infective and nutritional components combined with growth factors, enzymes that aid in digestion and

absorption of nutrients, and fatty acids that promote brain growth and development. Infant formulas are usually adequate in providing nutrition to maintain infant growth and development within normal limits, but they are not equivalent to human milk.

Breastfeeding is defined as the transfer of human milk from the mother to the infant; the infant receives milk directly from the mother's breast. *Exclusive breastfeeding* means that the infant receives no other liquid or solid food (Health Canada, Canadian Paediatric Society [CPS], Dietitians of Canada and Breastfeeding Committee for Canada [BCC], 2012). If the infant is fed expressed breast milk from the mother or a donor milk bank, it is called *human milk feeding.*

Whether the parents choose breastfeeding, human milk feeding, or formula-feeding, nurses provide support and ongoing education. Parent education and care management are necessarily based on current research findings and standards of practice. Nurses and lactation consultants (who are often nurses) provide education, assistance, and support for mothers,

720

infants, and families. After hospital discharge, nurses and lactation consultants in primary care and community health settings provide ongoing support and assistance to promote optimal feeding practices and positive health outcomes.

This chapter focuses on meeting the nutritional needs for normal growth and development from birth to 6 months of age, with an emphasis on the newborn period, when feeding practices and patterns are established. Both breastfeeding and formula-feeding are addressed. Information on breastfeeding is focused on the direct transfer of milk from mother to infant.

RECOMMENDED INFANT NUTRITION

The World Health Organization (WHO), Health Canada, Canadian Paediatric Society (CPS), Dieticians of Canada, and Breastfeeding Committee for Canada recommend exclusive breastfeeding for the first 6 months of life for healthy, term infants (Health Canada et al., 2012; WHO, 2011). Breast milk is recognized as the normal and optimal food for infants. Nutrient-rich complementary foods, with particular attention to iron, should be introduced at 6 months with continued partial breastfeeding for 2 years or longer. Breastfed babies should also receive a daily vitamin D supplement until their diet provides a reliable source or until they reach 1 year of age. If weaned before 12 months, infants should receive iron-fortified infant formula (Health Canada et al., 2012).

Breastfeeding Rates

The rate of breastfeeding initiation in Canada has increased from 84.6% in 2003 to 90.3% in 2012 (Statistics Canada, 2014). The rate of women who exclusively breastfeed (no water, other liquids, or solid food) for 6 months or longer has increased from 16.8% in 2003 to 24.4% in 2012 (Statistics Canada, 2014).

Although there are reports that breastfeeding is low among Indigenous families (Best Start Resource Centre, 2013), in some Indigenous communities 43% of children were breastfed longer than 6 months (UNICEF, 2009). Breastfeeding patterns vary across Canada and across communities, with a trend toward higher initiation rates in the west and among women over 25 years of age (Public Health Agency of Canada [PHAC], 2013).

Benefits of Breastfeeding

Human milk is designed specifically for human infants and is nutritionally superior to any alternative. Breast milk is considered a living tissue because it contains almost as many live cells as blood. It is bacteriologically safe and is always fresh. The nutrients in breast milk are more easily absorbed than those in formula.

Benefits of breastfeeding for the infant include the following:

- Breast milk enhances maturation of the gastrointestinal tract and contains immune factors that contribute to a lower incidence of gastroenteritis, necrotizing enterocolitis in preterm infants, childhood obesity as well as obesity in adolescence

and adulthood, Crohn's disease, and celiac disease (Oddy, 2012; Pound, Unger, & CPS, 2012/2015).
- Breastfed infants receive specific antibodies and cell-mediated immunological factors that help protect against otitis media, respiratory illnesses such as respiratory syncytial virus and pneumonia, urinary tract infections, bacteremia, and bacterial meningitis (Denne, 2015; Pound et al., 2012/2015).
- There is a lower incidence of certain allergies among breastfed infants, particularly for families at high risk. Allergic manifestations occur at a greater rate and are more severe in formula-fed infants (Iyengar & Walker, 2012).
- Breastfed infants are less likely to die from sudden infant death syndrome (SIDS) (Pound et al., 2012/2015).
- Breast milk may have a protective effect against childhood lymphoma and type 1 and type 2 diabetes mellitus (Geddes & Prescott, 2013; Horta & Victora, 2013).
- Breast milk may enhance cognitive development for term and preterm infants (Horta & Victora, 2013; Kramer, Aboud, Mironova, et al., 2008).
- Breastfeeding has been shown to provide pain relief for newborns undergoing painful procedures such as venipuncture and heel stick (Johnston, Campbell-Yeo, Fernandes, et al., 2014; Shah, Herbozo, Aliwalas, et al., 2012).

Maternal benefits include the following:
- Women who have breastfed have a decreased risk of ovarian cancer, uterine cancer, breast cancer, rheumatoid arthritis, type II diabetes, hypertension hypercholesterolemia, and cardiovascular disease (Pikwer, Bergström, Nilsson, et al., 2009; Pound et al., 2012/2015; Stuebe & Swartz, 2010).
- Breastfeeding promotes uterine involution and is associated with a decreased risk of postpartum hemorrhage (Lawrence & Lawrence, 2011).
- Mothers who are breastfeeding tend to return to their prepregnancy weight more quickly (Pound et al., 2012/2015).
- Breastfeeding may provide some protection against the development of osteoporosis and risk for hip fractures (Chapman, 2012).
- Breastfeeding provides a unique bonding experience, enhances development of the maternal role, and may provide protection against postpartum depression, when breastfeeding difficulties are appropriately addressed (Kendall-Tackett, 2007, 2015; Lawrence & Lawrence, 2011).

Benefits to families and society include the following:
- Breastfeeding is convenient; there are no bottles or other equipment to purchase, clean, or dispose of (a benefit to the community by not having to dispose of formula bottles and equipment used in manufacture).
- Breastfed babies are portable; when travelling, there are fewer supplies to take along.
- Parental absenteeism from work is decreased (Abdulwadud & Snow, 2012).
- Breastfeeding saves money. The cost of formula far exceeds the cost of extra food for the lactating mother. Because breastfed babies have a lower incidence of illness and infection, health care costs are lower for families and for federal and provincial governments (Pound et al., 2012/2015).

Contraindications to Breastfeeding

Contraindications to breastfeeding include the following (Lawrence & Lawrence, 2015; Pound et al., 2012/2015; WHO, 2015):

- Maternal cancer therapy or diagnostic and therapeutic radioactive isotopes
- Active tuberculosis not under treatment in the mother
- Human immunodeficiency virus (HIV) infection in the mother, in high-income countries
- Maternal herpes simplex lesion on a breast
- Galactosemia (classic) in the infant
- Maternal substance use (e.g., cocaine, methamphetamines, marijuana)
- Maternal human T-cell leukemia virus type 1
- Some medications (although rare) that may exert an untoward effect on the breastfeeding infant; use of these requires consultation of the practitioner and available references such as Hale and Rowe (2014) or Motherisk (http://www.motherisk.org)

Conditions that are not considered contraindications to breastfeeding are as follows (Lawrence & Lawrence, 2015; Pound et al., 2012/2015):

- Maternal infection with hepatitis A or C
- Hepatitis B surface antigen (HBsAg)–positive status
- Maternal fever
- Mothers who are cytomegalovirus (CMV) positive

Baby-Friendly Hospital Initiative

All parents are entitled to a birthing environment in which breastfeeding is promoted and supported. To that end, the Baby-Friendly Hospital Initiative (BFHI) is a joint effort of the WHO and the United Nations Children's Fund (UNICEF) to promote and support worldwide breastfeeding as the model for optimum infant nutrition, through the Ten Steps to Successful Breastfeeding.

The Breastfeeding Committee for Canada (BCC) is the national authority for the BFHI in Canada, which is called the Baby-Friendly Initiative (BFI). To reflect the continuum of care between hospitals and communities, the BCC describes the international standards within the Canadian context and has developed a set of 10 practice outcome indicators (Box 27-1). These integrated steps are the basis for the process by which hospitals and communities can achieve the Baby-Friendly™ designation, an internationally recognized accomplishment confirming that the 10 BFHI outcomes have been achieved and that there is adherence to the WHO International Code of Marketing of Breastmilk Substitutes (BCC, 2012).

The number of BFI-designated facilities in Canada is steadily increasing. The BCC 2014 annual report noted that the BFI designation has been achieved by 10 hospitals, 7 birthing centres, 109 Community Health Services, and 1 Indigenous health centre across the provinces of British Columbia, Saskatchewan, Manitoba, Ontario, and Quebec (BCC, 2014). The BFI is an important step toward re-establishing a culture that supports breastfeeding in Canada. Meanwhile, the BFI requires time and resources to implement and is not without its critics. Some women may not be willing or able to breastfeed

---

BOX 27-1   TEN STEPS TO BABY-FRIENDLY DESIGNATION

Step 1. Have a written breastfeeding policy that is routinely communicated to all health care providers and volunteers.

Step 2. Ensure that all health care providers have the knowledge and skills necessary to implement the breastfeeding policy.

Step 3. Inform pregnant women and their families about the importance and process of breastfeeding.

Step 4. Place babies in skin-to-skin contact with their mothers immediately following birth for at least an hour or until completion of the first feeding or as long as the mother wishes; encourage mothers to recognize when their babies are ready to feed, offering help as needed.

Step 5. Assist mothers in breastfeeding and maintaining lactation should they face challenges, including separation from their infants.

Step 6. Infants are not offered food or drink other than human milk for the first 6 months, unless *medically* indicated.

Step 7. Facilitate 24-hour rooming-in for all mothers; mothers and infants remain together.

Step 8. Encourage baby-led or cue-based breastfeeding. Encourage sustained breastfeeding beyond 6 months with appropriate introduction of complementary foods.

Step 9. Support mothers to feed and care for their breastfeeding babies without the use of artificial teats or pacifiers (dummies or soothers).

Step 10. Provide a seamless transition between the services provided by the hospital, community health services, and peer support programs.

From Breastfeeding Committee for Canada. (2010). *Summary Integrated 10 steps practice outcome indicators for hospitals and community health services.* Retrieved from <http://www.breastfeedingcanada.ca/BFI.aspx>.

---

and may experience pressure to conform to the new breastfeeding norms. Some health providers interpret the BFI as eliminating discussions with families about formula and the practicalities of formula-feeding. One of the key messages of the BFI, however, is that health care providers have the responsibility to inform parents of safe and alternative feeding methods when a baby needs to be supplemented or when an informed decision to use infant formula has been made (Best Start Resource Centre & Baby-Friendly Initiative Ontario, 2013). Application of the BFI 10 steps involves using effective communication skills in a supportive and nonjudgemental manner to promote informed decision making about infant feeding. Nursing care includes respecting parents' feeding choices and supporting their learning about responding to infant needs.

CHOOSING AN INFANT FEEDING METHOD

For most women there is a clear choice to either breastfeed or formula-feed. In some cases women decide to combine breastfeeding and formula-feeding. However, this practice may be associated with a shorter duration of breastfeeding (Holmes,

Auinger, & Howard, 2011). In some instances women want their infants to receive breast milk but prefer not to feed directly from their breasts.

Choosing to Breastfeed

Women most often choose to breastfeed because they are aware of the benefits to the infant (Nelson, 2012). This reinforces the importance of prenatal education about the numerous benefits of breastfeeding. Breastfeeding is a natural extension of pregnancy and childbirth; it is much more than simply a means of supplying nutrition for infants. Many women seek the unique bonding experience between mother and infant that is characteristic of breastfeeding. The support of the partner and family is a major factor in a mother's decision to breastfeed and in her ability to do so successfully. Women who perceive their partners to prefer breastfeeding are more likely to breastfeed. Women are more likely to breastfeed successfully when partners and family members have a positive view of breastfeeding and have the skills to support it. Ideally, prenatal preparation includes the woman's partner, who needs information about the benefits of breastfeeding and how he or she can participate in infant care and nurturing.

There appears to be a correlation between maternal weight and infant feeding decisions: women who are overweight or obese are less likely to breastfeed than women who are underweight or of average weight (Mehta, Siega-Riz, Herring, et al., 2011). Also, women tend to select the same method of infant feeding for each of their children. If the first child was breastfed, subsequent children will likely also be breastfed.

The decision to breastfeed exclusively is related to the mother's knowledge about the health benefits to the infant and her comfort level with breastfeeding in social settings (Stuebe & Bonuck, 2011). The likelihood that women will breastfeed exclusively may be greater if they made the decision to do so during pregnancy (Tenfelde, Finnegan, & Hill, 2011). In a meta-synthesis of 14 qualitative studies about decision making regarding infant feeding, Nelson (2012) reported that common barriers to breastfeeding included lack of comfort or uneasiness with breastfeeding, pain, lifestyle incompatibility, discomfort with public breastfeeding, and a lack of formal support.

Individualized, needs-based prenatal breastfeeding education has been used effectively to encourage the intention to breastfeed (Best Start Resource Centre, 2015; Dyson, McCormick, & Renfrew, 2005). Each encounter with an expectant parent is an opportunity to dispel myths, clarify misinformation, and address personal concerns. Connecting expectant mothers with women who are breastfeeding or who have successfully breastfed and are from similar backgrounds may be helpful for all involved. Peer counselling programs, such as those instituted by La Leche League, are beneficial, particularly in low socioeconomic groups, where formula-feeding is common. To provide effective support for the mother, health care providers must be knowledgeable about the benefits of breastfeeding, the basic process of breastfeeding, breastfeeding management, and interventions for common concerns (Box 27-2).

BOX 27-2 GUIDELINES FOR BREASTFEEDING SUPPORT

During pregnancy, perform an assessment that includes intent to breastfeed, breastfeeding history, access to breastfeeding support, a breast examination, and a medication use history.

Develop a prenatal care plan to prepare the woman for lactation.

Inform the mother and her family of the importance of early and frequent skin-to-skin contact after birth.

After birth, the nurse

- Encourages the mother to position her baby skin-to-skin on the mother's chest as soon as possible and until after the first feeding unless medically contraindicated.
- Assists with recognition of early feeding cues, latch-on, and positioning, as needed.
- Reinforces the need for frequent feedings of breast milk—at least 8–12 times per day (without supplementation).
- Encourages keeping mothers and infants in the same room during the entire postpartum stay.
- Gives discharge instructions emphasizing signs of successful breastfeeding.
- Provides information about community resources for breastfeeding support.
- Encourages breastfeeding, especially for preterm and low-birth-weight infants.
- Reinforces the recommendation for exclusive breastfeeding for the first 6 months, with the introduction of complementary foods at 6 months and continued breastfeeding up to 2 years and beyond.

Adapted from International Lactation Consultant Association. (2014). *Clinical guidelines for the establishment of exclusive breastfeeding* (3rd ed.). Morrisville, NC: Author; Registered Nurses' Association of Ontario (RNAO). (2003). *Breastfeeding best practice guidelines for nurses.* Toronto: Author; RNAO (2007). *Breastfeeding best practice guidelines revision supplement.* Toronto: Author. Retrieved from <http://rnao.ca/bpg/guidelines/breastfeeding-best-practice-guidelines-nurses>.

Choosing to Formula-Feed

Parents who choose to formula-feed often make this decision without complete information and understanding of the benefits of breastfeeding. Even women who are educated about the advantages of breastfeeding may still decide to formula-feed. Cultural beliefs and myths and misconceptions about breastfeeding influence women's decision making. Many women see bottle-feeding as more convenient or less embarrassing than breastfeeding. Some view formula-feeding as a way to ensure that the father, partner, or other family members, and day care providers can feed the baby. Some women lack confidence in their ability to produce breast milk of adequate quantity or quality. Women who have had previous unsuccessful breastfeeding experiences may choose to formula-feed subsequent infants. Some women see breastfeeding as incompatible with an active social life, or they think that it will prevent them from going back to work. Modesty issues and societal barriers exist against breastfeeding in public. A major barrier for many women is the influence of family and friends (Nelson, 2012).

Cultural Influences on Infant Feeding

Cultural beliefs and practices are significant influences on infant feeding methods. Many regional and ethnic cultures are found within Canada. Nurses need to be knowledgeable about and sensitive to the various cultural factors influencing infant feeding practices among their patients. At the same time, they must not assume that generalized observations about any cultural group hold true for all members of that group.

Breastfeeding beliefs and practices vary across cultures. For example, generally the historical tradition among Indigenous people was to only breastfeed infants until they were able to digest other food sources. These traditional practices shifted to bottle-feeding in the 1950s when infant formula was introduced to these communities. Since then the incidence of breastfeeding among this population had remained somewhat lower than that for the general population in Canada; however, there now appears to be a trend toward increased breastfeeding among Indigenous populations (UNICEF, 2009). Among Indigenous peoples are communities unique in culture, language, and history; thus, their breastfeeding practices and beliefs vary. For instance, among the Cree women of Northern Quebec, breastfeeding is the norm and is considered good for the health of the baby. These women accept the traditional view that, in order to make milk, they must eat a large amount and expect to have difficulty losing their pregnancy weight. The Cree concept of *miyupimaatisiiun*, or "being alive well," which places emphasis on quality of life rather than on aspects of the physical body, has been a starting point for community-based programs that support breastfeeding while addressing issues of obesity in this population. Current recommendations for promotion and support of breastfeeding for Indigenous women include careful attention to the social determinants of breastfeeding experiences and attitudes toward breastfeeding in communities (Best Start Resource Centre & Baby-Friendly Initiative Ontario, 2013; Eni, Phillips-Beck, & Mehta, 2014).

Because of beliefs about the harmful nature or inadequacy of colostrum, some cultures apply restrictions on breastfeeding for a period of days after birth. Such is the case for many cultures in Southern Asia, the Pacific Islands, and parts of sub-Saharan Africa. Before the mother's milk is deemed to be "in," babies are fed prelacteal food such as honey or clarified butter in the belief that these substances will help clear out meconium. Other cultures begin breastfeeding immediately after birth and offer the breast each time the infant cries.

A common practice among Mexican women is *las dos cosas* ("both things"). This refers to combining breastfeeding and commercial infant formula. It is based on the belief that, by combining the two methods, the mother and infant receive the benefits of breastfeeding, and the infant receives the additional vitamins from infant formula (Bartick & Reyes, 2012; Rios, 2009). This practice can result in problems with milk supply and babies refusing to latch on to the breast, which can lead to early termination of breastfeeding.

Some cultures have specific beliefs and practices related to the mother's intake of foods that foster milk production. Korean mothers often eat seaweed soup and rice to enhance milk production. Hmong women believe that boiled chicken, rice, and hot water are the only appropriate nourishments during the first postpartum month. The balance between energy forces, hot and cold, or yin and yang is integral to the diet of the lactating mother. Latin Americans, Vietnamese, Chinese, East Indians, and Arabs often use this principle in choosing foods for particular conditions. "Hot" foods are considered best for new mothers. This belief does not necessarily relate to the temperature or spiciness of foods; for example, chicken and broccoli are considered "hot," whereas many fresh fruits and vegetables are considered "cold." Families often bring desired foods into the health care setting.

Faith-based breastfeeding traditions are also evident in some cultures. For example, Muslim and Jewish cultures value breastfeeding of infants (Rassin, Klug, Nathanzon, et al., 2009). Some Muslim women practise the tradition of a 40-day rest period, during which the woman is relieved of housekeeping duties and other women help care for her. During this time, the mother may exclusively breastfeed. Breastfeeding for 2 years is recommended in the Qur'an; however, Muslim women typically cease exclusive breastfeeding early in infancy due to the cultural custom of prelacteal feedings (Jessri, Farmer, & Olson, 2013). For many Jewish women, breastfeeding is perceived as being important, but its practice is highly influenced by maternal education level, assimilated cultural values depending on geographic region of origin, and previous breastfeeding experience. The Talmud endorses the value of human milk and of breastfeeding for 2 to 4 years.

Cultural attitudes regarding modesty and breastfeeding are important considerations in whether a woman breastfeeds her baby. Language barriers may also prevent successful breastfeeding and counselling when women cannot connect with resources in their language. With the large percentage of immigrants in Canada, it is incumbent on nurses to consider the range of cultural values related to infant feeding and perceptions of the benefits of breastfeeding so that the mother can make an informed decision based on both knowledge and an approach that is personally acceptable. Breastfeeding support services need to be provided in a culturally sensitive manner and, where possible, in the family's native language. One of the goals of the Canada Prenatal Nutrition Program (CPNP) is to provide long-term funding to community groups to develop or enhance programs for breastfeeding education and support (PHAC, 2015).

Sociocultural values may preclude the mother from receiving adequate information on breastfeeding; for example, if the family is strongly patriarchal and the father is the only English-speaking person in the family and acts as translator, the necessary information being conveyed to the mother by the health care provider may not be correctly translated. Persons immigrating to North America often tend to acquire the local customs of their new home; although breastfeeding may have been common in their own country, they may abandon the practice in their new country, considering it "outdated."

225

Nurses need to be aware that many parenting and breast-feeding challenges are common across cultures for heterosexual and same-sex or queer families. At the same time, members of LGBTQ communities may have specific parenting and infant feeding questions and concerns related to co-nursing and induced lactation, chest-feeding versus breastfeeding, or breast-feeding after breast augmentation (transgender women). In feeding discussions with and physical examination of trans-gendered individuals, the nurse needs to be sensitive to the potential for processes of pregnancy and lactation to effect *gender dysphoria* (when an individual feels discomfort about parts of the body not matching the person's gender) (Farrow, 2015). Detailed information on LGBTQ breastfeeding concerns is available from Rainbow Health Ontario and Milk Junkies (see Additional Resources at the end of the chapter).

Overall, most parents want what is best for their children. This desire provides a focus for nursing discussions on infant feeding. Nurses need to clarify individual parental expectations of infant feeding and collaborate with parents to meet their goals.

Nutrient Needs

Fluids

During the first 2 days of life the fluid requirement for healthy infants (more than 1500 g) is 60 to 80 mL of water per kilogram of body weight per day. From day 3 to 7 the requirement is 100 to 150 mL/kg/day; from day 8 to day 30 it is 120 to 180 mL/kg/day (Dell, 2011). In general, neither breastfed nor formula-fed infants need to be given water, not even those living in very hot climates. Breast milk contains 87% water, which easily meets the infant's fluid requirements. Feeding water to infants can decrease caloric consumption at a time when they are growing rapidly.

Infants have room for little fluctuation in fluid balance and should be monitored closely for fluid intake and water loss. They lose water through excretion of urine and insensibly through respiration. Under normal circumstances they are born with some fluid reserve, and some of the weight loss during the first few days is related to fluid loss. However, in some cases they do not have this fluid reserve, possibly because of inadequate maternal hydration during labour or birth.

Juices are not necessary for proper nutrient intake. There is no evidence that juice intake provides better nutrients than human milk or fortified formula; on the contrary, there are data indicating that excess juice consumption may replace essential elements, leading to nutritional deficits (Health Canada et al., 2012). Juices may also cause significant dental decay, especially when consumed from a bottle.

Energy

Infants require adequate caloric intake to provide energy for growth, digestion, physical activity, and maintenance of organ metabolic function. Energy needs vary according to age, maturity level, thermal environment, growth rate, health status, and activity level. For the first 3 months, the infant needs 110 kcal/kg/day. From 3 months to 6 months, the requirement decreases to approximately 100 kcal/kg/day. This level decreases slightly to 95 kcal/kg/day from 6 to 9 months, and increases to 100 kcal/kg/day from 9 months to 1 year (American Academy of Pediatrics, Committee on Nutrition, 2009).

Human milk provides an average of 67 kcal/100 mL or 20 kcal/30 mL. The fat portion of the milk provides the greatest amount of energy. Infant formulas are made to simulate the caloric content of human milk. Usually a standard formula contains 20 kcal/30 mL, although the composition differs among brands.

Carbohydrates

According to the Institute of Medicine (2005), the recommended Adequate Intake (AI) for carbohydrates in the first 6 months of life is 60 g/day and 95 g/day for the second 6 months. Because newborns have only small hepatic glycogen stores, carbohydrates should provide at least 40 to 50% of the total calories in the diet. Moreover, newborns may have limited ability for gluconeogenesis (formation of glucose from amino acids and other substrates) and ketogenesis (formation of ketone bodies from fat), the mechanisms that provide alternative sources of energy.

As the primary carbohydrate in human milk and commercially prepared formula, lactose is the most abundant carbohydrate in the diet of infants up to 6 months of age. Lactose provides calories in an easily available form. Its slow breakdown and absorption probably also increase calcium absorption. Corn syrup solids or glucose polymers are added to infant formulas to supplement the lactose in cow's milk and provide sufficient carbohydrates.

Oligosaccharides, another form of carbohydrate found in breast milk, are critical in the development of microflora in the intestinal tract of the newborn. These prebiotics promote an acidic environment in the intestines, preventing the growth of Gram-negative and other pathogenic bacteria, thus increasing the infant's resistance to gastrointestinal (GI) illness.

Fat

Fats provide a major source of energy for infants, supplying as much as 50% of the calories in breast milk and formula. The recommended AI of fat for infants younger than 6 months is 31 g/day (Institute of Medicine, 2005). The fat content of human milk is composed of lipids, triglycerides, and cholesterol; cholesterol is an essential element for brain growth. Human milk contains the essential fatty acids (EFAs) linoleic acid and linolenic acid and the long-chain polyunsaturated fatty acids arachidonic acid (ARA) and docosahexaenoic acid (DHA). Fatty acids are important for growth, neurological development, and visual function. Cow's milk contains fewer of the EFAs and no polyunsaturated fatty acids. Most formula companies add DHA to their products, although there is a lack of evidence supporting the benefit (Lawrence & Lawrence, 2011).

Modified cow's milk is used to make most infant formulas, but the milk fat is removed and replaced by another fat source, such as corn oil, that can be more easily digested and absorbed by the infant. If whole milk or evaporated milk without added carbohydrate is fed to infants, the resulting fecal loss of fat (and therefore loss of energy) may be excessive because the milk moves through the infant's intestines too quickly for adequate absorption to take place. This can lead to poor weight gain. There is evidence that whole milk may also increase the infant's chances for developing allergies from exposure to cow's milk protein.

Protein

High-quality protein from breast milk, infant formula, or other complementary foods is necessary for infant growth. The protein requirement per unit of body weight is greater in the newborn than at any other time of life. For infants younger than 6 months the recommended AI for protein is 9.1 g/day (Institute of Medicine, 2005).

Human milk contains the two proteins whey and casein in a ratio of approximately 70:30, compared with the ratio of 20:80 in most cow's milk–based formula (Blackburn, 2013). This whey/casein ratio in human milk makes it more easily digestible and produces the soft stools seen in breastfed infants. The primary whey protein in human milk is alpha-lactalbumin; this protein is high in essential amino acids needed for growth. The whey protein lactoferrin in human milk has iron-binding capabilities and bacteriostatic properties, particularly against Gram-positive and Gram-negative aerobes, anaerobes, and yeasts. The casein in human milk enhances the absorption of iron, thus preventing iron-dependent bacteria from proliferating in the GI tract (Lawrence & Lawrence, 2015). The amino acid components of human milk are uniquely suited to the newborn's metabolic capabilities. For example, cystine and taurine levels are high, whereas phenylalanine and methionine levels are low.

Vitamins

With the exception of vitamin D, human milk contains all of the vitamins required for infant nutrition, with individual variations based on maternal diet and genetic differences (Kim & Froh, 2012). Vitamins are added to cow's-milk formulas to resemble levels found in breast milk. Although cow's milk contains adequate amounts of vitamin A and B complex, vitamin C (ascorbic acid), vitamin E, and vitamin D must be added.

Vitamin D facilitates intestinal absorption of calcium and phosphorus, bone mineralization, and calcium resorption from bone. Canadian recommendations regarding vitamin D supplementation are based on Canada's northern geographic latitude, current practices related to protection from the sun, prevalence of vitamin D–deficiency rickets, and history of safe use of vitamin D supplementation. Health Canada recommends that all breastfed, healthy term infants in Canada receive a daily vitamin D supplement of 10 mcg (400 IU). Supplementation should begin at birth and continue until the infant's diet includes at least 10 mcg (400 IU) per day of vitamin D from other dietary sources or until the breastfed infant reaches 1 year of age (Health Canada et al., 2012).

Vitamin K, required for blood coagulation, is produced by intestinal bacteria. However, the gut is relatively sterile at birth, and a few days are needed for intestinal flora to become established and to produce vitamin K. To prevent hemorrhagic problems in the newborn, an injection of vitamin K is routinely given within the first 6 hours after birth, following initial stabilization of the baby and family–baby interaction (McMillan, CPS, & College of Family Physicians of Canada, 1997/2016) (see Chapter 26, Medication Guide on vitamin K, p. 677).

The breastfed infant's vitamin B_{12} intake depends on the mother's dietary intake and stores. Mothers who are on strict vegetarian (vegan) diets and those who consume few dairy products, eggs, or meat are at risk for vitamin B_{12} deficiency. Breastfed infants of vegan mothers should be supplemented with vitamin B_{12} from birth.

Minerals

The mineral content of commercial infant formula is designed to reflect that of breast milk. Whole cow's milk is much higher in mineral content than human milk, which also makes it unsuitable for infants in the first year of life. Minerals are typically highest in human milk during the first few days after birth and decrease slightly throughout lactation.

The ratio of calcium to phosphorus in human milk is 2:1, an optimal proportion for bone mineralization. Although cow's milk is high in calcium, the calcium/phosphorus ratio is low, resulting in decreased resorption. Consequently, young infants (less than 12 months) fed whole cow's milk are at risk for hypocalcemia, tetany, and seizures. The calcium/phosphorus ratio in commercial infant formulas is between the ratios of human and cow's milk.

Milk of all types is low in iron; however, iron from human milk is better absorbed than that from cow's milk, iron-fortified formula, or infant cereals. Breastfed infants draw on iron reserves deposited in utero and benefit from the high lactose and vitamin C levels in human milk that facilitate iron absorption. The infant who is totally breastfed normally maintains adequate hemoglobin levels for at least the first 6 months of life. After that time, meat, meat alternatives, iron-fortified cereals, and other iron-rich foods may be added to the diet. Infants weaned from the breast before 6 months of age and all formula-fed infants should receive an iron-fortified commercial infant formula until 12 months of age. Infants should not be given low-iron formula (Health Canada et al., 2012).

Fluoride levels in human milk and commercial formulas are low. This mineral, which is important in the prevention of dental caries, can cause staining of the permanent teeth (fluorosis) in excess amounts. Fluoride supplementation should be considered for any child over age 6 months whose drinking water is deficient in fluoride or if other factors put the child at high risk for developing dental caries (Canadian Dental Association, 2012; Health Canada et al., 2012).

OVERVIEW OF LACTATION

Breast Anatomy

Each female breast is composed of approximately 15 to 20 segments (lobes) embedded in fat and connective tissues and well supplied with blood vessels, lymphatic vessels, and nerves (Fig. 27-1). Within each lobe is glandular tissue consisting of alveoli, the milk-producing cells, surrounded by myoepithelial cells that resume their usual feeding pattern as the mother's milk supply increases.

NURSING CARE

Supporting Breastfeeding Mothers and Infants

The key to encouraging mothers to breastfeed is education and anticipatory guidance, beginning as early as possible during and even before pregnancy. Each encounter with an expectant mother and her family is an opportunity to educate, dispel myths, clarify misinformation, and address concerns. Prenatal education and preparation for breastfeeding influence feeding decisions, breastfeeding success, and the amount of time that women breastfeed. Prenatal preparation ideally includes the father of the baby, partner, or another significant support person and provides information about benefits of breastfeeding and how he or she can participate in infant care and nurturing.

Connecting expectant mothers with women from similar backgrounds who are breastfeeding or have successfully breastfed is often helpful. Nursing mothers' support groups such as La Leche League provide information about breastfeeding along with opportunities for breastfeeding mothers to talk with one another and share concerns.

For some women the postpartum period may provide the first opportunity for education about breastfeeding. Even women who have indicated the desire to formula-feed can benefit from information about the benefits of breastfeeding. In offering these women the chance to try breastfeeding with the assistance of a nurse or lactation consultant they may change their infant feeding practices. Learning along with other new mothers can be encouraging (Fig. 27-4).

Promoting feelings of competence and confidence in the breastfeeding mother and reinforcing the unequalled contribution she is making toward the health and well-being of her infant are the responsibility of the nurse and other health care providers. The first 2 weeks of breastfeeding can be the most challenging, as mothers are adjusting to life with a newborn, the baby is learning to latch on and feed effectively, and the mother may be experiencing nipple or breast discomfort. This is a time when support is critical. Primiparous women are most likely to experience early breastfeeding problems, which often result in less exclusive breastfeeding and shorter duration of breastfeeding (Chantry, 2011). Anticipatory guidance during the prenatal period and especially during the hospital stay after birth can provide the mother with information and increase her confidence in her ability to successfully breastfeed her infant. New mothers need access to lactation support following discharge through primary care offices, health departments, or outpatient lactation services. Peer support is also helpful.

The most common reasons for breastfeeding cessation are insufficient milk supply, painful nipples, and problems getting the infant to feed (Lauwers & Swisher, 2011; Lawrence & Lawrence, 2015). Early and ongoing assistance and support from health care providers to prevent and address problems with breastfeeding can help promote a successful and satisfying

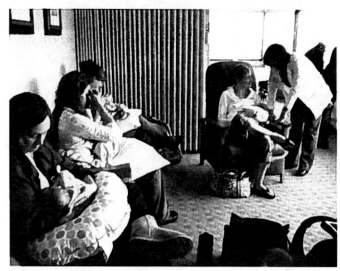

FIGURE 27-4 Breastfeeding mothers' support group with lactation consultant. (Courtesy Shannon Perry.)

breastfeeding experience for mothers and infants. Many health care agencies have certified lactation consultants on staff. These consultants, who are often nurses, have specialized training and experience in helping breastfeeding mothers and infants.

Care of the breastfeeding mother and infant requires that nurses and other health care providers be knowledgeable about the benefits and basic anatomical and physiological aspects of breastfeeding. They also need to know how to help the mother with feedings and discuss interventions for common problems. Ongoing support of the mother enhances her self-confidence and promotes a satisfying and successful breastfeeding experience. Mothers should be encouraged to ask for help with breastfeeding, especially while they are in the hospital. Primiparas are likely to need the most assistance and in many facilities are routinely seen by lactation consultants. The mother needs to understand infant behaviours in relation to breastfeeding and recognize signs that the baby is ready to feed. Infants exhibit feeding-readiness cues or early signs of hunger. Instead of waiting to feed until the infant is crying in a distraught manner or withdrawing into sleep, the mother should attempt to breastfeed when the baby exhibits feeding cues. Feeding cues are often easiest to recognize when the newborn is held skin-to-skin (see Research Focus box). Common newborn hunger cues are as follows:

- Hand-to-mouth or hand-to-hand movements
- Sucking motions
- *Rooting reflex*—infant moves toward whatever touches the area around the mouth and attempts to suck
- Mouthing
- Flexed arms and legs with clenched fists held over chest and tummy (sometimes called *hunger posture*)

In the postpartum period interventions focus on helping the mother and the newborn initiate successful breastfeeding. An important goal is to build maternal confidence in breastfeeding. Interventions to promote successful breastfeeding include educating and assisting mothers and their partners with basics such as latch-on and positioning, cue-based feeding, signs of adequate

RESEARCH FOCUS

Maternal Feeding Styles and Childhood Obesity   —*Pat Mahaffee Gingrich*

Ask the Question

Does caregiver responsiveness to infant feeding cues have an impact on overweight in early childhood and beyond?

Search for the Evidence
Search Strategies

English-language research-based publications on infant, feeding, satiety, breastfeeding, overweight, and obesity were included.

Databases Used

Cochrane Collaborative Database, National Guidelines Clearinghouse (AHRQ), CINAHL, PubMed, UpToDate

Critically Analyze the Evidence

- Childhood obesity can have its roots in the feeding patterns established in infancy. This research field for primary prevention of obesity is new, and many infant feeding studies are currently ongoing.
- Overfeeding can impair the infant's ability to self-regulate. Infants whose caregivers are responsive to an infant's hunger and satiety (full) cues are significantly less likely to be overweight (DiSantis, Hodges, Johnson, et al., 2011).
- Discordant responsiveness occurs when the caregiver perceives that the infant cannot recognize hunger or satiety. Restrictive feeding style is associated with maternal fear of causing obesity. Pressuring feeding style is associated with caregiver concern that the infant has poor appetite and will be underweight (Gross, Mendelsohn, Fierman, et al., 2011).
- In a Latin American population a pressuring feeding style emerged as a result of belief that all infant crying or hand sucking is caused by hunger and that babies should always finish their bottles. Pressuring style is more likely in foreign-born women and women with less than a high-school education (Gross, Fierman, Mendelsohn, et al., 2010).
- Low-income, food-insecure mothers are more likely to be discordant, either restrictive or pressuring, than food-secure mothers (Gross, Mendelsohn, Fierman, et al., 2012).

Apply the Evidence: Nursing Implications

- Parental education about infant hunger and satiety cues ideally should begin in prenatal education classes and be reinforced intensively during the postpartum period. The nurse should point out the infant cues and praise the parents for appropriate responsiveness.
- Videos and printed material and warm lines should be made available to new parents. Specific suggestions about how much formula to feed initially and how voiding and stool patterns and weight gain reflect adequate nutrition can provide education guidelines.
- Assessing for familial and cultural beliefs enables the nurse to address parental and extended-family concerns. The nurse can address how the new mother might respond to well-meaning but incorrect comments from family and strangers.
- Education regarding the various newborn cries and their possible causes can reassure parents and their extended families that feeding should not be the first and only option.
- Breastfeeding is the gold standard for infant feeding because it is more difficult to overfeed.
- Nurses can advocate on a local and national level to eliminate food insecurity.

References

DiSantis, K. I., Hodges, E. A., Johnson, S. L., et al. (2011). The role of responsive feeding in overweight during infancy and toddlerhood: A systematic review. *International Journal of Obesity (London), 35*(4), 480–492.

Gross, R. S., Fierman, A. H., Mendelsohn, A. L., et al. (2010). Maternal perceptions of infant hunger, satiety, and pressuring feeding styles in an urban Latina WIC population. *Academic Pediatrics, 10*(1), 29–35.

Gross, R. S., Mendelsohn, A. L., Fierman, A. H., et al. (2011). Maternal controlling feeding styles during early infancy. *Clinical Pediatrics, 50*(12), 1125–1133.

Gross, R. S., Mendelsohn, A. L., Fierman, A. H., et al. (2012). Food insecurity and obesogenic maternal infant feeding styles and practices in low-income families. *Pediatrics, 130*(2), 254–261.

---

feeding, and self-care measures such as prevention of engorgement. It is important to provide the parents with a list of resources that they can contact after discharge from the hospital.

The ideal time to begin breastfeeding is within the first hour after birth, when the infant is in the quiet, alert state (WHO, 2010). Newborns without complications should be allowed to remain in direct skin-to-skin contact with the mother until the baby is able to breastfeed for the first time (Pound et al., 2012/2015). This is true both for mothers who gave birth by Caesarean and for those who gave birth vaginally. Early skin-to-skin holding and delay of infant bathing for 12 to 24 hours after birth have both been linked to the successful initiation of breastfeeding and longer exclusive breastfeeding (Bramson, Lee, Moore, et al., 2010; Moore, Anderson, Bergman, et al., 2012; Preer, Pisegna, Cook, et al., 2013). Routine procedures such as vitamin K injection, eye prophylaxis, and weighing should be delayed until the newborn has completed the first feeding.

During feeding, the infant is assessed by direct observation for feeding cues, latch-on, position and alignment, and suckling and swallowing. A breastfeeding assessment tool known as LATCH was developed by Jensen, Wallace, and Kelsey in 1994.

Subsequent research has demonstrated that early LATCH scores are linked to breastfeeding success at 6 weeks of age (Kumar, Mooney, Wieser, et al., 2006; Mannel, 2011). Higher LATCH scores have been linked to higher milk intake (Altuntas, Kocak, Akkurt, et al., 2015). The tool involves assessing for the following:

L (characteristics of latch-on)

A (degree of audible swallowing)

T (type of nipple)

C (maternal comfort)

H (holding skills)

Systematic assessment of these five aspects can assist the mother and nurse to focus together on what is needed for extra support.

Positioning

For the initial feedings it can be advantageous to encourage and assist the mother to breastfeed in a semi-reclining position with the newborn lying prone, skin-to-skin on the mother's bare chest. Her body supports the baby. The mother is more relaxed, nipple pain is reduced or eliminated, and the mother has more freedom of movement to use her hands. The baby is able to use

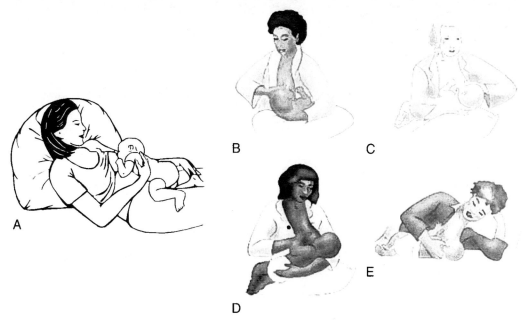

FIGURE 27-5 Breastfeeding positions. **A:** Laid-back breastfeeding (biological nurturing). **B:** Football hold. **C:** Cross-cradle. **D:** Cradling. **E:** Side-lying position. (Reprinted with permission by the Best Start Resource Centre.)

inborn reflexes to latch on to the breast and feed effectively. This approach to breastfeeding is based on the concept of "biological nurturing" (BN) (Colson, 2010, 2012). BN is described as a neurobehavioural approach to initiating breastfeeding (Colson, 2012; La Leche League International, 2014). There is no one "correct" position for BN: the mother assumes a comfortable semi-reclining position and the baby lies prone on top of the mother so that every part of the baby is facing and close to the mother; thus the term *laid-back breastfeeding* is sometimes applied to this approach (Fig. 27-5, A). Stimulation of primitive newborn reflexes occurs with this posture, aiding suckling. With BN, mothers are encouraged to be comfortable with responding to their own and their baby's natural breastfeeding instincts.

The four other positions for breastfeeding are the football or clutch hold (under the arm), cross-cradle or across the lap, cradle, and side-lying. The mother should be encouraged to use the position that most easily facilitates latch while allowing maximal comfort. The football or clutch hold is often recommended for early feedings because the mother can see the baby's mouth easily as she guides the infant on to the nipple.

Mothers who gave birth by Caesarean often prefer the football or clutch hold (Fig. 27-5, B). The cross-cradle or across-the-lap position works well for early feedings, especially with smaller babies (Fig. 27-5, C). The side-lying position allows the mother to rest while breastfeeding and is often preferred by women experiencing perineal pain and swelling (Fig. 27-5, E). Cradling is the most common breastfeeding position for infants who have learned to latch on easily and feed effectively (Fig. 27-5, D). Before discharge from the birth institution, the nurse can help the mother try all of the positions so that she will feel confident in her ability to vary positions at home.

During breastfeeding the mother should be as comfortable as possible. After arranging for privacy, the nurse might suggest that she empty her bladder and attend to other needs before

starting to feed the newborn. The nurse who is assisting with breastfeeding should be at the mother's eye level. The mother holds the infant securely at the level of the breast, supported by firm pillows or folded blankets, facing toward her ("belly-to-belly"). The newborn's nose should be pointing toward the mother's nipple, avoiding "centring" the mouth over the nipple. The mother should support the baby's neck and shoulders with her hand and not push on the occiput. The baby's body is held in alignment (ears, shoulders, and hips are in a straight line) during latch and feeding.

Latch

Latch, or latch-on, is defined as placement of the infant's mouth over the nipple, areola, and breast, making a seal between the mouth and breast to create adequate suction for milk removal. In preparation for latch during early feedings it may be helpful for the mother to manually express a few drops of colostrum or milk to spread over the nipple. This lubricates the nipple and may entice the baby to open the mouth as the milk is tasted.

To facilitate latch when in an upright position, the mother may support her breast in one hand with the thumb on top and four fingers underneath at the back edge of the areola; this may be called the *C hold* (Fig. 27-6, A). She may also compress the breast slightly so that an adequate amount of breast tissue is taken into the mouth with latch. Some mothers need to support the breast during feeding for at least the first few days until the infant is adept at feeding.

The mother holds the baby close to the breast and lightly touches the infant's upper lip with her nipple, stimulating the mouth to open (rooting reflex). When the mouth is open wide and the tongue is down, the mother brings the baby in close (Fig. 27-6, B), with the head slightly tilted so that the chin touches the breast first; if the infant does not move forward

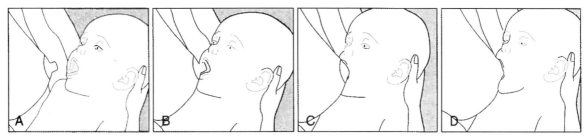

FIGURE 27-6 Latching on. **A:** When mouth is wide open, draw baby close. **B:** Nipple should be centred upward in infant's mouth. **C:** As baby latches on, draw infant closer to breast. Chin should be tucked in close to breast. **D:** Baby should be allowed to nurse until he or she stops swallowing. (Monica Schroeder/Science Source.)

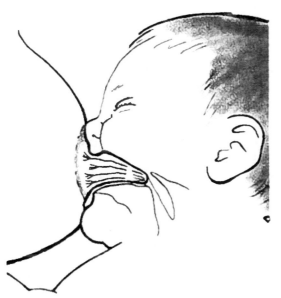

FIGURE 27-7 Correct attachment (latch-on) of infant at breast. (Courtesy Cumberland Health Authority.)

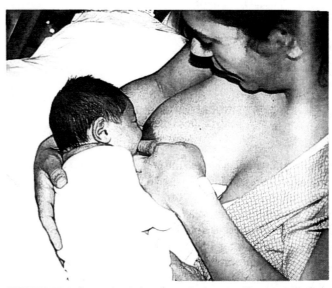

FIGURE 27-8 Removing infant from the breast. (Courtesy Marjorie Pyle, RNC, Lifecircle.)

independently, she can quickly pull the infant onto the nipple (Fig. 27-6, C). She should bring the infant to the breast, not the breast to the infant. If the breast is pushed into the infant's mouth, the infant often closes the mouth too soon and does not latch on.

The amount of the areola in the newborn's mouth with latch depends on the size of the newborn's mouth and the size of the areola and nipple. In general, the infant's mouth should cover the nipple and areola, with more of the areola visible above the baby's upper lip than below the lower lip (Fig. 27-7).

When the newborn is latched on effectively, the chin should be pressed into the breast, and the cheeks and nose may be lightly touching the breast. The mother should not pull the nipple out of the mouth when trying to create a breathing space for the newborn's nose. Depressing the breast tissue around the newborn's nose is not necessary. If the mother is worried about the infant's breathing, she can raise the newborn's hips slightly to change the angle of the infant's head at the breast. If the newborn cannot breathe, reflexes will prompt the newborn to move the head and pull back to breathe.

Once the newborn is latched on and sucking, there are signs that the feeding is going well: (1) the mother reports a firm

tugging sensation on her nipple, but feels no pinching or pain; (2) the baby sucks with cheeks rounded, not dimpled; (3) the baby's jaw glides smoothly with sucking; and (4) swallowing is usually audible. Sucking creates a vacuum in the intraoral cavity as the breast is compressed between the tongue and the palate. When the infant is latched on and sucking correctly, breastfeeding is not painful. If the mother feels pinching or pain after the initial sucks or does not feel a strong tugging sensation on the nipple, the latch and positioning are evaluated. If breastfeeding is painful, the baby likely has not taken enough of the breast into the mouth, and the tongue is pinching the nipple. Repositioning usually alleviates this problem. For a small number of infants *ankyloglossia* ("tongue-tie") may lead to difficulty latching effectively, resulting in low milk intake and maternal nipple pain and trauma.

Any time the signs of adequate latch and sucking are not present, the newborn should be taken off the breast and latch attempted again. To prevent nipple trauma as the newborn is taken off the breast, the mother is instructed to break the suction by inserting her finger in the side of the infant's mouth between the gums and keeping it there until the nipple is completely out of the newborn's mouth (Fig. 27-8) (see Nursing

Care Plan: Breastfeeding and Infant Nutrition, available on Evolve).

Milk Ejection, or Let-Down

As the newborn begins suckling on the nipple, the milk ejection, or let-down, reflex is stimulated. Two to three "let-downs" can occur with each feeding session. The following signs indicate that milk ejection has occurred:

- The mother may feel a tingling sensation in the nipples and breasts, although some women never feel when milk ejection (let-down) occurs.
- The newborn's suck changes from quick, shallow sucks to a slower, deeper, more drawing sucking pattern.
- Audible swallowing is present as the baby sucks.
- The mother may feel thirsty and relaxed or drowsy during feedings.
- In the early days the mother feels uterine cramping.
- The opposite breast may leak milk.

Frequency of Feedings

Babies normally consume small amounts of colostrum with frequent feedings during the first 3 days of life. As the mother's transitional milk is followed by mature milk, the baby adjusts to extrauterine life, and the digestive tract is cleared of meconium, the baby's fluid intake gradually increases. Feeding patterns vary because every mother–infant dyad is unique. Breastfeeding frequency is influenced by a variety of factors, including the infant's age and weight, the infant's stomach capacity and gastric emptying time, and the storage capacity of the breast (i.e., the milk available when the breast is full).

The feeding pattern should include cue-based feedings without time restrictions, on average at least 8 to 12 times per 24 hours (International Lactation Consultant Association [ILCA], 2014; Registered Nurses' Association of Ontario [RNAO], 2003) (see Critical Thinking Case Study). Some infants breastfeed every 2 to 3 hours throughout a 24-hour period. Others cluster-feed, breastfeeding every hour or so for three to five feedings and then sleeping for 3 to 4 hours between clusters. During the first 24 to 48 hours after birth, most newborns do not awaken this often to feed. Parents need to understand that they should awaken the sleepy infant to feed at least every 3 hours during the day and at least every 4 hours at night during the first few weeks of life. Feeding frequency is determined by counting from the beginning of one feeding to the beginning of the next. Once the newborn is feeding well and gaining weight adequately, going to *demand feeding* is appropriate, in which case the infant determines the frequency of feedings. With demand feeding the infant should still receive at least eight feedings in 24 hours.

Parents should be cautioned about attempting to place newborn infants on strict feeding schedules. Infants should be fed whenever they exhibit feeding cues such as hand-to-mouth movements, rooting, and mouth and tongue movements. Crying is a late sign of hunger, and infants may become frantic when they have to wait too long to feed. Some infants will shut down or go into a deep sleep when their needs are not met. Understanding and responding to an infant's states

CRITICAL THINKING CASE STUDY
Newborn Breastfeeding

Neide is a 27-year-old married woman from Costa Rica who recently moved to Canada and has a 5-day-old, 3180 g male infant. His birth weight was 3540 g. She is being seen in the clinic for a follow-up consultation on breastfeeding and jaundice. On examination the infant is alert, fussy, and visibly jaundiced. Neide states that breastfeeding has not been going as well and she is not certain the infant is receiving enough milk. She states, in tears, that all the baby does is cry and fuss when she places him to the breast, and she wants to try formula. She recalls that yesterday the baby had one or two greenish stools and three wet diapers.

1. Evidence—Is there sufficient evidence to draw conclusions about the effectiveness of the infant's breastfeeding pattern?
2. Assumptions—What assumptions can be made about the following factors?
   a. The infant's ability to latch on
   b. Adequacy of breast milk intake
   c. The need for additional infant assessments
   d. The mother's desire to give the infant formula
   e. The mother's physical and emotional status
3. What implications and priorities for nursing care can be drawn at this time?
4. Does the evidence objectively support your conclusion?

and cues (see Chapter 25) is essential to the infant feeding interaction.

Frequent skin-to-skin holding helps mothers to notice state changes and early hunger cues and thus provide the frequent feedings required at the breast in the first few days (see Research Focus box). One recommendation is that mother and breastfeeding infant sleep in close proximity (in the same room but not in the same bed) to promote breastfeeding. The issue of bed sharing has raised concerns because of the association between a higher incidence of SIDS and bed sharing with an adult. Health Canada recommends that the safest place for any infant to sleep is in a crib within arm's reach of where the parents sleep. This practice allows for more convenient breastfeeding and at the same time prevents continuous bed sharing (Health Canada, 2010). Room sharing is recommended for at least the first 6 months. (See Chapter 26 for more discussion on SIDS.)

Duration of Feedings

The duration of breastfeeding sessions is highly variable, as the timing of milk transfer differs for each mother–baby pair. The average time for early feedings is 30 to 40 minutes, or approximately 20 minutes per breast, although instructing mothers to feed for a set number of minutes is inappropriate. It is more effective to teach mothers how to determine when an infant has finished a feeding: the infant's suck-swallow pattern has slowed, and the newborn appears content and may fall asleep or release the nipple. Other, more subtle, satiation cues include extended and relaxed fingers, arms and legs extended, back arching, or pushing away (Spietz, Johnson-Crowley, Summer, et al., 2008). As infants grow they become more efficient at breastfeeding

RESEARCH FOCUS

Skin-to-Skin Contact for Full-Term Newborns

—*Maureen White*

Ask the Question

What is the evidence for recommending skin-to-skin (STS) contact for full-term newborns?

Search for Evidence

Search Strategies

Randomized controlled trials, meta-analyses, systematic reviews, experimental research, prospective studies, and guidelines from professional and international health organizations since 2008

Databases Searched

MedLine, PubMed, Ovid CINAHL, Cochrane, and websites for the Canadian Paediatric Society (CPS), Association of Women's Health, Obstetric and Neonatal Nurses (AWHONN), Association of Breastfeeding Mothers (ABM), World Health Organization (WHO), Breastfeeding Committee for Canada (BCC), World Alliance for Breastfeeding Action (WABA)

Critically Analyze the Evidence

Health care research concerning STS contact increased in the 1970s following "kangaroo mother care" (KMC) interventions with premature infants in Bogota, Colombia. Subsequent evidence for clinical, physiological, and psychological advantages of KMC led to KMC being regarded as safe and superior care for vulnerable infants worldwide. The term *KMC* is now used chiefly to describe a method of intensive care for preterm and very-low-birth-weight infants that involves extended STS, exclusive breastfeeding, and support of the mother–infant dyad. Recent research also focuses on the impact of STS contact on full-term newborns and their parents. STS contact involves holding the baby naked in a prone position against the skin of the mother's (or partner's) chest between the breasts. The baby wears only a diaper and, if needed, a hat. A blanket or shirt can cover baby and parent.

A 2012 Cochrane Database Systematic Review examined 34 studies involving 2177 healthy mother–infant dyads and concluded that, for full-term infants, STS contact with their mothers in the first 24 hours of life had a significant positive impact on breastfeeding initiation and duration for 1 to 4 months, improved cardiorespiratory stability, and less crying, with no short- or long-term negative effects (Moore, Anderson, Bergman, et al., 2012).

Several studies concluded that longer periods of STS contact lead to increased positive impact on breastfeeding for full-term infants. STS contact in the first 3 hours of life contributes to effective suckling and increased exclusive breastfeeding rates in hospitals (Bramson, Lee, Moore, et al., 2010; Cantrill, Creedy, Cooke, et al., 2014). In addition to breastfeeding outcomes, recent studies show that STS can be an effective means of maintaining the newborn's temperature, regulating sleep–wake cycles, and minimizing the impact of painful procedures. Parents report high levels of satisfaction with STS contact, and some evidence is emerging that parent–child interaction is enhanced by STS contact (Moore et al., 2012; Saloojee, 2008). Further research is required to examine more outcome measures and best practices in STS care.

Implications for Practice

There is compelling evidence to warrant giving support to breastfeeding families in initiating STS contact following birth and encouraging frequent and prolonged STS holding in the newborn period. Such support can be achieved through education of health care providers, discussion of STS care prenatally with expectant parents, and implementation of supportive policies. In hospitals, policies should include initiating STS contact as soon as possible after each birth and limiting unnecessary interruptions for care activities—for example, delaying infant weighing and the first newborn bath.

Studies show benefits of STS care across cultures and settings; in practice, nurses need to attend to the individual responses of parents related to modesty, culture, and personal feelings (Saloojee et al., 2008). Promoting discreet ways to manage STS contact and offering practical help in positioning the baby can increase the practice of STS care.

Caesarean birth is a common barrier to initiation of STS holding within the first hour following birth because of traditional operating room practices, although many institutions are changing practice so the newborn can be placed STS with the mother or her partner. While it is important to promote early STS contact and breastfeeding for the postoperative or ill mother, when feasible, encouraging her partner to hold the newborn STS can promote stabilization of infant temperature and parental attachment. Most studies focus on breastfeeding outcomes; however, the benefits of STS contact are not limited to breastfeeding families (Erlandsson, Dsilna, Fagerberg, et al., 2007; Gouchon, Gregori, Picotto, et al., 2010). Nurses should encourage parents who are formula-feeding to practise frequent STS holding so that parents and their infants have more opportunities for attachment and to promote stable infant physiological and behavioural states.

References

Bramson, L., Lee, J. W., Moore, E., et al. (2010). Effect of early skin-to-skin mother–infant contact during the first 3 hours following birth on exclusive breastfeeding during the maternity hospital stay. *Journal of Human Lactation, 26*(2), 130–137. doi:10.1177/0890334409355779.

Cantrill, R. M., Creedy, D. K., Cooke, M., & Dykes, F. (2014). Effective suckling in relation to naked maternal-infant body contact in the first hour of life: An observation study. *BMC Pregnancy and Childbirth, 14*, 20. doi:10.1186/1471-2393-14-20.

Erlandsson, K., Dsilna, A., Fagerberg, I., & Christensson, K. (2007). Skin-to-skin care with the father after Cesarean birth and its effect on newborn crying and prefeeding behaviour. *Birth (Berkeley, Calif.), 34*(2), 105–114.

Gouchon, S., Gregori, D., Picotto, A., et al. (2010). Skin-to-skin contact after Cesarean delivery: An experimental study. *Nursing Research, 59*(2), 78–84. doi:10.1097/NNR.0b013e3181d1a8bc.

Moore, E. R., Anderson, G. C., Bergman, N., & Dowswell, T. (2012). Early skin-to-skin contact for mothers and their healthy newborn infants. *The Cochrane Database of Systematic Reviews*, (5), doi:10.1002/14651858.CD003519.pub3.

Saloojee, H. (2008). *Early skin-to-skin contact for mothers and their healthy newborn infants: RHL commentary. WHO Reproductive Health Library*. Geneva: World Health Organization. Retrieved from <http://apps.who.int/rhl/archives/hsguide2/en/index.html>.

and, consequently, the length of feedings decreases. The amount of time an infant spends breastfeeding is not a reliable indicator of the amount of milk the infant consumes because some of the time at the breast is spent in non-nutritive sucking.

The amount of intake with each feeding reflects the size of the infant's stomach; approximate increases in stomach capacity for term infants are 5 to 7 mL on day 1; 22 to 27 mL on day 3; and 60 to 81 mL on day 10. Comparing these volumes to a cherry, a walnut, and a hen's egg is one way to help parents visualize the sizes (Fig. 27-9).

If a baby seems to be feeding effectively and the urine output is adequate but the weight gain is not satisfactory, the mother may be switching to the second breast too soon. Feeding on the first breast until it softens ensures that the baby receives the higher-fat hindmilk, which usually results in increased weight gain.

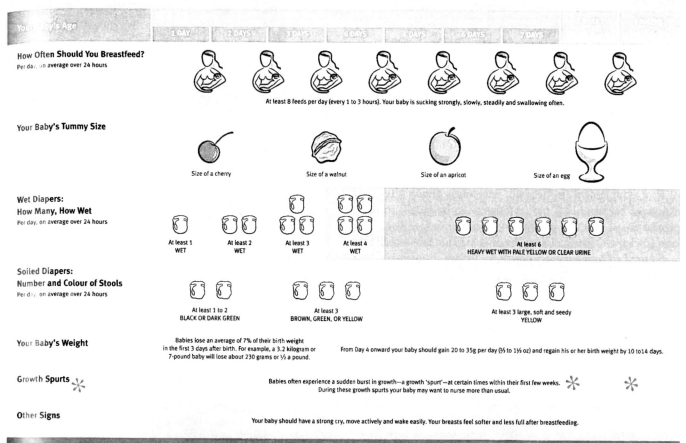

FIGURE 27-9 Guidelines for nursing mothers regarding how often to feed and how to know the baby is getting enough to eat. (Courtesy Best Start, http://beststart.org/resources/breastfeeding/pdf/breastfdeskref09.pdf. Reprinted with permission by the Best Start Resource Centre.)

Indicators of Effective Breastfeeding

One of the most common concerns of breastfeeding mothers is how to determine if the baby is getting enough milk. In the newborn period, when breastfeeding is becoming established, parents should be taught about the signs that breastfeeding is going well. Awareness of these signs helps them recognize when problems arise so they can seek appropriate assistance (see Fig. 27-9).

During the early days of breastfeeding, keeping a feeding diary can be helpful, recording the time and length of feedings and infant urine output and bowel movements. The data from the diary provide evidence of the effectiveness of breastfeeding and are useful to health care providers in assessing adequacy of feeding. Parents are instructed to take this feeding diary to the follow-up visit with the pediatric care provider.

The infant's output is highly indicative of feeding adequacy. It is important that parents are aware of the expected changes in the characteristics of urine output and bowel movements during the early newborn period. As the volume of breast milk increases, urine becomes more dilute and should be light yellow; dark, concentrated urine can be associated with inadequate intake and possible dehydration. (**Note**: Infants with jaundice often have darker urine as bilirubin is excreted.) Infants should have at least six sufficiently wet diapers (light yellow urine) every 24 hours after day 5. The first 1 to 2 days after birth newborns pass meconium stools, which are greenish black, thick, and sticky. By day 3 the stools become greener, thinner, and less sticky. If the mother's mature milk has come in by day 3 or 4, the stools start to appear greenish yellow and are looser. By the end of the first week breast milk stools are yellow, soft, and seedy (they resemble a mixture of mustard and cottage cheese) (see Fig. 25-5). If an infant is still passing meconium stool by day 3 or 4, breastfeeding effectiveness and milk transfer should be assessed.

Infant should have at least three stools (quarter-size or larger) per day for the first month. Some babies stool with every feeding. The stooling pattern gradually changes; breastfed infants can continue to stool more than once per day or they may stool only every 2 or 3 days or even longer. As long as the baby continues to gain weight and appears healthy, this decrease in the number of bowel movements is normal.

Other factors to assess include the presence of jaundice, weight loss greater than 10%, and whether the infant has regained birth weight by 10 to 14 days of age. See Box 28-2 for calculation of weight loss.

Supplementation

The Canadian Paediatric Society (Pound et al., 2012/2015) recommends that, unless a medical indication exists, no supplements be given to breastfeeding infants. With sound breastfeeding knowledge and practice, supplements are rarely needed. Early supplementation by hospital staff undermines a new mother's confidence and models behaviour that is counterproductive to prolonging breastfeeding.

If a supplement is deemed necessary, giving the baby expressed breast milk is best. Mothers can be taught to hand express breast milk and give this to the newborn (see discussion later in chapter). A small amount of colostrum is often all that is required to supplement a newborn. Before supplementation it is important to perform a careful evaluation of the mother–infant dyad.

Possible indications for supplementary feeding include infant factors such as hypoglycemia, dehydration, weight loss of more than 10% associated with delayed lactogenesis, or delayed passage of bowel movements or meconium stool continued to day 5.

Maternal indications for possible supplementation include severe illness, delayed lactogenesis, or taking medications that are incompatible with breastfeeding (Breastfeeding Committee for Canada [BCC], 2012; Pound et al., 2012/2015). Women who have had previous breast surgery such as augmentation or reduction may need to provide supplementary feedings for their infants.

Supplemental feedings may contribute to "nipple confusion" (i.e., difficulty knowing how to latch on to the breast or preferring the easy flow from an artificial nipple) and to low milk supply because the baby becomes overly full and does not breastfeed often enough. Supplementation interferes with the supply-meets-demand cycle of milk production. The parents may interpret the newborn's willingness to take a bottle to mean that the mother's milk supply is inadequate. They need to know that a newborn will automatically suck from a bottle, as the artificial nipple triggers the suck-swallow reflex.

Bottles and Pacifiers

Newborns may become confused going from breast to bottle or bottle to breast when breastfeeding is first initiated. Breastfeeding and bottle-feeding require different oral motor skills. The ways newborns use their tongues, jaw, and lips, as well as the swallowing patterns, are very different. It is recommended that parents avoid giving bottles until breastfeeding is well established, usually at least after 3 to 4 weeks.

If supplemental feeding is needed, nurses or lactation consultants can help parents use supplemental nursing devices. This allows the baby to be supplemented with expressed breast milk or infant formula while still breastfeeding (Fig. 27-10). Infants can also be fed with a spoon, dropper, cup, or syringe. If parents choose to use bottles, a slow-flow nipple is recommended. Although some parents combine breastfeeding and bottle-feeding, many babies never take a bottle and go directly from the breast to a cup.

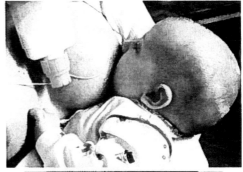
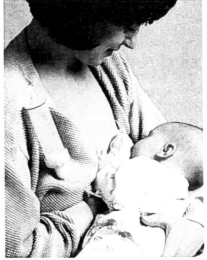

FIGURE 27-10 Supplemental nursing device. (Copyright © 2013 Medela.)

The Canadian Paediatric Society (Ponti & CPS, 2003/2016) recommends that health care providers recognize pacifier use as a parental choice determined by the needs of their child and that pacifier use be delayed until breastfeeding is established. Pacifier use should not replace actual feeding or suckling. Prohibiting early pacifier use will not ensure an increase in the length of breastfeeding, but it may help with promoting milk production (Jaafar, Jahanfar, Angolkar, et al., 2012). The emphasis should be on allowing the infant to control the pace, frequency, and termination of feeding, instead of allowing the pacifier (or anything else) to become the focus of the interaction. The CPS recommends that pacifiers not be routinely discouraged, as the current evidence suggests a decreased risk of SIDS associated with their use (Ponti & CPS, 2003/2016). The American Academy of Pediatrics (2011/2015) recommends that parents consider offering a pacifier at nap time and bedtime, as there is reported to be a protective effect against the incidence of SIDS that persists through the sleep period even if the pacifier falls out of the infant's mouth.

Special Considerations

Sleepy newborn. During the first few days of life, some newborns need to be awakened for feedings. If the infant is awakened from a sound sleep, attempts at feeding are more likely to be unsuccessful. Babies are more likely to feed if they are awakened from a light or active sleep state. Signs that the

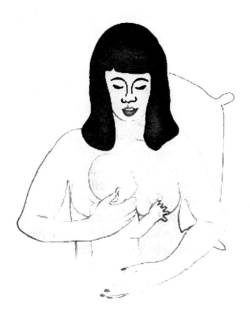

FIGURE 27-11 Infant and mother skin-to-skin. Infant is placed between the mother's breasts. (Reprinted with permission by the Best Start Resource Centre.)

infant is in this sleep state are movements of the eyelids, body movements, and making sounds while sleeping. Unwrapping or undressing the newborn, changing the diaper, sitting the infant upright, talking to the newborn with variable pitch, gently massaging the infant's chest or back, and stroking the arms, legs, palms, or soles may bring the newborn to an alert state. Placing the sleeping infant skin-to-skin with the mother's chest may also stimulate a state change; she can move the infant to the breast when feeding-readiness cues are apparent (Fig. 27-11).

Fussy newborn. In the early days at home some babies start crying soon after they are put in their beds and are asking to be comforted (see Patient Teaching box). Other infants sometimes awaken from sleep crying frantically. Although they may be hungry, they cannot focus on feeding until they are calmed. Calming techniques include holding him or her close, talking soothingly, and allowing the infant to suck on a clean finger until calm enough to latch on to the breast. Placing the baby skin-to-skin with the mother can be very effective in calming a fussy infant. Fussiness during feeding can be the result of birth injury, such as bruising of the head or fractured clavicle. Changing the feeding position can help alleviate this problem.

Infants who were suctioned extensively or intubated at birth can demonstrate an aversion to oral stimulation. The baby may scream and stiffen if anything approaches the mouth. Parents need to spend time holding and cuddling the baby before attempting to breastfeed.

An infant can become fussy and appear discontented when sucking if the nipple does not extend far enough into the mouth. The feeding can begin with well-organized sucks and swallows, but the infant soon begins to pull off the breast and cry. The mother should support her breast throughout the feeding so

PATIENT TEACHING
Baby's Second Night

You've made it through your first 24 hours as a new mom. Maybe you have other children, but you are a new mom all over again … and now it's your baby's second night.

All of a sudden, your little one discovers that he's no longer back in the warmth and comfort—though a bit crowded—womb where he spent the last 9 months—and it is SCARY out here! He isn't hearing your familiar heartbeat, the swooshing of the placental arteries, the soothing sound of your lungs, or the comforting gurgling of your intestines. Instead, he's in a crib, swaddled in a diaper, a tee-shirt, a hat, and a blanket. All sorts of people have been handling him, and he's not yet become accustomed to the new noises, lights, sounds, and smells. He has found one thing though, and that's his voice … and you find that each time you take him off the breast, where he comfortably drifted off to sleep, and put him in the bassinet—he protests, loudly!

In fact, each time you put him back on the breast he nurses for a little bit and then goes to sleep. As you take him off and put him back to bed—he cries again … and starts rooting around, looking for you. This goes on—seemingly for hours. A lot of moms are convinced it is because their milk isn't "in" yet, and the baby is starving. However, it isn't that, but the baby's sudden awakening to the fact that the most comforting and comfortable place for him to be is at the breast. It's the closest to "home" he can get. It seems that this is pretty universal among babies; lactation consultants all over the world have noticed the same thing.

So, what do you do? When he drifts off to sleep at the breast after a good feed, break the suction and take your nipple gently out of his mouth. Don't move him except to gently slide him into an upright neutral position with his head to the side. Don't try and burp him—just snuggle with him until he falls into a deep sleep where he won't be disturbed by being moved. Babies go into a light sleep state (REM) first, and then cycle in and out of REM and deep sleep about every half-hour or so. If he starts to root and act as though he wants to go back to breast, that's fine—this is his way of settling and comforting. During deep sleep, the baby's breathing is very quiet and regular, and there is no movement beneath his eyelids.

Another helpful hint: his hands were his best friends in utero … he could suck on his thumb or his fingers anytime he was the slightest bit disturbed or uncomfortable. And all of a sudden he's had them taken away from him and someone has put mittens on him! He has no way of soothing himself with those mittens on. Babies need to touch—to feel—and even his touch on your breast will increase your oxytocin levels, which will help boost your milk supply! So take the mittens off and loosen his blanket so he can get to his hands. He might scratch himself, but it will heal very rapidly—after all, he had fingernails when he was inside you, and no one put mittens on him then!

By the way—this might happen every once in a while at home too, particularly if you've changed his environment, such as going to the doctor's, to church, to the mall, or to the grandparents! Don't let it throw you—sometimes babies just need some extra snuggling at the breast, because for the baby, the breast is "home."

© 2016/Jan Barger RN, MA, IBCLC/Lactation Education Consultants.

the nipple stays in the same position as the feeding proceeds and the breast softens.

Fussiness may be related to GI distress (i.e., cramping and gas pains). It can occur in response to an occasional feeding of infant formula or be related to something the mother ingested. Most mothers are able to eat a normal diet without causing GI distress to the breastfeeding baby. Persistent crying or refusing

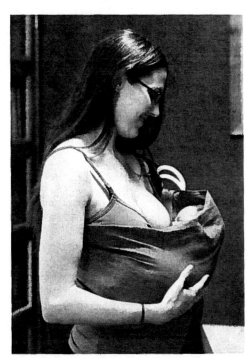

FIGURE 27-12 Baby breastfeeding while in sling. (Courtesy Julie Perry Nelson.)

to breastfeed can indicate illness. Parents should be instructed to notify the health care provider if either circumstance occurs (see Family-Centred Teaching box in Chapter 26, "The Period of PURPLE Crying®", p. 716).

Some mothers find that their babies are less fussy when placed in a sling or carrier. Some slings make it easy to breastfeed without removing the baby from the sling (Fig. 27-12).

Slow weight gain. Newborns may lose up to 10% of their birth weight during the first 3 to 5 days after birth; this is mostly water weight acquired in utero. Thereafter, they should begin to gain weight at the rate of 110 to 200 g/week, or 20 to 28 g/day. The breastfed infant who loses more than 10% of birth weight requires careful assessment regarding feeding behaviours and maternal milk supply. The infant who continues to lose weight after 5 days, does not regain birth weight by 2 weeks, or whose weight is below the tenth percentile by 1 month should be evaluated and closely monitored by a health care provider.

At times, slow weight gain is related to inadequate breastfeeding. Feedings can be short or infrequent, or the infant may be latching on incorrectly or sucking ineffectively or inefficiently. Other causes are illness, infection, malabsorption, or circumstances that increase the newborn's energy needs, such as congenital heart disease, cystic fibrosis, or simply being small for gestational age. However, newborns gain weight in differing patterns, and one should not assume that the newborn is ill just because weight gain is not the same as that of another breastfed or bottle-fed infant. Breastfed infants and formula-fed infants have different patterns of growth in the first year. Use of the WHO growth charts is recommended for appropriate growth monitoring (Denne, 2015; Health Canada

et al., 2012) (see Appendix C). Slow weight gain must be differentiated from failure to thrive; this can be a serious problem that warrants medical intervention. (See Chapter 35, Failure to thrive.)

Maternal factors may also contribute to slow infant weight gain. There may be inadequate milk supply, pain with feeding, or inappropriate timing of feedings. Inadequate glandular breast tissue or previous breast surgery may affect milk supply. Severe intrapartum or postpartum hemorrhage (Sheehan's syndrome), illness, or medications can decrease milk supply. Stress and fatigue also negatively affect milk production (Lauwers & Swisher, 2011; Lawrence & Lawrence, 2015).

In most instances the solution to slow weight gain is to increase feeding frequency and to improve the feeding technique. Positioning and latch are evaluated, and adjustments are made. Adding a feeding or two in a 24-hour period can help. If the problem is a sleepy baby, parents should be instructed in waking techniques.

Using alternate breast massage during feedings can help increase the amount of milk going to the infant. With this technique, the mother massages her breast from the chest wall to the nipple whenever the baby has sucking pauses. This technique also can increase the fat content of the milk, which aids in weight gain.

When newborns are calorie deprived and need supplementation, the extra breast milk or formula can be given with a spoon or cup, syringe, a supplemental nursing device (see Fig. 27-10), or a bottle. If there are latch-on problems, it is best to avoid bottles and pacifiers. In most cases, supplementation is needed only for a short time until the newborn gains weight and is feeding adequately. Most breastfeeding problems require simple solutions; a lactation consultant can help by developing a feeding plan with the mother.

Jaundice. Jaundice and hyperbilirubinemia in the newborn are discussed in detail in Chapter 26. Breastfeeding infants can develop *early-onset jaundice* or *breastfeeding-associated jaundice,* which is associated with insufficient feeding and infrequent stooling. Colostrum has a natural laxative effect and promotes early passage of meconium. Bilirubin is excreted from the body primarily through the intestines. Infrequent stooling allows bilirubin in the stool to be resorbed into the infant's system, thus increasing bilirubin levels (Blackburn, 2013). To prevent early-onset, breastfeeding-associated jaundice, newborns should be breastfed frequently during the first several days of life. Increased frequency of feedings is associated with decreased bilirubin levels.

To treat early-onset jaundice, breastfeeding is evaluated in terms of frequency and length of feedings, positioning, latch, and milk transfer. Factors such as a sleepy or lethargic infant or maternal breast engorgement can interfere with effective breastfeeding and should be corrected. If the infant's intake of milk needs to be increased, a supplemental feeding device can deliver additional breast milk or formula while the infant is nursing. Bilirubin levels should be closely monitored (see Chapter 26).

Late-onset jaundice or *breast milk jaundice* affects a small number of breastfed infants and develops between 5 and 10 days of age. Affected infants are typically thriving, gaining weight, and stooling normally; all pathological causes of jaundice have been ruled out. In the presence of other risk factors, hyperbilirubinemia can be severe enough to require phototherapy. In most cases of breast milk jaundice no intervention is necessary.

Any breastfeeding infant who develops jaundice should be evaluated carefully for weight loss greater than 7%, decreased milk intake, infrequent stooling (fewer than three stools per day by day 4), and decreased urine output (fewer than four to six wet diapers per day). Bilirubin levels should be assessed by serum testing or transcutaneous monitoring. The CPS recommendations on management of hyperbilirubinemia include professional breastfeeding support and continued exclusive breastfeeding during phototherapy treatment (Barrington, Sankaran, & CPS, 2007/2016) (see Chapter 26).

Preterm infants. Human milk is the ideal food for preterm infants, with benefits that are unique to the individual preterm infant in addition to those received by healthy term infants. Breast milk enhances retinal maturation in the preterm infant and improves neurocognitive outcomes; it also decreases the risk of necrotizing enterocolitis. Greater physiological stability occurs with breastfeeding than with bottle-feeding (Lawrence & Lawrence, 2015).

Initially, breast milk for preterm infants contains higher concentrations of energy, protein, sodium, chloride, potassium, iron, and magnesium than term milk. It is more similar to term milk by approximately 4 to 6 weeks. Depending on gestational age and physical condition, many preterm infants are capable of breastfeeding for at least some feedings each day. Mothers of preterm infants who are not able to breastfeed their infants should begin pumping their breasts as soon as possible after birth with a hospital-grade electric pump (Fig. 27-13). Pumping frequency depends on the mother's breastfeeding goals but may be recommended 8 to 10 times every 24 hours to establish the milk supply. These women must be taught proper handling and

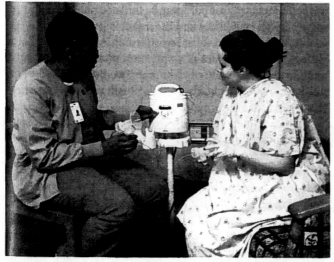

FIGURE 27-13 Nurse explains use of hospital-grade electric breast pump to new mother. (Courtesy Kathryn Alden.)

storage of breast milk to minimize bacterial contamination and growth. Kangaroo care (skin-to-skin contact) is advised until the baby is able to breastfeed and while breastfeeding is established because it enhances milk production (Hurst & Meier, 2010; Lauwers & Swisher, 2011).

Mothers of preterm infants often receive specific emotional benefits in breastfeeding or providing breast milk for their babies. They find reward in knowing that they can provide the healthiest nutrition for the infant and experience enhanced feelings of closeness to the infant through breastfeeding.

Late preterm infants. Newborns born at 34 0/7 to 36 6/7 weeks of gestation are categorized as *late preterm infants.* These newborns are at risk for feeding difficulties because of their low energy stores and high energy demands (ABM Protocol Committee, 2011a; Cooper, Holditch-Davis, Verklan et al., 2012). They tend to be sleepy, with minimal and short wakeful periods. Late preterm infants often tire easily while feeding and have a weak suck and low tone; these factors can contribute to inadequate milk intake. Early and extended skin-to-skin contact promotes breastfeeding and helps prevent hypothermia. Because these infants are more prone to positional apnea than term infants, mothers are advised to use the clutch (under the arm or football) hold for feeding and avoid flexing the head, which can impede breathing. Often supplementation is needed; expressed breast milk is the optimal supplement, preferably at the breast using a supplemental feeding device (see Fig. 27-10) (Cleveland, 2010).

Breastfeeding multiple infants. Breastfeeding is especially beneficial to twins, triplets, and other higher-order multiples because of the immunological and nutritional advantages and the opportunity for the mother to interact with each baby frequently. Most mothers are capable of producing an adequate milk supply for multiple infants. Parenting multiples can be overwhelming; mothers and their husbands or partners need extra support and help to learn how to manage feedings (Fig. 27-14).

Caring for twins takes planning and organization, but with breastfeeding feedings are always ready and no one has to wash bottles and prepare formula; some mothers can feed both babies at once. The mother with twins will need extra nourishment for herself (200 to 500 kcal/day for each infant).

A typical pattern is that each newborn feeds from one breast per feeding, usually for about 20 to 30 minutes. Some mothers assign each newborn a breast; others switch infants from one breast to the other, either on a schedule or randomly. The mother may find it easiest to use a modified demand feeding schedule; that is, feeding the first infant who wakes up and then waking the second infant for feeding.

During the early weeks, parents may find it helpful to keep a record of feeding times and of which breast was used first by which infant. If one twin nurses more vigorously than the other, that infant should be alternated between breasts to equalize breast stimulation.

If the mother wants to feed the newborns simultaneously, she may wish to experiment with positions. For example, one newborn can be held in the football hold and the other in the cradle hold, or the newborns can each be held in the football

Summary *of* Recommendations

	RECOMMENDATION	*LEVEL OF EVIDENCE
Practice Recommendations	1 Nurses endorse the Baby-Friendly™ Hospital Initiative (BFHI), which was jointly launched in 1992 by the World Health Organization (WHO) and the United Nations Children's Fund (UNICEF). The BFHI directs health care facilities to meet the "Ten Steps to Successful Breastfeeding".	III
	1.1 Nurses have a role in advocating for "breastfeeding friendly" environments by: ■ advocating for supportive facilities and systems such as day-care facilities, "mother and baby" areas for breastfeeding, public breastfeeding areas, 24-hour help for families having difficulties in breastfeeding; and ■ promoting community action in breastfeeding.	III
	2 Nurses and health care practice settings endorse the WHO recommendation for exclusive breastfeeding for the first six months, with introduction of complementary foods and continued breastfeeding up to two years and beyond thereafter.	I
	3 Nurses will perform a comprehensive breastfeeding assessment of mother/baby/family, both prenatally and postnatally, to facilitate intervention and the development of a breastfeeding plan.	III
	3.1 Key components of the prenatal assessment should include: ■ personal and demographic variables that may influence breastfeeding rates; ■ intent to breastfeed; ■ access to support for breastfeeding, including significant others and peers; ■ attitude about breastfeeding among health care providers, significant others and peers; and ■ physical factors, including breasts and nipples, that may effect a woman's ability to breastfeed.	III

*See page 14 for details regarding "Interpretation of the Evidence"

10

RECOMMENDATION		LEVEL OF EVIDENCE
Practice Recommendations (cont.)	3.2 Key components of the postnatal assessment should include: ■ intrapartum medications; ■ level of maternal physical discomfort; ■ observation of positioning, latching and sucking; ■ signs of milk transfer; ■ parental ability to identify infant feeding cues; ■ mother-infant interaction and maternal response to feeding cues; ■ maternal perception of infant satisfaction/satiety cues; ■ woman's ability to identify significant others who are available and supportive of the decision to breastfeed; ■ delivery experience; and ■ infant physical assessment.	III
	3.3 Practice settings are encouraged to develop, adopt or adapt assessment tools encompassing key components for assessment and that meet the needs of their local practice setting.	III
	4 Nurses will provide education to couples during the childbearing age, expectant mothers/couples/families and assist them in making informed decisions regarding breastfeeding. Education should include, as a minimum, the following: ■ benefits of breastfeeding (Level I); ■ lifestyle issues (Level III); ■ milk production (Level III); ■ breastfeeding positions (Level III); ■ latching/milk transfer (Level II-2); ■ prevention and management of problems (Level III); ■ medical interventions (Level III); ■ when to seek help (Level III); and ■ where to get additional information and resources (Level III).	
	5 Small, informal group health education classes, delivered in the antenatal period, have a better impact on breastfeeding initiation rates than breastfeeding literature alone or combined with formal, non-interactive methods of teaching.	I

11

 RNAO

	RECOMMENDATION	LEVEL OF EVIDENCE
Practice Recommendations (cont.)	5.1 Evaluation of education programs should be considered in order to evaluate the effectiveness of prenatal breastfeeding classes.	II-2
	6 Nurses will perform a comprehensive breastfeeding assessment of mother/baby prior to hospital discharge.	III
	6.1 If mother and baby are discharged within 48 hours of birth, there must be a face-to-face follow up assessment conducted within 48 hours of discharge by a qualified health care professional, such as a Public Health Nurse or Community Nurse specializing in maternal/newborn care.	III
	6.2 Discharge of mother and baby after 48 hours should be followed by a telephone call within 48 hours of discharge.	III
	7 Nurses with experience and expertise in breastfeeding should provide support to mothers. Such support should be established in the antenatal period, continued into the postpartum period and should involve face-to-face contact.	I
	7.1 Organizations should consider establishing and supporting peer support programs, alone or in combination with one-to-one education from health professionals, in the antenatal and postnatal periods.	I
Education Recommendations	8 Nurses providing breastfeeding support should receive mandatory education in breastfeeding in order to develop the knowledge, skill and attitudes to implement breastfeeding policy and to support breastfeeding mothers.	II-2
Organization & Policy Recommendations	9 Practice settings need to review their breastfeeding education programs for the public and, where appropriate, make the necessary changes based on recommendations in this best practice guideline.	III
	10 Practice settings/organizations should work towards being accredited by the Baby-Friendly™ Hospital Initiative.	III

12

RNAO

Appendix E :
Postpartum Assessment Tools

Postpartum Assessment Tool	Reference
Infant Breastfeeding Assessment Tool (IBFAT)	See next page. Matthews, M.K. (1988). Developing an instrument to assess infant breastfeeding behaviour in the early neonatal period. *Midwifery, 4*(4), 154-165.
LATCH – Breastfeeding Charting System©	Jensen, D., Wallace, S., & Kelsay, P. (1994). LATCH: A breastfeeding charting system and documentation tool. *Journal of Obstetric, Gynecologic and Neonatal Nursing, 23*(1), 27-32.
Mother-Baby Assessment (MBA) Form	Mulford, C. (1992). The mother-baby assessment (MBA): An "Apgar Score" for breastfeeding. *Journal of Human Lactation, 8*(2), 79-82.

86

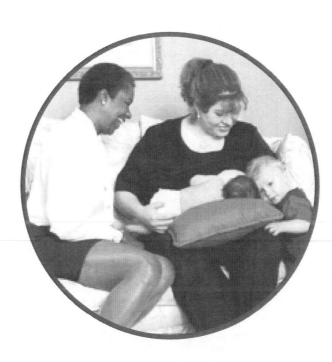
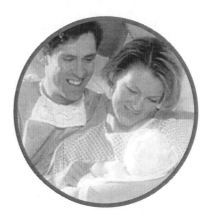

Infant Breastfeeding Assessment Tool (IBFAT)

Reprinted from: Matthews, M.K. (1988). Developing an instrument to assess infant breastfeeding behaviour in the early neonatal period. *Midwifery*, *4*(4), 154-165, with permission of Elsevier.

Infant Breastfeeding Assessment Tool (IBFAT)

Check the score which best describes the baby's feeding behaviours at this feed.

	3	2	1	0
In order to get baby to feed:	Placed the baby on the breast as no effort was needed.	Used mild stimulation such as unbundling, patting or burping.	Unbundled baby, sat baby back and forward, rubbed baby's body or limbs vigorously at beginning and during feeding.	Could not be aroused.
Rooting	Rooted effectively at once.	Needed coaxing, prompting or encouragement.	Rooted poorly even with coaxing.	Did not root.
How long from placing baby on breast to latch & suck?	0 – 3 minutes.	3 – 10 minutes.	Over 10 minutes.	Did not feed.
Sucking pattern	Sucked well throughout on one or both breasts.	Sucked on & off but needed encouragement.	Sucked poorly, weak sucking; sucking efforts for short periods.	Did not suck.

MOTHER'S EVALUATION
How do you feel about the way the baby fed at this feeding?
3 – Very pleased   2 – Pleased   1 – Fairly pleased   0 – Not pleased

IBFAT assigns a score, 0,1,2, or 3 to five factors. Scores range from 0 to 12.
The mother's evaluation score is not calculated in the IBFAT score.

87

▶ **RNAO**

Appendix F: Breastfeeding Positions

Cradle-Hold

This is a common position for breastfeeding. In order to latch the baby, the mother may support her breast with the hand opposite the side that the baby is nursing, with her thumb and fingers well back from the areola. Using the arm on the same side the baby is nursing on, the mother supports the baby's head and body and keeps the infant close. The baby should be at the level of the breast, and pillows are useful to provide additional support. The mother turns the baby towards her so that the infant's nose, chin, tummy and knees are touching her. The mother can tuck the infant's lower arm below her breast to keep it out of the way.

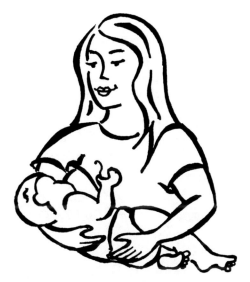

Modified Cradle-Hold

The mother should be seated comfortably with additional pillows as necessary to support her back and arms then tuck the baby under breast. Use of a footstool may be beneficial. The mother can support her breast with fingers positioned at the base of her breast well back from the areola. The baby should be held in the arm opposite to the breast being used. The baby's shoulder and neck are supported by her hand and the baby is turned facing the mother. Holding the back of the infant's head with her hand may cause the infant to pull away when being put onto the breast. The baby's head and neck should be in a slightly extended position to facilitate the chin touching the breast (Biancuzzo, 1999; Lothian, 1995).

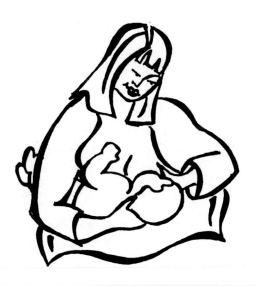

Illustrations reproduced with the permission of the City of Ottawa.

Side-Lying

The mother should lie on her side with one or two pillows supporting her head and her lower arm flexed up. Use pillows as necessary to support her back and legs. The baby should be positioned side-lying, facing the mother, with the head low enough that the mom's nipple is at the level of the baby's nose, and the neck extended so that eye contact with the mother is possible (Scarborough Breastfeeding Network, 1999; Society of Paediatric Nursing of the Royal College of Nursing, 1998). The mother's hand should be across baby's shoulder blades. The mother should pull the baby towards her abdomen, and wait. The baby will extend his head with a wide mouth and will latch onto the breast without assistance.

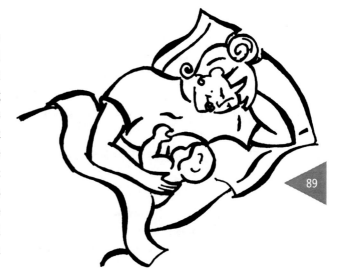

89

Football Hold (Clutch Hold)

The mother should be seated comfortably as per the 'cradle-hold' description. The baby should be positioned on a pillow at the mother's side, on the side of the breast to be used. Use extra pillows to raise baby to the level of the breast. The baby should be tucked in close to the mother's side and held like a football with the bottom against the back of the chair and the legs up behind mother's arm (Scarborough Breastfeeding Network, 1999; Society of Paediatric Nursing of the Royal College of Nursing, 1998). The baby's back should be supported with the mother's arm and his shoulders with mother's hand (avoid holding baby's head).

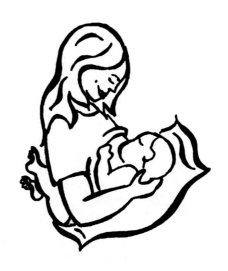

Illustrations reproduced with the permission of the City of Ottawa.

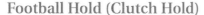

RNAO

Appendix G: *Latch, Milk Transfer and Effective Breastfeeding*

International Lactation Consultant Association (ILCA)
Association of Women's Health, Obstetric and Neonatal Nurses (AWHONN)

Latch (ILCA)

Observe infant for signs of correct latch-on:

- wide opened mouth
- flared lips
- nose, cheeks, and chin touching, or nearly touching, the breast

Milk Transfer (ILCA)

Observe infant for signs of milk transfer:

- sustained rhythmic suck/swallow patterns with occasional pauses
- audible swallowing
- relaxed arms and hands
- moist mouth
- satisfied after feedings

Observe mother for signs of milk transfer:

- strong tugging which is not painful
- thirst
- uterine contractions or increased lochia flow during or after feeding for the first 3-5 days
- milk leaking from the opposite breast while feeding
- relaxation or drowsiness
- breast softening while feeding
- nipple elongated after feeding but not pinched or abraded

90

RNAO

Infant Behaviours (AWHONN)

Infant feeding cues:

- Rooting
- Hand-to-mouth movements
- Sucking movements/sounds
- Sucking of fingers or hands
- Opening of mouth in response to tactile stimulation

Transition between behaviour states (sleep to drowsy and quietly alert)

Infant satisfaction/satiety cues including the following:

- During the feeding, a gradual decrease in number of sucks
- Pursed lips, pulling away from the breast and releasing the nipple
- Body relaxed
- Legs extended
- Absence of hunger cues
- Sleep, contented state
- Small amount of milk seen in mouth

Frequency and duration (ILCA)

Frequency and duration of feedings:

- Expect a minimum of 8-12 feedings in 24 hours
- Some infants will breastfeed every 3 hours day and night, others will cluster-feed, feeding every hour for 4-6 feeds then sleeping 4-6 hours
- Expect to feed 15-20 minutes on the first breast and 10-15 minutes on the second but do not be concerned if the infant is satisfied after one breast
- If necessary, wake a sleepy infant for feedings until an appropriate weight gain pattern is established
- Expect feeding frequency to decrease as the infant gets older

RNAO

Urine (AWHONN)

- One void by 24 hours
- 3 or more voids by next 24 hours
- 6 or more voids by day four

Stool (AWHONN, ILCA)

- One stool by 24 hours (AWHONN)
- 1-2 stools by day 3 (AWHONN)
- 3 or more stools by day 4 (AWHONN)
- Expect bowel movements to change from meconium to a yellow, soft, and watery consistency by day 4 (ILCA)

Weight (ILCA)

- Expect less than 7% weight loss the first week
- Expect return to birth weight by 14 days of age
- Expect weight gain of 4-8 ounces (120 – 240 grams) a week until the infant has doubled birth weight

Ineffective Breastfeeding (ILCA)

- Infant weight loss greater than 7%
- Continued weight loss after day 3
- Less than 3 bowel movements in 24 hours
- Meconium stools after day 4
- Less than 6 wet diapers in 24 hours after day 4
- Infant who is irritable and restless or sleepy and refusing to feed
- No audible swallowing during feedings
- No discernible change in weight or size of breasts and no discernible change in milk volume and composition by 3-5 days
- Persistent or increasingly painful nipples
- Engorgement unrelieved by feeding
- Infant who does not begin to gain weight by day 5
- Infant who has not returned to birth weight by day 14

RNAO

Appendix H:
Immediate Postpartum Decision Tree

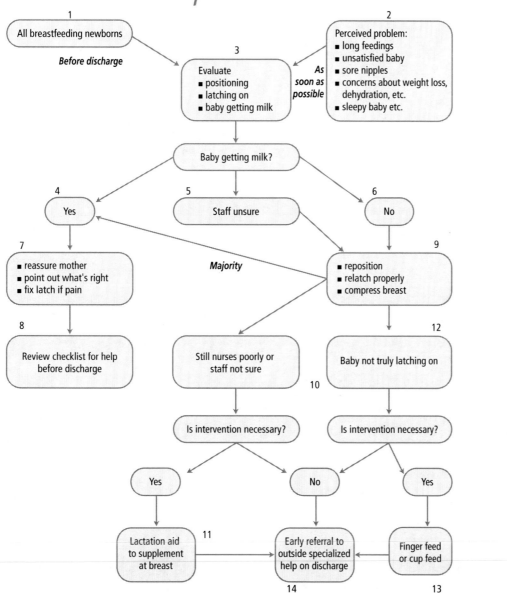

Immediate Postpartum Descision Tree. The same approach can be used to make decisions about breastfeeding at any age of the baby, but may require some modification depending on the age and problems encountered.

Reproduced with permission of Dr. J. Newman, Toronto, Ontario.

RNAO

Summary *of* Recommendations

RECOMMENDATION			*LEVEL OF EVIDENCE
Practice Recommendations			
Prevention	1.0	Nurses provide individualized, flexible postpartum care based on the identification of depressive symptoms and maternal preference.	Ia
	2.0	Nurses initiate preventive strategies in the early postpartum period.	Ia
Confirming Depressive Symptoms	3.0	The Edinburgh Postnatal Depression Scale (EPDS) is the recommended self-report tool to confirm depressive symptoms in postpartum mothers.	III
	4.0	The EPDS can be administered anytime throughout the postpartum period (birth to 12 months) to confirm depressive symptoms.	III
	5.0	Nurses encourage postpartum mothers to complete the EPDS by themselves in privacy.	III
	6.0	An EPDS cut-off score greater than 12 may be used to determine depressive symptoms among English-speaking women in the postpartum period. This cut-off criterion should be interpreted cautiously with mothers who: 1) are non-English speaking; 2) use English as a second language, and/or 3) are from diverse cultures.	III
	7.0	The EPDS must be interpreted in combination with clinical judgment to confirm postpartum mothers with depressive symptoms.	III
	8.0	Nurses should provide immediate assessment for self harm ideation/behaviour when a mother scores positive (e.g., from 1 to 3) on the EPDS self-harm item number 10.	IV
Treatment	9.0	Nurses provide supportive weekly interactions and ongoing assessment focusing on mental health needs of postpartum mothers experiencing depressive symptoms.	Ib
	10.0	Nurses facilitate opportunities for the provision of peer support for postpartum mothers with depressive symptoms.	IIb
General	11.0	Nurses facilitate the involvement of partners and family members in the provision of care for postpartum mothers experiencing depressive symptoms, as appropriate.	Ib
	12.0	Nurses promote self-care activities among new mothers to assist in alleviating depressive symptoms during the postpartum period.	IV
	13.0	Nurses consult appropriate resources for current and accurate information before educating mothers with depressive symptoms about psychotropic medications.	IV
Education Recommendations			
	14.0	Nurses providing care to new mothers should receive education on postpartum depression to assist with the confirmation of depressive symptoms and prevention and treatment interventions.	III

*Please refer to page 11 for details regarding "Interpretation of Evidence".

10

Background Context

The postpartum period is considered a time of increased risk for the onset of mood disorders. Research has shown that a woman is significantly more likely to be admitted to a psychiatric hospital within the first 4 weeks postpartum than at any other time in her life (Kendell, Chambers & Platz,1987; Paffenbarger, 1982; Brockington, Cernick, Schofield, Downing, Francis & Keelan, 1981) and up to 12.5% of all psychiatric hospital admissions of women occur during the postpartum period (Duffy, 1983). Postpartum affective disorders are typically divided into three categories: postpartum blues, postpartum depression, and puerperal psychosis. Postpartum blues is the most common postpartum mood disturbance with prevalence estimates ranging from 30% to 75%. Symptoms, which often begin within the immediate postpartum period and remit within days, include mood lability, irritability, tearfulness, generalized anxiety, and sleep and appetite disturbance. By definition, postpartum blues are transient, mild, time-limited, and do not require treatment other than reassurance (Kennerly & Gath, 1989). Conversely, postpartum psychosis is a very severe depressive episode characterized by the presence of psychotic features. This condition is the most severe and uncommon form of postpartum affective disorders, with rates of 1 to 2 episodes per 1000 deliveries (Kendell et al., 1987). The clinical onset is rapid, with symptoms presenting as early as the first 48 to 72 hours postpartum, and the majority of episodes develop within the first 2 weeks postpartum. The symptoms are typically depressed or elated mood (which can fluctuate rapidly), disorganized behaviour, mood lability, delusions, and hallucinations (Brockington et al., 1981).

Among these conditions is postpartum depression, a nonpsychotic depressive episode beginning in the postpartum period (Cox, Murray & Chapman, 1993; O'Hara,1994; Watson, Elliott, Rugg & Brough, 1984). At present, postpartum depression is not classified as a separate disease; it is diagnosed as part of affective or mood disorders in both the American Psychiatric Association's Diagnostic and Statistical Manual of Mental Disorders (DSM-IV) and the World Health Organization's International Classification of Diseases (ICD-10). According to the DSM-IV, postpartum depression is a depressive disorder with onset within the first 4 weeks postpartum. However to be comprehensive in the literature review and to be able to include the best evidence possible, for this practice guideline, postpartum depression is defined as any depressive episode that occurs within the first year postpartum.

The symptoms of postpartum depression are similar to depression unrelated to childbirth (Wisner, Parry & Piontek, 2002). However, despite these similarities, postpartum depression is frequently exacerbated by other indicators such as low self-esteem, inability to cope, loneliness, feelings of incompetence, and loss of self (Beck, Reynolds & Rutowski, 1992; Mills, Finchilescu & Lea, 1995; Righetti-Veltema, Conne-Perreard, Bousquet & Manzano, 1998; Ritter, Hobfoll, Lavin, Cameron & Hulsizer, 2000). Somatic symptoms of depression, including appetite and sleep disturbances, are often present in women with postpartum depression (Nonacs, & Cohen, 1998). Distinguishing between these depressive symptoms and the supposed 'normal' sequelae of childbirth can make postpartum depression potentially difficult to diagnose (Hostetter & Stowe, 2002). See *Apendix C* for the DSM-IV criteria for a major depressive episode.

Postpartum depression is a major health issue for many women (Affonso, De, Horowitz & Mayberry, 2000). A meta-analysis of 59 studies suggests that approximately 13% of women experience postpartum depression (O'Hara & Swain, 1996) with the inception rate greatest in the first 12 weeks postpartum (Goodman, 2004); these rates do not differ between primiparous and multiparous mothers. While up to 20% of women with postpartum blues will continue to develop postpartum depression (Campbell, Cohn, Flanagan, Popper & Meyers, 1992; O'Hara, Schlechte, Lewis & Wright, 1991b), other women enjoy a period of well-being after delivery followed by a gradual onset of depressive symptoms.

This hidden morbidity has well documented health consequences for the mother, child, and family. While women who have suffered from postpartum depression are twice as likely to experience future episodes of depression over a 5-year period (Cooper & Murray, 1995), infants and children are particularly vulnerable. Untreated postpartum depression can cause impaired maternal-infant interactions (Murray, Fiori-Cowley, Hooper & Cooper, 1996) and negative perceptions of infant behaviour (Mayberry & Affonso, 1993) which have been linked to attachment insecurity (Hipwell, Goossens, Melhuish, & Kumar, 2000; Murray, 1992), and emotional developmental delay (Cogill, Caplan, Alexandra, Robson & Kumar, 1986; Cummings & Davies, 1994; Hipwell et al., 2000; Murray, Sinclair, Cooper, Ducournau, Turner & Stein, 1999; Whiffen & Gotlib, 1989). Marital stress, resulting in separation or divorce (Boyce, 1994; Holden, 1991) is also a reported outcome.

The cause of postpartum depression remains unclear (Cooper & Murray, 1998), with extensive research suggesting a multifactorial aetiology (Ross, Gilbert Evans, Sellers & Romach, 2003). In particular, a variety of biological, psychological, and sociocultural variables likely interact to produce vulnerability to postpartum depression, and the causes or "triggers" of postpartum depression likely vary from woman to woman. Although researchers and health professionals have long speculated that postpartum depression may be linked to the dramatic hormone changes which accompany pregnancy and childbirth, to date no particular hormone has been consistently associated with postpartum depression, nor have any differences in hormones been identified between women with and without postpartum depression (Bloch et al., 2000).

To promote the identification of women experiencing postpartum depression, self-report measures have been developed specifically for use within a postpartum population. Self-report measures are easier and less costly to administer, and do not require the presence of trained specialists. The most well established self-report tool for the identification of postpartum depression is the Edinburgh Postnatal Depression Scale (EPDS), a 10 item self-report measure that has been translated into diverse languages. The EPDS has been rigorously validated against clinical diagnostic interviews (Cox, Holden & Sagovsky, 1987). English- and French-language versions of the EPDS are provided in *Appendices D & E*.

According to epidemiological studies and meta-analyses of predictive studies, the strongest predictors of postpartum depression are: antenatal depression and anxiety, personal and family history of depression, life stress (Beck, 2001; Bernazzani, Saucier, David & Borgeat, 1997; O'Hara & Swain, 1996; O'Hara, Schlechte, Lewis & Varner, 1991a), and the lack of social support (Beck, 2001; Brugha, Sharp, Cooper, Weisender, Britto & Shinkwin, 1998; Cooper & Murray, 1998; Mills et al., 1995; O'Hara & Swain, 1996; O'Hara et al., 1991a; Righetti-Veltema et al., 1998). Two meta-analyses also found a higher risk of postpartum depression among socially disadvantaged women (Beck, 2001; O'Hara & Swain, 1996).

To enhance our understanding of postpartum depression, numerous qualitative research studies have been conducted. To summarize this work, a meta-synthesis of 18 qualitative studies was conducted which identified several overarching themes including: 1) incongruity between expectations and reality of motherhood; 2) spiralling downward; and 3) pervasive loss (Beck, 2002).

Eight of the 18 studies in the meta-synthesis centred on the role that conflicting expectations and experiences of motherhood played in the development of postpartum depression. In particular, women often held unrealistic expectations which were inconsistent with their own experiences as mothers (Mauthner, 1999). This incongruity between expectations and lived experience was described in seven areas: labour and delivery, life with their infants, self as mother, relationship with partners, support from family and friends, life events and physical changes (Berggren-Clive, 1998). When women became disillusioned with motherhood and perceived they had failed to be the 'perfect mother' (Berggren-Clive, 1998), their emotions of despair and sadness started a spiral downward into postpartum depression.

Loss of control was identified as a central theme in 15 out of the 18 studies. Nicolson's (1999) study described how loss of autonomy and time were precursors to feeling out of control due to a lack of time to consider themselves or process their daily experiences. This in turn led to a loss of self-identify, including loss of former sense of self. Women also discussed how postpartum depression led to loss of relationships with their partners, children, and family members (Morgan, Matthey, Barnett & Richardson, 1997). Some women wanted their partners 'to be able to read their minds' and take some initiative in helping them, while others felt that admitting their feelings was a sign of personal inadequacy and failure as a mother (McIntosh, 1993). If they did admit to their feelings, women also risked being misunderstood, rejected, or stigmatized by their loved ones. Women with postpartum depression expressed feelings of being 'different' and 'abnormal' compared to other mothers. They consistently talked about a profound sense of isolation and loneliness. Mothers who were depressed frequently felt discomfort with being around others and believed that no one really understood what they were experiencing (Beck et al., 1992). Consequently, they socially withdrew to escape a potentially critical world (Semprevivo, 1996).

Although qualitative research cannot determine intervention effectiveness, it can provide valuable information such as determining which aspects of care women find most useful. In a variety of studies, mothers who were interviewed have identified the need for health professionals to be aware of and knowledgeable about postpartum depression (Mauthner, 1997). Community education to inform family members about the range of signs and symptoms of postpartum depression was also thought to be beneficial (Ugarizza, 2002). Mothers felt that postpartum depression should be openly discussed in antenatal classes so that women could be better informed. It was thought that this type of discussion may also help to reduce the stigma associated with postpartum depression. In addition, women felt antenatal classes provided an opportunity to develop social support networks (Mauthner, 1997). Mothers also identified 'talking therapies' as an option that should be made available (Chan, Levy, Chung & Lee, 2002). Health professionals who encouraged women to talk about their feelings and who spent time listening were highly valued (Mauthner, 1997). Telephone and web-based support groups have been suggested to assist mothers who are symptomatic in their homes (Ugariizza, 2002). Among ethnospecific populations, mothers felt nurses could foster connections with specific cultural groups by becoming aware of what was available in the community (Nahas, Hillege & Amasheh, 1999). There was also a stated need that nurses understand the cultural beliefs and values of new mothers in order to facilitate culturally sensitive care (Chan et al., 2002; Nahas et al., 1999; Nahas & Amasheh, 1999).

Appendix D: Edinburgh Postnatal Depression Scale (EPDS) English

Reproduction of the EPDS in it's entirety is restricted to print version only. The following is an excerpt of the EPDS for sample purposes.

How are you feeling?

As you have recently had a baby, we would like to know how you are feeling now. Please underline the answer which comes closest to how you have felt in the past 7 days, not just how you feel today. Here is an example, already completed.

I have felt happy:
Yes, most of the time
Yes, some of the time
No, not very often
No, not at all

This would mean: "I have felt happy some of the time during the past week". Please complete the other questions in the same way.

In the past 7 days

1. I have been able to laugh and see the funny side of things:
As much as I always could
Not quite so much now
Definitely not so much now
Not at all

Translations of the scale, and guidance as to its use, may be found in Cox, J. L. & Holden, J. (2003) Perinatal Mental Health: A Guide to the Edinburgh Postnatal Depression Scale. London: Gaskell.

The hard copy of the guideline Interventions for Postpartum Depression is available through the Registered Nurses' Association of Ontario. For more information and an order form, please visit the RNAO website at www.rnao.org/bestpractices.

Appendix F: Administration and Interpretation of the EPDS

The EPDS can be administered to mothers anytime from birth to 52 weeks that have been identified with depressive symptoms either subjectively or objectively.

Instructions for the administration of the EPDS

1. The EPDS may be administered in person.
2. Efforts should be make to have the mother complete the scale by herself, where she feels she can answer the questions honestly.
3. Mother's may need assistance with the EPDS if they have limited reading skills or understanding of the English language.
4. All 10 items on the questionnaire must be completed.
5. The mother or health care professional should underline the response that best describes the mother's feelings in the last week.
6. The EPDS can be administered anytime from 0 to 52 weeks.

Sample lead in statements

Please be as open and honest as possible when answering these questions. It is not easy being a new mother and it is OK to feel unhappy at times. As you have recently had a new baby, we would like to know how you are feeling. Please state the answer which comes closest to how you have felt during the past several days, not just how you are feeling today.

Scoring of the EPDS

Each response is scored 0, 1, 2 or 3 based on the increased severity of the symptoms. Calculate the total score by adding together each of the 10 items.

Interpretation of the EPDS

1. The EPDS score must be considered in combination with the assessment of the health care provider.
2. A score of 13 or greater indicates the presence of depressive symptoms.
3. The score does not reflect the severity of the symptoms.
4. Use caution when interpreting the score of mothers who are non-English speaking and/or use English as a second language or are multicultural.
5. If a mother scores positive (1, 2 or 3) on self-harm item number 10, further assessment should be done immediately for self-harm ideation (refer to *Appendix H & I* for examples of sample questions).
6. Follow agency/institution protocol regarding scores.
7. Remember that the EPDS is only a tool. If your clinical judgment indicates differently than the EPDS continue with the follow up as the assessment indicates.

Translations of the scale, and guidance as to its use, may be found in Cox, J. L. & Holden, J. (2003) Perinatal Mental Health: A Guide to the Edinburgh Postnatal Depression Scale. London: Gaskell.

Journal of Psychiatric and Mental Health Nursing, 2008, 15, 93–100

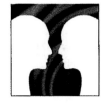

The Tidal Commitments: extending the value base of mental health recovery

P. BUCHANAN-BARKER[1] & P. J. BARKER[2] PhD FRCN

[1]Director, Clan Unity International, Fife, Scotland, and [2]Visiting Professor, Trinity College, Dublin, Ireland

Correspondence:
P. Buchanan-Barker
Clan Unity International
88 West Road
Newport on Tay
Fife DD6 8HP
Scotland
E-mail: tidalmodel@
btinternet.com

BUCHANAN-BARKER P. & BARKER P. J. (2008) *Journal of Psychiatric and Mental Health Nursing* 15, 93–100

The Tidal Commitments: extending the value base of mental health recovery

The emerging concept of recovery in mental health is often only loosely defined, but appears to be influenced more by specific human values and beliefs, than scientific research and 'evidence'. As a contribution to the further development of the philosophical basis of the concept of recovery, this paper reviews the discrete assumptions of the Tidal Model, describes the development of the Model's value base – the 10 Commitments – and illustrates the 20 Tidal Competencies, which aim to generate practice-based evidence for the process of recovery.

Key words: culture, mental health nursing, reclamation, recovery, Tidal Model, values

Accepted for publication: 25 September 2007

Problematizing recovery

Twentieth-century psychiatry focused mainly, although not exclusively, on the containment of mental *illness* – doing things *to* patients, or *for* them, to reduce disturbance, rather than working *with* people, to develop more personally meaningful ways of living. By the end of the 20th century, the assumption that professionals could 'fix' mental illness was waning and increasingly was overtaken by the view that people should participate in, if not actually lead, their own 'recovery' (Davidson & Strauss 1992). The concept of 'recovery' has become a key aspect of mental health policy in many Western countries, especially where mental health legislation or policy is under review, e.g. New Zealand (Mental Health Commission New Zealand 2001), England (Repper 2000), Scotland (Scottish Executive 2006) and Ireland (Mental Health Commission 2006). Government-led reviews of mental health nursing in England (Department of Health 2006) and Scotland (Scottish Executive 2006) proposed that nurses should adopt a 'recovery focus', with its attendant 'values', as part of the modernization of the discipline. However, the exact nature of these 'recovery values' seems unclear. O'Hagan (2004),

in New Zealand, acknowledged that, as another 'import from America', recovery tended to emphasize individual over social processes. Given that it had evolved from 'psychiatric rehabilitation (American recovery) was perhaps driven more by professionals than by service users' (O'Hagan 2004, p. 1) and that 'much of the American recovery literature accepted, at least implicitly, the biomedical model of "mental illness" (and) did not necessarily reflect all the values of the user/survivor movement' (O'Hagan 2004, p. 2). O'Hagan's reservations about pasting a recovery philosophy over traditional 'mental illness' values is well stated. People may well be 'ill at ease' with themselves or others, or 'ill-fitted' for the challenges that life presents. However, many might reject the idea that they are 'mentally ill', in any traditional medical sense (Buchanan-Barker & Barker 2002). This is neither a theoretical nor a semantic dispute. When people locate their problems within the world of their lived experience, the metaphorical nature of their 'illness' can become clear, with implications for any 'recovery journey'.

The contemporary mental health recovery literature appears to differ little from the philosophical assumptions of *Alcoholics Anonymous* (AA) and *Narcotics Anonymous*

93

(NA), from over 60 years ago (Frank 1996), which first promulgated ideas about empowerment, mutual support and self-help, common to today's mental health recovery literature. AA and NA recognized that, however useful professional help might be, recovery had to be pursued actively by the person.

Over the past 25 years, recovery has been proposed as an alternative to mainstream ideas of psychiatric care, especially for people with so-called 'serious' and/or 'enduring' forms of mental illness (Chamberlin 1978, Deegan 1988, Anthony 1993, Fitzpatrick 2002). At the same time, the passive 'patient' role has been transformed into the active 'user/consumer' of services (Barham & Hayward 1991, Deegan 1993), or what Manos called the 'prosumer' – someone directly influencing the help they required (Manos 1993).

Many of the significant descriptions of recovery were developed by people who had been (or still were) psychiatric 'patients' and who professed a more optimistic, empowering approach to identifying the help people might need to deal with problems of human living.

While the literature does include a few studies of recovery, from a psychiatric-medical perspective (Harding *et al.* 1987, Harrison *et al.* 2001), recovery *as a movement* appears to be based more on philosophical conviction than scientific evidence. Recovery proponents argued that people with serious mental illness *could* recover and described some of the social and interpersonal processes, which appeared to aid or enable recovery (Fisher 1999). These accounts, which emphasize *personal* experience, echo Samuel Smiles' ideas about 'living by example' when he first coined the term 'self-help' in the 19th century (Smiles 1996). How such accounts fit with the objective, unworldly 'evidence' beloved by researchers, politicians and professionals, is not at all clear (Goode 2000). However, mainstream services often assimilate alternative concepts, if only to become more 'consumer-friendly' (Barker & Buchanan-Barker 2003). Where government departments espouse recovery, while promoting ideas of 'compulsory treatment', or 'compliance', conflicts are inevitable (McLean 2003, Neuberger 2005). In part, this derives from the philosophical tension between the *person*-focus of recovery and the *patient* (or illness) focus of psychiatric medicine.

Sally Clay is a mental health advocate, and psychiatric survivor, with a 35-year-long experience of psychiatric 'care and treatment', with no illusions about the ephemeral nature of concepts like 'recovery' or how they might be used to meet political agendas. Almost a decade ago she wrote:

> Recovery is the latest buzz word in the mental health field. For the last year or so, I have been labelled 'recovered' from mental illness. (Clay 1999, p. 26)

When invited to discuss her 'recovery' with psychiatrists in New York State, she observed that the resulting discussions failed to address:

> the nature of mental illness itself. . . . If we are recovered, what is it that we have recovered from? If we are well now and were sick before, what is it that we have recovered to? . . . The psychiatrists in our dialogue become visibly uneasy when the subject arises, and they divert the discussion to less threatening lines of thought. 'Coping mechanisms' are just such a diversion, an attempt to regard the depth of madness as something that can be simply 'coped' with. (Clay 1999, pp. 26–27)

The concept of recovery may well be so deeply personal that it defies definition. However, it has also become an important social construct, which potentially might mean different things to different people.

Clarifying the value base of recovery

Any aspect of health or social care practice has a long developmental history and an even longer timeline of theoretical and philosophical influence. Today's popular 'evidence-based talking cure' – CBT – derives from the work of Beck (1952) and Ellis (1958), from 50 years ago, both of whom traced their philosophical influences centuries back. Notably, they devoted decades to describing and illustrating their discrete therapeutic processes, before beginning to study (research) their potential efficacy.

In this context the Tidal Model of Mental Health Recovery (Barker 1998, 2001, Barker & Buchanan-Barker 2005) is fairly young. Since its launch a decade ago, it has generated almost 100 projects in the UK, Ireland, Canada, Japan, Australia and New Zealand, from outpatient addictions, through acute and forensic units, to the care of older people with dementia (Buchanan-Barker 2004). Beyond the mental health field, practitioners in palliative care are exploring the Tidal Model as an alternative philosophy for death and dying. Here we aim to clarify the distinguishing philosophical assumptions of Tidal theory (Brookes 2006) by explicating the human values of the Tidal Model (the 10 Commitments) which provide a basis for auditing recovery-focused practice.

Although there are numerous models of 'recovery', Tidal was probably the first recovery model to be developed by nurses in practice (Brookes 2006) drawn mainly upon nursing research (Vaughn *et al.* 1995, Barker *et al.* 1999, Barker & Buchanan-Barker 2005). Tidal was originally described as a philosophical approach to the development of *practice-based evidence* in mental health care, inviting practitioners to ask: 'how do we tailor care to fit

94

the specific needs of the person and the person's story and unique lived experience, so that the person might begin, or advance further on the voyage of recovery?' (Barker 2000). In that sense, it focuses on enabling ways of living a *constructive life*, albeit under difficult circumstances.

The person is the key driver within the recovery process, but the practitioner can help unlock the person's potential for recovery.

The Tidal recovery attitude is expressed through six key philosophical assumptions:

1. A belief in the *virtue of curiosity*: the person is the world authority on their life and its problems. By expressing genuine curiosity, the professional can learn something of the 'mystery' of the person's story.
2. Recognition of the *power of resourcefulness*. Rather than focusing on problems, deficits and weaknesses, Tidal seeks to reveal the many resources available to the person – both personal and interpersonal – that might help on the voyage of recovery.
3. Respect for the *person's wishes*, rather than being paternalistic, and suggesting that we might 'know what is best' for the person.
4. Acceptance of the *paradox of crisis* as opportunity. Challenging events in our lives signal that something 'needs to be done'. This might become an opportunity for change in life direction.
5. Acknowledging that all goals must, obviously, *belong to the person*. These will represent the small steps on the road to recovery.
6. The virtue in *pursuing elegance*. Psychiatric care and treatment is often complex and bewildering. The simplest possible means should be sought, which might bring about the changes needed for the person to move forward.

Tidal developed from practice-based research conducted in the mid-1990s in England, Northern Ireland and the Republic of Ireland into what people *needed* nurses *for*, what people and their families *valued* in nursing, and what nurses *did* that appeared to make a difference (Barker *et al.* 1999). Over the past decade, other mental health professionals and consumers have helped further develop the model. Tidal is committed to compassionate caring and genuine 'nursing' – providing the conditions necessary for growth and development – but recognizes that this is not restricted to the professional discipline of nursing (Barker & Buchanan-Barker 2005). In particular, people with experience of psychiatric care, participated in the design, evaluation and development of the original model and, over the past 5 years, other 'user/consumer-consultants', from different countries, have helped refine the philosophical basis of Tidal, by helping clarify its value base.

The 10 Tidal Commitments and the 20 Tidal Competencies

The Tidal Model embraces specific assumptions about people, their experience of problems of human living and their capacity for change (Barker & Buchanan-Barker 2005). From these assumptions we have developed a set of related values, which provide practitioners with a philosophical focus for helping people make their own life changes, rather than trying to manage or control 'patient symptoms' (Barker & Buchanan-Barker 2005). The 10 Commitments remind us that although rules come from the head, reflecting our masculine selves (*animus*), commitment comes from the feminine heart (*anima*). To help judge the extent to which practitioners, in any setting, employ the 10 Commitments in 2002 we were invited to develop the 20 Tidal Competencies, which have since been used to audit recovery practice in several projects, notably in England (Gordon *et al.* 2005) and Scotland (Lafferty & Davidson 2006). Here, we present each Commitment accompanied by the respective Tidal Competencies.

Value the voice

The person's story represents the beginning and endpoint of the helping encounter, embracing not only an account of the person's distress, but also the hope for its resolution. The story is spoken by the voice of experience. We seek to encourage the true voice of the person – rather than enforce the voice of authority. Traditionally, the person's story is 'translated' into a third person, professional account, by different health or social care practitioners. This becomes not so much the person's story (my story) but the professional team's view of that story (history). Tidal seeks to help people develop their unique narrative accounts into a formalized version of 'my story', through ensuring that, all assessments and records of care are written in the person's own 'voice'. If the person is unable, or unwilling, to write in their own hand, then the nurse acts as secretary, recording what has been agreed, conjointly, is important – writing this in the 'voice' of the person.

> Competency 1: The practitioner demonstrates a capacity to *listen actively to the person's story.*
> Competency 2: The practitioner shows commitment to helping the person *record her/his story in her/his own words* as an ongoing part of the process of care.

Respect the language

People develop unique ways of expressing their life stories, representing to others that which only they can know. The language of the story – complete with its unusual grammar and personal metaphors – is the ideal medium for illuminating the way to recovery. We encourage people to speak their own words in their distinctive voice.

Stories written about patients by professionals are, traditionally, framed by the arcane, technical language of psychiatric medicine or psychology. Regrettably, many service users and consumers often come to describe themselves in the colonial language of the professionals who have diagnosed them (Buchanan-Barker & Barker 2002). By valuing – and using – the person's natural language, the Tidal practitioner conveys the simplest, yet most powerful, respect for the person.

> Competency 3: The practitioner helps the person express her/himself at all times in *her/his own language*.
> Competency 4: The practitioner helps the person express her/his *understanding* of particular experiences *through use of personal stories, anecdotes, similes or metaphors*.

Develop genuine curiosity

The person is writing a life story but is in no sense an 'open book'. No one can know another person's experience. Consequently, professionals need to express genuine interest in the story so that they can better understand the storyteller and the story.

Often, professionals are only interested in 'what is wrong' with the person, or in pursuing particular lines of professional inquiry – for example, seeking 'signs and symptoms'. Genuine curiosity reflects an interest in the person and the person's unique experience, as opposed to merely classifying and categorizing features, which might be common to many other 'patients'.

> Competency 5: The practitioner shows interest in the person's story by asking for clarification of particular points, and asking for further examples or details.
> Competency 6: The practitioner shows a willingness to help the person in *unfolding the story at the person's own rate*.

Become the apprentice

The person is the world expert on the life story. Professionals may learn something of the power of that story, but only if they apply themselves diligently and respectfully to the task by becoming apprentice-minded. We need to learn from the person, what needs to be done, rather than leading.

No one can ever know another person's experience. Professionals often talk 'as if' they might even know the person better than they know themselves. As Szasz noted: 'How can you know more about a person after seeing him

for a few hours, a few days or even a few months, than he knows about himself? He has known himself a lot longer! . . . The idea that the person remains entirely in charge of himself is a fundamental premise' (Szasz 2000).

> Competency 7: The practitioner develops a care plan based, *wherever possible*, on the *expressed needs, wants or wishes of the person*.
> Competency 8: The practitioner helps the person identify specific problems of living, and what might need to be done to address them.

Use the available toolkit

The story contains examples of 'what has worked' for the person in the past, or beliefs about 'what might work' for this person in the future. These represent the main tools that need to be used to unlock or build the story of recovery. The professional toolkit – commonly expressed through ideas such as 'evidence-based practice' – describes what has 'worked' for other people. Although potentially useful, this should only be used if the person's available toolkit is found wanting.

> Competency 9: The practitioner helps the person develop awareness of what works for or against them, in relation to specific problems of living.
> Competency 10: The practitioner shows interest in identifying what the person thinks specific people can or might be able to do to help them further in dealing with specific problems of living.

Craft the step beyond

The professional helper and the person work together to construct an appreciation of what needs to be done 'now'. Any 'first step' is a crucial step, revealing the power of change and potentially pointing towards the ultimate goal of recovery. Lao Tzu said that the journey of a thousand miles begins with a single step. We would go further: any journey begins in our *imagination*. It is important to imagine – or envision – moving forward. Crafting the step beyond reminds us of the importance of working with the person in the 'me now': addressing what needs to be done now, to help advance to the next step

> Competency 11: The practitioner helps the person identify what kind of change would represent a step in the direction of resolving or moving away from a specific problem of living.
> Competency 12: The practitioner helps the person identify what needs to happen in the immediate future, to help the person to begin to experience this 'positive step' in the direction of their desired goal.

Give the gift of time

Although time is largely illusory, nothing is more valuable. Time is the midwife of change. Often, professionals complain about not having enough time to work constructively with the person. Although they may not actually 'make' time, through creative attention to their work, professionals often find the time to do 'what needs to be done'. Here, it is the professional's relationship with the concept of time, which is at issue, rather than time itself (Jonsson 2005). Ultimately, any time spent in constructive interpersonal communion, is a gift – for both parties (Derrida 1992).

> Competency 13: The practitioner helps the person develop their awareness that dedicated time is being given to addressing their specific needs.
>
> Competency 14: The practitioner acknowledges the value of the time the person gives to the process of assessment and care delivery.

Reveal personal wisdom

Only the person can know him or herself. The person develops a powerful storehouse of wisdom through living the writing of the life story. Often, people cannot find the words to express fully the magnitude, complexity or ineffability of their experience, invoking powerful personal metaphors, to convey something of their experience (Barker 2002). A key task for the professional is to help the person reveal and come to value that wisdom, so that it might be used to sustain the person throughout the voyage of recovery.

> Competency 15: The practitioner helps the person identify and develop awareness of personal strengths and weaknesses.
>
> Competency 16: The practitioner helps the person develop self-belief, therefore promoting their ability to help themselves.

Know that change is constant

Change is inevitable for change is constant. This is the common story for all people. However, although change is inevitable, growth is optional. Decisions and choices have to be made if growth is to occur. The task of the professional helper is to develop awareness of how change is happening and to support the person in making decisions regarding the course of the recovery voyage. In particular, we help the person to steer out of danger and distress keeping on the course of reclamation and recovery.

> Competency 17: The practitioner helps the person develop awareness of the subtlest of changes – in thoughts, feelings or action.

> Competency 18: The practitioner helps the person develop awareness of how they, others or events have influenced these changes.

Be transparent

If the person and the professional helper are to become a team then each must put down their 'weapons'. In the story-writing process the professional's pen can all too often become a weapon: writing a story that risks inhibiting, restricting and delimiting the person's life choices. Professionals are in a privileged position and should model confidence by being transparent at all times, helping the person understand exactly what is being done and why. By retaining the use of the person's own language, and by completing all assessments and care plan records together (*in vivo*), the collaborative nature of the professional-person relationship becomes even more transparent.

> Competency 19: The practitioner aims to ensure that the person is aware, at all times, of the purpose of all processes of care.
>
> Competency 20: The practitioner ensures that the person is provided with copies of all assessment and care planning documents for their own reference.

Reclamation: in our own voice

Many psychotherapeutic models develop a special language that is awkward to use and patronizing to the uninitiated. In pursuit of the 10 Commitments, the Tidal Model eschews the use of jargon, valuing instead ordinary language, especially the everyday vernacular of the person, family or friends.

Traditionally, psychiatry has devalued the person's voice, by promoting diagnostic jargon (Kirk & Kutchins 1997). Given the power imbalance between professionals and their 'patients', many people end up describing their own experience in the technical language of psychiatry and psychology, as if their own story was inadequate (Furedi 2003), suggesting that the psychiatric narrative has colonized all our lives (Barker 2003). The Tidal Model asserts that 'lived experience' is understood best through use of natural language – using the metaphors and grammar that fit most easily with the way people talk naturally about their experiences. Consequently, Tidal focuses on helping people *reclaim* the story of their distress and, ultimately, their whole lives.

In human affairs, *reclamation* means the efforts necessary to *seek the return of one's property*. In the psychiatric context, reclamation means the return of one's personhood and its accompanying story. The Latin root (*reclamare*) means 'to cry out against'. Arguably, the emergence of the 'user/consumer' voice is one of the most powerful developments in mental health, worldwide, in the past 30 years. Such groups are reclaiming their story and personhood, through the act of 'speaking up' or 'speaking out', which is central to the act of reclamation within Tidal.

In Tidal terms, reclamation refers to the pursuit of a productive use of something that was lost or considered worthless. Typically, land submerged by the sea, is reclaimed for use as part of the mainland. In the same sense, that part of the person's life, which was submerged – and invalidated – by the effects of mental distress, is reclaimed to become part of the whole person. Like land reclamation, the reclaimed experience of mental distress is beyond value. Once brought (metaphorically) to the surface, it becomes (again) part of the person's *whole* lived experience.

The first Tidal step in facilitating reclamation, is to write all the main assessment 'stories' and subsequent descriptions of necessary care, in the person's own voice, rather than translate these into professional note-taking. This focus on 'my story' appeals to users and consumers, illustrating the practitioner's desire to work actively *with* the person, co-creating the story of the care. The psychiatric survivor and consumer advocate Sally Clay wrote:

> The Tidal Model makes authentic communication and the telling of our stories the whole focus of therapy. Thus the treatment of mental illness becomes a personal and human endeavour, in contrast to the impersonality and objectivity of treatment within the conventional mental health system. One feels that one is working with friends and colleagues rather than some kind of 'higher-up' providers. One becomes connected with oneself and others rather than isolated in a dysfunctional world of one's own. (Clay 2005)

Focusing on the person

The person's story describes not only the circumstances that led to the person's need for help, but holds the promise of what needs to be done to begin the process of recovery. Although influenced by different schools of psychotherapy, Tidal emphasizes ordinary conversation, which has a power that stands apart from that found in the therapeutic discourse (Zeldin 2000) and the 'narrative' of everyday 'story-telling' (Brunner 1990). As Fisher noted, human beings are *homo narrans*: natural story-tellers, constantly updated by the process of telling stories (Fisher 1987).

Commonly people with experience of Tidal say that 'it doesn't feel as if I am being treated; it just feels as if someone is listening to me' and want to tell a story about what it *was* like. A woman with a long history of psychi-

atric hospitalization recognized how this 'ordinary' experience could become 'extraordinary':

> Tidal has made room for my voice. I'm not just another patient who is mentally ill. I am a person with goals and dreams and a life worth living. I get to discover and learn and make changes. Now I can think, decide and act for myself. I don't need someone else to save me anymore, because I have been given the opportunity to save myself.

To emphasize the centrality of practical action within Tidal, we borrowed the term – 'doing what needs to be done' – from the work of Shoma Morita, the Japanese psychiatrist who developed a form of 'constructive living' therapy, in the 1920s (Morita *et al.* 1998). Working within the 'me-now' of the story, the conjoint work of the professional and the person in care involves negotiating what needs to be done, which might begin to address or respond to a current problem of human living.

Problematizing Tidal

Within a decade the Tidal Model has progressed from a local solution for mental health nursing to an international model of mental health recovery, recognized and practised in several different countries. Those developing Tidal-focused services appear to derive something personally or professionally satisfying from the Tidal Model itself, many noting that its inherent values remind them why they 'came into the field in the first place'. They often complain that they had no ambition to 'carry out observation protocols', 'implement control and restraint procedures', 'attend endless meetings' or 'shuffle paper'. Instead, they took up caring to help people address, manage or otherwise 'recover' from whatever problems have overtaken them in their lives. By embracing Tidal, they appear to be reclaiming their original caring vocation.

As Tidal practice has evolved over the past decade, we felt an increasing obligation to clarify its philosophical – or value – base. We have reflected greatly on what we value – as persons and professionals – and also have learned much, over several decades, about what other people value. In helping others introduce Tidal into their practice we have tried to clarify what the Tidal Model 'stands for' and how it might be pursued. In so doing we have favoured the kind of everyday language that characterizes the model itself. No philosophical system will satisfy everyone, but the values embraced by the 10 Commitments appear to have a broad constituency, across nations, societies and cultures.

However, for some, 'the only way to genuinely test . . . whether (the Tidal model) . . . makes a real difference' would be through 'a carefully planned and fairly large-scale clinical trial' (Gamble & Wellman 2002, p. 743). We are not averse to others undertaking such 'scientific' studies, but this is not one of our priorities. The major social movements, which have blossomed in our lifetime – feminism, black power and gay rights – did not reshape social attitudes and behaviour through the use of the randomized control trial, or any other 'scientific' method. Instead, they employed the ancient philosophical method of rhetoric. The 'success' of recovery movements, like AA, and the continued rise of the user/consumer 'movement' worldwide is also based on rhetoric and organized social action, seeking to communicate the beliefs and values of the group.

Gordon *et al.* (2005) argued that ample evidence existed for the impact of Tidal on practice. However, we would still urge caution. People often ask: 'does the Tidal model work?' We wonder what, exactly, they mean. All theories are merely 'suppositions or systems of ideas, explaining something' (Oxford English Dictionary). Models represent highly simplified descriptions of the 'thing' itself – in this case the process for enabling recovery. Therefore, we find it more appropriate to ask: '*in what way*, does the Tidal Model "work" *for whom* and *to what particular purpose?*' At least in human affairs, ultimately, no 'model' and its supporting 'theory' can be shown to 'work'. Only the individual practitioners and the organizational systems which support practice, might be viewed as 'working'. However, we need also to ask: 'working to what particular purpose?'

Here we have attempted to clarify the Tidal 'purpose', by re-framing its original philosophical assumptions and describing how, through ongoing collegiate dialogue we developed the 10 Commitments, which attempt to clarify the Tidal values and, the 20 Tidal Competencies, which might contribute to the study of recovery practice. We recognize that Tidal – as a developing theory of the recovery process and model for its practice – distils many thousands of voices of people who helped us to develop the model and who are the real 'guardians' of Tidal theory and practice. Many nurses take this guardianship role very seriously since it appears to extend their passion for reclaiming the practice of caring in its myriad forms. It seems appropriate to end with the voices and the values of Brookes *et al.* (2006):

> We valued the nurses' stories. Now we collect stories that tell of their successes and their frustrations practising Tidal . . . We continue to strive to transform nursing practice and contribute to person's journeys of recovery. There is ebb and flow in the process of implementing the model. Sometimes we faced setbacks, or at times we felt becalmed. There would also be times of success, great celebration and breakthroughs. We are sustained by our passion for excellence in psychiatric and mental health nursing and care – and by the stories. (pp. 462–463)

References

Anthony W.A. (1993) Recovery from mental illness: the guiding vision of the mental health system in the 1990s. *Psychosocial Rehabilitation Journal* 16, 11–23.

Barham P. & Hayward R. (1991) *From the Mental Patient to the Person*. Routledge, London.

Barker P. (1998) It's time to turn the tide. *Nursing Times* 18, 70–72.

Barker P. (2000) The Tidal Model: the lived experience in person-centred mental health care. *Nursing Philosophy* 2, 213–223.

Barker P. (2001) The Tidal Model: a radical approach to person-centred care. *Perspectives in Psychiatric Care* 37, 79–87.

Barker P. (2002) The Tidal Model: the healing potential of metaphor within the patient's narrative. *Journal of Psychosocial Nursing and Mental Health Services* 40, 42–50.

Barker P. (2003) The Tidal Model: psychiatric colonization, recovery and the paradigm shift in mental health care. *International Journal of Mental Health Nursing* 12, 96–102.

Barker P. & Buchanan-Barker P. (2003) Death by assimilation. *Asylum* 13, 10–13.

Barker P. & Buchanan-Barker P. (2005) *The Tidal Model: A Guide for Mental Health Professionals*. Brunner-Routledge, London.

Barker P., Jackson S. & Stevenson C. (1999) The need for psychiatric nursing: towards a multidimensional theory of caring. *Nursing Inquiry* 6, 103–111.

Beck A.T. (1952) Successful outpatient psychotherapy of a chronic schizophrenic with a delusion based on borrowed guilt. *Psychiatry* 15, 305–312.

Brookes N. (2006) Phil Barker: the Tidal Model of mental health recovery, Chapter 32. In: *Nursing Theorists and Their Work*, 6th edn (eds Tomey, A.M. & Alligood, M.R.), pp. 696–725. Mosby, New York.

Brookes N., Murata L. & Tansey M. (2006) Guiding practice development using the Tidal Commitments. *Journal of Psychiatric and Mental Health Nursing* 13, 460–463.

Brunner J. (1990) *Acts of Meaning*. Harvard University Press, Cambridge, MA.

Buchanan-Barker P. (2004) Uncommon sense: the Tidal Model of mental health recovery. *Mental Health Nursing* 23, 12–15.

Buchanan-Barker P. & Barker P. (2002) Lunatic language. *Openmind* 115, 23.

Chamberlin J. (1978) *On Our Own: Patient Controlled Alternatives to the Mental Health System*. Hawthorn Books, New York.

Clay S. (1999) Madness and reality, Chapter 2. In: *From the Ashes of Experience: Reflections on Madness, Survival and Growth* (eds Barker, P., Campbell, P. & Davidson, B.), pp. 16–36. Whurr, London.

Clay S. (2005) *A View from the USA. Foreword in P Barker and P Buchanan-Barker the Tidal Model: A Guide for Mental Health Professionals*. Brunner-Routledge, London.

Davidson L. & Strauss J. (1992) Sense of self in recovery from severe mental illness. *British Journal of Medical Psychology* 65, 131–145.

Deegan P. (1988) Recovery: the experience of rehabilitation. *Psychosocial Rehabilitation Journal* 11, 11.

Deegan P. (1993) Recovering our sense of value after being labelled. *Journal of Psychosocial Nursing* 31, 7–11.

Department of Health (2006) *From Values to Action: The Chief Nursing Officer's Review of Mental Health Nursing*. Department of Health, London.

Derrida J. (1992) *Given Time: I, Counterfeit Money* (translated by Kamuf Peggy). Chicago University Press, Chicago.

Ellis A. (1958) Rational psychotherapy. *Journal of General Psychology* 59, 35–49.

Fisher D. (1999) Hope, humanity and voice in recovery from mental illness. In: *From the Ashes of Experience: Reflections on Madness Survival and Growth* (eds Barker, P., Campbell, P. & Davidson, B.), pp. 127–133. Whurr, London.

Fisher W.R. (1987) *Human Communication as Narration: Toward a Philosophy of Reason, Value, and Action.* University of South Carolina Press, Columbia, SC.

Fitzpatrick C. (2002) A new word in serious mental illness: recovery. *Behavioural Healthcare Tomorrow* August, 2–5.

Frank D. (1996) *The Annotated AA Handbook: A Companion to the Big Book Fort Lee.* Barricade Books, Fort Lee, NJ.

Furedi F. (2003) *Therapy Culture: Cultivating Vulnerability in an Uncertain Age.* Routledge, London.

Gamble C. & Wellman N. (2002) Judgement impossible. *Journal of Psychiatric and Mental Health Nursing* 9, 741–743.

Goode C.J. (2000) What constitutes the 'evidence' in evidence-based practice? *Applied Nursing Research* 13, 222–225.

Gordon W., Morton T. & Brooks G. (2005) Launching the Tidal Model: evaluating the evidence. *Journal of Psychiatric and Mental Health Nursing* 12, 703–712.

Harding C.M., Brooks G.W., Ashikaga T., *et al.* (1987) The Vermont longitudinal study of persons with severe mental illness: 1 methodology, study sample and overall status 32 years later. *American Journal of Psychiatry* 144, 718–726.

Harrison G., Hopper K., Craig T., *et al.* (2001) Recovery from psychotic illness: a 15 and 25 year follow-up study. *British Journal of Psychiatry* 178, 506–517

Jonsson B. (2005) *Ten Thoughts about Time.* Constable and Robinson, London.

Kirk S.A. & Kutchins H. (1997) *Making Us Crazy: The Psychiatric Bible and the Creation of Mental Disorders.* Free Press, New York.

Lafferty S. & Davidson R. (2006) Person-centred care in practice an account of the experience of implementing the Tidal Model in an adult acute admission ward in Glasgow. *Mental Health Today* March, 31–34.

McLean A. (2003) Recovering consumers and a broken mental health system in the United States: ongoing challenges for consumers/survivors and the new freedom commission on mental health. *International Journal of Psychosocial Rehabilitation* 8, 47–68.

Manos E. (1993) Speaking out. *Psychosocial Rehabilitation Journal* 16, 117–120.

Mental Health Commission (2006) *A Vision for a Recovery Model in Irish Mental Health Services: Discussion Paper.* MHC, Dublin.

Mental Health Commission New Zealand (2001) *Recovery Competencies for New Zealand Mental Health Workers.* MHC, Wellington, NZ.

Morita M., Kondo A., Levine P., *et al.* (1998) *Morita Therapy and the True Nature of Anxiety-Based Disorders (Shinkeishitsu).* University of New York, Princeton, NJ.

Neuberger J. (2005) *The Moral State We're in.* Harper/Collins, London.

O'Hagan M. (2004) Recovery in New Zealand: lessons for Australia. *Australian E-Journal for the Advancement of Mental Health* 3, 1–3.

Repper J. (2000) Adjusting the focus of mental health nursing: incorporating service users' experiences of recovery. *Journal of Mental Health* 9, 575–587.

Scottish Executive (2006) *Rights, Relationships and Recovery – The Report of the National Review of Mental Health Nursing in Scotland.* Scottish Executive, Edinburgh.

Smiles S. (1996) [Orig 1859] *Self Help – with Illustrations of Conduct and Perseverance.* IEA Health and Welfare Unit, London.

Szasz T.S. (2000) Curing the therapeutic state: Thomas Szasz on the medicalisation of American life. Interviewed by Jacob Sullum. *Reason* 20 July 2000, pp. 27–34.

Vaughn K., Webster D., Orahood S., *et al.* (1995) Brief inpatient psychiatric treatment: finding solutions. *Issues in Mental Health Nursing* 16, 519–531.

Zeldin T. (2000) *Conversation: How Talk Can Change Our Lives.* Paulist Press, Mahwah, NJ.

16

Schizophrenia Spectrum and Other Psychotic Disorders

Edward A. Herzog, Elizabeth M. Varcarolis
Adapted by Wilma Schroeder

KEY TERMS AND CONCEPTS

abnormal motor behaviour, 286
acute dystonia, 304
affective symptoms, 291
akathisia, 304
anosognosia, 296
anticholinergic-induced delirium, 306
associative looseness, 293
boundary impairment, 293
circumstantiality, 293
cognitive symptoms, 291
command hallucinations, 294
concrete thinking, 292
delusions, 286
depersonalization, 293
derealization, 293
disorganized thinking, 286
echolalia, 293

echopraxia, 294
extrapyramidal side effects (EPS), 304
hallucinations, 286
ideas of reference, 309
illusions, 293
negative symptoms, 286
neologisms, 293
neuroleptic malignant syndrome (NMS), 304
paranoia, 306
positive symptoms, 291
pseudoparkinsonism, 304
reality testing, 292
recovery model, 297
stereotyped behaviours, 294
tangentiality, 293
tardive dyskinesia (TD or TDK), 304
word salad, 293

OBJECTIVES

1. Describe the progression of symptoms, focus of care, and intervention needs for the prepsychotic through maintenance phases of schizophrenia.
2. Discuss at least three of the neurobiological–anatomical–genetic findings that indicate that schizophrenia is a brain disorder.
3. Differentiate among the positive and negative symptoms of schizophrenia in terms of psychopharmacological treatment and effect on quality of life.
4. Discuss the concept of recovery for people living with schizophrenia.
5. Discuss how to deal with common reactions the nurse may experience while working with a person with schizophrenia.

6. Develop teaching plans for people taking conventional antipsychotic drugs (e.g., haloperidol [Haldol]) and atypical antipsychotic drugs (e.g., risperidone [Risperdal]).
7. Compare and contrast the conventional antipsychotic medications with atypical antipsychotics.
8. Identify nonpharmacological interventions that may be used to address symptoms of schizophrenia.
9. Create a nursing care plan that incorporates evidence-informed interventions for key areas of dysfunction in schizophrenia, including hallucinations, delusions, paranoia, cognitive disorganization, anosognosia, and impaired self-care.
10. Role-play intervening with a person who is hallucinating, delusional, and exhibiting disorganized thinking.

evolve WEBSITE

Visit the Evolve website for Flashcards, Case Studies, and additional testing resources related to the content in this chapter: http://evolve.elsevier.com/Canada/Varcarolis/psychiatric/   Pre-Test interactive review

Schizophrenia spectrum and other psychotic disorders are potentially devastating brain disorders that affect a person's thinking, language, emotions, social behaviour, and ability to perceive reality accurately. The most severe disorder in this category is schizophrenia, which is the major focus of this chapter. It affects 1 in every 100 people (over 300 000 people in Canada) and is among the most disruptive and disabling of mental disorders. Unfortunately, people with this disorder are often misunderstood and stigmatized not only by the general population but even by the medical community. Negative attitudes toward people can interfere with recovery and impair their quality of life (Crowe, Deane, Oades, et al., 2006). For example, many believe that people with schizophrenia are likely to be violent, but the overall rate of violence among those with schizophrenia is no greater than that of the general public. In fact, stranger homicide by persons with psychosis is extremely rare—1 incident per 14.3 million people per year (Nielssen, Bourget, Laajasalo, et al., 2009).

- The following How a Nurse Helped Me story demonstrates the four elements of the LEAP approach (Amador, 2000), which is based on the belief that trusting relationships are key to healing partnerships:
- Listen—Both nurses listened with compassion and genuineness.
- Empathize—It is clear that both nurses were able to convey that they understood what Tammy was feeling.

HOW A NURSE HELPED ME

They Helped Me to Believe in Myself

I live with schizoaffective disorder. I am 30 now, and I was diagnosed with a mental illness when I was 15. I experience both the psychotic symptoms often present in schizophrenia and a mood component often in the form of rapid cycling. For the first five to ten years of coping with my mental illness, the hospital was like a revolving door for me. It took me numerous years to find the right medications.

Through the dedication of nurses like Cheryl and Rhonda, I have been able to overcome my intense symptoms by finding balance in my chaotic moods and a decrease in my delusional symptoms and paranoia. Cheryl is a nurse who goes out of her way to be there for her patients. She uses compassion and humour to communicate with us. I have worked with Cheryl for ten years. From the very beginning, I felt a close connection with her and have felt privileged to work with her. She has had such a positive impact on my life. She believed in me even when I didn't believe in myself. She treats us each with the utmost respect. She has a gentle spirit, and she brings cheerfulness to the ward. If you are depressed or not feeling well, she is most often able to cheer you up. (That is no matter how bad you feel or how painful your day has been.) She has a fun-loving nature, and she is loved by all. Cheryl relates well to everyone. She is full of energy and enthusiasm. She truly cares. She is genuine, and even if she herself is struggling that day, she is still full of kindness and empathy. Her dedication to her patients never wavers. Cheryl is definitely one of a kind.

Rhonda is one of the most dedicated and compassionate nurses I have ever met. She has had a tremendous influence on my life. She often works long hours to offer full support to her patients. Sometimes I have called her past 6:00 in the evening thinking I would leave a message, yet to my surprise, she is still there, and she makes time to answer my call. She is very efficient and does her job extremely well. She treats us all equally with dignity and respect. I have never felt like I have been looked down upon or judged. She has an open mind and her compassion has supported me through many rough and painful times. Rhonda has always believed in me, and this has helped me on my road to recovery. I look forward to appointments with Rhonda because she always allows me to see life situations from a positive perspective, and she provides me with ongoing encouragement. Rhonda is an awesome nurse.

Rhonda and Cheryl are an asset to the health care system. If all psychiatric nurses were like them, the mental health system would be amazing.

Source: Story written by Tammy L. and reproduced with her permission.

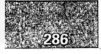

- Agree—Both nurses believed in Tammy and supported her in her goals, never looking down on her or judging her but helping her on her own road to recovery.
- Partner—Clearly, both nurses respected Tammy and worked with her as partners.

LEAP is described as a technique; however, inherent in that description is the risk of seeing it only technically. The LEAP approach must be underpinned by genuineness and caring. Cheryl and Rhonda invited Tammy into a trusting and therapeutic relationship. They did not apply these components as "techniques"; instead, it appears that the LEAP principles flowed naturally out of genuine caring. Tammy's story demonstrates how empowering and healing it is to experience being truly listened to, empathized with, and collaborated with.

CLINICAL PICTURE

Adding to observations made by Emil Kraepelin (1856–1926), Eugen Bleuler (1857–1939) coined the term *schizophrenia*. He first proposed that schizophrenia was not one illness but a heterogeneous group of illnesses with different characteristics and clinical courses. Five key features are associated with psychotic disorders:

1. Delusions: Alterations in *thought content* (what a person thinks about). Delusions are false fixed beliefs that cannot be corrected by reasoning or evidence to the contrary. "Unusual" beliefs maintained by one's culture or subculture are not delusions..
2. Hallucinations: Perception of a sensory experience for which no external stimulus exists (e.g., hearing a voice when no one is speaking).
3. Disorganized thinking: The loosening of associations, manifested as jumbled and illogical speech and impaired reasoning.
4. Abnormal motor behaviour: Alterations in behaviour, including bizarre and agitated behaviours (e.g., stilted, rigid demeanour or eccentric dress, grooming, and rituals). Grossly disorganized behaviours may include mutism, stupor, or catatonic excitement.
5. Negative symptoms: The absence of something that should be present but is not—for example, the ability to make decisions or to follow through on a plan. Negative symptoms contribute to poor social functioning and social withdrawal.

VIGNETTE

Samuel, a 25-year-old man soon to be discharged from the hospital, constantly tells the social worker he wants his own apartment. When Samuel is told that an apartment has been found for him, he asks, "But who will take care of me?" Samuel is acting out his ambivalence between his desire to be independent and his desire to be taken care of.

Clinicians in Canada use the criteria of the *Diagnostic and Statistical Manual of Mental Disorders*, fifth edition, for the diagnosis of schizophrenia spectrum and other psychotic disorders.

All those diagnosed with schizophrenia exhibit at least one psychotic symptom, such as delusions, hallucinations, or disorganized thinking, speech, or behaviour. The person experiences extreme difficulty with or an inability to function in family, social, or occupational realms and frequently neglects basic needs such as nutrition or hygiene. Over a period of six months, there may be times when the psychotic symptoms are absent, and in their place, the person may experience apathy or depression.

Other psychotic disorders (e.g., schizophreniform and schizoaffective disorders) are described in Box 16-1.

BOX 16-1   PSYCHOTIC DISORDERS OTHER THAN SCHIZOPHRENIA

Schizophreniform Disorder
The features of schizophreniform disorder are similar to schizophrenia, but the total duration of the illness is less than six months. This disorder may or may not develop into schizophrenia; people who do not develop schizophrenia have a good prognosis.

Brief Psychotic Disorder
This disorder involves a sudden onset of psychosis or grossly disorganized or catatonic behaviour lasting less than one month. It is often precipitated by extreme stressors and is followed by a return to premorbid functioning.

Schizoaffective Disorder
Schizoaffective disorder is characterized by a major depressive, manic, or mixed-mood episode presenting concurrently with symptoms of schizophrenia. The symptoms are not due to any substance use or to a medical condition.

Delusional Disorder
Delusional disorder is characterized by nonbizarre delusions (i.e., situations that could occur in real life, such as being followed, being deceived by a spouse, or having a disease). The person's ability to function is not markedly impaired, nor is behaviour otherwise odd or psychotic. A related disorder, Capgras syndrome, involves a delusion about a significant other (e.g., family member or pet) being replaced by an imposter; this disorder may be a result of psychiatric or organic brain disease (Denes, 2007).

Substance- or Medication-Induced Psychotic Disorder
Psychosis may be induced by substances such as drugs of abuse, alcohol, medications, or toxins (Mauri, Volonteri, De Gaspari, et al., 2006).

Psychosis or Catatonia Associated With Another Medical Condition or Another Mental Disorder
Psychoses may also be caused by a medical condition (delirium, neurological or metabolic conditions, hepatic or renal diseases, and many others). Medical conditions and substance abuse must always be ruled out before a diagnosis of schizophrenia or other psychotic disorder can be made.

Sources: Denes, G. (2007). Capgras delusion. *Neurological Sciences, 28,* 163–164. doi:10.1007/s10072-007-0813-1; Mauri, M.C., Volonteri, L.S., De Gaspari, I.F., et al. (2006). Substance abuse in first-episode schizophrenic patients: A retrospective study. *Clinical Practice and Epidemiology in Mental Health, 2,* 1–8. doi:10.1186/1745-0179-2-4.

EPIDEMIOLOGY

The lifetime prevalence of schizophrenia is 1% worldwide, with no differences related to race, social status, or culture. It is more common in males (1.4:1) and among persons growing up in urban areas (Tandon, Keshavan, & Nasrallah, 2008). Schizophrenia usually develops during the late teens and early twenties, although onset before the age of 10 has been reported (Masi, Mucci, & Pari, 2006). Childhood schizophrenia, although rare, does exist, occurring in 1 out of 40,000 children. Early onset (18 to 25 years) occurs more often in males and is associated with poor functioning before onset, more structural brain abnormality, and increased levels of apathy. Individuals with a later onset (25 to 35 years) are more likely to be female, have less structural brain abnormality, and have better outcomes.

CO-MORBIDITY

Substance abuse disorders occur in nearly 50% of persons with schizophrenia (Green, Noordsy, Brunette, et al., 2008). When substance abuse occurs in people with schizophrenia, it is associated with treatment nonadherence, relapse, incarceration, homelessness, violence, suicide, and a poorer prognosis (Mauri, Volonteri, De Gaspari, et al., 2006). Nicotine dependence rates in schizophrenia range from 70% to 90% and contribute to an increased incidence of cardiovascular and respiratory disorders (Green, Noordsy, Brunette, et al., 2008).

Anxiety, depression, and suicide co-occur frequently in schizophrenia. Anxiety may be a response to symptoms (e.g., hallucinations) or circumstances (e.g., isolation, overstimulation) and may worsen schizophrenia symptoms and prognosis (Mauri, Moliterno, Rossattini, et al., 2008). Almost half of all persons with schizophrenia attempt suicide at some point in their lives, and approximately 10% succeed (Hayashi, Ishida, Miyashita, et al., 2005). Both depression and suicide attempts can occur at any point in the illness (Osborn, Levy, Nazareth, et al., 2008).

Polydipsia can lead to fatal water intoxication (indicated by hyponatremia, confusion, worsening psychotic symptoms, and ultimately coma). It is characterized by a seemingly insatiable thirst that results in a dangerous intake of water. It occurs in 7% of inpatients with schizophrenia (Gonzalez & Perez, 2008). Factors that contribute to excess water intake include taking antipsychotic medication (causes dry mouth), compulsive behaviour, and neuroendocrine abnormalities (Bralet, Ton, & Falissard, 2007).

Physical illnesses are more common among people with schizophrenia than in the general population. Even after adjusting for demographics and socioeconomic status, the death rate for people with mental illness is close to 70% higher than for the general population, and this risk of premature death is even greater for people with schizophrenia (Kisely, 2010). On average, persons with schizophrenia die 28 years prematurely due to disorders such as hypertension (22%), obesity (24%), cardiovascular disease (21%), diabetes (12%), chronic obstructive pulmonary disease (COPD) (10%), and trauma (6%) (Miller, Paschall, & Svendsen, 2007). Disturbingly, this disparity in risk has actually increased in the past 20 to 30 years (Kisely, 2010).

People with psychotic disorders may be at greater risk due to apathy, poor health habits, medications (see the discussion of metabolic syndrome later in this chapter), or failure to recognize signs of illness. Communication problems or difficulties with informed consent may also be factors (Kisely, 2010). Owing to poverty, stigma, or stereotyping (e.g., emergency department personnel assuming that because a person has a psychotic disorder, his chest pain is imaginary), they may not receive adequate health care. Despite having more contact with family physicians than the general population, persons with psychiatric disorders are less likely to be assessed and treated for conditions such as hypertension or to receive preventive care such as smoking cessation (Kisely, 2010).

Incentives and barriers to engaging people with severe mental illness in lifestyle interventions have not been extensively studied, though there is some evidence that these interventions can be effective (Roberts & Bailey, 2011). Barriers that are reported in the literature include illness symptoms, treatment effects, lack of support, and negative staff attitudes; incentives include peer and staff support, staff participation, reduction of symptoms, knowledge, and personal attributes (Roberts & Bailey, 2011).

ETIOLOGY

Schizophrenia typically manifests in late adolescence or early adulthood. It becomes chronic or recurrent in at least 80% of those who develop it; on average, everyone has about a 0.7% chance of developing schizophrenia (Tandon, Keshavan, & Nasrallah, 2008).

Schizophrenia is a complicated disorder. In fact, what we call "schizophrenia" actually may be a group of disorders with common but varying features and multiple, overlapping etiologies. What is known is that brain chemistry, structure, and activity are different in a person with schizophrenia from those in a person who does not have the disorder.

The scientific consensus is that schizophrenia occurs when multiple inherited gene abnormalities combine with nongenetic factors (e.g., viral infections, birth injuries, prenatal malnutrition), altering the structures of the brain, affecting the brain's neurotransmitter systems, injuring the brain directly, or doing all three (Tandon, Keshavan, & Nasrallah, 2008). This effect is called the *diathesis–stress model of schizophrenia* (Walker & Tessner, 2008).

Biological Factors
Genetic Factors
Schizophrenia and schizophrenia-like symptoms, such as eccentric thinking, are more prevalent in relatives of individuals with schizophrenia. According to Smoller, Finn, and Gardner-Schuster (2008):

- Compared to the usual 1% risk in the population, having a first-degree relative with schizophrenia increases the risk to 10%.

- There is variability of expression of schizophrenia, depending upon environmental factors; schizoaffective disorder and cluster-A personality disorders are more common in relatives of people with schizophrenia.
- Concordance rates in twins (how often one twin will have the disorder when the other one has it) is about 50% for identical twins and about 15% for fraternal twins.

Evidence suggests that multiple genes on different chromosomes interact with each other in complex ways to create vulnerability to schizophrenia. Genes potentially linked to schizophrenia continue to be identified, suggesting a high degree of complexity (Tandon, Keshavan, & Nasrallah, 2008).

Neurobiological Factors

Dopamine theory. The dopamine theory of schizophrenia is derived from the study of the action of the first antipsychotic drugs, collectively known as *conventional* (or *first-generation*) *antipsychotics* (e.g., haloperidol [Haldol] and chlorpromazine [Largactil]). These drugs block the activity of dopamine-2 (D_2) receptors in the brain, limiting the activity of dopamine and reducing some of the symptoms of schizophrenia. However, because the dopamine-blocking agents do not alleviate all the symptoms of schizophrenia, it is recognized that there are other neurochemicals involved in generating the symptoms of schizophrenia. Amphetamines, cocaine, methylphenidate (Ritalin), and levodopa increase the activity of dopamine in the brain and, in biologically susceptible people, may precipitate schizophrenia's onset. If schizophrenia is already present, they may also exacerbate its symptoms.

Other neurochemical hypotheses. A newer class of drugs, collectively known as *atypical* (or *second-generation*) *antipsychotics*, block serotonin as well as dopamine, which suggests that serotonin may play a role in schizophrenia as well. A better understanding of how atypical agents modulate the expression and targeting of 5-hydroxytryptamine 2A (5-HT2A) and its receptors would likely lead to a better understanding of schizophrenia.

Researchers have long been aware that phenylcyclohexyl piperidine (PCP) induces a state closely resembling schizophrenia. This observation led to interest in the N-methyl-D-aspartate (NMDA) receptor complex and the possible role of glutamate in the pathophysiology of schizophrenia. Glutamate is a crucial neurotransmitter during periods of neuromaturation; abnormal maturation of the central nervous system (CNS) is considered to be a central contributing factor in schizophrenia (Goff, 2005).

Brain Structure Abnormalities

Disruptions in communication pathways in the brain are thought to be severe in schizophrenia. Therefore, it is conceivable that structural abnormalities cause disruption of the brain's functioning. Using brain imaging techniques—computed tomography (CT), magnetic resonance imaging (MRI), and positron emission tomography (PET)—researchers have provided substantial evidence that some people with schizophrenia have structural brain abnormalities (Broome, Woolley, Tabraham, et al., 2005), including:

- Enlarged lateral cerebral ventricles, a dilated third ventricle, ventricular asymmetry, or a combination of these
- Reduced cortical, frontal lobe, hippocampal, or cerebellar volumes
- Increased size of the sulci (fissures) on the surface of the brain

In addition, MRI and CT scans demonstrate lower brain volume and more cerebrospinal fluid in people with schizophrenia. PET scans also show a lowered rate of blood flow and glucose metabolism in the frontal lobes, which govern planning, abstract thinking, social adjustment, and decision making, all of which are affected in schizophrenia. (Figure 4-5 in Chapter 4 shows a PET scan demonstrating reduced brain activity in the frontal lobe of a person with schizophrenia.) Such structural changes may worsen as the disorder continues. Postmortem studies on individuals with schizophrenia reveal a reduced volume of grey matter in the brain, especially in the temporal and frontal lobes; those with the most tissue loss had the worst symptoms (e.g., hallucinations, delusions, bizarre thoughts, depression).

Psychological and Environmental Factors

A number of stressors, particularly those occurring during vulnerable periods of neurological development, are believed to combine with genetic vulnerabilities to produce schizophrenia. Reducing such stressors is believed to have the potential to reduce the severity of the disorder or even prevent it (Compton, 2004).

Prenatal Stressors

A history of pregnancy or birth complications is associated with an increased risk for schizophrenia. Prenatal risk factors include viral infection, poor nutrition, hypoxia, and exposure to toxins. Psychological trauma to the mother during pregnancy (e.g., the death of a relative) can also contribute to the development of schizophrenia (Khashan, Abel, McNamee, et al., 2008). Other risk factors include a father older than 35 at the child's conception and being born during late winter or early spring (Tandon, Keshavan, & Nasrallah, 2008).

Psychological Stressors

Although there is no evidence that stress alone causes schizophrenia, stress increases cortisol levels, impeding hypothalamic development and causing other changes that may precipitate the illness in vulnerable individuals. Schizophrenia often manifests at times of developmental and family stress, such as beginning college or moving away from one's family. Social, psychological, and physical stressors may play a significant role in both the severity and course of the disorder and the person's quality of life. Other factors increasing the risk of schizophrenia include cannabis use and exposure to psychological trauma or social defeat (Tandon, Keshavan, & Nasrallah, 2008).

Environmental Stressors

Environmental factors are also believed to contribute to the development of schizophrenia in vulnerable people. These include exposure to social adversity (e.g., living in chronic

CULTURAL CONSIDERATIONS

The Stigma of Schizophrenia

Mrs. Chou, a 25-year-old woman, left China for North America six months ago to join her husband. In China, she lived with her parents and had learned English. She was shy and looked to her parents, and later to her husband, for guidance and support. Shortly after arrival in her new country, her mother developed pneumonia and died. Mrs. Chou later told her husband that if she had stayed in China, her mother would not have become ill and that evil would now come to their 1-year-old child because Mrs. Chou had not taken proper care of her mother.

Mrs. Chou became increasingly lethargic, staring into space and mumbling to herself. When Mr. Chou asked who she was talking to, she answered, "My mother."

Mr. Chou realized that something was terribly wrong with his wife, yet he was reluctant to ask either relatives or professionals for assistance since mental illness is strongly stigmatized in the Chinese culture. In fact, mental illness may be believed to be a punishment for personal failings.

Mrs. Chou was finally admitted to a psychiatric unit when Mr. Chou noticed she had quit eating and taking care of herself and was certainly unable to care for their child. During her admission assessment, she sat motionless and mute. Mr. Nolan, her primary nurse, noticed that after he checked her pulse, her arm remained in midair until he lowered it for her. Mrs. Chou was unkempt and pale, and her skin turgor was poor.

Mr. Nolan also spoke with Mr. Chou, who was visibly distressed by his wife's condition. He discovered that Mr. Chou blamed himself for his wife's illness because his relocation prevented her from caring for her ailing mother. He agreed with his wife that their mutual failings placed their child at risk of retribution. He conceded that coming to the hospital had been very difficult, owing to embarrassment both about his wife's mental illness and his own belief that he should not burden others with the care of himself and his wife. Mr. Nolan helped Mr. Chou recognize that in North American culture, family members shared caregiving burdens, professional help was more available, and stigmatization was less intense.

Gradually, Mr. Chou's distress lessened as he came to appreciate that he would not have to carry the level of burden he had anticipated. As Mrs. Chou's psychosis abated, both she and Mr. Chou came to ascribe more culpability for the illness to fate, reducing their burden of self-blame. They agreed to meet with a healer who helped them integrate the beliefs and resources of their original and adopted cultures, further reducing their guilt and distress.

Source: Wong, D.F.K., Tsui, H.K.P., Pearson, V., et al. (2004). Family burdens, Chinese health beliefs, and the mental health of Chinese caregivers in Hong Kong. *Transcultural Psychiatry, 4,* 497–513.

poverty or high-crime environments) and migration to or growing up in a foreign culture (Tandon, Keshavan, & Nasrallah, 2008; Broome, Woolley, Tabraham, et al., 2005). O'Mahony and Donnelly (2007) found that immigrant women face many difficulties accessing mental health services. These authors suggest that although knowledge and cultural practices have an influence on such access, it is necessary for health care providers to be aware of social and economic diversity among immigrant groups, as they may face challenges different from those of the dominant cultural group. Although this was a small study, its results deserve consideration.

Course of the Disorder

The onset of symptoms or forewarning (prodromal) symptoms may appear a month to a year before the first psychotic break or full-blown manifestations of the illness; such symptoms represent a clear deterioration in previous functioning. The course thereafter typically includes recurrent exacerbations separated by periods of reduced or dormant symptoms. Some people will have a single episode of schizophrenia without recurrences or have several episodes and none thereafter. A recent study of over 2000 persons found four patterns of the course of the illness. Although the course of schizophrenia varied, all showed an initial deterioration followed by improvement (Levine, Lurie, Kohn, et al., 2011). Remission and recovery are increasingly common outcomes with early detection, appropriate treatment, and social support. For many people, however, schizophrenia is a chronic or recurring disorder that, like diabetes or heart disease, is managed but rarely cured.

Frequently, the history of a person with schizophrenia reveals that, prior to the illness, the person was socially awkward, lonely, and perhaps depressed and expressed himself or herself in vague, odd, or unrealistic ways. In this prodromal phase, complaints about anxiety, phobias, obsessions, dissociative features, and compulsions may be noted. As anxiety mounts, indications of a thought disorder become evident. Concentration, memory, and completion of school- or job-related work deteriorate. Intrusive thoughts, "mind wandering," and the need to devote more time to maintaining one's thoughts are reported.

The person may feel that something "strange" or "wrong" is happening. Events are misinterpreted, and mystical or symbolic meanings may be given to ordinary events. For example, the person may think that certain colours have special powers or that a song on the radio is a message from God. Discerning others' emotions becomes more difficult, and other people's actions or words may be mistaken for signs of hostility or evidence of harmful intent (Chung, Kang, Shin, et al., 2008).

Prognosis

Studies have shown that most of the deterioration occurs within the first two to five years after onset of psychosis, followed by a plateau in impairment and symptoms (Srihari, Shah, & Keshavan, 2012). For the majority of people, most symptoms can be at least somewhat controlled through medications and psychosocial interventions. With support and effective treatments, many people with schizophrenia experience a good quality of life and success within their families, occupations, and other roles. Associates may not even realize the person has schizophrenia.

In other cases, schizophrenia does not respond fully to available treatments, leaving residual symptoms and causing varying degrees of disability. Some cases require repeated or lengthy inpatient care or institutionalization. An abrupt onset of symptoms is usually a favourable prognostic sign, and those with good premorbid social, sexual, and occupational functioning have a greater chance for a good remission or a complete recovery. A slow, insidious onset over two to three years is more ominous, and the younger one is at the onset of schizophrenia, the more discouraging the prognosis. A childhood history of withdrawn, reclusive, eccentric, and tense behaviour is also an unfavourable diagnostic sign, as is a preponderance of negative symptoms (Möller, 2007).

Phases of Schizophrenia

Schizophrenia usually progresses through predictable phases, although the presenting symptoms during a given phase and the length of the phase can vary widely. The phases of schizophrenia are as follows (Chung, Kang, Shin, et al., 2008):

- **Phase I—Acute:** Onset or exacerbation of florid, disruptive symptoms (e.g., hallucinations, delusions, apathy, withdrawal) with resultant loss of functional abilities; increased care or hospitalization may be required.
- **Phase II—Stabilization:** Symptoms are diminishing, and there is movement toward one's previous level of functioning (baseline); day hospitalization or care in a residential crisis centre or a supervised group home may be needed.
- **Phase III—Maintenance:** The person is at or nearing baseline (or premorbid) functioning; symptoms are absent or diminished; level of functioning allows the person to live in the community. Ideally, recovery with few or no residual symptoms has occurred. Most people in this phase live in their own residences. Although this phase has been termed *maintenance*, current literature shows a trend toward reframing it with a greater emphasis on recovery. Some clinicians and people with schizophrenia contend that maintenance and recovery are opposing concepts, "maintenance" being a pessimistic view, and "recovery" being more optimistic. In a maintenance model, the goal of treatment is stability, while in a recovery model, the goal is to extend improvement beyond stability (Manschreck, Duckworth, Halpern, et al., 2008). This new way of looking at this final phase requires recognition that progress is not a linear process and that recovery-focused therapy may be at odds with stability-focused therapy; that is, the health care providers must be able to tolerate instability such as setbacks and struggles in the recovery process (Lysecker & Buck, 2006).

Some clinicians also designate an earlier prodromal (or prepsychotic) phase, in which subtle symptoms or deficits associated with schizophrenia are present; such symptoms may or may not herald the onset of schizophrenia. Detection and treatment programs in most major Canadian cities aim to detect psychosis in the prodromal phase and prevent acute episodes of schizophrenia. Strategies of early intervention include reducing the duration of untreated psychosis (DUP), reducing delay in treatment, and providing interventions adapted for younger people and their families in the early course of the illness (Srihari, Shah, & Keshavan, 2012). A list of Canadian programs can be found on the website of the International Early Psychosis Association at www.iepa.org.au.

There is controversy as to whether the benefits of early intervention can be maintained over time. However, a study at the Prevention and Early Intervention Program for Psychosis (PEPP) in London, Ontario, found symptom improvement was not only maintained at the five-year follow-up but increased for an additional two to five years (Norman, Manchanda, Malia, et al., 2011). This program provides continuity of care for five years, with more intense intervention in the initial two years and a gradual, individualized transfer to usual services. When compared to programs that provide only two years of treatment, the PEPP approach demonstrates better durability of benefit (Srihari, Shah, & Keshavan, 2012).

APPLICATION OF THE NURSING PROCESS

ASSESSMENT

Nursing assessment of people who have or may have a psychotic disorder focuses largely on symptoms, coping, functioning, and safety. Assessment involves interviewing the person and observing behaviour and other outward manifestations of the disorder. It also should include mental status and spiritual, cultural, biological, psychological, social, and environmental elements. Sound therapeutic communication skills, an understanding of the disorder and the ways the person may be experiencing the world, and the establishment of trustworthiness and a therapeutic nurse–patient relationship all strengthen the assessment. Indeed, the therapeutic relationship is of critical importance. A helping partnership between the nurse and the person with schizophrenia facilitates recovery (Anthony, 2008). Early engagement between the nurse and a person with schizophrenia is an important factor in predicting recovery and continued disease remission (Bertolote & McGorry, 2005). For example, a small study of health care providers working with immigrant women found that the care provider–patient relationship had a great influence on how these women sought mental health care (O'Mahony & Donnelly, 2007).

One effective approach to developing this trusting relationship is the LEAP approach described by Amador (2000) and referenced at the beginning of this chapter. It consists of four steps: (1) listen—try to put yourself in the other person's shoes to gain a clear idea of his or her experience; (2) empathize—seriously consider and empathize with the other person's point of view; (3) agree—find common ground and identify facts you can both agree upon; (4) partner—collaborate on accomplishing the agreed-upon goals (Amador, 2000, pp. 56–58). In this way, trust can be gained and an alliance formed.

During the Prepsychotic Phase

Experts believe that detection and treatment of symptoms that may warn of schizophrenia's onset lessen the risk of developing the disorder or decrease the severity of the disorder if it does develop. A delay in diagnosis and treatment allows the psychotic process to become more entrenched; it can also result in relational, work, housing, and school problems (Riecher-Rössler, Gschwandtner, Borgwardt, et al., 2006).

Therefore, early assessment plays a key role in improving the prognosis for persons with schizophrenia (Chung, Kang, Shin, et al., 2008). This form of primary prevention involves

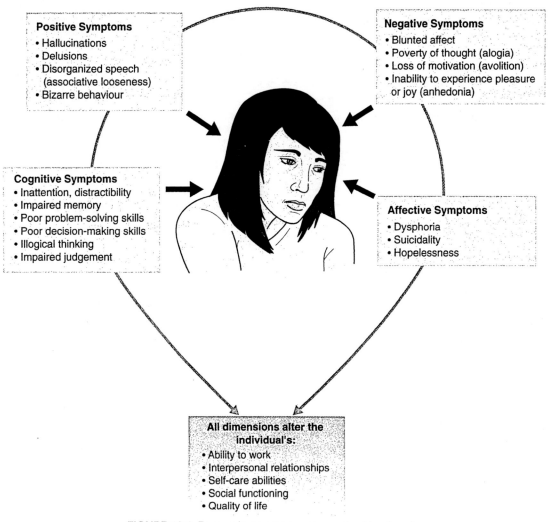

Positive Symptoms
- Hallucinations
- Delusions
- Disorganized speech (associative looseness)
- Bizarre behaviour

Negative Symptoms
- Blunted affect
- Poverty of thought (alogia)
- Loss of motivation (avolition)
- Inability to experience pleasure or joy (anhedonia)

Cognitive Symptoms
- Inattention, distractibility
- Impaired memory
- Poor problem-solving skills
- Poor decision-making skills
- Illogical thinking
- Impaired judgement

Affective Symptoms
- Dysphoria
- Suicidality
- Hopelessness

All dimensions alter the individual's:
- Ability to work
- Interpersonal relationships
- Self-care abilities
- Social functioning
- Quality of life

FIGURE 16-1 Four main symptom groups of schizophrenia.

monitoring those at high risk (e.g., children of parents with schizophrenia) for symptoms such as abnormal social development and cognitive dysfunction. Intervening to reduce stressors (i.e., reduce or avoid exposure to triggers), enhancing social and coping skills (e.g., build resiliency), and administering prophylactic antipsychotic medication may also be of benefit (Bechdolf, Phillips, Francey, et al., 2006).

Similarly, in people who have already developed the disorder, minimizing the onset and duration of relapses is believed to improve the prognosis. Research suggests that with each relapse of psychosis, there is an increase in residual dysfunction and deterioration. Recognition of the early warning signs of relapse, such as reduced sleep and concentration, followed by close monitoring and intensification of treatment is essential (van Meijel, van der Gaag, Sylvain, et al., 2004). For this reason, adherence to a drug regimen of antipsychotics can be more important than the risk of adverse effects because most adverse effects are reversible, whereas the consequences of relapse may not be.

General Assessment

Not all people with schizophrenia have the same symptoms, and some of the symptoms of schizophrenia are also found in other disorders. Figure 16-1 describes the four main symptom groups of schizophrenia:

1. Positive symptoms: the presence of something that is not normally present
2. Negative symptoms: the absence of something that should be present but is not
3. Cognitive symptoms: abnormalities in how a person thinks
4. Affective symptoms: symptoms involving emotions and their expression

Positive Symptoms

The positive symptoms usually appear early in the illness, and their dramatic nature captures our attention and often precipitates hospitalization. They are also the symptoms most laypeople associate with insanity, making schizophrenia the disorder most associated with being "crazy." However, positive psychotic symptoms are perhaps less important prognostically and usually respond to antipsychotic medication. Positive symptoms are associated with:

- Acute onset
- Normal premorbid functioning
- Normal social functioning during remissions

- Normal CT findings
- Normal neuropsychological test results
- Favourable response to antipsychotic medication

The positive symptoms presented here are categorized as alterations in thinking, speech, perception, and behaviour.

Alterations in thinking. All people experience occasional and momentary errors in thinking (e.g., "Why are all these lights turning red when I'm already late? Someone must be trying to slow me down!"), but most can catch and correct the error by using intact reality testing—the ability to determine accurately whether or not an experience is based in reality. People with impaired reality testing, however, maintain the error, which contributes to delusions, or alterations in *thought* content. A person experiencing delusions is convinced that what he or she believes to be real *is* real. Student nurses sometimes try unsuccessfully to argue a person out of delusions by offering evidence of reality; this approach may irritate the person and slow the development of a therapeutic relationship. Table 16-1 provides definitions and examples of frequent types of delusions.

About 75% of people with schizophrenia experience delusions at some time. The most common delusions are persecutory or grandiose or those involving religious or hypochondriacal ideas. A delusion may be a response to anxiety or may reflect areas of concern for a person; for example, someone with poor self-esteem may believe he is Beethoven or an emissary of God, allowing him to feel more powerful or important. Looking for and addressing such underlying themes or needs can be a key nursing intervention. At times, delusions hold a kernel of truth. One person repeatedly told the staff that the Mafia was out to kill him. Later, staff learned that he had been selling drugs, had not paid his contacts, and gang members *were* trying to find him to hurt or even kill him.

Concrete thinking refers to an impaired ability to think abstractly. The person interprets statements literally. For example, the nurse might ask what brought the person to the hospital, and the person might answer, concretely, "a cab" (rather than explaining that he had attempted suicide). Traditionally, concreteness has been assessed through the patient's interpretation of proverbs. However, this assessment is not accurate if the person is from another culture or is otherwise unfamiliar with the proverb (Haynes & Resnick, 1993). It is preferable to use the *similarities test*, which involves asking the person to explain how two things are similar, such as an orange and an apple, a chair and a table, or a child and an adult. A description of physical characteristics ("apples and oranges are

TABLE 16-1   SUMMARY OF DELUSIONS

DELUSION	DEFINITION	EXAMPLE
Thought insertion	Believing that another person, group of people, or external force controls thoughts	Bruce always wears a hat so that aliens don't insert thoughts into his brain.
Thought withdrawal	Believing that others are taking thoughts out of a person's mind	Bernadette covers her windows with foil so the police can't empty her mind.
Thought broadcasting	Believing that one's thoughts are being involuntarily broadcasted to others	Marcel was convinced that everyone could hear what he was thinking at all times.
Ideas of reference	Giving personal significance to trivial events; perceiving events as relating to you when they do not	When Maria saw staff talking, she believed they were plotting against her.
Ideas of influence	Believing that you have somehow influenced events that are, in fact, out of your control	Jean Pierre is convinced that he caused the flooding in Manitoba.
Persecution	Believing that one is being singled out for harm by others; this belief often takes the form of a plot by people in power	Saed believed that the RCMP was planning to kill him by poisoning his food. Therefore, he would eat only food he bought from machines.
Grandeur	Believing that one is a very powerful or important person	Sam believed he was a famous playwright and tennis pro.
Somatic	Believing that the body is changing in an unusual way (e.g., rotting inside)	David told the doctor that his heart had stopped and his insides were rotting away.
Erotomanic	Believing that another person desires you romantically	Although he barely knew her, Mary insisted that Mr. Johansen would marry her if only his current wife would stop interfering.
Jealousy	Believing that one's mate is unfaithful	Harry wrongly accused his girlfriend of going out with other men. His proof was that she came home from work late twice that week, even though the girlfriend's boss explained that everyone had worked late.

both round") would be a concrete answer, while an abstract answer recognizes ideas such as classifications ("apples and oranges are fruit"). Concreteness reduces one's ability to understand and address abstract concepts such as love or the passage of time or to reality-test delusions or other symptoms. Educational strategies need to take into account a person's ability to think abstractly.

Alterations in speech. Alterations in speech demonstrate difficulties with *thought process* (how a person thinks). *Associations* are the threads that tie one thought logically to another. In associative looseness, these threads are interrupted or illogically connected; thinking becomes haphazard, illogical, and difficult to follow:

Nurse: "Are you going to the picnic today?"

Patient: "I'm not an elephant hunter; no tiger teeth for me."

At times, the nurse may be able to decipher or decode the patient's messages and begin to understand the patient's feelings and needs. Any exchange in which a person feels understood is useful. Therefore, the nurse might respond to the patient in this way:

Nurse: "Are you saying that you're afraid to go out with the others today?"

Patient: "Yeah, no tiger getting me today."

Sometimes it is not possible to understand the person's meaning because his or her speech is too fragmented. For example:

Patient: "I sang out for my mother .:. for this to hell I went. These little hills hop aboard, share the Christmas mice spread … the devil will be washed away."

If the nurse does not understand what the patient is saying, it is important that he or she let the patient know. Clear messages and honesty are a vital part of working effectively in psychiatric mental health nursing. An honest response lets the person know that the nurse does not understand, would like to understand, and can be trusted to be honest.

Other alterations in speech that can make communication challenging are *circumstantiality, tangentiality, neologisms, echolalia, clang association,* and *word salad*:

- Circumstantiality refers to the inclusion of unnecessary and often tedious details in one's conversation (e.g., describing your breakfast when asked how your day is going).
- Tangentiality is a departure from the main topic to talk about less important information; the patient goes off on tangents in a way that takes the conversation off-topic.
- Neologisms are made-up words (or idiosyncratic uses of existing words) that have meaning for the person but a different or nonexistent meaning to others (e.g., "I was going to tell him the *mannerologies* of his hospitality won't do"). This eccentric use of words represents disorganized thinking and interferes with communication.
- Echolalia is the pathological repeating of another's words and is often seen in catatonia.
- *Nurse:* "Mary, come get your medication."
- *Mary:* "Come get your medication."
- *Clang association* is the choosing of words based on their sound rather than their meaning, often rhyming and sometimes having a similar beginning sound (e.g., "On the track,

have a Big Mac," "Click, clack, clutch, close"). Clanging may also be seen in neurological disorders.
- Word salad is a jumble of words that is meaningless to the listener—and perhaps to the speaker as well—because of an extreme level of disorganization.

Alterations in perception. Alterations in perception are errors in one's view of reality. The most common form of altered perception in psychosis is hallucination, but depersonalization, derealization, and boundary impairment are sometimes experienced as well:

- Depersonalization is a nonspecific feeling that a person has lost his or her identity and that the self is different or unreal. People may feel that body parts do not belong to them or may sense that their body has drastically changed. For example, a person may see her fingers as snakes or her arms as rotting wood.
- Derealization is the false perception that the environment has changed. For example, everything seems bigger or smaller, or familiar surroundings have become somehow strange and unfamiliar. Both depersonalization and derealization can be interpreted as *loss of ego boundaries* (sometimes called *loose ego boundaries*).
- Boundary impairment is an impaired ability to sense where one's self ends and others' selves begin. For example, a person might drink another's beverage, believing that because it is in his vicinity, it is his.
- Hallucinations result from perceiving a sensory experience for which no external stimulus exists (e.g., hearing a voice when no one is speaking). Hallucinations differ from illusions in that illusions are misperceptions or misinterpretations of a real experience; for example, a man sees his coat on a coat rack and believes it is a bear about to attack. He does see something real but misinterprets what it is.

Causes of hallucinations include psychiatric disorders, drug abuse, medications, organic disorders, hyperthermia, toxicity (e.g., digitalis), and other conditions. Hallucinations can involve any of the five bodily senses. Table 16-2 provides definitions and examples of these types of hallucinations.

Auditory hallucinations are experienced by up to 15% of people without psychotic disorders and 60% of people with schizophrenia at some time during their lives (Hubl, Koenig, Strik, et al., 2004). Voices typically seem to come from outside the person's head, and auditory processing areas of the brain are activated during auditory hallucinations just as they are when a genuine external sound is heard (Hubl, Koenig, Strik, et al., 2004). This abnormal activation may cause hallucinations, but another leading theory is that "voices" are a misperception of one's internally generated conversation (Hoffman & Varanko, 2006). John Nash (n.d.), the world-renowned mathematician portrayed in the 2001 film *A Beautiful Mind*, described the voices he heard during the acute phase of his illness: "I thought of the voices as … something a little different from aliens. I thought of them more like angels. … It's really my subconscious talking, it was really that. … I know that now."

Voices may be of people familiar or unknown, single or multiple. They may be perceived as supportive and pleasant or

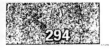

TABLE 16-2 SUMMARY OF HALLUCINATIONS

HALLUCINATION	DEFINITION	EXAMPLE
Auditory	Hearing voices or sounds that do not exist in the environment but are misperceptions of inner thoughts or feelings	Juan hit the ambulance attendant when a voice told him the attendant was taking him to a concentration camp.
Visual	Seeing a person, object, animal, colours, or visual patterns that do not exist in the environment	Antoine became very frightened and screamed, "There are rats coming at me!"
Olfactory	Smelling odours that do not exist	Theresa "smells" her insides rotting.
Gustatory	Tasting sensations that do not exist	Simon will not eat his food because he "tastes" the poison they are putting in it.
Tactile	Feeling strange sensations on the skin where no external objects stimulate such feelings; common in delirium tremens	Jack "feels" electrical impulses tingling as they control his mind, and he covers his walls in tinfoil to block them out.

derogatory and frightening. Voices commenting on the person's behaviour or conversing with the person are most common. A person who hears voices when no one is present often struggles to understand the experience, sometimes developing related delusions to explain the voices (e.g., the person may believe the voices are from God, the devil, or deceased relatives). People with chronic hallucinations may attempt to cope by drowning them out with loud music or competing with them by talking loudly (Farhall, Greenwood, & Jackson, 2007).

Command hallucinations are "voices" that direct the person to take an action. All hallucinations must be assessed and monitored carefully, because the voices may command the person to hurt self or others. For example, voices might command a person to "jump out the window" or "take a knife and kill my child." Command hallucinations are often terrifying and may herald a psychiatric emergency. In all cases, it is essential to assess what the person hears, the person's ability to recognize the hallucination as real or not real, and the person's ability to resist any commands. A person may falsely deny hallucinations, requiring behavioural assessment to support (validate) or refute the person's report. Outward indications of possible hallucinations include turning or tilting the head as if to listen to someone, suddenly stopping current activity as if interrupted, and moving the lips silently.

Visual hallucinations occur less frequently in schizophrenia and are more likely to occur in organic disorders such as acute alcohol withdrawal or dementia. Olfactory, tactile, or gustatory hallucinations are unusual; when present, other physical causes should be investigated (Sadock & Sadock, 2008).

Alterations in behaviour. Alterations in behaviour include bizarre and agitated behaviours involving such things as stilted, rigid demeanour or eccentric dress, grooming, and rituals. Other behavioural changes seen in schizophrenia include the following:
- Catatonia, a pronounced increase or decrease in the rate and amount of movement. The most common form is stuporous behaviour, in which the person moves little or not at all.

- Psychomotor retardation, a pronounced slowing of movement. It is important to differentiate the slowed movements secondary to schizophrenia from those seen in depression; careful assessment of thought content and thought processes is essential for making this determination.
- Psychomotor agitation, excited behaviour such as running or pacing rapidly, often in response to internal or external stimuli. Psychomotor agitation can pose a risk to others and to the person, who is at risk for exhaustion, collapse, and even death.
- Stereotyped behaviours, repeated motor behaviours that do not presently serve a logical purpose.
- Automatic obedience, the performance by a catatonic person of all simple commands in a robotlike fashion.
- Waxy flexibility, the extended maintenance of posture usually seen in catatonia. For example, the nurse raises the person's arm, and the person retains this position in a statuelike manner.
- Negativism, akin to resistance but may not be intentional. In *active negativism*, the person does the opposite of what he or she is told to do; *passive negativism* is a failure to do what is requested.
- Impaired impulse control, a reduced ability to resist one's impulses. Examples include performing socially inappropriate behaviours such as grabbing another's cigarette, throwing food on the floor, pushing others around, and changing TV channels while others are watching.
- Echopraxia, the mimicking of the movements of another. It is also seen in catatonia.

Behaviours such as agitation and impaired impulse control are likely to bring the person into contact with the police and justice system. One consequence of deinstitutionalization is that behaviours previously managed in psychiatric settings are increasingly brought to the attention of police, resulting in criminal charges rather than hospitalization (Jansman-Hart, Seto, Crocker, et al., 2011). As a result, the criminal justice system is becoming the entry point to mental health services for increasing numbers of people (Jansman-Hart et al., 2011).

Unfortunately, though, the prison system is not designed for mental health treatment, and the conditions there are neither therapeutic nor rehabilitative for people with mental health concerns (Zinger, 2012).

Negative Symptoms

Negative symptoms develop slowly and are those that most interfere with a person's adjustment and ability to cope. They tend to be persistent and crippling because they render the person inert and unmotivated. Negative symptoms impede one's ability to:

- Initiate and maintain conversations and relationships
- Obtain and maintain a job
- Make decisions and follow through on plans
- Maintain adequate hygiene and grooming

Negative symptoms contribute to poor social functioning and social withdrawal. During the acute phase, they are difficult to assess because positive symptoms (such as delusions and hallucinations) dominate. Selected negative symptoms are outlined in Table 16-3.

In schizophrenia, affect—the external manifestation of feeling or emotion that is manifested in facial expression, tone of voice, and body language—may not always coincide with inner emotions. Affect in schizophrenia can usually be categorized in one of four ways:

- Flat—immobile or blank facial expression
- Blunted—reduced or minimal emotional response
- Inappropriate—emotional response incongruent with the tone or circumstances of the situation (e.g., a man laughs when told that his father has died)
- Bizarre—odd, illogical, emotional state that is grossly inappropriate or unfounded; especially prominent in disorganized schizophrenia and includes grimacing and giggling

Cognitive Symptoms

Cognitive symptoms represent the third symptom group and are evident in most people with schizophrenia. They include difficulty with attention, memory, information processing, cognitive flexibility, and executive functions (e.g., decision making, judgement, planning, and problem solving) (Braw, Bloch, Mendelovich, et al., 2008). These impairments can leave the person unable to manage personal health care, hold a job, initiate or maintain a support system, or live alone.

Affective Symptoms

Affective symptoms, the fourth symptom group, are common and increase a person's suffering. Assessment for depression is crucial because depression:

- May herald an impending relapse
- Increases substance abuse
- Increases suicide risk
- Further impairs functioning

This assessment can be done by inquiring into mood and the presence of depressive thoughts or suicidal ideation.

Self-Assessment

Working with individuals with schizophrenia produces strong emotional reactions in most health care workers. The acutely ill person's intensely anxious, lonely, dependent, and distrustful presentation evokes similarly intense, uncomfortable, and frightening emotions in others. The chronicity, repeated exacerbations, and slow response to treatment that many people experience can lead to feelings of helplessness and powerlessness in staff. Some behaviour (especially violent behaviour) can produce strong emotional responses (called *counter-transference*) such as fear or anger (see Chapter 10).

Ironically, knowledge that schizophrenia is a brain disease may contribute to stigmatizing attitudes and feelings of hopelessness. Early research suggests that when public education focuses on illness without including personal contact or information about recovery, stigma actually increases or becomes entrenched (Martin & Johnson, 2008). Nurses who do not see recovering people or learn about recovery may be subject to this effect. Inpatient nurses, in particular, tend to see only the most ill people, and so it is important for them to avoid a skewed and hopeless view by staying aware of the growing numbers of people who are living well with schizophrenia. The importance of hope in the nursing of people with schizophrenia and their families is well documented, and being hopeful is an essential characteristic of mental health providers in this field (Koehn & Cutliffe, 2007).

At the same time, it is necessary to be realistic about the length of time that it may take for a patient to recover from an acute episode. It can be helpful to remember that the person

TABLE 16-3	SELECTED NEGATIVE SYMPTOMS OF SCHIZOPHRENIA
NEGATIVE SYMPTOM	**DESCRIPTION**
Affective blunting	A reduction in the expression, range, and intensity of affect (in *flat affect*, no facial expression is present)
Anergia	Lack of energy; passivity, lack of persistence at work or school; may also be a symptom of depression, so needs careful evaluation
Anhedonia	Inability to experience pleasure in activities that usually produce it; result of profound emotional barrenness
Avolition	Reduced motivation; inability to initiate tasks such as social contacts, grooming, and other activities of daily living (ADLs)
Poverty of content of speech	While adequate in amount, speech conveys little information because of vagueness or superficiality
Poverty of speech (alogia)	Reduced amount of speech—responses range from brief to one-word answers

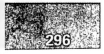

has essentially had a brain injury, to set realistic, achievable goals, and to acknowledge small steps. Negative symptoms, in particular, can be very slow to resolve. It may also take a long time to gain trust, so the nurse can expect the orientation phase of the helping relationship to be prolonged.

Without support and the opportunity and willingness to explore feelings with more experienced staff, the nurse may adopt nontherapeutic behaviours—denial, withdrawal, avoidance, and anger most commonly. These behaviours thwart the patient's progress and undermine the nurse's self-esteem. Comments such as "These patients are hopeless," and "All you can do is babysit these people" are indications of unrecognized or unresolved counter-transference that, if left uncorrected, interfere with both treatment and work satisfaction. Canadian nurse Jan Landeen, cited by Koehn and Cutliffe

(2007), found that strategies for increasing hope include getting to know the patient as a person, sharing patient successes, learning about treatments and research, and keeping expectations realistic.

People living with schizophrenia may experience fear, self-stigma, or shame related to their mental illness, leading them to conceal some aspects of their experience. Negativism and alogia (reduced verbalization) can also limit the person's responses. Many people with schizophrenia experience anosognosia, an inability to realize they are ill, which is caused by the illness itself. The resulting lack of insight can make assessment (and treatment) challenging, delaying completion of a full assessment and requiring additional skills on the part of the nurse. Selected techniques that may help you overcome these challenges can be found in Table 16-4.

TABLE 16-4 INTERVENTIONS FOR OVERCOMING OBSTACLES TO ASSESSMENT

INTERVENTION	RATIONALE	EXAMPLE
Use empathic comments and observations to prompt the patient to provide information.	Empathy conveys understanding and builds trust and rapport.	*Nurse:* "It must be difficult to find yourself in a psychiatric hospital." *Patient:* "Yes…I'm frightened."
Minimize questioning, especially closed-ended questioning. Seek data conversationally, using prompts and open-ended questions.	Extended questioning can increase suspiciousness, and closed questions elicit minimal information. Both become wearying and off-putting.	"Could you please tell me more about … ?" "Tell me what life has been like for you lately."
Use short, simple sentences and introduce only one idea at a time. Allow time for responses to questions.	Long sentences or rambling questions can confuse a person who has difficulty processing auditory information or is actively hallucinating. Also, a person with alogia requires more time to respond to questions.	*Therapeutic:* "Would you like to join us for a basketball game?" *Nontherapeutic:* "Would you like to join us for a basketball game? Sports can be very good for you, you know, and you seem very lonely, so it would help you a lot. I really hope you will come play a game"
Directly but supportively seek the needed information, explaining the reasons for the assessment.	Being direct but supportive conveys genuineness, builds rapport, and helps reduce anxiety.	"You seem very sad. Sometimes sad people think about hurting themselves. Have you ever thought about hurting yourself?"
Judiciously use indirect, supportive (therapeutic) confrontation. Seek other data to support (validate) the person's report (obtain further history from third parties, past medical records, and other treatment providers when possible), preferably with the person's permission.	Blunt contradiction or premature confrontation increases resistance. Patients may be unable or unwilling to provide information fully and reliably. Validating their reports assures the validity of the assessment.	"I realize admitting to hearing voices might be difficult to do. I notice you talking as if to others when no one is there." "Your brother reports he works at a factory. Is that your understanding?"
Prioritize the data you seek, and avoid seeking nonessential data.	Patients may have limited tolerance for the assessment interview and answer only a limited number of inquiries. Seeking nonessential information does not benefit the person or assessment.	*Patient:* "I hate school! I wish they'd all die!" *Nurse:* (less therapeutic) "Which school do you go to?" *Nurse:* (more therapeutic) "Things would be better if they were dead. …" *(Paraphrasing prompts elaboration and confirmation or refutation of the comment.)*

ASSESSMENT GUIDELINES

Schizophrenia and Other Psychotic Disorders

1. Determine if the patient has had a medical workup. Are there any indications of physical medical problems that might mimic psychosis (e.g., digitalis or anticholinergic toxicity, brain trauma, drug intoxication, delirium, fever)?
2. Assess whether the person abuses or is dependent on alcohol or drugs.
3. Assess for risk to self or others.
4. Assess for command hallucinations (e.g., voices telling the patient to harm self or another). If present, ask the person:
   - Do you recognize the voices?
   - Do you believe the voices are real?
   - Do you plan to follow the command? (A positive response to any of these questions suggests an increased risk that the person will act on the commands.)
5. Assess the patient's belief system. Is it fragmented or poorly organized? Is it systematized? Are the beliefs delusional? If yes, then ask:
   - Do you feel that you or loved ones are being threatened or are in danger?
   - Do you feel the need to act against a person or organization to protect or avenge yourself or loved ones? (A positive response to either of these questions suggests an increased risk of danger to others.)
6. Assess for suicide risk (see Chapter 25).
7. Assess for ability to ensure self safety, addressing:
   - Adequacy of food and fluid intake
   - Hygiene and self-care
   - Handling of potentially hazardous activities, such as smoking and cooking
   - Ability to transport self safely
   - Impulse control and judgement
   - Appropriate dress for weather conditions
8. Assess for coexisting disorders:
   - Depression
   - Anxiety
   - Substance abuse or dependency
   - Medical disorders (especially brain trauma, toxicity, delirium, cardiovascular disease, obesity, and diabetes)
9. Assess medications the patient has been prescribed, whether and how the patient is taking the medications, and what factors (e.g., costs, mistrust of staff, adverse effects) are affecting adherence.
10. Assess for the presence and severity of positive and negative symptoms. Complete a mental status examination, noting which symptoms are present, how they affect functioning, and how the patient is managing them.
11. Assess the patient's insight, knowledge of the illness, relationships and support systems, other coping resources, and strengths.
12. Assess the family's knowledge of and response to the patient's illness and its symptoms. Are family members overprotective? Hostile? Anxious? Are they familiar with family support groups and respite resources?

The Unpleasant Voices Scale has been designed for assessment of the risk of harm related to command hallucinations and can be used in conjunction with the Harm Command Safety Protocol (Gerlock, Buccheri, Buffum, et al., 2010). The Inventory of Voice Experiences, a nursing tool developed in Canada, offers increased accuracy of assessment of voices (England, 2007).

DIAGNOSIS

People with schizophrenia have multiple disturbing and disabling symptoms that require a multifaceted approach to care and treatment of both the patient and the family. Table 16-5 lists potential nursing diagnoses for a person with schizophrenia.

OUTCOMES IDENTIFICATION

Desired outcomes vary with the phase of the illness. *Nursing Outcomes Classification (NOC)* (Moorhead, Johnson, Maas, et al., 2008) is a useful guide. Ideally, outcomes should focus on enhancing strengths and minimizing the effects of the patient's deficits and symptoms. Outcomes should be consistent with the recovery model (see Chapter 31), which stresses hope, living a full and productive life, and eventual recovery rather than focusing on controlling symptoms and adapting to disability.

Phase I—Acute

During the acute phase, the overall goal is the person's safety and medical stabilization. Therefore, if the person is at risk for violence to self or others, initial outcome criteria address safety issues (e.g., *Person refrains from self harm*). Another outcome is *Person consistently labels hallucinations as "not real—a symptom of an illness."* Table 16-6 gives selected short-term and intermediate indicators for the outcome *Distorted thought self-control.*

Phase II—Stabilization

Outcome criteria during phase II focus on helping the patient adhere to treatment, become stabilized on medications, and control or cope with symptoms. The outcomes target the negative symptoms and may include ability to succeed in social, vocational, or self-care activities.

Phase III—Maintenance

Outcome criteria for phase III focus on maintaining achievement, preventing relapse, and achieving independence and a satisfactory quality of life.

TABLE 16-5   POTENTIAL NURSING DIAGNOSES FOR SCHIZOPHRENIA

SYMPTOM	NURSING DIAGNOSES
Positive Symptoms	
Hears voices that others do not (*auditory hallucinations*)	*Disturbed sensory perception: auditory**
Hears voices telling him or her to hurt self or others (*command hallucinations*)	*Risk for self-directed violence* *Risk for other-directed violence*
Delusions†	*Disturbed thought processes‡*
Shows loose association of ideas (*associative looseness*)	*Disturbed thought processes‡*
Conversation is derailed by unnecessary and tedious details (*circumstantiality*)	*Impaired verbal communication*
Negative Symptoms	
Uncommunicative, withdrawn	*Social isolation*
Expresses feelings of rejection or aloneness (lies in bed all day, positions back to door)	*Impaired social interaction* *Risk for loneliness*
Talks about self as "bad" or "no good"	*Chronic low self-esteem*
Feels guilty because of "bad thoughts"; extremely sensitive to real or perceived slights	*Risk for self-directed violence*
Shows lack of energy (*anergia*)	*Ineffective coping*
Shows lack of motivation (*avolition*), unable to initiate tasks (social contact, grooming, and other aspects of daily living)	*Self-care deficit (bathing, dressing, feeding, toileting)* *Constipation*
Other	
Families and significant others become confused or overwhelmed, lack knowledge about disorder or treatment, feel powerless in coping with the patient	*Compromised family coping* *Caregiver role strain* *Deficient knowledge*
Stops taking medication (because of anosognosia, adverse effects, drugs costs, mistrust of staff), stops going to therapy, is not supported in treatment by significant others	*Nonadherence*

*Diagnosis retired from Herdman, T.H. (Ed.). (2012). *NANDA International nursing diagnoses: Definitions & classification, 2012–2014.* Oxford, UK: Wiley-Blackwell.

†Although NANDA has always classified these as "disturbed thought process," in fact, delusions are a problem of thought *content* and are classified as such in the standard mental status examination.

‡Diagnosis retired from Herdman, T.H. (Ed.). (2012). *NANDA International nursing diagnoses: Definitions & classification, 2012–2014.* Oxford, UK: Wiley-Blackwell.

TABLE 16-6   *NOC* OUTCOMES RELATED TO DISTORTED THOUGHT SELF-CONTROL

NURSING OUTCOME AND DEFINITION	INTERMEDIATE INDICATORS	SHORT-TERM INDICATORS
Distorted thought self-control: Self-restraint of disruptions in perception, thought processes, and thought content	Maintains affect consistent with mood Interacts appropriately Perceives environment and the ideas of others accurately Exhibits logical thought flow patterns Exhibits reality-based thinking Exhibits appropriate thought content	Recognizes that hallucinations or delusions are occurring Refrains from attending to and responding to hallucinations or delusions Describes content of hallucinations or delusions Reports decrease in hallucinations or delusions Asks for validation of reality

Source: Moorhead, S., Johnson, H., Maas, M., et al. (2008). *Nursing outcomes classification (NOC)* (4th ed.). St. Louis, MO: Mosby.

PLANNING

The planning of appropriate interventions is guided by the phase of the illness and the strengths and needs of the patient. It is influenced by cultural considerations, available resources, and the patient's preferences.

Phase I—Acute

Hospitalization is indicated if the patient is considered a danger to self or others, refuses to eat or drink, or is too disorganized or otherwise impaired to function safely in the community without supervision. The planning process focuses on the best strategies to ensure the person's safety and provide symptom stabilization. Additionally, during the patient's hospitalization, this process also includes discharge planning.

In discharge planning, the patient and interprofessional treatment team identify aftercare needs for follow-up and support. Discharge planning considers not only external factors, such as the person's living arrangements, economic resources, social supports, and family relationships, but also internal factors, such as resilience and repertoire of coping skills. Because relapse can be devastating to the person's circumstances (resulting in loss of employment, housing, and relationships) and worsen the long-term prognosis, vigorous efforts are made to connect the person and family with (and not simply refer them to) community resources that provide therapeutic programming and social, financial, and other needed support.

Phase II—Stabilization/Phase III—Maintenance

Planning during the stabilization and maintenance phases includes providing individual and family education and skills training (psychosocial education). Relapse prevention skills are vital. Planning identifies interpersonal, coping, health care, and vocational needs and addresses how and where these needs can best be met within the community.

IMPLEMENTATION

Interventions are geared toward the phase of schizophrenia the person is experiencing. For example, during the acute phase, the clinical focus is on crisis intervention, medication for symptom stabilization, and safety. Interventions are often hospital-based; however, people in the acute stage are increasingly being treated in the community.

Phase I—Acute

Settings

A number of factors that affect the choice of treatment setting include the following:

- Level of care and restrictiveness needed to protect the person from harm to self or others
- Person's needs for external structure and support
- Person's ability to cooperate with treatment
- Need for a particular treatment available only in particular settings
- Need for treatment of a coexisting medical condition
- Availability of supportive others who can provide critical information and treatment history to staff and permit stabilization in less restrictive settings

The use of less restrictive and more cost-effective alternatives to hospitalization that work for many people include:

- Partial hospitalization: Patients sleep at home and attend treatment sessions (similar to what they would receive if admitted) during the day or evening.
- Residential crisis centres: Patients who are unable to remain in the community but do not require full in-person services can be admitted (usually for 1 to 14 days) to receive increased supervision, guidance, and medication stabilization.
- Group homes: Patients live in the community with a group of other people, sharing expenses and responsibilities. Staff

are present in the house 24 hours a day, 7 days a week to provide supervision and therapeutic activities.
- Day treatment programs: Patients reside in the community and attend structured programming during the day.

These programs may include group and individual therapy, supervised activities, and specialized skill training. It is vital that staff be aware of these and other community resources and make this information available to discharged people and their families, ideally by directly connecting them with these resources. Patients and family members should be given telephone numbers and addresses of local support groups such as their provincial Schizophrenia Society. Northern and rural communities, however, may not have local support groups.

Other community resources include community mental health centres (usually providing medication services, day treatment, access to 24-hour emergency services, psychotherapy, psychoeducation, and case management); home health services; supported employment programs, offering services from job training to on-site coaches, who help people to learn to succeed in the work environment, often via peer-led services (e.g., drop-in centres, sometimes called "clubhouses," that offer social contact, constructive activities, and sometimes employment opportunities); family educational and skills groups (e.g., the Schizophrenia Society of Canada's "Strengthening Families Together" program); and respite care for caregivers.

Interventions

Acute phase interventions include the following:
- Psychiatric, medical, and neurological evaluation
- Psychopharmacological treatment
- Support, psychoeducation, and guidance
- Supervision and limit setting in the milieu

Due to a shortage of inpatient beds, there is pressure to keep the length of hospitalization short. This situation may create an ethical dilemma for treatment teams, as short initial hospital stays have been found to be related to high rates of readmission and shorter intervals between hospitalizations (Canadian Institute for Health Information, 2008). Typically, as soon as the acute symptoms are adequately stabilized, the patient is discharged to the community, where appropriate treatment can be continued during the stabilization and maintenance phases. However, in some cases, discharge may be delayed while appropriate housing and supports are sought.

Phase II—Stabilization/Phase III—Maintenance

Effective long-term care of an individual with schizophrenia relies on a three-pronged approach: medication administration and adherence, nursing intervention, and community support. Family psychoeducation, a key role of the nurse, is an essential intervention. All interventions and strategies are geared to the patient's strengths, culture, personal preferences, and needs.

Milieu Management

Effective hospital care provides (1) protection from stressful or disruptive environments and (2) structure. People in the acute phase of schizophrenia show greater improvement in a structured milieu than on an open unit that allows more freedom. A therapeutic milieu is consciously designed to maximize safety,

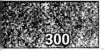

opportunities for learning skills, therapeutic activities, and access to resources. The milieu also provides guidance, supportive peer contact, and opportunities for practising conflict resolution, stress reduction techniques, and dealing with symptoms.

Activities and Groups

Participation in activities and groups appropriate to the patient's level of functioning may decrease withdrawal, enhance motivation, modify unacceptable behaviours, develop friendships, and increase social competence. Activities such as drawing, reading poetry, and listening to music may be used to focus conversation and promote the recognition and expression of feelings. Self-esteem is enhanced as patients experience successful task completion. Recreational activities such as picnics and outings to stores and restaurants are not simply diversions; they teach constructive leisure skills, increase social comfort, facilitate growth in social concern and interactional skills, and enhance the ability to develop boundaries and set limits on self and others. After discharge, group therapy can provide necessary structure within the patient's community milieu.

Safety

A small percentage of people with schizophrenia, especially during the acute phase, may exhibit a risk for physical violence, typically in response to hallucinations, delusions, paranoia, impaired judgement or impulse control, or self-referentiality (believing neutral, everyday occurrences carry special personal meaning). Concurrent substance use disorders are a greater risk factor for violence than is schizophrenia alone (Fazel, Gulati, Linsell, et al., 2009). When the potential for violence exists, measures to protect the patient and others become the priority. Interventions include increasing staff supervision, reducing stimulation (e.g., noise, crowds), addressing paranoia and other contributing symptoms, providing constructive diversion and outlets for physical energy, teaching and practising coping skills, implementing cognitive-behavioural approaches (to correct unrealistic expectations or selectively extinguish aggression), de-escalating tension verbally, and, when necessary, using seclusion, chemical (i.e., medication) or physical restraints. The Harm Command Safety Protocol provides guidelines for how to respond when a person indicates intent to harm someone else (Gerlock, Buccheri, Buffum, et al., 2010). Refer to Chapter 26 for more detailed discussions of caring for the aggressive person, seclusion, and restraints.

Counselling and Communication Techniques

Therapeutic communication techniques for patients with schizophrenia aim to lower the person's anxiety, build trust, encourage clear communication, decrease defensiveness, encourage interaction, enhance self-esteem, and reinforce skills such as reality testing and assertiveness. It is important to remember that people with schizophrenia may have memory impairment and require repetition. They may also have limited tolerance for interaction, owing to the stimulation it creates. Therefore, shorter (<30 minutes) but more frequent interactions may be more therapeutic. Interventions for paranoia and other selected presentations are discussed later in this chapter.

Hallucinations

When a patient is having a hallucination, the nursing focus is on understanding the person's experiences and responses. Suicidal or homicidal themes or commands necessitate appropriate safety measures. For example, "voices" that tell a patient a particular individual plans to harm him or her may lead to aggressive actions against that person; one-to-one supervision of the patient or transfer of the potential victim to another unit is often essential.

Hallucinations are real to the patient who is experiencing them and may be distracting during nurse–patient interactions. Call the person by name, speak simply but in a louder voice than usual, approach the person in a nonthreatening and nonjudgemental manner, maintain eye contact, and redirect the person's focus to the conversation as needed (Farhall, Greenwood, & Jackson, 2007). The following Guidelines for Communication box lists other techniques for communicating with patients experiencing hallucinations.

◆ GUIDELINES FOR COMMUNICATION
With People Experiencing Hallucinations

- Ask the person directly about the hallucinations (e.g., "Are you hearing voices?" followed by "What are you hearing?").
- Watch the person for cues that he or she is hallucinating, such as darting the eyes to one side, muttering, appearing distracted, or watching a vacant area of the room.
- Avoid reacting to hallucinations as if they are real. Do not address the voices.
- Do not negate the person's experience, but offer your own perceptions (e.g., "I don't see the devil standing over you, but I understand how upsetting that must be for you").
- Focus on reality-based, "here-and-now" diversions such as conversations or simple projects. Tell the person, "The voice you hear is part of your illness; it cannot hurt you. Try to listen to me and the others you can see around you."
- Be alert to signs of anxiety in the person, which may indicate that hallucinations are increasing.

Source: Farhall, J., Greenwood, K.M., & Jackson, H.J. (2007). Coping with hallucinated voices in schizophrenia: A review of self-initiated strategies and therapeutic interventions. *Clinical Psychology Review, 27,* 476–493. doi:10.1016/j.cpr.2006.12.002.

Delusions

Delusions may be the patient's attempts to understand confusion and distorted experiences. They reflect the misperception of one's circumstances, which go uncorrected in schizophrenia due to impaired reality testing. When, as a nurse, you attempt to see the world through the eyes of the patient, it is easier to understand his or her delusional experience. For example:

Patient: "You people are all alike … all in on the RCMP plot to destroy me."

Nurse: "I don't want to hurt you, Tom. Thinking that people are out to destroy you must be very frightening."

In this example, the nurse acknowledges the patient's experience, conveys empathy about the patient's fearfulness, and avoids focusing on the content of the delusion (RCMP and plot to destroy) but labels the patient's feelings so they can be explored, as tolerated. Note that talking about the feelings is helpful, but extended focus on delusional material is not.

It is *never* useful to debate or attempt to dissuade the patient regarding the delusion. Doing so can intensify the patient's retention of irrational beliefs and cause him or her to view you as rejecting or oppositional. However, it *is* helpful to clarify misinterpretations of the environment and gently suggest, as tolerated, a more reality-based perspective. For example:

Patient: "I see the doctor is here; he is out to destroy me."

Nurse: "It is true the doctor wants to see you, but he just wants to talk to you about your treatment. Would you feel more comfortable talking to him in the day room?"

Focusing on specific reality-based activities and events in the environment helps to minimize the focus on delusional thoughts. The more time the patient spends engaged in activities or with people, the more opportunities there are to receive feedback about and become comfortable with reality.

Work with the patient to find out which coping strategies succeed and how the patient can make the best use of them. The following Guidelines for Communication box lists techniques for communicating with people experiencing delusions, and the subsequent Patient and Family Teaching box presents patient and family teaching topics for coping with hallucinations and delusions.

GUIDELINES FOR COMMUNICATION

With People Experiencing Delusions

- To build trust, be open, honest, and reliable.
- Respond to suspicions in a matter-of-fact, empathic, supportive, and calm manner.
- Ask the person to describe the delusions. Example: "Tell me more about someone trying to hurt you."
- Avoid debating the delusional content, but interject doubt where appropriate. Example: "It seems as though it would be hard for that petite girl to hurt you."
- Focus on the feelings that underlie or flow from the delusions. Example: "You seem to wish you could be more powerful" or "It must feel frightening to think others want to hurt you."
- Once it is understood and addressed, do not dwell further on the delusion. Instead, focus on more reality-based topics. If the person obsesses about delusions, set firm limits on the amount of time you will talk about them, and explain your reason.
- Observe for events that trigger delusions. If possible, help the person find ways to reduce or manage them.
- Validate a part of the delusion that is real. Example: "Yes, there was a man at the nurse's station, but I did not hear him talk about you."

Source: Data from Farhall, J., Greenwood, K.M., & Jackson, H.J. (2007). Coping with hallucinated voices in schizophrenia: A review of self-initiated strategies and therapeutic interventions. *Clinical Psychology Review, 27*, 476–493. doi:10.1016/j.cpr.2006.12.002.

Associative Looseness

Associative looseness often mirrors the person's abnormal thoughts and reflects poorly organized thinking. An increase in associative looseness often indicates that the person is feeling increased anxiety or is overwhelmed by internal and external stimuli. The person's ramblings may also produce confusion and frustration in the nurse. The following guidelines are useful for intervention with a patient whose speech is confused and disorganized:

- Do *not* pretend you understand the patient's words or meaning when you do not; tell the person you are having difficulty understanding.

PATIENT AND FAMILY TEACHING

Coping With Auditory Hallucinations or Delusions

Distraction
- Listening to music
- Reading (aloud may help more)
- Counting backwards from 100
- Watching television

Interaction
- Looking at others—if they do not seem to be hearing or fearing what you are, ignore the voices or thoughts
- Talking with another person

Activity
- Walking
- Cleaning the house
- Having a relaxing bath
- Playing the guitar or singing
- Going to the gym (or anyplace you enjoy being, where others will be present)

Talking to Yourself
- Telling the voices or thoughts to go away
- Telling yourself that the voices and thoughts are a symptom and not real
- Telling yourself that no matter what you hear, voices can be safely ignored

Social Action
- Talking to a trusted friend or member of the family
- Calling a help line or going to a drop-in centre
- Visiting a favourite place or a comfortable public place

Physical Action
- Taking extra medication when ordered (call your prescriber)
- Going for a walk or doing other exercise
- Using breathing exercises and other relaxation methods

Sources: Farhall, J., Greenwood, K.M., & Jackson, H.J. (2007). Coping with hallucinated voices in schizophrenia: A review of self-initiated strategies and therapeutic interventions. *Clinical Psychology Review, 27*, 476–493. doi:10.1016/j.cpr.2006.12.002.; Jenner, J.A., Neinhuis, F.J., van de Willige, G., et al. (2006). "Hitting" voices of schizophrenia patients may lastingly reduce persistent auditory hallucinations and their burden: 18-month outcome of a randomized controlled trial. *Canadian Journal of Psychiatry, 51*(3), 169–177.

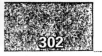

- Place the difficulty in understanding on yourself, *not* on the patient. Example: "I'm having trouble following what you are saying," *not* "You're not making any sense."
- Look for recurring topics and themes in the patient's communications, and tie these to events and timelines. Example: "You've mentioned trouble with your brother several times, usually after your family has visited. Tell me about your brother and your visits with him."
- Summarize or paraphrase the patient's communications to role-model more effective ways of making his or her point and to give the person a chance to correct anything you may have misunderstood.
- Reduce stimuli in the vicinity, and speak concisely, clearly, and concretely.
- Tell the person what you *do* understand, and reinforce clear communication and accurate expression of needs, feelings, and thoughts.

Health Teaching and Health Promotion

Education is an essential strategy and includes teaching the patient and family about the illness, including possible causes, medications and medication adverse effects, coping strategies, what to expect, and prevention of relapse. Understanding these things helps the patient and family to recognize the impact of stress, enhances their understanding of the importance of treatment to a good outcome, encourages involvement in (and support of) therapeutic activities, and identifies resources for consultation and ongoing support in dealing with the illness.

Including family members in any strategies aimed at reducing psychotic symptoms reduces family anxiety and distress and enables the family to reinforce the staff's efforts. The family plays an important role in the stability of the patient. The patient who returns to a warm, concerned, and supportive environment is less likely to experience relapse. An environment in which people are critical or their involvement in the patient's life is intrusive is associated with relapse and poorer outcomes.

Lack of understanding of the disease and its symptoms can lead others to misinterpret the patient's apathy and lack of drive as laziness, fostering a hostile response by family members, caregivers, or community. Thus, public education about the symptoms of schizophrenia can reduce tensions in families, as well as communities. The most effective education occurs over time and is available when the family is most receptive (Weisman, Duarte, Koneru, et al., 2006). The following Patient and Family Teaching box offers guidelines for patient and family teaching about schizophrenia.

Pharmacological Interventions

Drugs used to treat psychotic disorders, antipsychotics, first became available in the 1950s. Before that time, the available medications provided only sedation, not treatment of the disorder itself. Until the 1960s, people who had even one episode of schizophrenia usually spent months or years in provincial mental health hospitals. Psychotic episodes resulted in great emotional burdens to families and people with schizophrenia. The advent of antipsychotic drugs at last provided symptom control and allowed people to live in the community.

PATIENT AND FAMILY TEACHING
Schizophrenia

1. Learn all you can about the illness.
   - Attend psychoeducational and support groups.
   - Join the National Network for Mental Health.
   - Contact your provincial Schizophrenia Society.
2. Develop a relapse prevention plan.
   - Know the early warning signs of relapse (e.g., avoiding others, trouble sleeping, troubling thoughts).
   - Know whom to call, what to do, and where to go when early signs of relapse appear. Make a list and keep it with you.
   - Relapse is part of the illness, not a sign of failure.
3. Take advantage of all psychoeducational tools.
   - Participate in family, group, and individual therapy.
   - Learn new ways to act and coping skills to help handle family, work, and social stress. Get information from your nurse, case manager, doctor, self-help group, community mental health group, or hospital.
   - Have a plan, on paper, of what to do to cope with stressful times.
   - Recognize that everyone needs a place to address their fears and losses and to learn new ways of coping.
4. Adhere to treatment.
   - People who adhere to treatment that works for them do the best in coping with the disorder.
   - Engaging in struggles over adherence does not help, but tying adherence to the patient's own goals does. ("Staying in treatment will help you keep your job and avoid trouble with the police.")
   - Share concerns about troubling adverse effects or concerns (e.g., sexual problems, weight gain, "feeling funny") with your nurse, case manager, doctor, or social worker; most adverse effects can be helped.
   - Keeping adverse effects a secret or stopping medication can prevent you from having the life you want.
5. Avoid alcohol and drugs; they can act on the brain and cause a relapse.
6. Keep in touch with supportive people.
7. Keep healthy—stay in balance.
   - Taking care of one's diet, health, and hygiene helps prevent medical illnesses.
   - Maintain a regular sleep pattern.
   - Keep active (hobbies, friends, groups, sports, job, special interests).
   - Nurture yourself, and practise stress-reduction activities daily.

Source: Data from Tandon, R., Harvey, P.D., & Nasrallah, H.A. (2003, October). *Beyond symptom control: Moving towards positive patient outcomes.* Paper presented at the American Psychiatric Association 55th Institute on Psychiatric Services Boston. Retrieved from http://www.medscape.com/viewprogram/2835_pnt.
Further information can be found in the pamphlet *For Consumers: Schizophrenia and Substance Abuse*, available at http://www.schizophrenia.ca/SSC_for_Consumers.pdf. or via the Your Recovery Journey Web site (Schizophrenia Society of Canada), http://www.your-recovery-journey.ca/.

INTEGRATIVE THERAPY

Yoga as an Adjunctive Treatment for Schizophrenia

Social and occupational functioning is a problem for people with schizophrenia. Studies indicate that yoga, in conjunction with conventional medical treatment, may improve symptoms of schizophrenia, social and occupational functioning, and quality of life. Yoga is based on an ancient Indian spiritual practice that has been reported to improve the connection among the mind, body, and spirit.

In a randomized controlled study by Duraiswamy and colleagues (2007), 61 people with a diagnosis of schizophrenia participated in a trial that compared the efficacy of physical exercise (stretching and aerobic) and yoga. Participants were supervised as they performed one or the other and also practised independently for one hour each day. After four months, both groups experienced symptom reduction, but subjects who had practised yoga showed greater improvement of both negative symptoms of schizophrenia and psychological quality of life.

Machleidt and Ziegenbein (2008) found that yoga together with traditional medical treatment improved not only quality of life but also occupational and social functioning. Yoga, therefore, is a promising adjunctive treatment for schizophrenia that provides participants with an essential experience of grounding, especially in distinguishing themselves from the outside world. It may be the centring quality of the breathing work, in particular, that improves the interrelationship of mind, body, and spirit.

A subsequent systematic review and meta-analysis by Cramer, Lauche, Klose, et al. (2013) found moderate evidence of short-term benefits of yoga on quality of life. However, these researchers caution that yoga should be considered on an individual patient basis and not prescribed as a routine intervention.

Sources: Cramer, H., Lauche, R., Klose, P., et al. (2013). Yoga and schizophrenia: A systematic review and meta-analysis. *BioMed Central, 13*(1), 1–12. doi: 10.1186/1471-244X-13-32.; Duraiswamy, G., Thirhalli, J., Nagendra, H.R., et al. (2007). Yoga therapy as an add-on treatment in the management of patients with schizophrenia—A randomized controlled trial. *Acta Psychiatrica Scandinavica, 3*, 226–232. doi:10.1111/j.1600-0447.2007.01032.x.; Machleidt, W., & Ziegenbein, M. (2008). An appreciation of yoga-therapy in the treatment of schizophrenia. *Acta Psychiatrica Scandinavica, 117*, 397–398. doi:10.1111/j.1600-0447.2008.01159.x.

Two groups of antipsychotic drugs exist: conventional antipsychotics (traditional dopamine antagonists [D_2 dopamine receptor antagonists]), also known as *typical* or *first-generation antipsychotics*, and atypical antipsychotics (serotonin–dopamine antagonists [$5\text{-}HT_{2A}$ receptor antagonists]), also known as *second-generation antipsychotics*. Newer "third-generation" drugs (aripiprazole [now available] and bifeprunox [pending]) give hope for enhanced effectiveness and adverse-effect reduction (Wadenberg, 2007). Other drugs, such as anticonvulsants and antiparkinsonian drugs, are used to augment antipsychotics for patients who do not respond fully. For example, D-serine—an amino acid that enhances NMDA activity—has been shown to increase the effectiveness of selected antipsychotics (Heresco-Levy, Javitt, Ebstein, et al., 2005).

All antipsychotics are effective for most exacerbations of schizophrenia and for reduction or mitigation of relapse. The conventional antipsychotics affect primarily the positive symptoms of schizophrenia (e.g., hallucinations, delusions, disordered thinking). The atypical antipsychotics can improve negative symptoms (e.g., asociality, blunted affect, lack of motivation) as well.

Antipsychotic agents usually take effect two to six weeks after the regimen is started. Only about 10% of people with schizophrenia fail to respond to antipsychotic drug therapy; these patients should not continue to take medication that holds only risks and no benefit for them.

Polypharmacy is an issue for patients with severe and persistent symptoms that do not respond easily to a single medication. It is not unusual to find patients being prescribed a combination of antipsychotic medications, sometimes both oral and depot or both typical and atypical. These individuals may also be taking antiparkinsonian agents and other medications to combat adverse effects. It is important in these cases to have the medication regime carefully and regularly reviewed by both the physician and a pharmacist and to monitor closely for adverse effects. These patients would be at high risk of anticholinergic toxicity, a potentially life-threatening situation (see Table 16-9).

Atypical Antipsychotics

Atypical antipsychotics first emerged in the early 1990s with clozapine (Clozaril). Unfortunately, clozapine produces agranulocytosis in 0.8% to 1% of those who take it and also increases the risk for seizures. Clozapine produced dramatic improvement in some patients whose disorder had been resistant to the earlier antipsychotics. Due to the risk for agranulocytosis, however, people taking clozapine must have weekly white blood cell counts for the first six months, then frequent monitoring thereafter, to obtain the medication. As a result, clozapine use is declining.

Atypicals are often chosen as first-line antipsychotics because they treat both the positive and negative symptoms of schizophrenia. Furthermore, they produce minimal to no extrapyramidal side effects (EPSs) or tardive dyskinesia in most people, although these effects may still occur for some patients. Adverse effects tend to be significantly less, resulting in greater adherence to treatment.

Atypical antipsychotics include risperidone (Risperdal), lurasidone (Latuda), olanzapine (Zyprexa), quetiapine (Seroquel), ziprasidone (Zeldox), and aripiprazole (Abilify), the last of which is technically a third-generation drug. These atypicals are free of the potential hematological adverse effects of clozapine and are all first-line agents because of their lower adverse-effect profile.

One significant disadvantage of the atypicals, with the exception of ziprasidone and aripiprazole, is that they have a tendency to cause significant weight gain. Metabolic syndrome—which includes weight gain, dyslipidemia, and altered glucose metabolism—is a significant concern with the administration of most atypicals and increases the risk of diabetes, hypertension, and atherosclerotic heart disease (Tschoner, Engl, Laimer, et al., 2007). An additional disadvantage of atypicals is cost: they are more expensive than conventional antipsychotics. Table 16-7 lists the classification, route, and adverse-effect profile of the antipsychotic drugs.

Conventional Antipsychotics

Conventional antipsychotics are antagonists at the D_2 dopamine receptor site in both the limbic and motor centres. This blockage of D_2 dopamine receptor sites in the motor areas causes extrapyramidal side effects (EPS), which include akathisia, acute dystonias, pseudoparkinsonism, and tardive dyskinesia. Other adverse reactions include anticholinergic effects, orthostasis, photosensitivity, and lowered seizure threshold.

Specific drugs are often chosen for their adverse-effect profiles. For example, chlorpromazine is the most sedating agent and has fewer EPSs than do other antipsychotic agents, but it causes significant hypotension. Haloperidol (Haldol) is less sedating and induces less hypotension but has a high incidence of EPSs. As a result, haloperidol has value for treating hallucinations because of its effectiveness in controlling positive symptoms with minimal hypotension and sedation. People taking these medications may prefer less sedating drugs, but those who are agitated or excitable may do better with a more sedating medication.

Conventional antipsychotics are becoming less common in the treatment of schizophrenia because of their minimal impact on negative symptoms and their adverse effects. However, conventional antipsychotics are effective against positive symptoms, are much less expensive than atypicals, and come in a depot (long-acting injectable) form, which is given once or twice a month. (*Note:* Risperidone, an atypical antipsychotic, is also available in a depot form [Risperdal Consta].) For people who respond to them and can tolerate their adverse effects, conventional antipsychotics remain an appropriate choice (Swartz, Perkins, Stroup, et al., 2007), especially when metabolic syndrome or cost are concerns.

The conventional antipsychotics are often divided into low-potency and high-potency drugs on the basis of their anticholinergic (ACh) adverse effects, EPSs, and sedative profiles:

Low potency = high sedation + high ACh + low EPSs
High potency = low sedation + low ACh + high EPSs

Conventional antipsychotics must be used cautiously in people with seizure disorders; they can lower the seizure threshold. Three of the more common EPSs are acute dystonia (acute sustained contraction of muscles, usually of the head and neck), akathisia (psychomotor restlessness evident as pacing or fidgeting, sometimes pronounced and very distressing to patients), and pseudoparkinsonism (a medication-induced, temporary constellation of symptoms associated with Parkinson's disease: tremor, reduced accessory movements, impaired gait, and stiffening of muscles). Most patients develop tolerance to these EPSs after a few months.

EPSs can usually be minimized by lowering dosages or adding antiparkinsonian drugs, especially centrally acting anticholinergic drugs such as trihexyphenidyl and benztropine

mesylate (Cogentin). Diphenhydramine hydrochloride (Benadryl) is also useful. Lorazepam, a benzodiazepine, may be helpful in reducing akathisia. Table 16-8 identifies some of the drugs most commonly used to treat EPSs.

Unfortunately, antiparkinsonian drugs can cause significant anticholinergic adverse effects and worsen the anticholinergic adverse effects of conventional antipsychotics and other anticholinergic medications. These adverse effects include anticholinergic syndrome, which is seen in the peripheral nervous system (tachycardia, hyperthermia, hypertension, dry skin, urinary retention, functional ileus) and central nervous system (mydriasis, hallucinations, delirium, seizures, and, in some cases, coma) (Ramjan, Williams, Isbister, et al., 2007). Other troubling adverse effects of conventional antipsychotics include weight gain, sexual dysfunction, endocrine disturbances (e.g., galactorrhea), drooling, and tardive dyskinesia, discussed in the following section. Weight gain, frequently a problem for women, can be more than 45 kilograms; therefore, changing the antipsychotic may be necessary. Impotence and sexual dysfunction are occasionally reported (but frequently experienced) by men and may also necessitate a medication change.

Table 16-9 identifies common adverse effects of the conventional antipsychotic medications, their usual times of onset, and related nursing and medical interventions.

Tardive dyskinesia (TD or TDK) is a persistent EPS that usually appears after prolonged treatment and persists even after the medication has been discontinued. TD is evidenced by involuntary tonic muscular contractions that typically involve the tongue, fingers, toes, neck, trunk, or pelvis. This potentially serious EPS is most frequently seen in women and older persons and affects up to 50% of individuals receiving long-term, high-dose therapy. TD varies from mild to moderate and can be disfiguring or incapacitating; a common presentation is a guppylike mouth movement sometimes accompanied by tongue protrusion. Its appearance can contribute to the stigmatization of people with mental illness.

Early symptoms of tardive dyskinesia are fasciculations of the tongue (described as looking like a bag of worms) or constant smacking of the lips. These symptoms can progress into uncontrollable biting, chewing, or sucking motions; an open mouth; and lateral movements of the jaw. No reliable treatment exists for tardive dyskinesia. The National Institute of Mental Health (NIMH) developed the Abnormal Involuntary Movement Scale (AIMS), a brief test for the detection of tardive dyskinesia and other involuntary movements (Figure 16-2 on pp. 309–310). It examines facial, oral, extremity, and trunk movement. Regularly administering the AIMS exam to detect TD as early as possible is a key nursing role.

Potentially Dangerous Responses to Antipsychotics

Nurses need to know about some rare—but serious and potentially fatal—effects of antipsychotic drugs, including neuroleptic malignant syndrome, agranulocytosis, liver impairment, and anticholinergic-induced delirium.

Neuroleptic malignant syndrome (NMS) occurs in about 0.2% to 1% of people who have taken conventional antipsychotics, although it can occur with atypicals as well. Acute

TABLE 16-7 ANTIPSYCHOTIC DRUGS: CLASSIFICATION, ROUTE, AND ADVERSE-EFFECT PROFILE

GENERIC (BRAND)	ROUTE	EPSS	SEDATION	ORTHOSTATIC HYPOTENSION	ANTICHOLINERGIC	WEIGHT GAIN	DIABETES
Atypical Antipsychotics—Treat Positive and Negative Symptoms							
Aripiprazole (Abilify)	PO	Very low	Low	Low	None	Low	Low
Clozapine (Clozaril)	PO	Very low	High	Moderate	High	High	High
Olanzapine (Zyprexa)	PO, IM	Very low	High	Moderate	High	High	High
Paliperidone (Invega)	PO	Moderate	Low	Low	None	Moderate	*
Quetiapine (Seroquel)	PO	Very low	Moderate	Moderate	None	Moderate	Moderate
Risperidone (Risperdal)	PO, IM	Very low	Low	Low	None	Moderate	Moderate
Ziprasidone (Zeldox)	PO, IM	Moderate	Moderate	Moderate	None	Low	Low
Conventional Antipsychotics—Treat Positive Symptoms							
Low Potency							
Chlorpromazine (generic only)	PO, IM, IV, R	Moderate	High	High	Moderate	Moderate	—
Medium Potency							
Loxapine (Loxapac)	PO	Moderate	Moderate	Low	Low	Low	—
Perphenazine (generic only)	PO	Moderate	Moderate	Low	Low	—	—
High Potency							
Thiothixene (Navane)	PO	High	Low	Moderate	Low	Moderate	—
Fluphenazine (Modecate)	PO, IM	High	Low	Low	Low	—	—
Haloperidol (Haldol)	PO, IM	High	Low	Low	Low	Moderate	—
Pimozide (Orap)	PO	High	Moderate	Low	Moderate	—	—
Conventional Antipsychotics for Which Limited Data Is Available							
Flupentixol (Fluanxol, Fluanxol Depot)	PO, IM	High	Low	Moderate	Low	—	—
Zuclopenthixol (Clopixol, Clopixol Depot, Clopixol Acuphase)	PO IM	—	—	—	May potentiate ACh effects of other drugs	—	—

*Data unavailable.
ACh = Anticholinergic adverse effects; *EPSs* = extrapyramidal side effects.
Sources: Canadian Pharmacists Association. (2011). *Electronic compendium of pharmaceuticals and specialties (eCPS)*. Retrieved from https://www.e-therapeutics.ca/; Centre for Addiction and Mental Health. (2009). *Types of antipsychotics*. Retrieved from http://www.camh.net/Care_Treatment/Resources_clients_families_friends/psych_meds/antipsychotics/upm_antipsychotics_types%20.html; Lehne, R.A. (2010). *Pharmacology for nursing care* (7th ed.). St. Louis, MO: Saunders; Martinez, M., Marangell, L.B., & Martinez, J.M. (2008). Psychopharmacology. In R.E. Hales, S.C. Yudofsky, & G.O. Gabbard (Eds.), *Textbook of psychiatry*. Arlington, VA: American Psychiatric Publishing.

TABLE 16-8	ANTIPARKINSONIAN AND ANTICHOLINERGIC AGENTS FOR TREATMENT OF EXTRAPYRAMIDAL SIDE EFFECTS

Note: All anticholinergic agents (ACAs) can contribute to the risk of anticholinergic toxicity. Practise caution when using multiple ACA agents. After one to six months of long-term maintenance antipsychotic therapy, most ACAs can be withdrawn.

GENERIC (TRADE) NAME	CHEMICAL TYPE
Trihexyphenidyl (Apo-Trihex, Artane)*	ACA
Benztropine mesylate (Cogentin)*	ACA
Diphenhydramine hydrochloride (Benadryl)	Antihistamine (used for its anticholinergic properties)

*Antiparkinsonian agent.
Source: Tirgobov, E., Wilson, B.A., Shannon, M.T., et al. (2005). *Psychiatric drug guide.* Upper Saddle River, NJ: Pearson/Prentice Hall.

reduction in brain dopamine activity plays a role in its development. NMS is a life-threatening medical emergency and is fatal in about 10% of cases. It usually occurs early in therapy but has been reported in people after 20 years of treatment.

NMS is characterized by reduced consciousness, increased muscle tone (muscular rigidity), and autonomic dysfunction—including hyperpyrexia, labile hypertension, tachycardia, tachypnea, diaphoresis, and drooling. Treatment consists of early detection, discontinuation of the antipsychotic, management of fluid balance, temperature reduction, and monitoring for complications. Mild cases of neuroleptic malignant syndrome may be treated with benzodiazepines, vitamins E and B6, or bromocriptine. More severe cases may even be treated with electroconvulsive therapy (ECT) (Agar, 2010; Haddad & Dursun, 2007). Dantrolene, recommended in much of the literature, carries a black box warning (the most serious medication warning required by the Food and Drug Administration) for hepatotoxicity in the United States (Agar, 2010) and is not available in Canada.

Agranulocytosis is a serious, potentially fatal, adverse effect. Liver impairment may also occur. Nurses need to be aware of the prodromal signs and symptoms of these adverse effects and teach them to patients and their families (see Table 16-9).

Anticholinergic-induced delirium is a potentially life-threatening adverse effect usually seen in older adults, although it can occur in younger people as well. It is also seen in patients taking multiple antipsychotic drugs. See Table 16-9 for symptoms and treatment of this serious adverse effect.

Adjuncts to Antipsychotic Drug Therapy

Antidepressants are recommended along with antipsychotic agents for the treatment of depression, which is common in schizophrenia. Refer to Chapter 14 for a more detailed discussion of depression and antidepressant drugs.

Antimanic (mood-stabilizing) agents have been helpful in enhancing the effectiveness of antipsychotics. Valproic acid (Epival, Valproate) is used during acute exacerbations of psychosis to hasten response to antipsychotics (Freudenreich, Weiss, & Goff, 2008). Lamotrigine may be given along with clozapine to improve therapeutic effects.

Augmentation with benzodiazepines (e.g., clonazepam) can reduce anxiety and agitation and contribute to improvement in positive and negative symptoms (Tirgobov, Wilson, Shannon, et al., 2005).

When to Change an Antipsychotic Regimen

The following circumstances suggest a need to adjust or change the antipsychotic agent or add supplemental medications (e.g., lithium, carbamazepine, valproate):
- Inadequate improvement in target symptoms despite an adequate trial of the drug
- Persistence of dangerous or intolerable adverse effects

Specific Interventions for Paranoia, Catatonia, and Disorganization

The following sections discuss paranoia, catatonia, and disorganization in psychoses and identify pertinent communication guidelines, self-care needs, and milieu needs.

Paranoia

Any intense and strongly defended irrational suspicion can be regarded as **paranoia**. Paranoia is evident, at least intermittently, in many people without psychotic disorders but is verified as irrational and discarded by the reality-testing process. This process fails in people experiencing paranoia concomitant with psychotic disorders. For them, paranoid ideas cannot be corrected by experiences or modified by facts or reality. *Projection* is the most common defence mechanism used in paranoia: when individuals with paranoia feel angry (or self-critical), they project the feeling onto others and believe others are angry with (or harshly critical toward) them—as if to say, "I'm not angry—you are!"

Schizophrenia with predominantly paranoid symptoms usually has a later age of onset (late 20s to 30s), develops rapidly in individuals with good premorbid functioning, tends to be intermittent during the first five years of the illness, and, in some cases, is associated with a good outcome or complete recovery. People with paranoia are usually frightened and may behave defensively (e.g., a delusion that another person is planning to kill the patient can result in the patient attacking or killing that person first). The paranoia is often a defence against painful feelings of loneliness, despair, helplessness, and fear of abandonment. Useful nursing strategies are outlined in the following sections.

Communication guidelines. Because people with paranoia have difficulty trusting those around them, they are usually guarded, tense, and reserved. To ensure interpersonal distance, they may adopt a superior, aloof, hostile, or sarcastic attitude, disparaging and dwelling on the shortcomings of others to maintain their self-esteem. Although they may shun interpersonal contact, functional impairment other than paranoia may

TABLE 16-9   ADVERSE EFFECTS OF CONVENTIONAL ANTIPSYCHOTICS AND RELATED NURSING INTERVENTIONS

ADVERSE EFFECT	NURSING INTERVENTIONS
Dry mouth	Provide frequent sips of water, ice chips, and sugarless candy or gum; if severe, provide moisture spray
Urinary retention and hesitancy	Check voiding Try warm towel on abdomen, and consider catheterization if no result
Constipation	Usually short term May use stool softener Ensure adequate fluid intake Increase fibre intake Use dietary laxatives (e.g., prune juice)
Blurred vision	Usually abates in 1 to 2 weeks May require use of reading or magnifying glasses If intolerable, consider consult regarding change in medication
Photosensitivity	Encourage person to wear sunglasses, sunscreen, and sun-blocking clothing Limit exposure to sunlight
Dry eyes	Use artificial tears
Inhibition of ejaculation or impotence in men	Consult prescriber: person may need alternative medication
Anticholinergic-induced delirium: dry mucous membranes; reduced or absent peristalsis; mydriasis; nonreactive pupils; hot, dry, red skin; hyperpyrexia without diaphoresis; tachycardia; agitation; unstable vital signs; worsening of psychotic symptoms; delirium; urinary retention; seizure; repetitive motor movements	***Potentially life-threatening medical emergency*** Consult prescriber immediately Hold all medications Implement emergency cooling measures as ordered (cooling blanket, alcohol, or ice bath) Implement urinary catheterization as needed Administer benzodiazepines or other sedation as ordered Physostigmine may be ordered
Pseudoparkinsonism: masklike facies, stiff and stooped posture, shuffling gait, drooling, tremor, "pill-rolling" phenomenon *Onset:* 5 hours–30 days	Administer prn antiparkinsonian agent (e.g., trihexyphenidyl or benztropine) If intolerable, consult prescriber regarding medication change Provide towel or handkerchief to wipe excess saliva
Acute dystonic reactions: acute contractions of tongue, face, neck, and back (usually tongue and jaw first) Opisthotonos: tetanic heightening of entire body, head and belly up Oculogyric crisis: eyes locked upward Laryngeal dystonia: could threaten airway (rare) Cogwheel rigidity: stiffness and clicking in elbow joints felt by the examiner during passive range of motion (early indicator of acute dystonia) *Onset:* 1–5 days	Administer antiparkinsonian agent as above—give IM for more rapid effect and because of swallowing difficulty Also consider diphenhydramine hydrochloride (Benadryl) 25–50 mg IM or IV Relief usually occurs in 5–15 minutes Prevent further dystonias with antiparkinsonian agent (see Table 16-8) Experience can be frightening, and person may fear choking Accompany to quiet area to provide comfort and support Assist person to understand the event and avert distortion or mistrust of medications Monitor airway
Akathisia: motor inner-driven restlessness (e.g., tapping foot incessantly, rocking forward and backward in chair, shifting weight from side to side) *Onset:* 2 hours–60 days	Consult prescriber regarding possible medication change Give antiparkinsonian agent Tolerance to akathisia does not develop, but akathisia disappears when neuroleptic is discontinued Propranolol (Inderal), lorazepam (Ativan), or diazepam (Valium) may be used In severe cases, may cause great distress and contribute to suicidality

Continued

TABLE 16-9 ADVERSE EFFECTS OF CONVENTIONAL ANTIPSYCHOTICS AND RELATED NURSING INTERVENTIONS—cont'd

ADVERSE EFFECT	NURSING INTERVENTIONS
Tardive dyskinesia (TD): *Face:* protruding and rolling tongue, blowing, smacking, licking, spastic facial distortion, smacking movements *Limbs:* Choreic: rapid, purposeless, and irregular movements Athetoid: slow, complex, and serpentine movements *Trunk:* neck and shoulder movements, dramatic hip jerks and rocking, twisting pelvic thrusts *Onset:* Months to years	No known treatment Discontinuing the drug rarely relieves symptoms Possibly 20% of people taking these drugs for >2 years may develop TD Nurses and doctors should encourage people to be screened for TD at least every 3 months Onset may merit reconsideration of meds Changes in appearance may contribute to stigmatizing response Teach patient actions to conceal involuntary movements (purposeful muscle contraction overrides involuntary tardive movements)
Hypotension and postural hypotension	Check blood pressure before giving agent: a systolic pressure of 80 mm Hg when standing is indication not to give the current dose Advise person to rise slowly to prevent dizziness and hold on to railings or furniture while rising to reduce falls Effect usually subsides when drug is stabilized in 1 to 2 weeks Elastic bandages may prevent pooling If condition is dangerous, consult prescriber regarding medication change, volume expanders, or pressure agents
Tachycardia	Always evaluate patients with existing cardiac problems before antipsychotic drugs are administered Haloperidol (Haldol) is usually the preferred drug because of its low ACh effects
Agranulocytosis (a rare occurrence, but a possibility the nurse should be aware of): symptoms include sore throat, fever, malaise, and mouth sores; any flulike symptoms should be carefully evaluated *Onset:* During the first 12 weeks of therapy, occurs suddenly	***A potentially dangerous blood dyscrasia*** Blood work usually done every week for 6 months, then every 2 months Physician may order blood work to determine presence of leukopenia or agranulocytosis If test results are positive, the drug is discontinued, and reverse isolation may be initiated Mortality is high if the drug is not ceased and if treatment is not initiated Teach person to observe for signs of infection
Cholestatic jaundice: rare, reversible, and usually benign if caught in time; prodromal symptoms are fever, malaise, nausea, and abdominal pain; jaundice appears 1 week later	Consult prescriber regarding possible medication change Bed rest and high-protein, high-carbohydrate diet if ordered Liver function tests should be performed every 6 months
Neuroleptic malignant syndrome (NMS): rare, potentially fatal *Severe extrapyramidal:* severe muscle rigidity, oculogyric crisis, dysphasia, flexor-extensor posturing, cogwheeling *Hyperpyrexia:* elevated temperature (over 39°C or 103°F) *Autonomic dysfunction:* hypertension, tachycardia, diaphoresis, incontinence *Delirium, stupor, coma* *Onset:* Variable, progresses rapidly over 2–3 days *Risk factors:* Concomitant use of psychotropics, older age, female, presence of a mood disorder, and rapid dose titration (increase)	***Acute, life-threatening medical emergency*** Stop neuroleptic Transfer stat to medical unit Bromocriptine can relieve muscle rigidity and reduce fever Cool body to reduce fever (cooling blankets, alcohol, cool water, or ice bath as ordered) Maintain hydration with oral and IV fluids; correct electrolyte imbalance Arrhythmias should be treated Small doses of heparin may decrease possibility of pulmonary emboli Early detection increases patient's chance of survival

Source: Kemmerer, D.A. (2007). Anticholinergic syndrome. *Journal of Emergency Nursing, 33*, 76–78. doi:10.1016/j.jen.2006.10.013.

be minimal. These people frequently misinterpret the intent or actions of others, perceiving oversights as personal rejection. They also may personalize unrelated events (ideas of reference, or *referentiality*). For example, a patient might see a nurse talking to the psychiatrist and believe the two are talking about her.

During care, a patient suffering from paranoia may make offensive yet accurate criticisms of staff and of unit policies. It is important that responses focus on reducing the patient's anxiety and fear and not be defensive reactions or rejections of the patient. Staff conferences and clinical supervision help

---

ABNORMAL INVOLUNTARY MOVEMENT SCALE (AIMS)

Public Health Service
Alcohol, Drug Abuse, and Mental Health Administration
National Institute of Mental Health

Name: _____
Date: _____
Prescribing Practitioner: _____

Code: 0 = None
1 = Minimal, may be extreme normal
2 = Mild
3 = Moderate
4 = Severe

Instructions: Complete Examination Procedure before making ratings.

Movement ratings: Rate highest severity observed. Rate movements that occur upon activation one *less* than those observed spontaneously. Circle movement as well as code number that applies.		Rater Date	Rater Date	Rater Date	Rater Date
Facial and Oral Movements	**1. Muscles of facial expression** (e.g., movements of forehead, eyebrows, periorbital area, cheeks, including frowning, blinking, smiling, grimacing)	0 1 2 3 4	0 1 2 3 4	0 1 2 3 4	0 1 2 3 4
	2. Lips and perioral area (e.g., puckering, pouting, smacking)	0 1 2 3 4	0 1 2 3 4	0 1 2 3 4	0 1 2 3 4
	3. Jaw (e.g., biting, clenching, chewing, mouth opening, lateral movement)	0 1 2 3 4	0 1 2 3 4	0 1 2 3 4	0 1 2 3 4
	4. Tongue: Rate only increases in movement both in and out of mouth — *not* inability to sustain movement. Darting in and out of mouth.	0 1 2 3 4	0 1 2 3 4	0 1 2 3 4	0 1 2 3 4
Extremity Movements	**5. Upper (arms, wrists, hands, fingers):** Include choreic movements (i.e., rapid, objectively purposeless, irregular, spontaneous) and athetoid movements (i.e., slow, irregular, complex, serpentine). *Do not include tremor* (i.e., repetitive, regular, rhythmic).	0 1 2 3 4	0 1 2 3 4	0 1 2 3 4	0 1 2 3 4
	6. Lower (legs, knees, ankles, toes) (e.g., lateral knee movement, foot tapping, heel dropping, foot squirming, inversion and eversion of foot)	0 1 2 3 4	0 1 2 3 4	0 1 2 3 4	0 1 2 3 4
Trunk Movements	**7. Neck, shoulder, hips** (e.g., rocking, twisting, squirming, pelvic gyrations)	0 1 2 3 4	0 1 2 3 4	0 1 2 3 4	0 1 2 3 4
Global Judgments	**8. Severity of abnormal movements overall**	0 1 2 3 4	0 1 2 3 4	0 1 2 3 4	0 1 2 3 4
	9. Incapacitation due to abnormal movements	0 1 2 3 4	0 1 2 3 4	0 1 2 3 4	0 1 2 3 4
	10. Patient's awareness of abnormal movements: Rate only patient's report. No awareness　　　　　0 Aware, no distress　　　1 Aware, mild distress　　2 Aware, moderate distress　3 Aware, severe distress　4	0 1 2 3 4	0 1 2 3 4	0 1 2 3 4	0 1 2 3 4
Dental Status	**11. Current problems with teeth and/or dentures**	No　Yes	No　Yes	No　Yes	No　Yes
	12. Are dentures usually worn?	No　Yes	No　Yes	No　Yes	No　Yes
	13. Edentia	No　Yes	No　Yes	No　Yes	No　Yes
	14. Do movements disappear in sleep?	No　Yes	No　Yes	No　Yes	No　Yes

FIGURE 16-2 Abnormal Involuntary Movement Scale (AIMS).

Continued

AIMS Examination Procedure

Either before or after completing the Examination Procedure, observe the patient unobtrusively, at rest (e.g., in waiting room).

The chair to be used in this examination should be a hard, firm one without arms.

1. Ask patient to remove shoes and socks.
2. Ask patient whether there is anything in his or her mouth (e.g., gum, candy) and, if there is, to remove it.
3. Ask patient about the *current* condition of his or her teeth. Ask patient if he or she wears dentures. Do teeth or dentures bother the patient *now*?
4. Ask patient whether he or she notices any movements in mouth, face, hands, or feet. If yes, ask to describe and to what extent they *currently* bother patient or interfere with his or her activities.
5. Have patient sit in chair with hands on knees, legs slightly apart, and feet flat on floor. Look at entire body movements while in this position.
6. Ask patient to sit with hands hanging unsupported: if male, between legs; if female and wearing a dress, hanging over knees. Observe hands and other body areas.
7. Ask patient to open mouth. Observe tongue at rest within mouth. Do this twice.
8. Ask patient to protrude tongue. Observe abnormalities of tongue movement. Do this twice.
9. Ask patient to tap thumb, with each finger, as rapidly as possible for 10 to 15 seconds, separately with right hand, then with left hand. Observe each facial and leg movement.
10. Flex and extend patient's left and right arms (one at a time). Note any rigidity.
11. Ask patient to stand up. Observe in profile. Observe all body areas again, hips included.
12. Ask patient to extend both arms outstretched in front with palms down. Observe trunk, legs, and mouth.
13. Have patient walk a few paces, turn, and walk back to chair. Observe hands and gait. Do this twice.

FIGURE 16-2, cont'd

maintain objectivity and a therapeutic perspective about the patient's motivation and behaviour, increasing professional effectiveness.

Self-care needs. People with paranoia usually have stronger ego resources than do individuals in whom other symptoms predominate; this is particularly evident in occupational functioning and capacity for independent living. Grooming, dress, and self-care may not be problems and may, in fact, be meticulous. Nutrition, however, may be affected by a delusion, such as that the food is poisoned. Providing foods in commercially sealed packaging—for example, peanut butter and crackers or nutritional drinks in cartons—can improve nutrition. If people worry that others will harm them when they are asleep, they may be fearful of going to sleep—a problem that impairs restorative rest and warrants nursing intervention.

Milieu needs. A person with paranoia may become physically aggressive in response to his or her paranoid hallucinations or delusions. The person projects hostile drives onto others and then acts on these drives. Homosexual urges are projected onto others as well, and fear of sexual advances from others may stimulate aggression. An environment that provides a sense of security and safety minimizes anxiety and environmental distortions. Activities that distract the patient from ruminating on paranoid themes also decrease anxiety.

Case Study and Nursing Care Plan 16-1 on pages 313–315 discusses a person with paranoia.

Catatonia: Withdrawn Phase

The essential feature of catatonia is abnormal levels of motor behaviour, either extreme motor agitation or extreme motor retardation. Other associated behaviours include posturing, waxy flexibility (described below), stereotyped behaviour,

muteness, extreme negativism or automatic obedience, echolalia, and echopraxia (discussed earlier in this chapter). The onset of catatonia is usually abrupt, and the prognosis favourable. With pharmacotherapy and improved individual management, severe catatonic symptoms are rarely seen today. Useful nursing strategies for intervening in catatonia are discussed in the following sections.

Communication guidelines. People with catatonia can be so withdrawn they appear stuporous or comatose. They can be mute and may remain so for hours, days, or even weeks or months if untreated. Although such patients may not appear to pay attention to events going on around them, they are acutely aware of the environment and may accurately remember events at a later date. Developing skill and confidence in working with withdrawn patients takes practice. The person's inability or refusal to cooperate or participate in activities challenges staff to work to remain objective and avert frustration and anger.

Self-care needs. In extreme withdrawal, a person may need to be hand- or tube-fed to maintain adequate nutritional status. Aspiration is a risk. Normal control over bladder and bowel functions may be interrupted, so the assessment and management of urinary or bowel retention or incontinence is essential. When physical movements are minimal or absent, range-of-motion exercises can reduce muscular atrophy, calcium depletion, and contractures. Dressing and grooming usually require direct assistance.

Milieu needs. The catatonic person's appearance may range from decreased spontaneous movement to complete stupor. Waxy flexibility is often seen; for example, if the patient raises arms over the head, he or she may maintain that position for hours or longer. Caution is advised because, even after holding a single posture for long periods, the patient may suddenly and without provocation show brief outbursts of gross motor activity in response to inner hallucinations, delusions, and changes in neurotransmitter levels.

Catatonia: Excited Phase

Communication guidelines. During the excited stage of catatonia, the patient is in a state of greatly increased motor activity. He or she may talk or shout continually and incoherently, requiring the nurse's communication to be clear, direct, and loud (enough to focus the patient's attention on the nurse) and to reflect concern for the safety of the patient and others.

Self-care needs. A person who is constantly and intensely hyperactive can become completely exhausted and even die if medical attention is not available. Patients with coexisting medical conditions (e.g., congestive heart failure) are most at risk. Intramuscular administration of a sedating antipsychotic is often required to reduce psychomotor agitation to a safer level. During heightened physical activity, the patient requires stimulation reduction and additional fluids, calories, and rest. It is not unusual for the agitated person to be destructive or aggressive to others in response to hallucinations or delusions or inner distress. Many of the concerns and interventions are the same as those for mania. See Chapter 15 for more information about bipolar disorders.

Disorganization

Disorganization represents the most regressed and socially impaired form of schizophrenia. A person with disorganization may have marked associative looseness, grossly inappropriate affect, bizarre mannerisms, and incoherence of speech and may display extreme social withdrawal. Delusions and hallucinations are fragmentary and poorly organized. Behaviour may be considered odd, and a giggling or grimacing response to internal stimuli is common.

Disorganization has an earlier age of onset (early to middle teens), often develops insidiously, is associated with poor premorbid functioning and a significant family history of psychiatric disorders, and carries a poor prognosis. Often, these people reside in long-term care facilities and can live safely in the community only in a structured, well-supervised setting or with intensive follow-up such as a PACT (Program for Assertive Community Treatment) service. Families of patients living at home need significant community support, respite care, and access to day hospital services. Unfortunately, a good portion of these people become homeless. See the Case Study and Nursing Care Plan for Disorganized Thinking on the Evolve Web site.

Communication guidelines. People with disorganization experience persistent and severe perceptual and communication problems. Communication should be concise, clear, and concrete. Tasks should be broken into discrete tasks that are performed one at a time. Repeated refocusing may be needed to keep the patient on topic or to allow task completion. This repetition can be frustrating to the nurse and others, requiring special effort to identify and correct counter-transference and nontherapeutic responses.

Self-care needs. In people with disorganization, grooming is neglected; hair is often dirty and matted, and clothes are unclean and often inappropriate for the weather (presenting a risk to self). Cognition, memory, and executive function are grossly impaired, and the person is frequently too disorganized to carry out simple activities of daily living (ADLs). Areas of nursing focus include encouraging optimal levels of functioning, preventing further regression, and offering alternatives for inappropriate behaviours whenever possible. Significant direct assistance for ADLs is also needed.

Milieu needs. People with disorganization need assistance to conform their behaviour to social expectations. Nurses should provide for the patient's privacy needs. Peer education about the disorder may reduce peer frustration and acting out.

VIGNETTE

Martin, a 36-year-old man, is accompanied to the mental health centre by his mother. Ms. Lam, Martin's nurse, obtains background information from his mother. According to her, he had been in a long-term care facility for treatment of schizophrenia for three months and, after his discharge, had been doing well at home until recently. His only employment history was five months as a janitor after high school graduation. His mother states that, as a teenager, Martin was an excellent athlete and received average grades. At age 17, he had his first psychotic break, when he took various street drugs. His behaviour became markedly bizarre (e.g., eating cat food and swallowing a rubber-soled heel, which precipitated an emergency laparotomy).

Ms. Lam meets with Martin. He is unshaven and dishevelled. He is wearing a headband that holds Popsicle sticks and paper scraps. He chain-smokes, paces, and frequently changes position. He reports that he is Alice from Alice in the Underground and that people from space hurt him with needles. His speech is marked by associative looseness and occasional blocking, and he often stops in the middle of a phrase and giggles to himself.

He starts to giggle, and Ms. Lam asks what he is thinking about. He states, "You interrupted me." He then begins to shake his head while repeating in a singsong voice, "Shake them tigers ... shake them tigers. ..." He denies suicidal or homicidal ideation. Ms. Lam notes that Martin has great difficulty accurately perceiving what is going on around him. He exhibits regressed social behaviours (e.g., eating with his hands and picking his nose in public). He has no apparent insight into his problems, telling Ms. Lam that his biggest problem is the people in space.

Advanced-Practice Interventions

Services that may be provided by advanced-practice nurses and nurse therapists include psychotherapy, cognitive-behavioural therapy (CBT), group therapy, medication administration, social skills training, cognitive remediation, and family therapy. Family therapy is one of the most important interventions the advanced-practice nurse or nurse therapist can implement for the patient with schizophrenia.

Family Therapy

Family therapy is a service usually delivered by health care providers with specific education in this area, including advanced-practice nurses, nurse therapists, master's-prepared social workers, and registered marriage and family therapists. The field of family therapy was actually originally developed as a treatment for schizophrenia. Families of people with schizophrenia, particularly direct caregivers, often endure considerable hardships while coping with the psychotic and residual symptoms of the illness. The patient and family may become isolated from other relatives, communities, and support systems. In fact, until the 1970s (and sometimes even today), families were often blamed for causing schizophrenia in the affected family member.

Family education and family therapy improve the quality of life for the person with schizophrenia and reduce the relapse rate for many.

The following example shows how a family came to distinguish between "Martha's problem" and "the problem caused by schizophrenia":

> It was a good idea, us all meeting in our own home to discuss my sister's illness. We were all able to say how it felt, and for the first time I realized that I knew very little about what she was suffering or how much—the word *schizophrenia* meant nothing to me before. I used to think she was just being lazy until she told me what it was really like. (Gamble & Brennan, 2000, p. 192)

Programs that provide support, education, coping skills training, and social network development are extremely effective. This psychoeducational approach brings educational and behavioural approaches into family treatment and does not blame families but, rather, recognizes them as secondary victims of a biological illness. In family therapy sessions, fears, faulty communication patterns, and distortions are identified; problem-solving skills are taught; healthier alternatives to conflict are explored; and guilt and anxiety can be lessened.

EVALUATION

Evaluation is especially important in planning care for people who have psychotic disorders. Outcome expectations that are unrealistic discourage the patient and staff alike. It is critical for staff to remember that change is a process that occurs over time. For a person with schizophrenia, progress may occur erratically, and gains may be difficult to discern in the short term.

Chronically ill people must be reassessed regularly so that new data can be considered and treatment adjusted when needed. Questions to be asked include the following:

- Is the patient not progressing because a more important need is not being met?
- Is the staff making the best use of the patient's strengths and interests to promote treatment and achieve desired outcomes?
- Are other possible interventions being overlooked?
- Are new or better interventions available?
- How is the patient responding to existing or recently changed medications or other treatments?

┌─────────────────────────────────┐
RESEARCH HIGHLIGHT
└─────────────────────────────────┘

Cognitive Interventions for Auditory Hallucinations

Source: England, M. (2007). Efficacy of cognitive nursing intervention for voice hearing. *Perspectives in Psychiatric Care, 43*, 69–76. doi:10.1111/j.1744-6163.2007.00114.x.

Problem
Medications alone do not always fully relieve hallucinations. Research has suggested that cognitive interventions can reduce distress stemming from residual hallucinations.

Purpose of Study
This study sought to determine whether structured cognitive nursing interventions would produce significant improvement in a population of people who hear voices.

Methods
Patients were divided into a usual-care control group and an experimental structured-cognitive-interventions group. Symptom reports, treatment adherence, and other parameters were measured before and after intervention. A clinical nurse specialist provided twelve 90-minute, individual cognitive sessions focusing on patients' thoughts about their hallucinations and alternative ways of thinking about their hallucinations that would be more reality-based and less distressing.

Key Findings
The cognitive-intervention group demonstrated significant improvement in self-esteem and reduced distress related to symptoms. This outcome is consistent with research showing that hearing voices is tied to poor self-esteem and the nature of one's relationship with the voices.

Implications for Nursing Practice
Existing cognitive interventions, when added to traditional psychopharmacology, can significantly enhance symptom management. Although within the scope of practice for nurses, such interventions are not consistently used at present. Training nurses in their use and providing other support to increase their use has the potential to contribute to a higher quality of life for patients with residual hallucinations.

- Is the patient becoming discouraged, anxious, or depressed?
- Is the patient participating in treatment? Are adverse effects controlled or troubling?
- Is functioning improving or regressing?
- What is the patient's quality of life, and is it improving?
- Is the family involved, supportive, and knowledgeable regarding the patient's disorder and treatment?

Active staff involvement and interest in the patient's progress communicate concern and caring, help the patient to maximize progress, promote participation in treatment, and reduce staff feelings of helplessness and burnout. Input from the patient can offer valuable information about why a certain desired outcome has not occurred.

CASE STUDY AND NURSING CARE PLAN 16-1

Paranoia in Schizophrenia

Tom, a 32-year-old man, is an inpatient at a Veterans Affairs Canada hospital. He has been separated from his wife and four children for three years. His records state that he has been in and out of hospitals for 13 years. Tom is a former master seaman who first "heard voices" at the age of 19 while he was serving in the Gulf War. He subsequently received a medical discharge.

The hospitalization was precipitated by an exacerbation of auditory hallucinations. "I thought people were following me. I hear voices, usually a woman's voice, and she's tormenting me. People say that it happens because I don't take my medications. The medications make me tired, and I can't have sex." Tom also uses marijuana, which he knows increases his paranoia. "It makes me feel good, and not much else does." Tom finished 11 years of school but did not graduate. He says he has no close friends. He spent five years in prison for manslaughter and was abusing alcohol and drugs when the crime occurred. Drug abuse has also been a contributing factor to Tom's psychiatric hospitalizations.

Ms. Lally is Tom's nurse. Tom is dressed in T-shirt and jeans, his hygiene is good, and he is well nourished. He reports that "the voices get worse at night, and I can't sleep." Ms. Lally notes in Tom's medical record that he has had two episodes of suicidal ideation, during which the voices were telling him to jump "off

rooftops" and "in front of trains." During the first interview, Tom rarely makes eye contact and speaks in a low monotone. At times, he glances about the room as if distracted, mumbles to himself, and appears upset.

Nurse: "Tom, my name is Ms. Lally. I will be your nurse today and every day that I am here. If it is okay with you, we will meet every day for 30 minutes at 10 in the morning. We can talk about areas of concern to you."

Tom: "Well, don't believe what they say about me. I want to start. ... Are you married?"

Nurse: "This time is for you to talk about your concerns."

Tom: "Oh ..." (Looks furtively around the room, then lowers his eyes) "I think someone is trying to kill me. ..."

Nurse: "You seem to be focusing on something other than our conversation."

Tom: "The voices tell me things ... I can't say ..."

Nurse: "It seems like the voices are upsetting to you. I can't hear them. What kinds of things are they saying?"

Tom: "The voices tell me bad things."

Ms. Lally stays with Tom and encourages him to communicate with her. As Tom focuses more on the conversation, his anxiety appears to lessen. His thoughts become more connected, he is able to concentrate more, and he mumbles to himself less.

ASSESSMENT

Self-Assessment

On the first day of admission, Tom assaults another male patient, stating that the other person accused him of being a homosexual and touched him on the buttocks. After assessing the incident, the staff agrees that Tom's provocation came more from his own projections (Tom's sexual attraction to the other person) than from anything the other person did or said.

Tom's difficulty with impulse control frightens Ms. Lally. She has concerns regarding Tom's ability to curb his impulses and the possibility of Tom's striking out at her, especially when Tom is hallucinating and highly delusional. Ms. Lally mentions her concerns to the nursing coordinator, who suggests that Ms. Lally meet with Tom in the day room until he demonstrates more control and less suspicion of others. After five days, Tom is less excitable, and the sessions are moved to a room reserved for private interviews. Ms. Lally also speaks with a senior staff nurse regarding her fears. By talking to the senior nurse and understanding more clearly her own fear, Ms. Lally is able to manage her fear and identify interventions to help Tom regain a better sense of control.

Objective Data	Subjective Data
Speaks in low monotone	"I hear voices."
Makes poor eye contact	"I think someone is trying to kill me. ..."
Weight appropriate for height	"I don't take my medications. [They] make me tired, and I can't
Clean, bathed, clothes match	have sex."
Impaired reality testing	"The voices get worse at night and I can't sleep."
Has a history of drug abuse (marijuana), which appears to	"[Marijuana] makes me feel good, and not much else does."
contribute to relapses	Voices have told him to jump "off rooftops" and "in front of
Has no close friends, separated from wife and children	trains."
Was first hospitalized at age 19 and has not worked since that	
time	
Has had suicidal impulses twice, both associated with command	
hallucinations	
Was imprisoned for five years for violence (manslaughter) and	
assaulted a peer in the hospital	
Thoughts scattered when anxious	

DIAGNOSIS

1. *Disturbed thought processes* related to alteration in neurological function, as evidenced by persecutory hallucinations and paranoia

Continued

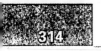

CASE STUDY AND NURSING CARE PLAN 16-1—cont'd

Paranoia in Schizophrenia

Supporting Data
- Voices have told him to jump "off rooftops" and "in front of trains."
- "I think someone is trying to kill me."
- Abuses marijuana (although it increases paranoia) because "it makes me feel good."

2. *Nonadherence to medication regimen* related to adverse effects of therapy, as evidenced by verbalization of nonadherence and persistence of symptoms

Supporting Data
- Failure to take prescribed medications because "they make me tired, and I can't have sex."
- Chronic history of relapse of symptoms

OUTCOMES IDENTIFICATION

1. Tom consistently refrains from acting on his "voices" and suspicions.
2. Tom consistently adheres to treatment regimen.

PLANNING

The nurse plans intervention that will (1) help Tom deal with his disturbing thoughts and (2) minimize drug abuse and adverse effects of medication to increase adherence and decrease the potential for relapse and violence.

IMPLEMENTATION

1. **Nursing diagnosis:** Disturbed thought processes
   Outcome: Tom consistently refrains from acting on his "voices" and suspicions when they occur.

Short-Term Goal	Intervention	Rationale	Evaluation
1. By the end of the first week, Tom will recognize the presence of hallucinations and identify one or more contributing factors, as evidenced by telling his nurse when they occur and what preceded them.	1a. Meet with Tom each day for 30 minutes to establish trust and rapport. 1b. Explore those times when voices are most threatening and disturbing, noting the circumstances that precede them. 1c. Provide noncompetitive activities that focus on the here and now.	1a. Short, consistent meetings help decrease anxiety and establish trust. 1b. Identifying events that increase anxiety and trigger "voices" and then learning to manage triggers, hallucinations can be reduced. 1c. Increased time spent in reality-based activities decreases focus on hallucinations.	**GOAL MET** By the end of the first week, Tom tells the nurse when he is experiencing hallucinations.
2. By the end of the first week, Tom will recognize hallucinations as "not real" and ascribe them to his illness.	2a. Explore content of hallucinations with Tom. 2b. Educate Tom about the nature of hallucinations and ways to determine if "voices" are real.	2a. Exploring hallucinations identifies suicidal or aggressive themes or command hallucinations. 2b. Education improves Tom's reality testing and helps him begin to attribute his experiences to schizophrenia.	**GOAL MET** Tom identifies that the voices tell him he is a loser and he needs to be careful "because someone is after me." He identifies that the voices are worse at nighttime. He notes that others do not seem to hear what he hears and also states that smoking marijuana produces very threatening voices.
3. By discharge, Tom will consistently report a decrease in hallucinations.	3. Explore with Tom possible actions that can minimize anxiety and reduce hallucinations, such as whistling or reading aloud.	3. Such activities offer alternatives while anxiety level is relatively low.	**GOAL MET** Tom states that he is hearing voices less often, and they are less threatening to him. Tom identifies that if he whistles or sings, he stays calm and can control the voices.

Continued

CASE STUDY AND NURSING CARE PLAN 16-1—cont'd

Paranoia in Schizophrenia

2. **Nursing diagnosis:** Nonadherence to medication regimen
   Outcome: Tom consistently adheres to medication regimen.

Short-Term Goal	Intervention	Rationale	Evaluation
1. By the end of week 1, Tom will discuss his concerns about medication with staff.	1a. Evaluate medication response and adverse-effect issues. 1b. Initiate medication change to olanzapine (Zyprexa). Administer a large dose at bedtime to increase sleep and a small dose during the day to decrease fatigue. 1c. Educate Tom regarding adverse effects—how long they last and what actions can be taken.	1a. Such evaluation identifies drugs and dosages that have increased therapeutic value and decreased adverse effects. 1b. Olanzapine causes no known sexual difficulties. 1c. This knowledge can give an increased sense of control over symptoms.	**GOAL MET** Tom identifies the reasons for stopping his medication. He agrees to try olanzapine because he trusts staff's assurances that the adverse effects will be reduced. Tom states that he sleeps better at night but is still tired during the day.
2. By the end of week 2, Tom will describe two ways to reduce or cope with adverse effects and two ways the medications help him meet his goals (e.g., avoiding jail and reducing fear).	2a. Connect Tom with the local Schizophrenia Society support group.	2a. Being part of a group provides peer support and a chance to hear from others (further along in recovery) how medications can be helpful and adverse effects can be managed. The peer group can also offer suggestions for dealing with his loneliness and other problems.	**GOAL MET** **Week 1:** Tom attends meeting. **Week 2:** He speaks in the group about "not feeling good." Several group members say they understand and try to help him figure out why he is not feeling good. Peers tell him how taking medication has helped them feel better.

EVALUATION

By discharge, Tom expresses hope that the medications will help him feel better and avoid problems like jail. He has a better understanding of his medications and what to do for adverse effects. He knows that marijuana increases his symptoms and explains that when he gets lonely, he now has ideas of things other than drugs he can do to "feel good." Tom continues with the support group and outpatient counselling, stating that his reason for doing so is "because Ms. Lally really cared about me"; her caring made him want to get better and led him to trust what staff told him. He reports sleeping much better and says that he has more energy during the day.

■ KEY POINTS TO REMEMBER

- Schizophrenia is a biological disorder of the brain. It is not one disorder but a group of disorders with overlapping symptoms and treatments.
- Recovery is increasingly possible with early identification, new treatments, and adequate social supports.
- The primary differences among subtypes involve the spectrum of symptoms that dominate their severity, the impairment in affect and cognition, and the impact on social and other areas of functioning.
- Psychotic symptoms are often more pronounced and obvious than are symptoms found in other disorders, making schizophrenia more likely to be apparent to others and increasing the risk of stigmatization.
- Neurochemical (catecholamines and serotonin), genetic, and neuroanatomical findings help explain the symptoms of schizophrenia. However, no one theory accounts fully for the complexities of schizophrenia.

- There are four categories of symptoms of schizophrenia: positive, negative, cognitive, and affective. Symptoms vary considerably among people and fluctuate over time.
- The positive symptoms of schizophrenia (e.g., hallucinations, delusions, associative looseness) are more pronounced and respond best to antipsychotic drug therapy.
- The negative symptoms of schizophrenia (e.g., social withdrawal and dysfunction, lack of motivation, reduced affect) respond less well to antipsychotic therapy and tend to be more debilitating.
- The degree of cognitive impairment (cognitive symptom) warrants careful assessment and active intervention to increase the patient's ability to adapt, function, and maximize his or her quality of life.
- Coexisting depression (affective symptom) must be identified and treated to reduce the potential for suicide, substance abuse, nonadherence, and relapse.

- Some applicable nursing diagnoses include *Disturbed sensory perception, Disturbed thought processes, Impaired communication, Ineffective coping, Risk for self-directed or other-directed violence,* and *Impaired family coping.*
- Outcomes are chosen based on the type and phase of schizophrenia and the person's individual needs, strengths, and level of functioning. Short-term and intermediate indicators are also developed to better track the incremental progress typical of schizophrenia.
- Interventions for people with schizophrenia include trust building, therapeutic communication techniques, support, assistance with self-care, promotion of independence, stress management, promotion of socialization, psychoeducation to promote understanding and adaptation, milieu management, cognitive-behavioural interventions, cognitive

enhancement or remediation techniques, and medication administration.
- Because antipsychotic medications are essential in the care of people with schizophrenia, the nurse must understand the properties, adverse and toxic effects, and dosages of conventional and atypical antipsychotics and other medications used to treat schizophrenia. The nurse helps the patient and family understand and appreciate the importance of medication to recovery.
- Schizophrenia can produce counter-transference responses in staff; clinical supervision and self-assessment help the nurse remain objective and therapeutic.
- Hope is closely tied to recovery; it is essential for nurses to hold hope for people with schizophrenia.

CRITICAL THINKING

1. Jasmine, a 24-year-old woman, is hospitalized after an abrupt onset of psychosis and is diagnosed with paranoid schizophrenia. Jasmine is recently divorced and works as a legal secretary. Her work had become erratic, and her suspiciousness was attracting negative responses. Jasmine is being discharged in two days to her mother's care until she is able to resume her job. Jasmine's mother is overwhelmed and asks the nurse how she is going to cope: "I can hardly say anything to Jasmine without her getting upset. She is still mad at me because I called 911 and had her admitted. She says there is nothing wrong with her, and I'm worried she'll stop her medication once she is home. What am I going to do?"
   a. Explain Jasmine's behaviour and symptoms to a classmate as you would to Jasmine's mother.

   b. How would you respond to the mother's immediate concerns?
   c. What are some of the priority concerns the nurse should address before discharge?
   d. Identify interventions that are based on the concepts of the recovery model.
   e. What are some community resources that can help support this family? Describe how each could be helpful to this family.
   f. What do you think of the prognosis for Jasmine? Support your position with data regarding Jasmine's diagnosis and the treatment you have planned.

CHAPTER REVIEW

1. A person is found in a closet with an empty two-litre bottle of cola taken from the staff refrigerator. The bottle was full but now is empty. Recently, staff have noticed an increase in this person's response to auditory hallucinations and the recent addition of confusion to his symptoms. For the past several days, the person has been seen drinking from the hallway water cooler and taking items from his peers' dinner trays. Which response is most appropriate for decreasing these behaviours?
   1. Place the person on every-15-minute checks to identify any further deterioration.
   2. Restrict his access to fluids, and evaluate for water intoxication via daily weights.
   3. Attempt to distract the person from excess fluid intake and other bizarre behaviour.
   4. Request an increase in antipsychotic medication, owing to the worsening of his psychosis.

2. Jim is sometimes seen moving his lips silently or murmuring to himself when he does not realize others are watching. Sometimes when he is conversing with others, he suddenly stops, appears distracted for a moment, and then resumes. Based on these observations, which symptom or set of symptoms is Jim most likely experiencing? Select all that apply.
   1. Illusions
   2. Paranoia
   3. Delusional thinking
   4. Auditory hallucinations
   5. Impaired reality testing
   6. Stereotyped behaviours

3. Maricel, a person diagnosed with schizophrenia, is encouraged to attend groups but stays in her room instead. Staff and peers encourage her participation, but her hygiene remains poor. She does not seem to care that others wish that she would behave differently. Which is the most likely explanation for Maricel's failure to respond to others' efforts to help her behave in a more adaptive fashion? Select all that apply.
   1. She is avolitional.
   2. She is displaying anergia.
   3. She is displaying negativism.
   4. She is exhibiting paranoid delusions.
   5. She is being resistant or oppositional.
   6. She is experiencing social withdrawal.
   7. She is apathetic due to her schizophrenia.

4. The nurse is attempting to interview Mr. Jones, a newly admitted involuntary person with schizophrenia. Mr. Jones seems evasive and uncomfortable and gives one-word responses that are minimally informative. Which response would be most useful for facilitating the interview?
   1. "Why did you come to the hospital today?"
   2. "It must be difficult to be admitted to a hospital against your will."
   3. "If you could cooperate for just a few minutes, we could get this done."
   4. "Did your schizophrenia get worse because you stopped taking your medication?"

5. A week later, Mr. Jones has begun to take the conventional antipsychotic haloperidol. You approach him with his bedtime dose and notice that he is sitting very stiffly and immobile. When you approach, you notice that he is diaphoretic, and when you ask if he is okay he seems unable to turn towards you or to respond verbally. You also notice that his eyes are aimed sharply upward and he seems frightened. How should the nurse respond to reduce the symptoms displayed by Mr. Jones? Select all that apply.

   1. Begin to wipe him with a washcloth wet with cold water or alcohol.
   2. Hold his medication, stat page his doctor, and check his temperature.
   3. Administer a medication such as benztropine IM to correct his dystonic reaction.
   4. Reassure him that although there is no treatment for his tardive dyskinesia, it will pass.
   5. Explain that he has anticholinergic toxicity, hold his meds, and give IM physostigmine.
   6. Hold his medication tonight, and consult his doctor after completing medication rounds.

6. The nurse is planning a cognitive intervention group for auditory hallucinations. According to the study by England (2007), what does the evidence show regarding this type of intervention?
   1. Improving self-esteem will reduce auditory hallucinations
   2. Cognitive intervention for hallucinations also improves attention deficits
   3. People with schizophrenia are too ill to benefit from cognitive therapy
   4. Providing alternate ways of thinking about hallucinations reduces distress

⊝volve WEBSITE

Post-Test interactive review

Visit the Evolve Web site for Chapter Review Answers and Rationales, Critical Thinking Answer Guidelines, and additional resources related to the content in this chapter: http://evolve.elsevier.com/Canada/Varcarolis/psychiatric/

REFERENCES

Agar, L. (2010). Recognizing neuroleptic malignant syndrome in the emergency department: A case study. *Perspectives in Psychiatric Care, 46*(2), 143–151. doi:10.1111/j.1744-6163.2010.00250.x.

Amador, X. (2000). *I'm not sick, I don't need help!* New York: Vida Press.

Anthony, K.H. (2008). Helping partnerships that facilitate recovery from severe mental illness. *Journal of Psychosocial Nursing, 46*(7), 25–33.

Bechdolf, A., Phillips, L.J., Francey, S.M., et al. (2006). Recent approaches to psychological interventions for people at risk of psychosis. *European Archive of Psychiatry and Clinical Neuroscience, 256*, 159–173. doi:10.1007/s00406-006-0623-0.

Bertolote, J., & McGorry, P. (2005). Early intervention and recovery for young people with early psychosis: Consensus statement. *British Journal of Psychiatry, 187*, S116–S119. doi:10.1192/bjp.187.48.s116.

Bralet, M., Ton, T., & Falissard, B. (2007). Schizophrenic patients with polydipsia and water intoxication more often have a form of schizophrenia first described by Kraepelin. *Psychiatry Research, 152*, 267–271. doi:10.1016/j.psychres.2006.11.009.

Braw, Y., Bloch, Y., Mendelovich, S., et al. (2008). Cognition in young schizophrenia outpatients: Comparison of first episode with multiepisode patients. *Schizophrenia Bulletin, 34*, 544–554. doi:10.1093/schbul/sbm115.

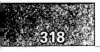

Broome, M.R., Woolley, J.B., Tabraham, P., et al. (2005). What causes the onset of psychosis? *Schizophrenia Research, 79*(1), 23–34.

Canadian Institute for Health Information (CIHI). (2008). *Hospital length of stay and readmission for individuals diagnosed with schizoprhenia: Are they related?* Retrieved from https://secure.cihi.ca/estore/productSeries.htm?pc=PCC410.

Chung, Y.S., Kang, D., Shin, N.Y., et al. (2008). Deficit of theory of mind in individuals at ultra-high risk for schizophrenia. *Schizophrenia Research, 99*, 111–118.

Compton, M.T. (2004). Considering schizophrenia from a prevention perspective. *American Journal of Preventive Medicine, 26*, 178–185. Retrieved from http://www.ajpmonline.org/.

Crowe, T.P., Deane, F.P., Oades, L.G., et al. (2006). Effectiveness of a collaborative recovery training program in Australia in promoting positive views about recovery. *Psychiatric Services, 57*, 1497–1500. doi:10.1176/appi.ps.57.10.1497.

England, M. (2007). Accuracy of nurses' perceptions of voice hearing and psychiatric symptoms. *Journal of Advanced Nursing, 58*, 103–109. doi:10.1111/j.1744-6163.2007.00114.x.

Farhall, J., Greenwood, K.M., & Jackson, H.J. (2007). Coping with hallucinated voices: A review of self-initiated strategies and therapeutic interventions. *Clinical Psychology Review, 27*, 476–493. doi:10.1016/j.cpr.2006.12.002.

Fazel, S., Gulati, G., Linsell, L., et al. (2009). Schizophrenia and violence: A systematic review and meta-analysis. *PLOS Medicine, 6*(8), 1–15. doi:10.1371/journal.pmed.1000120.

Freudenreich, O., Weiss, A.P., & Goff, D.C. (2008). Psychosis and schizophrenia. In T.A. Stern, J.F. Rosenbaum, M. Fava, et al. (Eds.), *Massachusetts General Hospital comprehensive clinical psychiatry* (pp. 371–389). St. Louis, MO: Mosby.

Gamble, C., & Brennan, G. (2000). Working with families and informed careers. In C. Gamble & G. Brennan (Eds.), *Working with serious mental illness: A manual for clinical practice.* London, UK: Baillière Tindall.

Gerlock, A.A., Buccheri, R., Buffum, M.D., et al. (2010). Responding to command hallucinations to harm self and others: The Unpleasant Voices Scale and Harm Command Safety Protocol. *Journal of Psychosocial Nursing and Mental Health Services, 48*(5), 26–33. doi:10.3928/02793695-20100304-03.

Goff, D.C. (2005). Pharmacologic implications of neurobiological models of schizophrenia. *Harvard Review of Psychiatry, 13*, 352–359. doi:10.1080/10673220500433262.

Gonzalez, I., & Perez, N. (2008). High risk of polydipsia and water intoxication in schizophrenia patients. *Schizophrenia Research, 99*(1–3), 377–378.

Green, A.I., Noordsy, D.L., Brunette, M.F., et al. (2008). Substance abuse and schizophrenia: Pharmacotherapeutic intervention. *Journal of Substance Abuse Treatment, 34*, 61–71. doi:10.1016/j.jsat.2007.01.008.

Haddad, P.M., & Dursun, S.M. (2007). Neurological complications of psychiatric drugs: Clinical features and management. *Human Psychopharmacology, 23*, 15–26. doi:10.1002/hup.918.

Hayashi, T., Ishida, Y., Miyashita, T., et al. (2005). Fatal water intoxication in a schizophrenia patient—an autopsy case. *Journal of Clinical Forensic Medicine, 12*, 157–159. doi:10.1016/j.jcfm.2005.01.009.

Haynes, R.M., & Resnick, P.J. (1993). Proverb familiarity and the mental status exam. *Bulletin of the Menninger Clinic, 57*(4), 523–529.

Heresco-Levy, U., Javitt, D.C., Ebstein, R., et al. (2005). D-serine efficacy as add-on pharmacotherapy to risperidone and olanzapine for treatment-refractory schizophrenia. *Biological Psychiatry, 57*, 577–585. doi:10.1016/j.biopsych.2004.12.037.

Hoffman, R.E., & Varanko, M. (2006). Seeing voices: Fused visual/auditory verbal hallucinations reported by three persons with schizophrenia-spectrum disorder. *Acta Psychiatrica Scandinavica, 114*, 290–293.

Hubl, D., Koenig, T., Strik, W., et al. (2004). Pathways that make voices: White matter changes in auditory hallucinations. *Archives of General Psychiatry, 61*(7), 658–668.

Jansman-Hart, E.M., Seto, M.C., Crocker, A.G., et al. (2011). International trends in demand for forensic mental health services. *International Journal of Forensic Mental Health, 10*(4), 326–336. doi:10.1080/14999013.2011.625591.

Khashan, A.S., Abel, K.M., McNamee, R., et al. (2008). Higher risk of offspring schizophrenia following antenatal maternal exposure to severe adverse life events. *Archives of General Psychiatry, 65*(2), 146–152.

Kisely, S. (2010). Excess mortality from chronic physical disease in psychiatric patients: The forgotten problem. *Canadian Journal of Psychiatry, 55*(12), 749–751.

Koehn, C.V., & Cutliffe, J.R. (2007). Hope and interpersonal psychiatric/mental health nursing: A systematic review of the literature: Part one. *Journal of Psychiatric and Mental Health Nursing, 14*, 134–140. doi:10.1111/j.1365-2850.2007.01054.x.

Levine, S.Z., Lurie, I., Kohn, R., et al. (2011). Trajectories of the course of schizophrenia: From progressive deterioration to amelioration over three decades. *Schizophrenia Research, 126*, 184–191. doi:10.1016/j.schres.2010.10.026.

Lysecker, P., & Buck, K. (2006). Moving toward recovery within clients' personal narratives: Directions for a recovery-focused therapy. *Journal of Psychosocial Nursing, 44*(1), 29–35.

Manschreck, T.C., Duckworth, K.S., Halpern, L., et al. (2008). Recovery: Time for optimism? *Current Psychiatry, 7*(5), 41–58.

Martin, V., & Johnson, C. (2008). *A time for action: Tackling stigma and discrimination.* Calgary: Mental Health Commission of Canada.

Masi, G., Mucci, M., & Pari, C. (2006). Children with schizophrenia: Clinical picture and pharmacological treatment. *CNS Drugs, 20*(10), 841–866.

Mauri, M.C., Moliterno, D., Rossattini, M., et al. (2008). Depression in schizophrenia: Comparison of first- and second-generation antipsychotic drugs. *Schizophrenia Research, 99*, 7–12. doi:10.1016/j.schres.2007.10.020.

Mauri, M.C., Volonteri, L.S., De Gaspari, I.F., et al. (2006). Substance abuse in first-episode schizophrenic patients: A retrospective study. *Clinical Practice and Epidemiology in Mental Health, 2*, 1–8. doi:10.1186/1745-0179-2-4.

Miller, B.J., Paschall, C.B., & Svendsen, D.P. (2007, March). *Mortality and medical co-morbidity in patients with serious mental illness.* Poster presentation at the 8th Annual All-Ohio Institute on Community Psychiatry, Beachwood, OH.

Möller, H.J. (2007). Clinical evaluation of negative symptoms in schizophrenia. *European Psychiatry, 22*, 380–386. doi:10.1016/j.eurpsy.2007.03.010.

Moorhead, S., Johnson, M., Maas, M.L., et al. (2008). *Nursing outcomes classification (NOC)* (4th ed.). St. Louis, MO: Mosby.

Nash, J. (n.d.) *John Nash quotes.* Retrieved from http://thinkexist.com/quotes/john_nash/.

Nielssen, O., Bourget, D., Laajasalo, T., et al. (2009). Homicide of strangers by people with a psychotic illness. *Schizophrenia Bulletin, 37*, 572–579. doi:10.1093/schbul/sbp112.

Norman, R.M., Manchanda, R., Malla, A.K., et al. (2011). Symptom and functional outcomes for a 5-year early intervention program for psychoses. *Schizophrenia Research, 129*(2–3), 111–115. doi:10.1016/j.schres.2011.04.006.

O'Mahony, J.M., & Donnelly, T.T. (2007). The influence of culture on immigrant women's mental health care experiences from the perspectives of health care providers. *Issues in Mental Health Nursing, 28*, 453–471. doi:10.1080/01612840701344464.

Osborn, D., Levy, G., Nazareth, I., et al. (2008). Suicide and severe mental illnesses. *Schizophrenia Research, 99*(1–3), 134–138.

Ramjan, K.A., Williams, A.J., Isbister, G.K., et al. (2007). "Red as a beet and blind as a bat": Anticholinergic delirium in adolescents: Lessons for the paediatrician. *Journal of Paediatrics and Child Health, 43*(11), 773-780. doi:10.1111/j.1440-1754.2007.01220.x.

Riecher-Rössler, A., Gschwandtner, U., Borgwardt, S., et al. (2006). Early detection and treatment of schizophrenia: How early? *Acta Psychiatrica Scandinavica, 113*, 73–80. doi:10.1111/j.1600-0447.2005.00722.x.

Roberts, S.H., & Bailey, J.E. (2011). Incentives and barriers to lifestyle interventions for people with severe mental illness: A narrative synthesis of quantitative, qualitative, and mixed method studies. *Journal of Advanced Nursing, 67*, 690–708. doi:10.1111/j.1365-2648.2010.05546.x.

Sadock, B.J., & Sadock, V.A. (2008). *Concise textbook of clinical psychiatry* (3rd ed.). Philadelphia: Lippincott Williams & Wilkins.

Smoller, J.W., Finn, C.T., & Gardner-Schuster, E.E. (2008). Genetics and psychiatry. In T.A Stern, J.F. Rosenbaum, M. Fava, et al. (Eds.),

303

Massachusetts General Hospital comprehensive clinical psychiatry (pp. 853–883). St. Louis, MO: Mosby.

Srihari, V.H., Shah, J., & Keshavan, M.S. (2012). Is early intervention for psychosis feasible and effective? *Psychiatric Clinics of North America, 35*(3), 613–631. doi:10.1016/j.psc.2012.06.004.

Swartz, M.S., Perkins, D.O., Stroup, T.S., et al. (2007). Effects of antipsychotic medications on psychosocial functioning in patients with chronic schizophrenia: Findings from the NIMH CATIE study. *American Journal of Psychiatry, 164*, 428–436. doi:10.1176/appi.ajp.164.3.428.

Tandon, R., Keshavan, M.S., & Nasrallah, H.A. (2008). Schizophrenia, "just the facts": What we know in 2008. 2. Epidemiology and etiology. *Schizophrenia Research, 102*, 1–18. doi:10.1016/j.schres.2008.04.011.

Tirgobov, E., Wilson, B.A., Shannon, M.T., et al. (2005). *Psychiatric drug guide.* Upper Saddle River, NJ: Pearson/Prentice Hall.

Tschoner, A., Engl, J., Laimer, M., et al. (2007). Metabolic side effects of antipsychotic medication. *International Journal of Clinical Practice, 61*, 1356–1370. doi:10.1111/j.1742-1241.2007.01416.x.

van Meijel, B., van der Gaag, M., Sylvain, R.K., et al. (2004). Recognition of early warning signs in patients with schizophrenia: A review of the literature. *International Journal of Mental Health Nursing, 13*, 107–116. doi:10.1111/j.1440-0979.2004.00314.x.

Wadenberg, M.G. (2007). Bifeprunox: A novel antipsychotic agent with partial agonist properties at dopamine D_2 and serotonin $5\text{-}HT_{1A}$ receptors. *Future Neurology, 2*, 153–165. doi:10.2217/14796708.2.2.153.

Walker, E., & Tessner, K. (2008). Schizophrenia. *Perspectives on Psychological Science, 3*, 30–37. doi:10.1111/j.1745-6916.2008.00059.x.

Weisman, A., Duarte, E., Koneru, V., et al. (2006).The development of a culturally informed, family-focused treatment for schizophrenia. *Family Process, 45*, 171–186. doi:10.1111/j.1545-5300.2006.00089.x.

Zinger, I. (2012). Mental health in federal corrections: Reflections and future directions. *Health Law Review, 20*(2), 22–25. Retrieved from http://www.cashra2012.ca/documents/presentation_ivan_zinger.pdf.

SOCIAL WORK IN MENTAL HEALTH
2016, VOL. 14, NO. 6, 607–624
http://dx.doi.org/10.1080/15332985.2015.1100153

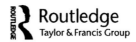

The lived experience of schizophrenia: A systematic review and meta-synthesis

Joseph Walsh, PhD, Rebecca Hochbrueckner, MPT, Jacqueline Corcoran, PhD, and Rachel Spence, BA

School of Social Work, Virginia Commonwealth University, Richmond, Virginia, USA

ABSTRACT

Schizophrenia is a serious mental illness characterized by abnormal patterns of thought and perception. What has been studied less often is the personal experience of having schizophrenia. Qualitative studies have been illuminating in this regard, and the purpose of this meta-synthesis is to determine the themes that can be identified across those studies. The inclusion criteria required that the studies employed qualitative methods, that participants had been diagnosed with schizophrenia, and the studies focused on their "lived experience." After applying search criteria to databases, 27 studies were included in the meta-synthesis. Five major themes were identified in the results, including: (1) the experience of symptoms; (2) the process of acceptance; (3) personal relationships; (4) treatment experiences; and (5) spiritual practices and faith. Implications of these results are explored.

KEYWORDS

Schizophrenia; qualitative research; meta-synthesis

Schizophrenia is a mental disorder characterized by abnormal patterns of thought and perception. It includes two types of symptoms (American Psycholagical Association [APA], 2013). *Positive* symptoms represent exaggerations of normal behavior, and include hallucinations, delusions, disorganized thought processes, and tendencies toward agitation. The *negative* symptoms of schizophrenia represent the diminution of what would be considered normal behavior, and include flat affect (the absence of expression), social withdrawal, non-communication, anhedonia (blandness), passivity, and ambivalence in decision making. Complete and permanent remission in schizophrenia is relatively uncommon. A person with the disorder may experience a chronic course, with symptoms being more or less florid but never really disappearing, or one in which periods of psychosis are interspersed with periods of remission (van Os, Rutten, Bart, & Poulton, 2008). The average life span of persons with schizophrenia is variously reported as 16 to 22 years shorter than the national average in the United States due to lifestyle factors such as diet, physical health, and risks related to

CONTACT Jacqueline Corcoran, PhD ✉ jcorcora@vcu.edu ▣ School of Social Work, Virginia Commonwealth University, 907 Floyd Avenue, Richmond, VA 23284.

poverty (Cohen, 2012). Suicide is the leading cause of premature death in schizophrenia, as 20–40% of persons attempt suicide at some point in their lives and 5–10% succeed (Johnson, Gooding, & Tarrier, 2008).

The nature of schizophrenia has been a major research topic in the health sciences for more than a century, but most studies have focused on its causes and treatment. What has been studied less often is the personal experience of having schizophrenia. Qualitative studies have been illuminating in this regard, and the purpose of this meta-synthesis is to determine the themes that can be identified across those studies.

Method

Inclusion criteria and search

The inclusion criteria required that the studies employed qualitative methods, the participants had been diagnosed with schizophrenia, and the studies focused on the "lived experience," in other words, what it is like to live with a diagnosis of schizophrenia, rather than honing in on specific aspects of the disorder. A database search was completed by a PhD-level research assistant at Virginia Commonwealth University. The search was based on terms and appropriate Boolean operatives provided by a reference librarian that included the following keywords: *personal reflection, lived experience, qualitative, phenomenology, schizophrenia, schizoaffective disorders, schizotypal, schizoid personality disorder, schizophreniform, personal experience,* and *psychotic disorder.* Searches were conducted using the following databases: CINAHL, Social Work Abstracts, Psychology & Behavioral Sciences, PsycARTICLES, PsycINFO, PsycEXTRA, Academic Search Complete, and Dissertations ProQuest. Search criteria did not specify a beginning date and extended to May, 2014. The initial searches produced a list of 4,298 potential studies.

The three-step process of study selection developed by Meade and Richardson (1997) was used to narrow the results of the search based first on title alone, then including the abstract, and finally the entire text of the study. The research assistant submitted the studies he believed fit the inclusion criteria to the principal investigator, who made final determinations. Primary reasons for excluding studies were that they focused narrowly on a specific aspect of schizophrenia, focused on families rather than the individuals with the disorder, or were quantitative as opposed to qualitative (mixed method designs were included as long as there was qualitative data that was analyzed). Through this process, the original list of articles was narrowed to 43 studies, of which 27 met all inclusion criteria.

Table 1. Primary studies: methodological details and themes.

Study	Design/theory	Sample	Themes
Anderson (2011)	Interviews Interpretive phenomenology	N = 5 African American males	Experience of symptoms Process of acceptance
Baier (1995)	Interviews Naturalistic inquiry	N = 26 18 males, 8 females 22 Caucasians, 4 African Americans	Experience of symptoms Process of acceptance Personal relationships Treatment/medication
Baker (1996)	Interviews Interpretative interactionism	N = 15 10 males, 5 females Canadian study	Experience of symptoms Personal relationships Treatment/provider interaction
Eklund et al. (2012)	Interviews Content analysis	N = 10 5 males, 5 females Swedish study	Experience of symptoms Process of acceptance Personal relationships
Evenson et al. (2008)	Interviews Interpretative phenomenology	N = 10 Biological fathers with schizophrenia All Caucasian	Experience of symptoms Process of acceptance Personal relationships Treatment/medication
Fernandes (2009)	Interviews Psychodynamic	N = 4 2 males, 2 females Ethnicity not noted	Experience of symptoms Process of acceptance Personal relationships Treatment/provider interactions
Flanagan et al. (2012)	Interviews Interpretive phenomenology	N = 17 71% female 77% African American, 17% White, 6% Native American	Experience of symptoms Personal relationships Treatment/provider interactions
Forchuk et al. (2003)	Interviews Leninger's phases of qualitative analysis	N = 10 7 males, 3 females All Caucasian/Canadian	Experience of symptoms Process of acceptance Personal relationships Treatment/provider interactions Medication
Gee, Pearce, and Jackson (2003)	Interviews Grounded theory	N = 6 3 males, 3 females Ethnicity not noted	Experience of symptoms Process of acceptance Personal relationships Treatment/medication
Gould et al. (2005)	Focus groups Constant comparative method	N = 4 All male Ethnicity not noted	Experience of symptoms Process of acceptance Personal relationships
Humberstone (2002)	Interviews Grounded theory	N = 13 10 males, 3 females New Zealand study	Experience of symptoms Process of acceptance Personal relationships Faith/spirituality Treatment/provider interactions Medication
Jarosinski (2006)	Interviews Herdeggaroam hermeneutic approach	N = 12 5 males, 7 females 6 African Americans, 6 Caucasians	Experience of symptoms Process of acceptance

(Continued)

Table 1. (Continued).

Study	Design/theory	Sample	Themes
Liu et al. (2012)	Interviews Comparative analysis	N = 16 5 males, 11 females Residents of Shanghai	Experience of symptoms Personal relationships Treatment/provider interactions
McCann and Clark (2004)	Interviews Descriptive phenomenology	N = 9 5 males, 4 females Australian study	Experience of symptoms Personal relationships Faith/spirituality Treatment/medication
Ng et al. (2008)	Focus group Grounded theory	N = 8 4 males, 4 females Chinese	Experience of symptoms Process of acceptance Personal relationships Treatment/provider interactions Medication
Phillips (2008)	Interviews Grounded theory	N = 8 6 males, 2 females 4 Caucasians, 1 Jamaican, 3 African Americans	Process of acceptance Personal relationships Faith/spirituality Treatment/provider interactions Medications
Phripp (1995)	Interviews Comparative analysis	N = 3 1 male, 2 females Canadian study	Experience of symptoms Process of acceptance Personal relationships Treatment/medication
Powell (1998)	Interviews Interpretive interactionist	N = 33 18 males, 15 females Caucasian 51%, African American 27%, Hispanic 22%	Experience of symptoms Process of acceptance Personal relationships Treatment/provider interactions Medication
Roe et al. (2004)	Interviews Open-coding case analysis	N = 41 25 males, 18 females Ethnicity not noted	Experience of symptoms Process of acceptance Faith/spirituality
Sanseeha, Chantawan, Sethabouppha, Disayavanish, and Turale (2009)	Interviews, reflective journaling, observation Heidegger's hermeneutic phenomenology	N = 18 individuals with schizophrenia N = 12 family members Thai study, all were Buddhists	Experience of symptoms Process of acceptance Personal relationships Faith/spirituality Treatment/medication
Shepherd, Depp, Harris, Palinkas, and Jeste (2012)	Interviews Grounded theory	N = 32 Approx. 41% females Ethnicity not noted	Process of acceptance Personal relationships
Sung and Puskar (2006)	Interviews Interpretive phenomenology	N = 21 13 males, 8 females Korean	Experience of symptoms Process of acceptance Personal relationships Treatment/medication
Suryani et al. (2013)	Interviews Colaizzi's (1973) phenomeno-logical approach	N = 13 6 males, 7 females Indonesian	Experience of symptoms Process of acceptance Personal relationships Treatment/provider interactions

(Continued)

Table 1. (Continued).

Study	Design/theory	Sample	Themes
Tooth et al. (2003)	Focus groups NUDIST program was used for analysis	$N = 57$ 42 males, 15 females Australian study	Process of acceptance Personal relationships Faith/spirituality Treatment/provider interactions Medication
Walton (1992, 2000)	Interviews Heideggerian phenomenology	$N = 10$ 7 males, 3 females Canadian study	Process of acceptance Personal relationships Faith/spirituality Treatment/provider interactions Medication
Yennari (2011)	Interviews Thematic analysis	$N = 7$ 5 males, 2 females 4 African Americans, 3 Caucasians	Experience of symptoms Process of acceptance Personal relationships Faith/spirituality Treatment/provider interactions Medication

Data extraction

A table was developed to organize the relevant information based on methodologies, participant demographics, and results of each study (see Table 1). Data extraction was completed by two master's-level research students and reviewed for accuracy by the principal investigator.

Data analysis

The studies were analyzed using the methodological framework provided by Noblit and Hare (1988) for meta-synthesis, which they refer to as meta-ethnography and is the oldest form of synthesizing qualitative research. The method involves seeing how studies are related, which involves identifying common themes across studies and checking or "translating" them against each other to ultimately create new third-order constructs (Ring, Ritchie, Mandava, & Jepson, 2011; Thomas & Harden, 2008). Initial themes were developed by a group of four trained research students and, through an iterative process with the primary investigator, involved discussion and review of tables and concepts, which yielded final themes and subthemes.

Results

After applying the selection criteria, a total of 27 studies published between 1992 and 2013 were included in our meta-synthesis, with a total of 408 participants, all with diagnoses of schizophrenia or schizoaffective disorder. About one third of the participants were women and two-thirds were men. Caucasians and African

Americans were the most represented ethnicities in this sample, although four studies focused on specific ethnic groups, including Thai, Indonesian, Chinese, and Korean populations. A wide variation existed in the marital and parenting status of participants as well as age range, with most falling between 18 and 50 years. Some had college degrees but the majority had obtained a high school diploma or less. Participants were recruited most often using purposive and convenience sampling methods and were frequently identified through local mental health facilities. Most were receiving some kind of mental health services for their condition, in both inpatient and outpatient settings. Most studies used individual interviews but a few (3 out of 26) involved focus groups. A majority of the studies (65%) were conducted outside the United States, with 35% within the United States. Thirty-one percent were dissertations with the rest of the studies published in refereed journals. The most commonly utilized theories for the approach and analysis were interpretive phenomenology and grounded theory.

Five major themes were identified in the results, including: (1) the experience of symptoms; (2) acceptance processes; (3) personal relationships; (4) spiritual practices and faith; and (5) treatment experiences.

The experience of symptoms

The experience of symptoms was discussed in 22 of the 27 studies. Themes that emerged within the rubric of "symptoms" included the experience of hallucinations, disorientation, and the loss of a sense of self.

Hallucinations

The onset of hallucinations, considered in 14 studies, was described as gradual by some and immediate by others (Fernandes, 2009). In general the experience of hallucinations was described as frightening, confusing, and exhausting (Flanagan et al., 2012; Forchuk, Jewell, Tweedell, & Steinnagel, 2003; Humberstone, 2002; Jarosinski, 2006; Yennari, 2011). The common experience of hearing voices was often associated with violence, negativity, and yelling (Forchuk et al., 2003; Humberstone, 2002; Walton, 2000). Participants in Suryani, Welch, and Cox's (2013) study reported feeling the need to comply with orders given by the voices. One participant noted, "'The voices seemed to command my brain.... In my mind I felt as if I was under their command" (p. 315). Not uncommonly, participants experienced the voices as coming from electronic media, such as television or radio (Baier, 1995). Participants noted the importance of gaining some level of control or understanding of the voices as an important step in learning to cope with schizophrenia (Roe, Chopra, & Rudnick, 2004).

Disorientation

Disorientation, described as not knowing what was real or unreal, was noted in 14 of the studies (e.g., Anderson, 2011; Baier, 1995; Baker, 1996; Phripp,

1995; Roe et al., 2004; Sung & Puskar, 2006). Experiences of hallucinations, both visual and auditory, as well as delusions, left individuals constantly questioning reality. Multiple studies noted that participants made use of reality testing (ways to evaluate one's sensory impressions) to distinguish symptoms from reality (Anderson, 2011; Roe et al., 2004). A participant in Anderson's study (2011), who expressed concern that others could read his mind, reportedly asked the researcher, his psychiatrist, his counselor, and his case manager if they could in fact hear his thoughts.

Another aspect of schizophrenia that leads to disorientation stems from difficulties with concentrating and problems with memory (Evenson, Rhodes, Feigenbaum, & Solly, 2008; Fernandes, 2009; Forchuk et al., 2003; Liu, Ma, & Zhao, 2012; Sung & Puskar, 2006). Participants described confusion and difficulty with remembering and tracking information (Fernandes, 2009). The combination of unpredictable symptoms, being out of touch with reality, and difficulty thinking and remembering work together to increase anxiety (Liu et al., 2012). As one participant noted, "'For me, the future is unrealistic and unpredictable. The only thing I can do now is just to take care of my daily life" (Liu et al., 2012, p. 1711).

Loss of sense of self

Loss of sense of self was discussed in 12 of the 27 studies. In general, participants found that the symptoms of schizophrenia were so overwhelming that they experienced a lost "sense of self" (Phripp, 1995, p. 30), defined as a loss of self-control or personal agency (Baker, 1996; Phripp, 1995), and a loss of identity (Fernandes, 2009; Humberstone, 2002; Jarosinski, 2006; Phripp, 1995). Jarosinski described participants as wondering, "Are they who they are?" (2006, p. ix). Participants in Fernandes' (2009) study expressed feeling fragmented rather than whole. Jarosinski's (2006) participants reported on the difficulties of finding a sense of self separate from the hallucinations, which was consistent with Yennari's (2011) study, finding that participants struggled to find a sense of identity. A young man from one study explained it this way:

> There was nowhere I could go for—for a sense of privacy because I felt that everyone was understanding everything that I was thinking and it didn't matter where I was. And uh just the sense of being absolutely out of control and having absolutely no control in your life. No control for your thoughts, no control of your actions no control of anything. Just being completely manipulated by exterior forces. No sense of self. (Phripp, 1995, p. 144)

Process of acceptance

The second major theme, the process of acceptance, was covered in 22 studies. This theme considers the progress that individuals make in living with and managing schizophrenia. In general, participants did not feel that "recovery" was an appropriate description of their reality (Phripp, 1995; Tooth, Kalyanasundaram, Glover, & Momenzadah, 2003). Due to the long-term nature of schizophrenia, recovery was seen as something that was never complete but an ongoing process better described as coping. As one participant noted: "It's like a brand new car and a repaired car that was crashed, the prices are very different. The chassis was all bent and you straightened it up, but it is still different" (Ng et al., 2008, p. 125).

The subthemes considered in this section include feelings of shame and loss, regaining a sense of self, acceptance (as a continuum), and reengagement.

Shame and loss

The subtheme of shame and loss was noted in 13 studies. As symptoms appeared and individuals first became aware of their diagnosis, their feelings of shame and loss could be overwhelming. Many study participants reported feeling like failures (Baker, 1996; Evenson et al., 2008; Sung & Puskar, 2006), with a sense of shame at being diagnosed with schizophrenia and not being able to maintain control of their lives (Evenson et al., 2008; Fernandes, 2009; Sanseeha, Chantawan, Sethabouppha, Disayavanish, & Turale, 2009; Suryani et al., 2013). Feelings of shame were frequently connected with internalized stigma (Flanagan et al., 2012) and negative self-thoughts (Forchuk et al., 2003). Participants described feelings of low self-confidence and poor self-image (Liu et al., 2012; McCann & Clark, 2004).

These negative feelings were associated with a sense of loss. Participants expressed that they had lost the chance to have a normal life (Baker, 1996; Gould, DeSouza, & Rebeiro-Gruhl, 2005), lost relationships (Baker, 1996), and lost tangible resources, such as jobs and homes (Humberstone, 2002). One participant stated this simply as, "'I remember when I was normal'" (Gould et al., 2005, p. 469), which, in turn, led to feelings of isolation, hopelessness, and depression (Fernandes, 2009; Forchuk et al., 2003; Liu et al., 2012; Ng et al., 2008; Sung & Puskar, 2006). For some, this led to thoughts of suicide, "'I feel like a suicide. I feel like taking a knife and putting it right through my chest'" (Baker, 1996, p. 27). As the symptoms they experienced were unpredictable and difficult to understand, participants were also filled with worry, anxiety, and fear for the future (Baker, 1996; Evenson et al., 2008; Fernandes, 2009). Confusing, overwhelming, and erratic symptoms left the individuals in these studies feeling shame and loss.

Regaining a sense of self

This subtheme was discussed in 13 studies. Participants reported regaining a sense of self as they began to feel some level of control over their symptoms (Eklund, Hermansson, & Håkansson, 2012; Phripp, 1995; Roe et al., 2004). As one person described, "'I feel like a human being again. I've got my emotions back. I've got my long-term memory. I've got my short-term memory. I'm just coping and doing fine'" (Forchuk et al., 2003, p. 147). This control enabled them to feel safer and to move forward in other areas such as reengagement (Eklund et al., 2012). Participants noted that gaining this control was hard work and required determination (Fernandes, 2009; Tooth et al., 2003). The new sense of identity that formed tended to include the diagnosis of schizophrenia, which was incorporated and accepted as one part of the self (Baier, 1995; Phripp, 1995; Sung & Puskar, 2006). Some participants felt pride in their new sense of self and considered themselves to be survivors. One participant stated, "'You might notice that I'm very individual. I know that. I, myself, it's up to me, this person behind the face here. I know it's a bit fleshy, a bit funny, but that person that I am behind this face is responsible for all kinds of freedom'" (Humberstone, 2002, p. 370).

Acceptance (as a continuum)

The participants in these studies fell along a continuum of acceptance, that was particularly considered in nine studies. Some refused to accept their diagnosis or identify as mentally ill (Liu et al., 2012; Sung & Puskar, 2006). Others accepted the diagnosis and were able to incorporate it into their identity without being defined by it (Yennari, 2011).

Acceptance had more meanings beyond acceptance of the diagnosis, including coming to terms with the long-term nature of the disorder (Baier, 1995), the many losses inherent in the diagnosis, and acknowledging the need for support (Gould et al., 2005). Psychosocial support and psychoeducation sometimes helped individuals gain a level of acceptance (Phripp, 1995; Tooth et al., 2003), which generally enabled them to cope better and to move on with their lives, as this participant described: "But ah, so I think that I've come a long way in dealing with the schizophrenia so that I know it's not a healthy thing to have but it's not life threatening and it's not um, it doesn't have to control your life" (Phripp, 1995, p. 84)

Reengagement

Reengagement was specifically considered in 13 studies. Participants who were coping well with their schizophrenia showed signs of reengagement, most commonly involving social interactions (Baier, 1995; Phripp, 1995; Sung & Puskar, 2006; Tooth et al., 2003) but also in setting goals (Eklund et al., 2012; Jarosinski, 2006), such as having a job and living independently (Forchuk et al., 2003; Ng et al., 2008; Phillips, 2008). One participant, a young man, commented, "'Yeah, I want to get out of the system. . . . I'd get me a job, my own apartment, and a car and maybe even get married. . . . I'm gonna walk out that door. I'm getting discharged soon'" (Phillips, 2008, p. 60).

Personal relationships

The third major theme, personal relationships, dominated the narratives in 23 studies. Participants consistently expressed the belief that their ability to develop and maintain interpersonal relationships was profoundly affected by the disorder. Stigma and discrimination from others, as well as the necessity of support, were also indicated.

Deterioration of existing relationships

Deterioration of relationships was discussed in 10 studies. Individuals expressed that they had lost relationships, both by being rejected due to their symptoms and due to their own emotional disengagement and resentment (Baker, 1996; Evenson et al., 2008; McCann & Clark, 2004; Suryani et al., 2013; Yennari, 2011). The effect of the disorder on one father's relationship with his children is apparent in the following quote: "'Well because you alienated them from your mind ... they're my children but they're not my children ... it's a horrible feeling'" (Evenson et al., 2008, p. 634). Some expressed anger and resentment towards family members who they believed had betrayed them by participating in their involuntary hospitalizations (Baker, 1996).

When relationships with friends and family members were maintained, they were often described as being limited or superficial (Baker, 1996; Forchuk et al., 2003; Humberstone, 2002; Liu et al., 2012; Shepherd et al., 2012; Sung & Puskar, 2006). Participants often described feelings of loneliness and isolation as a result of this deterioration in relationships. One woman described this as an inherent feature of schizophrenia, noting: "'That's the thing about schizophrenia, it leaves you alone emotionally and alone physically.... . I got really lonely. People my own age left me alone ... the trouble with schizophrenia was loneliness'" (Humberstone, 2002, p. 7).

Difficulty establishing new relationships

Difficulty relating to others, referenced in 13 studies, often prevented individuals from establishing relationships that mattered to them (Baker, 1996; Gee, Pearce, & Jackson, 2003; McCann & Clark, 2004; Sung & Puskar, 2006). Difficulty connecting was related to paranoia, anxiety, fear regarding other people's motivations, and fear of being considered abnormal or psychotic (Baker, 1996; Liu et al., 2012; Suryani et al., 2013; Walton, 1992, 2000). As one woman noted, "You can't ever feel comfortable. I'm always nervous and tense with people" (Baker, 1996, p. 26). As a result, some individuals came to accept the idea of being alone, or limited their relationships to others with the diagnosis (Humberstone, 2002; Ng et al., 2008; Phillips, 2008). Some reported that they were eventually able to establish relationships with others, but only by utilizing a "false self" and hiding their true feelings and emotions

(Fernandes, 2009; Yennari, 2011). As one man explained, "[Regarding relationships] suppose people go out with you and are willing to be your friends. You don't really tell them too much. You'd be afraid of how they might look at you after you tell them" (Ng et al., 2008, p. 125). Others reported that the sense of discomfort never truly disappeared, but eased somewhat as they made progress toward recovery (Forchuk et al., 2003).

Stigma and discrimination

Individuals spoke of facing alienation and stigma from their families, friends, and their communities in 12 studies, based on both their diagnosis and actual symptoms (Gee et al., 2003; Humberstone, 2002; Jarosinki, 2006; Powell, 1998; Tooth et al., 2003; Yennari, 2011). Many expressed that this stigma led to feelings of shame, isolation, rejection, and distrust, and was a major contributor to voluntary isolation (Flanagan et al., 2012; Liu et al., 2012; Sanseeha et al., 2009). When discussing even brief encounters with the outside world, themes of paranoia often permeated the narrative: "But I remember I used to walk around, and I'd know that these people were looking at me. I used to get really paranoid, and they were all dressed in black, and I thought ... that's why I used to freak out so much, because I used to think someone was after me" (Walton, 2000, p. 3).

Many discussed the ways in which discrimination led to major consequences, such as difficulty finding housing. As a result, participants often concealed their diagnosis (McCann & Clark, 2004; Walton, 1992, 2000). While some individuals expressed a sense of injustice regarding being treated or judged negatively, many expressed the belief that these experiences were an inevitable part of living with the diagnosis of schizophrenia (Walton, 1992, 2000).

The importance of social support in coping

The final subtheme under relationships, noted in 16 studies, was the importance of social support in coping with the illness. Individuals described depending on others for basic survival, including necessities such as food, clothing, and housing (Baker, 1996; Walton, 1992, 2000). Positive relationships enabled them to cope with their illness and make progress in recovery (Baier, 1995; Evenson et al., 2008; Forchuk et al., 2003; Humberstone, 2002; Liu et al., 2012; Ng et al., 2008; Phillips, 2008; Sanseeha et al., 2009; Sung & Puskar, 2006; Tooth et al., 2003; Walton, 1992, 2000). One individual noted, "I believe that friends are very important. Don't have to keep talking about your illness. Just hanging out and interacting with friends is quite good" (Ng et al., 2008, p. 126). Many discussed the ways in which helping others suffering from schizophrenia was beneficial to their own recovery (Eklund et al., 2012; McCann & Clark, 2004; Phillips, 2008). In order to develop these relationships, many sought out support groups so they could maintain contact with other persons with schizophrenia and maintain awareness regarding their illness (Phripp, 1995).

Faith/spirituality

Another coping mechanism, in addition to social support, was the use of faith and spirituality (a theme present in 11 of 27 studies). Faith and spirituality were frequently listed as factors that helped participants cope with schizophrenia. Humberstone (2002) reported that participants found hope and meaning in God, as well as feeling that God was the only thing more powerful than their psychosis. Liu et al. (2012) noted the use of traditional Chinese spiritual methods, and Sanseeha et al. (2009) described participants using Buddhist teachings, mindfulness, meditation, and prayer for coping. Roe et al. (2004) also noted the use of mindfulness for coping. Faith and spirituality in general were used to instill hope (Phillips, 2008) and as a means of support (Walton, 2000). One participant noted, "'Well, I go to church and pray and all that. It made me more confident that I'll go to heaven in a good way … it gives me reassurance … it makes me feel sure that I have a spot in heaven'" (Phillips, 2008, p. 49). Participants found that faith and spirituality were tools they could use to transcend the daily challenges of coping with schizophrenia.

Treatment

Participant views on treatment, our fourth major theme, were discussed in 19 studies, with two subthemes emerging of contact with the mental health system and medication.

Interactions with providers

This subtheme was present in 12 studies, falling into two categories: issues of control and negative contact with staff. Many individuals expressed concern that their illness had caused them to lose control over both their lives and their behaviors (Baker, 1996; Forchuk et al., 2003; Suryani et al., 2013). Many who were interviewed within an inpatient setting had fears related to being controlled by others, which had been exacerbated by non-voluntary hospitalizations and being forced to take medications (Baier, 1995; Forchuk et al., 2003; Humberstone, 2002; Liu et al., 2012; Phillips, 2008; Yennari, 2011). One man encapsulated this feeling of helplessness regarding treatment options by noting, "'I was put on various drugs. I don't know if I can remember them all. . . . Then I was told that I wasn't allowed to leave the hospital unless I agreed to six months of injections outside the hospital. I was never all right there'" (Baker, 1996, p. 29). Some reported they were not well informed about their illness by doctors and staff, and, as a result, felt subject to the will of seemingly arbitrary decisions related to policies and treatment methods (Ng et al., 2008). Many expressed frustration at not being consulted regarding treatment decisions (Baker, 1996; Forchuk et al., 2003; Liu et al., 2012; Phillips, 2008). This lack of knowledge regarding their illness, combined with a lack of agency and control over decisions related to their health, often resulted in fear, discomfort, and disempowerment (Powell, 1998; Walton, 1992, 2000).

The second category under encounters with the mental health system was negative contact with staff. Many individuals expressed the belief that providers did not fully appreciate what it was like to experience a mental illness, and, consequently, failed to understand the impact of treatment decisions on clients' lives (Forchuk et al., 2003; Liu et al., 2012; Walton, 1992, 2000). Some complained about staff members who were not well informed about schizophrenia and invalidated their psychotic experiences (Forchuk et al., 2003; Powell, 1998; Yennari, 2011). Others complained that staff members treated them like children (Forchuk et al., 2003), which, at times, resulted in a desire to fight the system. As one woman noted, "She [nurse] never really lets go, you know, she sort of always treats you like a patient or something like that and you just, you want to rebel, or that's how I felt" (Walton, 2000, p. 80). Many respondents believed that staff did not always know what was best for them, and some expressed doubt that providers even had their best interest in mind (Baker, 1996; Fernandes, 2009; Liu et al., 2012; Ng et al., 2008; Tooth et al., 2003; Walton, 1992, 2000). As a result, some avoided communication with staff, "I keep my mouth shut.... I want to keep it a short stay" (Forchuk et al., 2003, p. 148). Even when some trust was developed, many emphasized that their relationships with staff continued to be largely superficial, "I know what the doctors are thinking about. They just take me as a patient. I mean, they just want to treat me like a client" (Liu et al., 2012, p. 1712).

Medications

The sub-theme of medication was present in 17 studies and divided into two categories of acceptance of medications and adverse effects. While many were resistant to medications at first, a large number of respondents acknowledged their necessity (Humberstone, 2002; Liu et al., 2012; Sanseeha et al., 2009; Sung & Puskar, 2006; Walton, 1992, 2000). Some spoke of the beneficial aspects of medications in managing their symptoms, and even seemed to accept the idea of medication as a long-term solution (Evenson et al., 2008; Phillips, 2008). One man stated, "'I'm hoping the medication keeps working for the rest of my life'" (Forchuk et al., 2003, p. 146). Even for those who were unhappy with their medications, many expressed a willingness and desire to try new medications in hopes they would find something that would work (Forchuk et al., 2003). However, even when medications were accepted, many individuals expressed the belief that they would not be completely "recovered" from their illness until they were able to be free of them (Liu et al., 2012; Ng et al., 2008).

The second category under medications involved side effects. Individuals described a variety of concerning side effects including lack of energy, weight gain, concentration and memory problems, excessive sleeping, and impaired ability to show emotions (Baier, 1995; Evenson et al., 2008; Fernandes, 2009; Forchuk et al., 2003; Gee et al., 2003; McCann & Clark, 2004; Phripp, 1995; Sung & Puskar, 2006; Tooth et al., 2003). The effect on memory was often particularly troubling, as one man noted: "… when I have those slips of memory, which are part of my illness, something major will get lost " (Evenson et al., 2008, p. 635). Concern about over-medication was a frequent point of focus, as individuals were fearful that taking too many medications would negatively impact their ability to function normally (Forchuk et al., 2003). Opinions on the effectiveness of medications varied, as some described positive effects (symptom reduction), some described negative effects (anxiety, restlessness, etc.), and some noted no change (Forchuk et al., 2003). One man reported that when his side effects were at their worst, they were "sometimes worse than the actual illness" (Yennari, 2011, p. 102). When this was the case, side effects often resulted in noncompliance (Sung & Puskar, 2006; Yennari, 2011).

Discussion

There were some limitations associated with this study. There were the usual problems inherent in meta-synthesis, such as reliance on secondary data and combining data from different methodologies, phenomenologies, and quality. Specific to these studies, many participants were interviewed in an inpatient setting and might differ in important ways from individuals seeking services from outpatient settings; therefore, perspectives shared in this meta-synthesis might not generalize to all people with schizophrenia. Still, this meta-synthesis provides a rich, detailed portrait of individuals with schizophrenia and avoids reducing those persons to mere symptomology.

The onset of the disorder brings great loss that extends from one's own identity to an individual's grasp of reality. Because the experience of schizophrenia happens internally there is much misunderstanding of the disorder. Individuals can have difficulty conveying what they are experiencing, which is problematic for relationships, in general, but is especially evident in interactions with health care providers where individuals with schizophrenia consistently feel disempowered and misunderstood. While nursing and hospital staff are equipped to provide appropriate medical interventions, problems related to issues of trust and control suggest that poor therapeutic relationships can have a negative impact on recovery. Hewitt and Coffey (2005) conducted a meta-analysis of studies on the significance of the therapeutic relationship with persons who have schizophrenia and concluded that those who experience an empathic, positive, facilitative relationship have better outcomes. Professional development programs that aim to increase awareness of the relationship issues facing this population could help to combat their perceived stigma and prejudice.

Probably the largest loss that individuals with schizophrenia face, and the one most mentioned within the studies of this qualitative meta-synthesis, is that of social relationships. Relationships that were strong prior to the onset of this disorder are challenged by the strange and often frightening symptoms experienced. The symptoms and diagnosis lead to stigma and discrimination. These feelings are internalized by those who are diagnosed which leads to a vicious cycle of self-isolation. As these individuals attempt to repair existing relationships and develop new relationships, they feel the need to hide some or all of the truth concerning their symptoms/diagnosis, afraid of how others will view and react to them. The effects of stigma were borne out in a 27-nation quantitative study (Thornicroft, Brohan, Rose, Sartorius, & Leese, 2009). Negative discrimination was experienced by 47% of study participants in making or keeping friends, by 43% from family members, by 29% in finding a job, by 29% in keeping a job, and by 27% when pursuing intimate relationships. Almost three-quarters (72%) of respondents felt the need to conceal their diagnosis.

The importance of social relationships and the need for social support cannot be overemphasized. Strong, supportive relationships help individuals struggling with schizophrenia to cope and heal and even to meet basic necessities such as finding a job and housing. Participants in the meta-synthesis spoke about the need for social support, even though they tended to withdraw from others. Practitoners should understand that a moderate amount of interaction with significant others is optimal (Harley, Boardman, & Craig, 2012). They respond favorably to attitudes of acceptance, reasonable expectations, opportunities to develop social and vocational skills, and a relatively small number, but broad range, of social supports. These may include family members, friends, neighbors, work peers, school peers, informal community relations, and perhaps members of shared religious groups and organizations (Gunnmo & Bergman, 2011).

The process of acceptance of the disorder should be a topic explored with people with schizophrenia to give them hope. They begin to accept their diagnosis, the long-term nature of the disorder, and their continued need for support. Many of the individuals in these studies turned to faith and spirituality as a way to transcend their struggle with the disorder. As individuals form a new identity that includes schizophrenia as only one part of themselves rather than as what defines them, they are able to move forward with their lives. They begin to set goals and make plans for the future. This type of healing requires a level of control over their symptoms, a thorough understanding of their disorder, almost always the continued use of medications, and a strong and supportive social network.

Psychotropic medication is, of course, a primary intervention modality for persons with schizophrenia, and there is approximately a 66% chance that a person will respond positively to an antipsychotic medication (Stahl, 2013). A systematic review of 65 controlled trials has affirmed that all of the anti-psychotic drugs are effective in controlling the resurgence of symptoms in persons with schizophrenia, even though they tend to produce adverse effects of movement disorders, sedation, and weight gain (Leucht et al., 2012). Participants in the study worried about side effects and the number of medications they were on. Medications tend to demonstrate variable adverse effects with regard to extrapyramidal symptoms, anticholinergic effects, weight gain, insomnia, headache, and increased heart rate (Komossa et al., 2010a, 2010b, 2011; Lobos et al., 2010). The findings of this meta-synthesis support the idea that many consumers have serious reservations about taking medications due to these adverse effects and should be encouraged to be open about their experiences so that an appropriate regimen of medications can be determined.

References

American Psychiatric Association (APA). (2013). *Diagnostic and statistical manual of mental disorders* (5th ed.). Arlington, VA: Author.

Anderson, L. (2011). *African American males diagnosed with schizophrenia: A phenomenological study.* (Unpublished doctoral dissertation). Virginia Commonwealth University, Richmond, VA.

Baier, M. (1995). *The process of developing insight and finding meaning within persons with schizophrenia.* (Unpublished doctoral dissertation). Saint Louis University, Saint Louis, MO.

Baker, C. (1996). Subjective experience of symptoms in schizophrenia. *Canadian Journal of Nursing Research, 28*(2), 19–35.

Cohen, D. (2012). Reduced life-expectancy on schizophrenia: Does premature ageing contribute to premature death in schizophrenia? *European Psychiatry, 27*(Suppl. 1), 1. doi:10.1016/S0924-9338(12)74108-1

Colaizzi, P. F. (1973). *Reflection and research in psychology: A phenomenological study of learning.* Dubuque, IA: Kendall Hunt Publishing.

Eklund, M., Hermansson, A., & Håkansson, C. (2012). Meaning in life for people with schizophrenia: Does it include occupation? *Journal of Occupational Science, 19*(2), 93–105. doi:10.1080/14427591.2011.605833

Evenson, E., Rhodes, J., Feigenbaum, J., & Solly, A. (2008). The experiences of fathers with psychosis. *Journal of Mental Health, 17*(6), 629–642. doi:10.1080/09638230701506259

Fernandes, N. J. (2009). *The subjective experience of self in schizophrenia: A phenomenological study* (Doctoral dissertation). Retrieved from ProQuest Database (3405284).

Flanagan, E., Solomon, L., Johnson, A., Ridgway, P., Strauss, J., & Davidson, L. (2012). Considering DSM-5: The personal experience of schizophrenia in relation to the DSM-IV-TR criteria. *Psychiatry: Interpersonal and Biological Processes, 75*(4), 375–386. doi:10.1521/psyc.2012.75.4.375

Forchuk, C., Jewell, J., Tweedell, D., & Steinnagel, L. (2003). Reconnecting: The client experience of recovery from psychosis. *Perspectives in Psychiatric Care, 39*(4), 141–150. doi:10.1111/ppc.2003.39.issue-4

Gee, L., Pearce, E., & Jackson, M. (2003). Quality of life in schizophrenia: A grounded theory approach. *Health and Quality of Life Outcomes, 1*(1), 1–11. doi:10.1186/1477-7525-1-31

Gould, A., DeSouza, S., & Rebeiro-Gruhl, K. (2005). And then I lost that life: A shared narrative of four young men with schizophrenia. *The British Journal of Occupational Therapy, 68*(10), 467–473. doi:10.1177/030802260506801005

Gunnmo, P., & Bergman, H. F. (2011). What do individuals with schizophrenia need to increase their well-being. *International Journal of Qualitative Studies on Health and Well-being, 6*(11), 1–11.

Harley, E. W., Boardman, J., & Craig, T. (2012). Friendship in people with schizophrenia: A survey. *Social Psychiatry and Psychiatric Epidemiology, 47*(8), 1291–1299. doi:10.1007/s00127-011-0437-x

Hewitt, J., & Coffey, M. (2005). Therapeutic working relationships with people with schizophrenia: Literature review. *Journal of Advanced Nursing, 52*(5), 561–570. doi:10.1111/jan.2005.52.issue-5

Humberstone, V. (2002). The experiences of people with schizophrenia living in supported accommodation: A qualitative study using grounded theory methodology. *Australian & New Zealand Journal of Psychiatry, 36*(3), 367–372. doi:10.1046/j.1440-1614.2002.01034.x

Jarosinski, J. (2006). *A life disrupted: Still lived.* (Unpublished doctoral dissertation). Virginia Commonwealth University, Richmond, VA.

Johnson, J., Gooding, P., & Tarrier, N. (2008). Suicide risk in schizophrenia: Explanatory models and clinical implications, the Schematic Appraisal Model of Suicide (SAMS). *Psychology and Psychotherapy: Theory, Research and Practice, 81*(1), 55–77. doi:10.1348/147608307X244996

Komossa, K., Rummel-Kluge, C., Hunger, H., Schwarz, S., Bhoopathi, P. S., Kissling, W., & Leucht, S. (2010a). Ziprasidone versus other atypical antipsychotics for schizophrenia. *Cochrane Collaboration.* doi:10.1002/14651858.CD006624.pub2

Komossa, K., Rummel-Kluge, C., Schmid, F., Hunger, H., Schwarz, S., Srisurpanont, M., ... Leucht, S. (2010b). Quetiapine versus other atypical antipsychotics for schizophrenia. *Cochrane Collaboration.* doi:10.1002/14651858.CD006569.pub3

Komossa, K., Rummel-Kluge, C., Schwarz, S., Schmid, F., Hunger, H., Kissling, W., & Leucht, S. (2011). Risperidone versus other atypical antipsychotics for schizophrenia. *Cochrane Collaboration.* doi:10.1002/14651858.CD006626.pub2

Leucht, S., Tardy, M., Komossa, K., Heres, S., Kissling, W., & Davis, J. M. (2012). Maintenance treatment with antipsychotic drugs for schizophrenia. *The Cochrane Library.* doi:10.1002/14651858.CD008016.pub2

Liu, L., Ma, X., & Zhao, X. (2012). What do psychotic experiences mean to Chinese schizophrenia patients? *Qualitative Health Research, 22*, 1707–1716. doi:10.1177/1049732312460589

Lobos, C. A., Komossa, K., Rummel-Kluge, C., Hunger, H., Schmid, F., Schwarz, S., & Leucht, S. (2010). Clozapine versus other atypical antipsychotics for schizophrenia. *Cochrane Collaboration.* doi:10.1002/14651858.CD006633.pub2

McCann, T., & Clark, E. (2004). Embodiment of severe and enduring mental illness: Finding meaning in schizophrenia. *Issues in Mental Health Nursing, 25*, 783–798. doi:10.1080/01612840490506365

Meade, M. O., & Richardson, W. S. (1997). Selecting and appraising studies for systematic review. *Annals of Internal Medicine, 127*(7), 531–537. doi:10.7326/0003-4819-127-7-199710010-00005

Ng, R., Pearson, V., Lam, M., Law, C., Chiu, C., & Chen, E. (2008). What does recovery from schizophrenia mean? Perceptions of long-term patients. *International Journal of Social Psychiatry, 54*(2), 118–130. doi:10.1177/0020764007084600

Noblit, G. W., & Hare, R. D. (1988). *Meta-ethnography: Synthesizing qualitative studies.* Newbury Park, CA: Sage.

Phillips, J. K. (2008). *The experience of hope in those diagnosed with schizophrenia: A qualitative study.* (Doctoral dissertation). Retrieved from ProQuest Database (3338144).

Phripp, T. (1995). *Not like I might have been.* (Unpublished Masters Thesis). Queen's University, Kingston, Ontario, Canada.

Powell, J. (1998). *Living with schizophrenia outside mental health provider's conceptualizations: An abyss of misunderstanding and marginalization.* (Unpublished doctoral dissertation). University of Wisconsin-Milwaukee, Milwaukee, WI.

Ring, N. A., Ritchie, K., Mandava, L., & Jepson, R. (2011). A guide to synthesising qualitative research for researchers undertaking health technology assessments and systematic reviews. *NHS Quality Improvement Scotland.* Retrieved from http://hdl.handle.net/1893/3205

Roberts, A. R. (Ed.). (2009). *Social workers' desk reference* (2nd ed.). New York, NY: Oxford University Press.

Roe, D., Chopra, M., & Rudnick, A. (2004). Persons with psychosis as active agents interacting with their disorder. *Psychiatric Rehabilitation Journal, 28*(2), 122–128. doi:10.2975/28.2004.122.128

Sanseeha, L., Chontawan, R., Sethbouppha, H., Disayavanish, C., & Turale, S. (2009). Illness perspectives of Thais diagnosed with schizophrenia. *Nursing & Health Sciences, 11*, 306–311. doi:10.1111/nhs.2009.11.issue-3

Shepherd, S., Depp, C., Harris, G., Halpain, M., Palinkas, L., & Jeste, D. (2012). Perspectives on schizophrenia over the lifespan: A qualitative study. *Schizophrenia Bulletin, 38*(2), 295–303. doi:10.1093/schbul/sbq075

Stahl, S. M. (2013). *Stahl's essential psychopharmacology: Neuroscientific basis and practical application.* Cambridge, England: Cambridge University Press.

Sung, K., & Puskar, K. (2006). Schizophrenia in college students in Korea: A qualitative perspective. *Perspectives in Psychiatric Care, 42*(1), 21–32. doi:10.1111/ppc.2006.42.issue-1

Suryani, S., Welch, A., & Cox, L. (2013). The phenomena of auditory hallucination as described by Indonesian people living with schizophrenia. *Archives of Psychiatric Nursing, 27*, 312–318. doi:10.1016/j.apnu.2013.08.001

Thomas, J., & Harden, A. (2008). Methods for the thematic synthesis of qualitative research in systematic reviews. *BMC Medical Research Methodology, 8*, 45. doi:10.1186/1471-2288-8-45

Thornicroft, G., Brohan, E., Rose, D., Sartorius, N., & Leese, M. (2009). Global pattern of experienced and anticipated discrimination against people with schizophrenia: A cross-sectional survey. *The Lancet, 373*(9661), 408–415. doi:10.1016/S0140-6736(08)61817-6

Tooth, B., Kalyanasundaram, V., Glover, H., & Momenzadah, S. (2003). Factors consumers identify as important to recovery from schizophrenia. *Australasian Psychiatry, 11*, S70–77. doi:10.1046/j.1440-1665.11.s1.1.x

Van Manen, M. (1990). *Researching lived experiences.* Albany, NY: State University of New York Press.

Van Os, J., Rutten, B. P. F., & Poulton, R. (2008). Gene-environmental interactions in schizophrenia: Review of epidemiological findings and future directions. *Schizophrenia Bulletin, 34*(6), 1066–1082. doi:10.1093/schbul/sbn117

Walton, J. (1992). The lived experience of schizophrenia. *Rogerian Nursing Science News: Newsletter of the Society of Rogerian Scholars, 4*(3), 5–6.

Walton, J. (2000). Schizophrenia and life in the world of others. *Canadian Journal of Nursing Research, 32*(3), 69–84.

Yennari, A. (2011). *Living with schizophrenia: A phenomenological investigation.* (Doctoral dissertation). Retrieved from ProQuest Database (3465900).

Can J Diabetes 42 (2018) S80–S87

Contents lists available at ScienceDirect

Canadian Journal of Diabetes

journal homepage:
www.canadianjournalofdiabetes.com

ELSEVIER

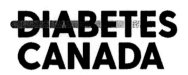

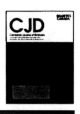

2018 Clinical Practice Guidelines

Glycemic Management in Adults With Type 1 Diabetes

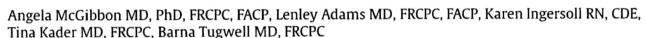

Diabetes Canada Clinical Practice Guidelines Expert Committee

Angela McGibbon MD, PhD, FRCPC, FACP, Lenley Adams MD, FRCPC, FACP, Karen Ingersoll RN, CDE,
Tina Kader MD, FRCPC, Barna Tugwell MD, FRCPC

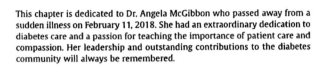

This chapter is dedicated to Dr. Angela McGibbon who passed away from a sudden illness on February 11, 2018. She had an extraordinary dedication to diabetes care and a passion for teaching the importance of patient care and compassion. Her leadership and outstanding contributions to the diabetes community will always be remembered.

- The insulin treatment your health-care provider prescribes will depend on your goals, lifestyle, meal plan, age and general health. Social and financial factors may also be taken into account.
- Learning to avoid and treat hypoglycemia (low blood glucose) is an important part of your education. The ideal balance is to achieve blood glucose levels that are as close to target as possible while avoiding hypoglycemia.

KEY MESSAGES

- Basal-bolus insulin therapies (i.e. multiple daily injections or continuous subcutaneous insulin infusion) are the preferred insulin management regimens for adults with type 1 diabetes.
- Insulin regimens should be tailored to the individual's treatment goals, lifestyle, diet, age, general health, motivation, hypoglycemia awareness status and ability for self-management.
- All individuals with type 1 diabetes should be counselled about the risk, prevention and treatment of hypoglycemia. Avoidance of nocturnal hypoglycemia may include changes in insulin therapy and increased monitoring.
- If glycemic targets are not met with optimized multiple daily injections, continuous subcutaneous insulin infusion may be considered. Successful continuous subcutaneous insulin infusion therapy requires appropriate candidate selection, ongoing support and frequent involvement with the health-care team.
- Continuous glucose monitoring may be offered to people not meeting their glycemic targets, who will wear the devices the majority of the time, in order to improve glycemic control.

KEY MESSAGES FOR PEOPLE WITH DIABETES

- Insulin therapy is required for the treatment of type 1 diabetes.
- There are a variety of insulins and methods of giving insulin to help manage type 1 diabetes.
- Insulin is injected by pen, syringe or insulin pump.
- Your health-care provider will work with you to determine such things as:
  - The number of insulin injections you need per day
  - The timing of your insulin injections
  - The dose of insulin you need with each injection
  - If and when an insulin pump is appropriate for you
  - Your pump settings if you are giving insulin that way.

Introduction

Insulin is lifesaving pharmacological therapy for people with type 1 diabetes. Insulin preparations are primarily produced by recombinant DNA technology and are formulated either as structurally identical to human insulin or as a modification of human insulin (insulin analogues) to alter pharmacokinetics. Human insulin and insulin analogues are preferred and used by most adults with type 1 diabetes; however, preparations of animal-sourced insulin are still accessible in Canada (1) although rarely required. Inhaled insulin is currently not approved for use in Canada.

Insulin preparations are classified according to their duration of action and are further differentiated by their time of onset and peak actions (see Appendix 6. Types of Insulin). For most adults with type 1 diabetes, premixed insulin preparations are not suitable as frequent adjustments of insulin are required. Insulin delivered by basal-bolus injection therapy or continuous subcutaneous insulin infusion (CSII, also called insulin pump therapy) as basal and bolus regimens are preferred. Avoidance of hypoglycemia with all regimens is a priority.

Achieving optimal glycemic targets, while avoiding hypoglycemia, can be challenging and requires individualized insulin regimens, which may include specialized insulin delivery devices and glucose monitoring often introduced in an escalating manner, starting with basal-bolus injection therapy then, in some cases, moving to CSII either with or without sensor augmentation. Continuous glucose monitoring (CGM) may be used with basal-bolus injection therapy or CSII. The role of adjuvant (noninsulin) injectable or oral antihyperglycemic medications in glycemic control is limited for most people with type 1 diabetes. Noninsulin pharmacotherapy for prevention of complications and treatment of risk factors is addressed in other chapters (see Cardiovascular Protection in People with Diabetes chapter, p. S162; Chronic Kidney Disease in Diabetes chapter, p. S201). Hypoglycemia as it relates to insulin therapy in type 1 diabetes is discussed here, and hypoglycemia in general is addressed in the Hypoglycemia chapter, p. S104.

Conflict of interest statements can be found on page S84.

1499-2671 © 2018 Canadian Diabetes Association.
The Canadian Diabetes Association is the registered owner of the name Diabetes Canada.
https://doi.org/10.1016/j.jcjd.2017.10.012

Insulin Therapy with Basal-Bolus Injection Therapy

People with type 1 diabetes are initiated on insulin therapy immediately at diagnosis. This requires both the selection of an insulin regimen and comprehensive diabetes education. Insulin regimens, usually with basal and bolus insulins, should be tailored to the individual's age, general health, treatment goals, lifestyle, diet, hypoglycemia awareness status, ability for self-management and adherence to treatment. Social and financial aspects also should be considered. After insulin initiation, some individuals experience a "honeymoon period," during which insulin requirements may be lower than expected; however, this period is transient (usually weeks to months), and insulin requirements typically increase and stabilize with time.

The Diabetes Control and Complications Trial (DCCT) conclusively demonstrated that intensive treatment of type 1 diabetes significantly delays the onset and slows the progression of microvascular and cardiovascular (CV) complications (2,3). The most successful management in the majority of adults with type 1 diabetes is based on basal-bolus injection therapy or CSII. Such regimens attempt to replicate normal pancreatic secretion of insulin.

Currently, new concentrated insulin preparations are available in basal and bolus formats. Sometimes they have identical pharmacokinetic and pharmacodynamic properties to the original preparation and other concentrated insulins have different pharmacological properties (see Appendix 6. Types of Insulin). These are further described below in the basal and bolus sections. In addition, biosimilar basal insulin is also available.

Basal insulin and basal-bolus injection therapy

Basal insulin refers to long- or intermediate-acting insulin, which provides control of glucose in the fasting state and between meals. Basal insulin is given once or twice a day and includes long-acting insulin analogues and intermediate-acting insulin neutral protamine Hagedorn (NPH). Insulin onset, peak and duration are shown in Appendix 6. Types of Insulin. Detemir insulin is available as a 100 units/mL formulation (U-100) (Levemir®). Glargine insulin is available as a 100 units/mL formulation (U-100) (Lantus™), a 300 units/mL formulation (U-300) (Toujeo®) and as a 100 units/mL biosimilar product (U-100) (Basaglar®). Degludec insulin is available as a 100 units/mL (U-100) and 200 units/mL (U-200) formulation (Tresiba®).

When used as a basal insulin in type 1 diabetes, the U-100 long-acting analogues, insulin detemir and insulin glargine (with rapid-acting insulin analogues for meals) resulted in lower fasting plasma glucose (FPG) levels and less hypoglycemia (4–7) or nocturnal hypoglycemia compared with once- or twice-daily NPH insulin (4,6–11). Given the potential severe consequences of nocturnal hypoglycemia, the avoidance of this complication is of great clinical importance.

Biosimilar insulin glargine has the identical amino acid sequence as glargine and is produced through a different manufacturing process. Biosimilar insulin glargine has been shown to have similar efficacy and safety outcomes in adults with type 1 diabetes maintained or switched from U-100 glargine (12).

Insulin glargine U-300 is a concentrated basal insulin, which appears to have a consistent, gradual and extended flat release from subcutaneous tissue with a longer duration of action (>30 hours) than U-100 glargine (13,14). Insulin glargine U-300 has been compared to insulin glargine U-100 in adults with type 1 diabetes and found to produce similar changes in A1C and similar or lower risk of hypoglycemia (13,15). Confirmed or severe nocturnal hypoglycemia was significantly lower in 1 study (16) but not in other shorter trials (15). Insulin glargine U-300 may require a higher dose than insulin glargine U-100 and may result in less weight gain (15,17).

Insulin degludec is a basal insulin with a long duration of action (42 hours) (14,18,19) in a once-daily injection that provides a consistent, flat glucose-lowering profile with low day-to-day variability (18,19). It provides similar glycemic control, but with less nocturnal hypoglycemia (20) and reduced basal and total insulin dose when compared to insulin glargine (21–23) and insulin detemir (24,25). The prolonged duration of action of insulin degludec allows for flexible timing of dosing without compromising metabolic control or safety (26). The 2 formulations of insulin degludec (U-100 and U-200) have similar glucose-lowering effects and half-lives (14).

Bolus insulin and basal-bolus injection therapy

Bolus insulin refers to rapid- or short-acting insulin given to control the glycemic rise at meals and to correct hyperglycemia. The prandial injection dose is decided based on carbohydrate content, carbohydrate-to-insulin ratio for each meal, planned exercise, time since last insulin dose and blood glucose level. Bolus insulins include rapid-acting insulin analogues (insulin aspart, insulin faster-acting aspart, insulin glargine, insulin lispro) and short-acting insulin (regular insulin).

Preprandial injections of rapid-acting insulin analogues result in a lower postprandial glucose and improved overall glycemic control (27–30). Insulin aspart, glulisine and lispro should be administered 0 to 15 minutes before the start of the meal while short-acting regular insulin should be administered 30 to 45 minutes before the start of the meal. Faster-acting insulin aspart may be administered at the start of the meal or, when necessary, up to 20 minutes after the start of the meal (31). When required, insulin aspart, glulisine and lispro can be administered from 0 to 15 minutes after the start of a meal although better control of postprandial hyperglycemia is seen with preprandial injections.

Insulin aspart and lispro have been associated with reduced nocturnal hypoglycemia, slightly lower A1C, improved postprandial glucose (30,32) and improved quality of life (33) when compared to short-acting insulin. Insulin glulisine has been shown to be equivalent to insulin lispro for glycemic control, with most effective A1C reduction when given before meals (27,34). Faster-acting insulin aspart has an earlier onset than insulin aspart (see Appendix 6. Types of Insulin). In type 1 diabetes, faster-acting insulin aspart demonstrated noninferiority with respect to A1C reduction and superior postprandial glucose control vs. insulin aspart (31).

Hypoglycemia and Insulin Therapy

Hypoglycemia is the most common adverse effect of insulin therapy in people with type 1 diabetes (for definitions see Hypoglycemia chapter, p. S104). In the DCCT, 35% of participants in the conventional treatment group and 65% in the intensive group experienced at least 1 episode of severe hypoglycemia (2,35,36). In a meta-analysis of 14 trials, the median incidence of severe hypoglycemia was 4.6 and 7.9 episodes per 100 patient-years in the conventionally treated and intensively treated people with type 1 diabetes, respectively (37). With adequate self-management education, appropriate glycemic targets, self-monitoring of blood glucose and support, intensive therapy may result in less hypoglycemia than reported in the DCCT (38–41), particularly with modern insulin formulations.

The frequency of hypoglycemic events is reduced with rapid-acting insulin analogues compared with regular insulin (8,42–44) although there are no differences in the magnitude and temporal pattern of the physiological, symptomatic and counterregulatory hormonal responses to hypoglycemia induced by regular human insulin or rapid-acting analogues (45,46).

Long-acting insulin analogues reduce the incidence of hypoglycemia and nocturnal hypoglycemia when compared to intermediate-acting insulin as the basal insulin (10,47–51). Lifestyle factors and changes from usual self-management behaviours (e.g. eating less food, taking more insulin, increased physical activity) account for 85% of hypoglycemic episodes (52,53). Adding bedtime snacks may be helpful to prevent nocturnal hypoglycemia among those taking NPH as the basal insulin or in those individuals at high risk of severe hypoglycemia (regardless of insulin type), particularly when bedtime plasma glucose (PG) levels are <7.0 mmol/L (54,55).

Knowledge of the acute effects of exercise is essential. Low- to moderate-intensity exercise lowers BG levels both during and after the activity, increasing the risk of a hypoglycemic episode. These effects on BG levels can be modified by altering diet, insulin, and the type and timing of physical activity. In contrast, high-intensity exercise raises BG levels during and immediately after the event but may result in hypoglycemia hours later. SMBG before, during and after exercise is important for establishing response to exercise and guiding the appropriate management of exercise. If ketosis is present, exercise should not be performed as metabolic deterioration can occur (56) (see Physical Activity and Diabetes chapter, p. S54).

Hypoglycemia prevention and treatment is discussed in more detail in the Hypoglycemia chapter, p. S104; however, it is the limiting factor in most treatment strategies for type 1 diabetes. Increased education, monitoring of blood glucose, changing insulins and insulin routines, and the use of new diabetes technologies may be required (57,58). An educational program for people with impaired hypoglycemia awareness in which participants were randomized to either CSII or basal-bolus injection therapy and to either SMBG or real-time CGM showed that severe hypoglycemia and hypoglycemia awareness were improved to a similar degree regardless of the insulin delivery method or monitoring method used, although treatment satisfaction was higher with CSII compared with basal-bolus injection therapy (59).

Continuous Subcutaneous Insulin Infusion Therapy

CSII or insulin pump therapy is a safe and effective method of intensive insulin delivery in type 1 diabetes. Both CSII and basal-bolus injection therapy are considered the standard of care for adults with type 1 diabetes. While many people with type 1 diabetes are on CSII due to personal preference, there are some medical indications for CSII therapy. In particular, CSII can be considered in people with type 1 diabetes who do not reach glycemic targets despite optimized basal-bolus injection therapy, as well as in the following individuals: those with significant glucose variability; frequent severe hypoglycemia and/or hypoglycemia unawareness; significant "dawn phenomenon" with rise of blood glucose early in the morning; very low insulin requirements; adequate glycemic control but suboptimal treatment satisfaction and quality of life or women contemplating pregnancy (60–63).

It is important to select the appropriate individual for pump therapy. Appropriate candidates should be motivated individuals, currently on optimized basal-bolus injection therapy, who are willing to frequently monitor BG, understand sick-day management and attend follow-up visits as required by the health-care team (62,63). The health-care team should ideally be interprofessional and include a diabetes educator and a physician/nurse practitioner with special interest and expertise in CSII therapy. Comprehensive preparation, initiation and follow up should be provided by the team and are critical for the success of CSII. The health-care team should periodically re-evaluate whether continued pump therapy is appropriate for the individual (62).

Rapid-acting insulin analogues have replaced short-acting insulin in CSII therapy for several reasons, including their demonstrated

safety, efficacy and more physiologic and rapid action (64). Although not recommended in Canada, insulin Humulin R® is still indicated for use in CSII while insulin Novolin Toronto® is not. The 3 rapid-acting insulin analogues approved for CSII are insulin lispro, aspart and glulisine. Faster-acting insulin aspart is not yet approved in Canada for use in CSII. Among people using CSII, insulin lispro has been demonstrated to provide similar (65) or superior (66,67) A1C lowering, overall improvement in postprandial hyperglycemia (66,67), and no increase in hypoglycemia (66,67) when compared to short-acting insulin. Insulin aspart provides a similar effect on A1C and hypoglycemia risk as short-acting insulin or lispro (65). Insulin glulisine has a similar effect on A1C when compared to aspart (68,69) and lispro (68); however, the rate of symptomatic hypoglycemia was higher with use of glulisine in 1 crossover study (68).

Clinical trial data on the rate of catheter occlusions among users of the 3 rapid-acting insulins do not show any consistent differences (68,69). In vitro studies have demonstrated some differences in product stability and catheter occlusions (64). Insulin glulisine is indicated to be changed at least every 48 hours in the infusion set and reservoir; aspart and lispro are to be changed according to the pump manufacturer's recommendations.

A1C benefit of CSII therapy

CSII treatment has gone through many advances since it was first introduced. Many studies using CSII have been limited by small numbers of participants, short duration and the inability to adequately blind participants. Interpretation of meta-analyses is difficult as some included trials with short-acting insulin in the CSII arm (70,71), and another included trials with only NPH-based basal-bolus injection therapy as the comparator (72). The most relevant meta-analyses included trials using rapid-acting insulin analogues in the CSII arms and NPH- or glargine-based basal-bolus injection therapy as the comparators (73–75). Trials using other basal analogues as the comparator were not identified. Use of CSII was shown to reduce A1C by 0.19% to 0.3% in adults (73,75) or in participants with a mean age over 10 years (74). An observational study of real-life outcomes using CSII therapy demonstrated that those who had a pre-CSII A1C of >9.0% had the greatest improvement in A1C after CSII initiation; people with a pre-CSII A1C of ≤7.0% were likely to maintain their A1C in the same range on CSII; and for all groups, A1C values slowly increased with time but remained below the pre-CSII levels (76).

A major advancement in CSII treatment has been the addition of continuous glucose monitoring systems (CGM) and sensor-augmented pumps (SAP) which is the use of CSII plus CGM. In people with type 1 diabetes with suboptimal control on basal-bolus injection therapy and SMBG, the introduction of CSII and CGM at the same time offers a more substantial A1C benefit over continuation of basal-bolus injection therapy with SMBG. In 2 major trials, participants suboptimally controlled on basal-bolus injection therapy were randomized to either continue basal-bolus injection therapy or to start SAP. One small trial in adults showed a mean difference in change in A1C of -1.21% in favour of the SAP arm (77), without an increase in hypoglycemia. In a larger trial of children and adults, end-of-trial mean difference in change in A1C was -0.6% in favour of the SAP arm, in all participants and in adults specifically (78) without an increase in hypoglycemia. Duration of sensor use was associated with the greatest decline in A1C in 1 trial (78) but not the other (77).

Further enhancement of sensor-augmented CSII technology has been the low glucose suspend function in which insulin delivery is stopped for a defined period of time if a critically low glucose threshold is detected on the CGM. To date, only 2 major trials have been published regarding this technology (79,80). Hypoglycemia benefit, rather than the change in A1C, was the primary focus of these trials and no conclusions can be made about A1C benefit of SAP with low glucose suspend.

CSII and hypoglycemia

The benefit of CSII with regard to hypoglycemia has been difficult to evaluate given that many studies were of short duration, had small numbers and rates of severe hypoglycemia were generally low. Severe hypoglycemia has not been significantly different between users of CSII and basal-bolus injection therapy, based on meta-analyses which included only rapid-acting insulin analogues in the CSII arms (73–75). However, in a meta-analysis of trials of participants with a high baseline rate of severe hypoglycemia (>10 episodes per 100 patient-years while on basal-bolus injection therapy), the use of CSII was associated with a reduction of severe hypoglycemia (81) when compared to basal-bolus injection regimens using older nonanalogue basal insulins.

Nonsevere hypoglycemia has been inconsistently defined and reported but, overall, CSII does not appear to reduce the frequency of nonsevere hypoglycemia. No differences have been found between CSII and basal-bolus injection therapy for nocturnal hypoglycemia (75). No consistent conclusions could be drawn regarding nonsevere hypoglycemia in 2 meta-analyses (73,74). In 1 meta-analysis, minor hypoglycemia, calculated as the mean number of mild episodes per patient per week, was found to be nonsignificantly lower in users of CSII in crossover trials of adolescents and adults (75).

When CSII has been introduced together with CGM (SAP), A1C has been consistently lowered without increasing the rate of hypoglycemia (77,78). Time spent in hypoglycemia and severe hypoglycemia was not consistently different (77,78) but hypoglycemia fear improved more in adults randomized to SAP compared to those randomized to continuation of basal-bolus injection therapy (82).

One large randomized controlled trial in adults compared the use of SAP with and without the low glucose suspend feature (80). Participants were randomized if they had demonstrated nocturnal hypoglycemia and high sensor compliance during the run-in phase. SAP with low glucose suspend led to a reduction in nocturnal hypoglycemia with no increase in A1C or ketoacidosis (80). In another trial of adults and children with hypoglycemia unawareness, the use of SAP with low glucose suspend, compared to the use of CSII and SMBG, was shown to reduce the rate of moderate and severe hypoglycemia (79) although this outcome lost significance when outliers were excluded. Overall, the use of SAP with low glucose suspend is promising for nocturnal hypoglycemia and hypoglycemia unawareness but more studies are needed.

CSII and quality of life

Several studies have demonstrated improved quality of life (QOL) or improved treatment satisfaction (TS) with CSII therapy whether due to improved glycemic control, flexibility in insulin administration, patient selection and/or motivation. The various studies used different measurement tools or older insulin regimens (70). Compared with basal-bolus injection therapy plus SMBG, CSII plus SMBG has been associated with improved diabetes-specific QOL (73) and TS (70). When compared with basal-bolus injection therapy plus SMBG, CSII plus CGM (SAP) has been associated with improved diabetes-specific health-related QOL (82), diabetes-related distress (77), TS (77,82), perceived frequency of hyperglycemia (77), fear of hypoglycemia (82), and general health and social functioning (77). Compared with CSII plus SMBG, SAP has been associated with improved TS (83,84), lower perceived frequency of hypoglycemia (83), less worry about hypoglycemia (83), and better treatment convenience and flexibility (84).

Data regarding long-term diabetes complications, adverse events, cost and mortality among users of CSII have been limited (70). An observational study of a large population-based Swedish national diabetes registry revealed lower cardiovascular (CV) mortality in users of CSII compared with users of basal-bolus injection therapy (85).

Continuous Glucose Monitoring

Adults with type 1 diabetes derive an A1C benefit from CGM, when compared to SMBG, regardless of the baseline level of A1C or the type of intensive insulin therapy and delivery. CGM may be done in a blinded manner ("professional" CGM), so that results are not immediately visible to the person with diabetes, or more commonly, in "real-time" where people with diabetes can immediately see values and take action if necessary. The discussion here refers to the studies using "real-time" CGM. The recommendations and findings presented here are consistent with those of the Endocrine Society Clinical Practice Guideline on this topic, which recommended the use of real-time CGM for adult patients with either A1C above target or who are well-controlled (at A1C target), provided that the devices are worn nearly daily (63).

In people with diabetes with a baseline A1C >7.0%, the use of CGM compared to SMBG results in an A1C reduction of approximately 0.4% to 0.6%. This A1C change has been demonstrated in adults using CSII (86), adults and children using either basal-bolus injection therapy or CSII (87), adults and children using CSII (88,89) and adults using basal-bolus injection therapy (90,91). In contrast, two trials in adults and children using CSII showed no A1C difference between users of CGM and SMBG (92,93) except in those who wore the sensor at least 70% of the time in 1 of the studies (92). Even with a baseline A1C <7.0%, in adults and children using basal-bolus injection therapy or CSII, the A1C benefit of CGM has been -0.27 to -0.34% (94,95). Meta-analyses of trials regardless of the baseline A1C have estimated the overall between-group change from baseline A1C to be approximately -0.2% to -0.3% in favour of CGM (73,96,97), and in adults specifically the A1C benefit has been -0.38% (73). The greatest A1C benefit has been demonstrated with the greatest duration of sensor use (97,73) and with the highest A1C at baseline (97).

The A1C benefits of CGM do not appear to be associated with excess hypoglycemia. Time spent in hypoglycemia was either lower in the CGM group (88,90,93,95) or was not significantly different between groups (86,92,94). Severe hypoglycemia was uncommon in these studies, and 1 study showed an increase in severe hypoglycemia with CGM (93) but this was not consistent in other trials.

People with type 1 diabetes with an A1C <7.0% may find that the use of CGM allows them to maintain their A1C at target without more hypoglycemia. One trial in patients with an A1C <7.5% (mean A1C at randomization, 6.9%) demonstrated shorter time in hypoglycemia with reduction of A1C in the CGM group compared with the SMBG group (95). In another trial of subjects with an A1C <7% (mean baseline A1C 6.4%-6.5%), while time in hypoglycemia was not significantly reduced, combined A1C and hypoglycemia endpoints favoured the CGM group, including the reduction of A1C without a substantial increase of hypoglycemia, and the reduction of hypoglycemia without worsening of A1C by 0.3% or more (94).

When CGM is introduced together with CSII therapy (SAP), the A1C benefit has been larger when compared to maintenance of basal-bolus injection therapy plus SMBG, without an increase of hypoglycemia (73,77,78,96).

Among adults with impaired hypoglycemia awareness, CGM has been shown to reduce severe hypoglycemia and increase time in normoglycemia in 1 trial of participants with high compliance of sensor use (98). In contrast, in another trial using a standardized education program, hypoglycemia awareness and severe hypoglycemia improved to a similar degree in participants randomized to CGM or SMBG, but sensor compliance was not high in this trial (59). This technology is, therefore, promising in this group but more studies are required.

Adjunctive Therapy for Glycemic Control

As the incidence of obesity and overweight increases in the population, including in those with type 1 diabetes, there is growing interest in the potential use of noninsulin antihyperglycemic agents that improve insulin sensitivity or work independently of insulin and may provide additional glucose-lowering benefits without increasing hypoglycemia risk (99,100). In several studies, the use of metformin in type 1 diabetes reduces insulin requirements and may lead to modest weight loss (101) without increased hypoglycemia. In the clinical trial setting, metformin does not result in improved A1C, fasting glucose or triglyceride (TG) levels (101) and changes do not persist long term (102).

Several small trials using SGLT2 inhibitors in type 1 diabetes demonstrated a reduction in mean glucose levels (103) and A1C (104,105). An increase in diabetic ketoacidosis (DKA) was also seen, which may be as high as 6% of participants in an 18-week study (105). DKA may have been precipitated by other factors, and several presented with glucose <13.9 mmol/L (106). A1C reduction and increased risk of ketosis was found when this class was added to insulin and liraglutide (107). Although early data are cautiously positive for the use of this class in type 1 diabetes, better understanding of the risk for euglycemic DKA is needed (99,100,108) and SGLT2 inhibitors do not have an indication for use in type 1 diabetes (see Hyperglycemic Emergencies in Adults chapter, p. S109).

GLP-1 receptor agonists have been studied as add-on therapy to insulin in type 1 diabetes (109–111). Addition of liraglutide allowed a reduction in insulin dose and weight (110,111) without consistent results on hypoglycemia risk or A1C reduction in normal weight (112) or overweight (113) people with type 1 diabetes. Liraglutide may be associated with hyperglycemia and ketosis with the 1.8 mg dose in some studies (110,111) but not others (109). There is no current indication for use of liraglutide in type 1 diabetes. Studies of other GLP-1 receptor agonists in type 1 diabetes have been limited (109).

RECOMMENDATIONS

1. In adults with type 1 diabetes, basal-bolus injection therapy or CSII as part of an intensive diabetes management regimen should be used to achieve glycemic targets [Grade A, Level 1A (2)].

2. In adults with type 1 diabetes using basal-bolus injection therapy or CSII, rapid-acting insulin analogues should be used in place of regular insulin to improve A1C and to minimize the risk of hypoglycemia [Grade B, Level 2 (30,32) for basal-bolus injection therapy; Grade B, Level 2 (66,67) for lispro in CSII; Grade B, Level 2 (65) for aspart in CSII; Grade D, Consensus, for glulisine in CSII] and to achieve postprandial BG targets [Grade B, Level 2 (32) for basal-bolus injection therapy; Grade B, Level 2 (66) for CSII].

3. In adults with type 1 diabetes on basal-bolus injection therapy:
   a. A long-acting insulin analogue may be used in place of NPH to reduce the risk of hypoglycemia [Grade B, Level 2 for detemir (7,50); Grade B, Level 2 for glargine U-100 (4,5,51); Grade D, Consensus for degludec and glargine U-300], including nocturnal hypoglycemia [Grade B, Level 2 (7) for detemir; Grade B, Level 2 (4) for glargine U-100; Grade D, Consensus for degludec, and glargine U-300].
   b. Degludec may be used instead of detemir or glargine U-100 to reduce nocturnal hypoglycemia [Grade B, Level 2 (24) compared to detemir; Grade C, Level 3 (20) compared to glargine U-100].

4. All individuals with type 1 diabetes and their support persons should be counselled about the risk and prevention of hypoglycemia, and risk factors for severe hypoglycemia should be identified and addressed [Grade D, Consensus].

5. In adults with type 1 diabetes and hypoglycemia unawareness, the following nonpharmacological strategies may be used to reduce the risk of hypoglycemia:
   a. A standardized education program targeting rigorous avoidance of hypoglycemia while maintaining overall glycemic control [Grade A, Level 1A (59)]
   b. Increased frequency of SMBG, including periodic assessment during sleeping hours [Grade D, Consensus]
   c. CGM with high sensor adherence in those using CSII [Grade C, Level 3 (98)]
   d. Less stringent glycemic targets with avoidance of hypoglycemia for up to 3 months [Grade C, Level 3 (15,16)].

6. In adults with type 1 diabetes on basal-bolus injection therapy who are not achieving glycemic targets, CSII with or without CGM may be used to improve A1C [Grade B, Level 2 (77,78) with CGM; Grade B, Level 2 (73–75) without CGM].

7. In adults with type 1 diabetes,
   a. CSII may be used instead of basal-bolus injection therapy to improve treatment satisfaction [Grade C, Level 3 (70)]
   b. CSII plus CGM may be used instead of basal-bolus injection therapy or CSII with SMBG to improve quality of life, treatment satisfaction and other health-quality-related outcomes [Grade B, Level 2 (77,84)].

8. Adults with type 1 diabetes on CSII should undergo periodic evaluation to determine whether continued CSII is appropriate [Grade D, Consensus].

9. In adults with type 1 diabetes and an A1C at or above target, regardless of insulin delivery method used, CGM with high sensor adherence may be used to improve or maintain A1C [Grade B, Level 2 (97)] without increasing hypoglycemia [Grade C, Level 3 (97)].

10. In adults with type 1 diabetes experiencing nocturnal hypoglycemia and using CSII and CGM, SAP with low glucose suspend may be chosen over SAP alone to reduce nocturnal hypoglycemia [Grade B, Level 2 (80)].

Abbreviations:
A1C, glycated hemoglobin; *BG,* blood glucose; *CGM,* continuous glucose monitoring; *CSII,* continuous subcutaneous insulin infusion; *DHC,* diabetes health care; *QOL,* quality of life; *RAIA,* rapid-acting insulin analogues; *SAP,* sensor augmented pump, *SMBG,* self-monitoring of blood glucose. *TS,* treatment satisfaction.

Other Relevant Guidelines

Targets for Glycemic Control, p. S42
Monitoring Glycemic Control, p. S47
Physical Activity and Diabetes, p. S54
Pharmacologic Glycemic Management of Type 2 Diabetes in Adults, p. S88
Hypoglycemia, p. S104
In-Hospital Management of Diabetes, p. S115
Management of Acute Coronary Syndromes, p. S190
Type 1 Diabetes in Children and Adolescents, p. S234
Type 2 Diabetes in Children and Adolescents, p. S247
Diabetes and Pregnancy, p. S255
Diabetes in Older People, p. S283

Relevant Appendix

Appendix 6. Types of Insulin

Author Disclosures

Dr. Adams reports personal fees from Novo Nordisk, Sanofi, Merck, AstraZeneca, Medtronic, Boehringer Ingelheim, Janssen, and Valeant,

327

outside the submitted work. Dr. Kader reports personal fees from Eli Lilly, Sanofi, Novo Nordisk, Merck, Janssen, Medtronic, and Hoffman Laroche, outside the submitted work. Dr. Tugwell reports grants from Sanofi-Aventis Canada, Inc., outside the submitted work; and contract research as investigator or sub-investigator with the following companies, for which she does not personally receive additional payment, but for which her institution does receive funding: GlaxoSmithKline, Novo Nordisk Canada, AMGEN, Sanofi-Aventis Canada, Ionis, Boehringer Ingelheim, Novartis, AstraZeneca, Bristol-Myers Squibb, Intarcia, Lexicon, Merck, Eli Lilly, Pfizer/Merck, Takeda, NPS Pharmaceuticals and Cerenis Pharmaceuticals. No other authors have anything to disclose.

References

1. Insulin products. It's your health. Ottawa: Health Canada, 2010. Report No.: # H13-7/80-2010E. http://www.hc-sc.gc.ca/hl-vs/alt_formats/pacrb-dgapcr/pdf/iyh-vsv/med/insulin-eng.pdf. Accessed November 15, 2017.
2. Diabetes Control and Complications Trial Research Group, Nathan DM, Genuth S, et al. The effect of intensive treatment of diabetes on the development and progression of long-term complications in insulin-dependent diabetes mellitus. N Engl J Med 1993;329:977–86.
3. Nathan DM, Cleary PA, Backlund JY, et al. Intensive diabetes treatment and cardiovascular disease in patients with type 1 diabetes. N Engl J Med 2005;353:2643–53.
4. Ratner RE, Hirsch IB, Neifing JL, et al. Less hypoglycemia with insulin glargine in intensive insulin therapy for type 1 diabetes. U.S. Study Group of Insulin Glargine in Type 1 Diabetes. Diabetes Care 2000;23:639–43.
5. Marra LP, Araujo VE, Silva TB, et al. Clinical effectiveness and safety of analog glargine in type 1 diabetes: a systematic review and meta-analysis. Diabetes Ther 2016;7:241–58.
6. Keating GM. Insulin detemir: a review of its use in the management of diabetes mellitus. Drugs 2012;72:2255–87.
7. Agesen RM, Kristensen PL, Beck-Nielsen H, et al. Effect of insulin analogues on frequency of non-severe hypoglycaemia in patients with type 1 diabetes prone to severe hypoglycaemia: the HypoAna trial. Diabetes Metab 2016;42:249–55.
8. DeWitt DE, Hirsch IB. Outpatient insulin therapy in type 1 and type 2 diabetes mellitus: scientific review. JAMA 2003;289:2254–64.
9. Warren E, Weatherley-Jones E, Chilcott J, et al. Systematic review and economic evaluation of a long-acting insulin analogue, insulin glargine. Health Technol Assess 2004;8(iii):1–57.
10. Szypowska A, Golicki D, Groele L, et al. Long-acting insulin analogue detemir compared with NPH insulin in type 1 diabetes: A systematic review and meta-analysis. Pol Arch Med Wewn 2011;121:237–46.
11. Home P, Bartley P, Russell-Jones D, et al. Insulin detemir offers improved glycemic control compared with NPH insulin in people with type 1 diabetes: A randomized clinical trial. Diabetes Care 2004;27:1081–7.
12. Hadjiyianni I, Dahl D, Lacaya LB, et al. Efficacy and safety of LY2963016 insulin glargine in patients with type 1 and type 2 diabetes previously treated with insulin glargine. Diabetes Obes Metab 2016;18:425–9.
13. Rosselli JL, Archer SN, Lindley NK, et al. U300 insulin glargine: A novel basal insulin for type 1 and type 2 diabetes. J Pharm Technol 2015;31:234–42.
14. Lamos EM, Younk LM, Davis SN. Concentrated insulins: the new basal insulins. Ther Clin Risk Manag 2016;12:389–400.
15. Dailey G, Lavernia F. A review of the safety and efficacy data for insulin glargine 300units/ml, a new formulation of insulin glargine. Diabetes Obes Metab 2015;17:1107–14.
16. Matsuhisa M, Koyama M, Cheng X, et al. Sustained glycaemic control and less nocturnal hypoglycaemia with insulin glargine 300 U/mL compared with glargine 100 U/mL in Japanese adults with type 1 diabetes (EDITION JP 1 randomised 12-month trial including 6-month extension). Diabetes Res Clin Pract 2016;122:133–40.
17. Wang F, Zassman S, Goldberg PA. rDNA insulin glargine U300 - a critical appraisal. Diabetes Metab Syndr Obes 2016;9:425–41.
18. Heise T, Hermanski L, Nosek L, et al. Insulin degludec: four times lower pharmacodynamic variability than insulin glargine under steady-state conditions in type 1 diabetes. Diabetes Obes Metab 2012;14:859–64.
19. Kerlan V, Gouet D, Marre M, et al. Use of insulin degludec, a new basal insulin with an ultra-long duration of action, in basal-bolus therapy in type 1 and type 2 diabetes. Annal Endocrinol 2013;74:487–90.
20. Russell-Jones D, Gall MA, Niemeyer M, et al. Insulin degludec results in lower rates of nocturnal hypoglycaemia and fasting plasma glucose vs. insulin glargine: A meta-analysis of seven clinical trials. Nutr Metab Cardiovasc Dis 2015;25:898–905.
21. Heller S, Buse J, Fisher M, et al. Insulin degludec, an ultra-longacting basal insulin, versus insulin glargine in basal-bolus treatment with mealtime insulin aspart in type 1 diabetes (BEGIN Basal-Bolus Type 1): A phase 3, randomised, open-label, treat-to-target non-inferiority trial. Lancet 2012;379:1489–97.
22. Bode BW, Buse JB, Fisher M, et al. Insulin degludec improves glycaemic control with lower nocturnal hypoglycaemia risk than insulin glargine in basal-bolus treatment with mealtime insulin aspart in Type 1 diabetes (BEGIN(®) Basal-Bolus Type 1): 2-year results of a randomized clinical trial. Diabet Med 2013;30:1293–7.
23. Dzygalo K, Golicki D, Kowalska A, et al. The beneficial effect of insulin degludec on nocturnal hypoglycaemia and insulin dose in type 1 diabetic patients: A systematic review and meta-analysis of randomised trials. Acta Diabetol 2014;52:231–8.
24. Davies M, Sasaki T, Gross JL, et al. Comparison of insulin degludec with insulin detemir in type 1 diabetes: A 1-year treat-to-target trial. Diabetes Obes Metab 2016;18:96–9.
25. Hirsch IB, Franek E, Mersebach H, et al. Safety and efficacy of insulin degludec/insulin aspart with bolus mealtime insulin aspart compared with standard basal-bolus treatment in people with Type 1 diabetes: 1-year results from a randomized clinical trial (BOOST® T1). Diabet Med 2016;34:167–73, Available from.
26. Mathieu C, Hollander P, Miranda-Palma B, et al. Efficacy and safety of insulin degludec in a flexible dosing regimen vs insulin glargine in patients with type 1 diabetes (BEGIN: Flex T1): a 26-week randomized, treat-to-target trial with a 26-week extension. J Clin Endocrinol Metab 2013;98:1154–62.
27. Garg SK, Rosenstock J, Ways K. Optimized Basal-bolus insulin regimens in type 1 diabetes: Insulin glulisine versus regular human insulin in combination with Basal insulin glargine. Endocr Pract 2005;11:11–17.
28. Schernthaner G, Wein W, Shnawa N, et al. Preprandial vs. postprandial insulin lispro-a comparative crossover trial in patients with Type 1 diabetes. Diabet Med 2004;21:279–84.
29. Jovanovic L, Giammattei J, Acquistapace M, et al. Efficacy comparison between preprandial and postprandial insulin aspart administration with dose adjustment for unpredictable meal size. Clin Ther 2004;26:1492–7.
30. Fullerton B, Siebenhofer A, Jeitler K, et al. Short-acting insulin analogues versus regular human insulin for adults with type 1 diabetes mellitus. Cochrane Database Syst Rev 2016;(6):CD012161.
31. Russell-Jones D, Bode BW, De Block C, et al. Fast-acting insulin aspart improves glycemic control in basal-bolus treatment for type 1 diabetes: Results of a 26-week multicenter, active-controlled, treat-to-target, randomized, parallel-group trial (Onset 1). Diabetes Care 2017 (in press).
32. Wojciechowski P, Niemczyk-Szechowska P, Olewinska E, et al. Clinical efficacy and safety of insulin aspart compared with regular human insulin in patients with type 1 and type 2 diabetes: A systematic review and meta-analysis. Pol Arch Med Wewn 2015;125:141–51.
33. Bott U, Ebrahim S, Hirschberger S, et al. Effect of the rapid-acting insulin analogue insulin aspart on quality of life and treatment satisfaction in patients with type 1 diabetes. Diabet Med 2003;20:626–34.
34. Dreyer M, Prager R, Robinson A, et al. Efficacy and safety of insulin glulisine in patients with type 1 diabetes. Horm Metab Res 2005;37:702–7.
35. The Diabetes Control and Complications Trial Research Group. Adverse events and their association with treatment regimens in the diabetes control and complications trial. Diabetes Care 1995;18:1415–27.
36. The Diabetes Control and Complications Trial Research Group. Hypoglycemia in the diabetes control and complications trial. Diabetes 1997;46:271–86.
37. Egger M, Davey Smith G, Stettler C, et al. Risk of adverse effects of intensified treatment in insulin-dependent diabetes mellitus: A meta-analysis. Diabet Med 1997;14:919–28.
38. Fanelli CG, Epifano L, Rambotti AM, et al. Meticulous prevention of hypoglycemia normalizes the glycemic thresholds and magnitude of most of neuroendocrine responses to, symptoms of, and cognitive function during hypoglycemia in intensively treated patients with short-term IDDM. Diabetes 1993;42:1683–9.
39. Bott S, Bott U, Berger M, et al. Intensified insulin therapy and the risk of severe hypoglycaemia. Diabetologia 1997;40:926–32.
40. Ahern J. Steps to reduce the risks of severe hypoglycemia. Diabetes Spectr 1997;10:39–41.
41. Bolli GB. How to ameliorate the problem of hypoglycemia in intensive as well as nonintensive treatment of type 1 diabetes. Diabetes Care 1999;22:B43–52.
42. Siebenhofer A, Plank J, Berghold A, et al. Short acting insulin analogues versus regular human insulin in patients with diabetes mellitus. Cochrane Database Syst Rev 2006;(2):CD003287.
43. Heller SR, Colagiuri S, Vaaler S, et al. Hypoglycaemia with insulin aspart: a double-blind, randomised, crossover trial in subjects with type 1 diabetes. Diabet Med 2004;21:769–75.
44. Plank J, Siebenhofer A, Berghold A, et al. Systematic review and meta-analysis of short-acting insulin analogues in patients with diabetes mellitus. Arch Intern Med 2005;165:1337–44.
45. Torlone E, Fanelli C, Rambotti AM, et al. Pharmacokinetics, pharmacodynamics and glucose counterregulation following subcutaneous injection of the monomeric insulin analogue [Lys(B28),Pro(B29)] in IDDM. Diabetologia 1994;37:713–20.
46. McCrimmon RJ, Frier BM. Symptomatic and physiological responses to hypoglycaemia induced by human soluble insulin and the analogue Lispro human insulin. Diabet Med 1997;14:929–36.
47. Monami M, Marchionni N, Mannucci E. Long-acting insulin analogues vs. NPH human insulin in type 1 diabetes. A meta-analysis. Diabetes Obes Metab 2009;11:372–8.
48. Garg SK, Gottlieb PA, Hisatomi ME, et al. Improved glycemic control without an increase in severe hypoglycemic episodes in intensively treated patients

with type 1 diabetes receiving morning, evening, or split dose insulin glargine. Diabetes Res Clin Pract 2004;66:49–56.

49. Garg SK, Paul JM, Karsten JI, et al. Reduced severe hypoglycemia with insulin glargine in intensively treated adults with type 1 diabetes. Diabetes Technol Ther 2004;6:589–95.

50. Goldman-Levine JD, Lee KW. Insulin detemir–a new basal insulin analog. Ann Pharmacother 2005;39:502–7.

51. Mullins P, Sharplin P, Yki-Jarvinen H, et al. Negative binomial meta-regression analysis of combined glycosylated hemoglobin and hypoglycemia outcomes across eleven Phase III and IV studies of insulin glargine compared with neutral protamine Hagedorn insulin in type 1 and type 2 diabetes mellitus. Clin Ther 2007;29:1607–19.

52. Clarke WL, Cox DJ, Gonder-Frederick LA, et al. The relationship between nonroutine use of insulin, food, and exercise and the occurrence of hypoglycemia in adults with IDDM and varying degrees of hypoglycemic awareness and metabolic control. Diabetes Educ 1997;23:55–8.

53. Fritsche A, Stumvoll M, Renn W, et al. Diabetes teaching program improves glycemic control and preserves perception of hypoglycemia. Diabetes Res Clin Pract 1998;40:129–35.

54. Kaufman FR, Halvorson M, Kaufman ND. A randomized, blinded trial of uncooked cornstarch to diminish nocturnal hypoglycemia at diabetes camp. Diabetes Res Clin Pract 1995;30:205–9.

55. Kalergis M, Schiffrin A, Gougeon R, et al. Impact of bedtime snack composition on prevention of nocturnal hypoglycemia in adults with type 1 diabetes undergoing intensive insulin management using lispro insulin before meals: A randomized, placebo-controlled, crossover trial. Diabetes Care 2003;26:9–15.

56. Berger M, Berchtold P, Cüppers HJ, et al. Metabolic and hormonal effects of muscular exercise in juvenile type diabetics. Diabetologia 1977;13:355–65.

57. Cox DJ, Kovatchev B, Koev D, et al. Hypoglycemia anticipation, awareness and treatment training (HAATT) reduces occurrence of severe hypoglycemia among adults with type 1 diabetes mellitus. Int J Behav Med 2004;11:212–18.

58. de Zoysa N, Rogers H, Stadler M, et al. A psychoeducational program to restore hypoglycemia awareness: The DAFNE-HART pilot study. Diabetes Care 2014;37:863–6.

59. Little SA, Leelarathna L, Walkinshaw E, et al. Recovery of hypoglycemia awareness in long-standing type 1 diabetes: A multicenter 2 × 2 factorial randomized controlled trial comparing insulin pump with multiple daily injections and continuous with conventional glucose self-monitoring (HypoCOMPaSS). Diabetes Care 2014;37:2114–22.

60. Pozzilli P, Battelino T, Danne T, et al. Continuous subcutaneous insulin infusion in diabetes: Patient populations, safety, efficacy, and pharmacoeconomics. Diabetes Metab Res Rev 2016;32:21–39.

61. Marcus AO. Continuous subcutaneous insulin infusion therapy with rapid-acting insulin analogs in insulin pumps: Does it work, how does it work, and what therapies work better than others? Open Diabetes J 2013;6:8–19. https://benthamopen.com/ABSTRACT/TODIAJ-6-8.

62. Grunberger G, Abelseth JM, Bailey TS, et al. Consensus statement by the american association of clinical endocrinologists/american college of endocrinology insulin pump management task force. Endocr Pract 2014;20:463–89.

63. Peters AL, Ahmann AJ, Battelino T, et al. Diabetes technology-continuous subcutaneous insulin infusion therapy and continuous glucose monitoring in adults: an endocrine society clinical practice guideline. J Clin Endocrinol Metab 2016;101:3922–37.

64. Cengiz E, Bode B, Van Name M, et al. Moving toward the ideal insulin for insulin pumps. Expert Rev Med Devices 2016;13:57–69.

65. Bode B, Weinstein R, Bell D, et al. Comparison of insulin aspart with buffered regular insulin and insulin lispro in continuous subcutaneous insulin infusion: A randomized study in type 1 diabetes. Diabetes Care 2002;25:439–44.

66. Zinman B, Tildesley H, Chiasson JL, et al. Insulin lispro in CSII: Results of a double-blind crossover study. Diabetes 1997;46:440–3.

67. Radermecker RP, Scheen AJ. Continuous subcutaneous insulin infusion with short-acting insulin analogues or human regular insulin: Efficacy, safety, quality of life, and cost-effectiveness. Diabetes Metab Res Rev 2004;20:178–88.

68. van Bon AC, Bode BW, Sert-Langeron C, et al. Insulin glulisine compared to insulin aspart and to insulin lispro administered by continuous subcutaneous insulin infusion in patients with type 1 diabetes: A randomized controlled trial. Diabetes Technol Ther 2011;13:607–14.

69. Hoogma RP, Schumicki D. Safety of insulin glulisine when given by continuous subcutaneous infusion using an external pump in patients with type 1 diabetes. Horm Metab Res 2006;38:429–33.

70. Misso ML, Egberts KJ, Page M, et al. Continuous Subcutaneous Insulin Infusion (CSII) versus multiple insulin injections for type 1 diabetes mellitus. Cochrane Database Syst Rev 2010;(1):CD005103.

71. Pickup J, Mattock M, Kerry S. Glycaemic control with continuous subcutaneous insulin infusion compared with intensive insulin injections in patients with type 1 diabetes: meta-analysis of randomised controlled trials. BMJ 2002;324:705.

72. Retnakaran R, Hochman J, DeVries JH, et al. Continuous subcutaneous insulin infusion versus multiple daily injections: The impact of baseline A1c. Diabetes Care 2004;27:2590–6.

73. Yeh HC, Brown TT, Maruthur N, et al. Comparative effectiveness and safety of methods of insulin delivery and glucose monitoring for diabetes mellitus: A systematic review and meta-analysis. Ann Intern Med 2012;157:336–47.

74. Monami M, Lamanna C, Marchionni N, et al. Continuous subcutaneous insulin infusion versus multiple daily insulin injections in type 1 diabetes: A meta-analysis. Acta Diabetol 2010;47:77–81.

75. Fatourechi MM, Kudva YC, Murad MH, et al. Clinical review: hypoglycemia with intensive insulin therapy: A systematic review and meta-analyses of randomized trials of continuous subcutaneous insulin infusion versus multiple daily injections. J Clin Endocrinol Metab 2009;94:729–40.

76. Orr CJ, Hopman W, Yen JL, et al. Long-term efficacy of insulin pump therapy on glycemic control in adults with type 1 diabetes mellitus. Diabetes Technol Ther 2015;17:49–54.

77. Hermanides J, Norgaard K, Bruttomesso D, et al. Sensor-augmented pump therapy lowers HbA(1c) in suboptimally controlled type 1 diabetes; a randomized controlled trial. Diabet Med 2011;28:1158–67.

78. Bergenstal RM, Tamborlane WV, Ahmann A, et al. Effectiveness of sensor-augmented insulin-pump therapy in type 1 diabetes. N Engl J Med 2010;363:311–20.

79. Ly TT, Nicholas JA, Retterath A, et al. Effect of sensor-augmented insulin pump therapy and automated insulin suspension vs standard insulin pump therapy on hypoglycemia in patients with type 1 diabetes: A randomized clinical trial. J Am Med Assoc 2013;310:1240–7.

80. Bergenstal RM, Klonoff DC, Garg SK, et al. Threshold-based insulin-pump interruption for reduction of hypoglycemia. N Engl J Med 2013;369:224–32.

81. Pickup JC, Sutton AJ. Severe hypoglycaemia and glycaemic control in Type 1 diabetes: Meta-analysis of multiple daily insulin injections compared with continuous subcutaneous insulin infusion. Diabet Med 2008;25:765–74.

82. Rubin RR, Peyrot M. STAR 3 Study Group. Health-related quality of life and treatment satisfaction in the sensor-augmented pump therapy for A1C reduction 3 (STAR 3) trial. Diabetes Technol Ther 2012;14:143–51.

83. Nørgaard K, Scaramuzza A, Bratina N, et al. Routine sensor-augmented pump therapy in type 1 diabetes: The INTERPRET Study. Diabetes Technol Ther 2013;15:273–80.

84. Hommel E, Olsen B, Battelino T, et al. Impact of continuous glucose monitoring on quality of life, treatment satisfaction, and use of medical care resources: Analyses from the SWITCH study. Acta Diabetol 2014;51:845–51.

85. Steineck I, Cederholm J, Eliasson B, et al. Insulin pump therapy, multiple daily injections, and cardiovascular mortality in 18 168 people with type 1 diabetes: Observational study. BMJ 2015;350:h3234.

86. Juvenile Diabetes Research Foundation Continuous Glucose Monitoring Study Group, Tamborlane WV, Beck RW, et al. Continuous glucose monitoring and intensive treatment of type 1 diabetes. N Engl J Med 2008;359:1464–76.

87. Deiss D, Bolinder J, Riveline J-P, et al. Improved glycemic control in poorly controlled patients with type 1 diabetes using real-time continuous glucose monitoring. Diabetes Care 2006;29:2730–2.

88. Battelino T, Conget I, Olsen B, et al. The use and efficacy of continuous glucose monitoring in type 1 diabetes treated with insulin pump therapy: A randomised controlled trial. Diabetologia 2012;55:3155–62.

89. O'Connell MA, Donath S, O'Neal DN, et al. Glycaemic impact of patient-led use of sensor-guided pump therapy in type 1 diabetes: A randomised controlled trial. Diabetologia 2009;52:1250–7.

90. Beck RW, Riddlesworth T, Ruedy K, et al. Effect of continuous glucose monitoring on glycemic control in adults with type 1 diabetes using insulin injections: the DIAMOND randomized clinical trial. JAMA 2017;317:371–8.

91. Lind M, Polonsky W, Hirsch IB, et al. Continuous glucose monitoring vs conventional therapy for glycemic control in adults with type 1 diabetes treated With multiple daily insulin injections: The GOLD randomized clinical trial. JAMA 2017;317:379–87.

92. Raccah D, Sulmont V, Reznik Y, et al. Incremental value of continuous glucose monitoring when starting pump therapy in patients with poorly controlled type 1 diabetes: The RealTrend study. Diabetes Care 2009;32:2245–50.

93. Hirsch IB, Abelseth J, Bode BW, et al. Sensor-augmented insulin pump therapy: Results of the first randomized treat-to-target study. Diabetes Technol Ther 2008;10:377–83.

94. Juvenile Diabetes Research Foundation Continuous Glucose Monitoring Study Group, Beck RW, Hirsch IB, et al. The effect of continuous glucose monitoring in well-controlled type 1 diabetes. Diabetes Care 2009;32:1378–83.

95. Battelino T, Phillip M, Bratina N, et al. Effect of continuous glucose monitoring on hypoglycemia in type 1 diabetes. Diabetes Care 2011;34:795–800.

96. Langendam M, Luijf YM, Hooft L, et al. Continuous glucose monitoring systems for type 1 diabetes mellitus. Cochrane Database Syst Rev 2012;(1):CD008101.

97. Pickup JC, Freeman SC, Sutton AJ. Glycaemic control in type 1 diabetes during real time continuous glucose monitoring compared with self monitoring of blood glucose: Meta-analysis of randomised controlled trials using individual patient data. BMJ 2011;343:d3805.

98. van Beers CA, DeVries JH, Kleijer SJ, et al. Continuous glucose monitoring for patients with type 1 diabetes and impaired awareness of hypoglycaemia (IN CONTROL): A randomised, open-label, crossover trial. Lancet Diabetes Endocrinol 2016;4:893–902.

99. Bode BW, Garg SK. The emerging role of adjunctive noninsulin antihyperglycemic therapy in the management of type 1 diabetes. Endocr Pract 2016;22:220–30.

100. Frandsen CS, Dejgaard TF, Madsbad S. Non-insulin drugs to treat hyperglycaemia in type 1 diabetes mellitus. Lancet Diabetes Endocrinol 2016;4:766–80.

101. Liu C, Wu D, Zheng X, et al. Efficacy and safety of metformin for patients with type 1 diabetes mellitus: A meta-analysis. Diabetes Technol Ther 2015;17:142–8.

329

102. Staels F, Moyson C, Mathieu C. Metformin as add-on to intensive insulin therapy in type 1 diabetes mellitus. Diabetes Obes Metab 2017 (in press).
103. Famulla S, Pieber TR, Eilbracht J, et al. Glucose exposure and variability with empagliflozin as adjunct to insulin in patients with type 1 diabetes: Continuous glucose monitoring data from a 4-week, randomized, placebo-controlled trial (EASE-1). Diabetes Technol Ther 2017;19:49–60, Available from.
104. Pieber TR, Famulla S, Eilbracht J, et al. Empagliflozin as adjunct to insulin in patients with type 1 diabetes: A 4-week, randomized, placebo-controlled trial (EASE-1). Diabetes Obes Metab 2015;17:928–35.
105. Henry RR, Thakkar P, Tong C, et al. Efficacy and safety of canagliflozin, a sodium-glucose cotransporter 2 inhibitor, as add-on to insulin in patients with type 1 diabetes. Diabetes Care 2015;38:2258–65.
106. Peters AL, Henry RR, Thakkar P, et al. Diabetic ketoacidosis with canagliflozin, a sodium-glucose cotransporter 2 inhibitor, in patients with type 1 diabetes. Diabetes Care 2016;39:532–8.
107. Kuhadiya ND, Ghanim H, Mehta A, et al. Dapagliflozin as additional treatment to liraglutide and insulin in patients with type 1 diabetes. J Clin Endocrinol Metab 2016;101:3506–15.
108. Comee M, Peters A. The changing therapeutic armamentarium for patients with type 1 diabetes. Curr Opin Endocrinol Diabetes Obes 2016;23:106–10.
109. Dejgaard TF, Frandsen CS, Holst JJ, et al. Liraglutide for treating type 1 diabetes. Expert Opin Biol Ther 2016;16:579–90.
110. Mathieu C, Zinman B, Hemmingsson JU, et al. Efficacy and safety of liraglutide added to insulin treatment in type 1 diabetes: The ADJUNCT ONE Treat-To-Target randomized trial. Diabetes Care 2016;39:1702–10.
111. Ahren B, Hirsch IB, Pieber TR, et al. Efficacy and safety of liraglutide added to capped insulin treatment in subjects with type 1 diabetes: The adjunct two randomized trial. Diabetes Care 2016;39:1693–701.
112. Frandsen CS, Dejgaard TF, Holst JJ, et al. Twelve-week treatment with liraglutide as add-on to insulin in normal-weight patients with poorly controlled type 1 diabetes: A randomized, placebo-controlled, double-blind parallel study. Diabetes Care 2015;38:2250–7.
113. Dejgaard TF, Frandsen CS, Hansen TS, et al. Efficacy and safety of liraglutide for overweight adult patients with type 1 diabetes and insufficient glycaemic control (Lira-1): A randomised, double-blind, placebo-controlled trial. Lancet Diabetes Endocrinol 2016;4:221–32.
114. Moher D, Liberati A, Tetzlaff J, et al. Preferred reporting items for systematic reviews and meta-analyses: The PRISMA statement. PLoS Med 2009;6:e1000097.

Literature Review Flow Diagram for Chapter 12: Glycemic Management in Adults with Type 1 Diabetes

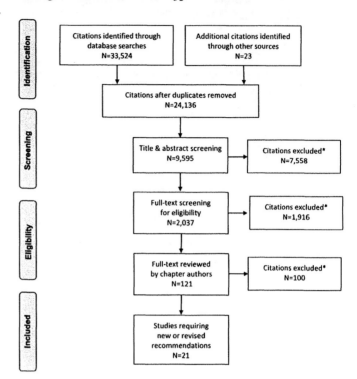

*Excluded based on: population, intervention/exposure, comparator/control or study design.

From: Moher D, Liberati A, Tetzlaff J, Altman DG, The PRISMA Group (2009). *Preferred Reporting Items for Systematic Reviews and Meta-Analyses: The PRISMA Statement.* PLoS Med 6(6): e1000097. doi:10.1371/journal.pmed1000097 (114).

For more information, visit www.prisma-statement.org.

Can J Diabetes 42 (2018) S234–S246

Contents lists available at ScienceDirect

Canadian Journal of Diabetes

journal homepage:
www.canadianjournalofdiabetes.com

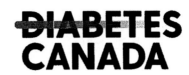 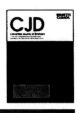

2018 Clinical Practice Guidelines

Type 1 Diabetes in Children and Adolescents

Diabetes Canada Clinical Practice Guidelines Expert Committee

Diane K. Wherrett MD, FRCPC, Josephine Ho MD, MSc, FRCPC, Céline Huot MD, MSc, FRCPC,
Laurent Legault MD, FRCPC, Meranda Nakhla MD, MSc, FRCPC,
Elizabeth Rosolowsky MD, MPH, FAAP, FRCPC

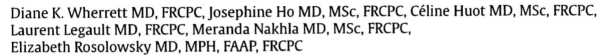

KEY MESSAGES

- Suspicion of diabetes in a child should lead to immediate confirmation of the diagnosis and initiation of treatment to reduce the likelihood of diabetic ketoacidosis.
- Management of pediatric diabetic ketoacidosis differs from diabetic ketoacidosis in adults because of the increased risk for cerebral edema. Pediatric protocols should be used.
- Children should be referred for diabetes education, ongoing care and psychosocial support to a diabetes team with pediatric expertise.

KEY MESSAGES FOR PEOPLE WITH CHILDREN AND ADOLESCENTS WITH DIABETES

- When a child is diagnosed with type 1 diabetes, the role of a caregiver becomes more important than ever. Family life and daily routines may seem more complicated in the beginning but, over time, and with the support of a diabetes team, these improve. Families discover that a child can have a healthy and fulfilling life with diabetes.

Note: Unless otherwise specified, the term "child" or "children" is used for individuals 0 to 18 years of age, and the term "adolescent" for those 13 to 18 years of age.

Introduction

Diabetes mellitus is the most common endocrine disease and one of the most common chronic conditions in children. Type 2 diabetes and other types of diabetes, including genetic defects of beta cell function, such as monogenic and neonatal diabetes, are being increasingly recognized in children and should be considered when clinical presentation is atypical for type 1 diabetes (for additional details see Definition, Classification and Diagnosis of Diabetes, Prediabetes and Metabolic Syndrome chapter, p. S10). This section addresses those areas of type 1 diabetes management that are specific to children.

Education

Children with new-onset type 1 diabetes and their families require intensive diabetes education by an interprofessional pediatric diabetes health-care (DHC) team that should include either a pediatric endocrinologist or pediatrician with diabetes expertise, dietician, diabetes nurse educator, social worker and mental health professional to provide them with the necessary skills and knowledge to manage this disease. The complex physical, developmental and emotional needs of children and their families necessitate specialized care to ensure the best long-term outcomes (1,2). Education topics must include insulin action, administration and dosage adjustment; blood glucose (BG) and ketone monitoring; sick-day management and prevention of diabetic ketoacidosis (DKA); nutrition therapy; physical activity; and prevention, detection and treatment of hypoglycemia.

Anticipatory guidance and healthy behaviour counselling should be part of routine care, especially during critical developmental transitions (e.g. daycare, school entry, adolescence). Health-care providers should regularly initiate discussions with children and their families about school, diabetes camp, psychological issues, fear of hypoglycemia, substance use, obtaining a driver's license and career choices. Behavioural interventions that have been applied broadly to clinic-based populations with a focus on improving self-efficacy and self-management skills have shown little benefit on improving glycemic control, but may improve caregiver coping skills and reduce parent-child conflict, emphasizing the need for a continuing programme of education (3–5).

Children with new-onset diabetes who present with DKA require a short period of hospitalization to stabilize the associated metabolic derangements and to initiate insulin therapy. Outpatient education for children with new-onset diabetes has been shown to be less expensive than inpatient education and associated with similar or slightly better outcomes when appropriate interprofessional resources to provide outpatient education on basic diabetes management are available (6,7).

Glycemic Targets

Improved metabolic control reduces both the onset and progression of diabetes-related complications in adults and adolescents with type 1 diabetes (8,9). Knowledge of glycemic targets by

Conflict of interest statements can be found on page S242.

1499-2671 © 2018 Canadian Diabetes Association.
The Canadian Diabetes Association is the registered owner of the name Diabetes Canada.
https://doi.org/10.1016/j.jcjd.2017.10.036

Table 1
Recommended glycemic targets for children and adolescents with type 1 diabetes

Age (years)	A1C (%)	Fasting/ preprandial PG (mmol/L)	2-hour postprandial PG* (mmol/L)	Considerations
<18	≤7.5	4.0–8.0	5.0–10.0	Caution is required to minimize severe or excessive hypoglycemia. Consider preprandial targets of 6.0–10.0 mmol/L as well as higher A1C targets in children and adolescents who have had severe or excessive hypoglycemia or have hypoglycemia unawareness.

A1C, glycated hemoglobin; *PG*, plasma glucose.
  * Postprandial monitoring is rarely done in young children except for those on continuous subcutaneous insulin infusion (CSII) therapy for whom targets are not available.

the child with diabetes and parents and consistent target setting by the diabetes health-care team have been shown to be associated with improved metabolic control (10). Aggressive attempts should be made to reach the recommended glycemic target outlined in Table 1; however, clinical judgement is required to determine which children can reasonably and safely achieve these targets without severe or recurrent hypoglycemia. Results from a large multicentre observational study found that glycated hemoglobin (A1C) targets of ≤7.5% can be safely achieved without an increase in the risk of severe hypoglycemia in children less than 6 years of age (11). In some follow-up studies, episodes of severe hypoglycemia have been associated with poorer cognitive function, such as with memory and learning, whereas other studies have found that chronic hyperglycemia and glycemic variability in young children (ages 4 to 10 years) are associated with white matter structural changes and poorer overall cognitive performance (12–15). Young age at diabetes onset (under 7 years of age) has also been associated with poorer cognitive function (16). Treatment goals and strategies must be tailored to each child, with consideration given to individual risk factors.

Insulin Therapy

Insulin therapy is the mainstay of medical management of type 1 diabetes. A variety of insulin regimens can be used, but few have been studied specifically in children with new-onset diabetes. The choice of insulin regimen depends on many factors, including the child's age, duration of diabetes, family lifestyle, school support, socioeconomic factors, and family, patient, and physician preferences. Regardless of the insulin regimen used, all children should be treated to meet glycemic targets.

The honeymoon period, which can last up to 2 years after diagnosis, is characterized by target glycemic control and low insulin requirements (<0.5 units/kg/day). At the end of this period, more intensive management may be required to continue meeting glycemic targets. Two methods of intensive diabetes management have been used: basal-bolus regimens (long-acting basal insulin analogues and rapid-acting bolus insulin analogues) and continuous subcutaneous insulin infusion (CSII) therapy. Basal-bolus therapy has resulted in improved control over traditional twice-daily neutral protamine Hagedorn (NPH) and rapid-acting bolus analogue therapy in some but not all studies (17–19).

CSII is safe and effective and can be initiated at any age (20–22). A Cochrane review found that CSII resulted in slightly improved

metabolic control over basal-bolus therapy (23). Some clinic-based studies of CSII in school-aged children and adolescents have shown a significant reduction in A1C with reduced hypoglycemia 12 to 24 months after initiation of CSII when compared to pre-CSII levels (24) or in the longer term when compared to controls on injections (25). Young age, A1C at CSII initiation and number of daily boluses may be associated with improved or sustained near-normal metabolic outcome (26). The Sensor-Augmented Pump Therapy for A1C Reduction (STAR) 3 study demonstrated that sensor-augmented insulin-pump therapy was more effective in lowering A1C levels than multiple daily injections (MDI) in children with poorly controlled type 1 diabetes mellitus (27).

Most, but not all, pediatric studies of the long-acting basal insulin analogues (detemir, glargine and degludec) have demonstrated improved fasting blood glucose (FBG) levels and fewer episodes of nocturnal hypoglycemia with a reduction in A1C (17,28–32). Two large population-based observational studies have not found improved A1C in children with diabetes using basal-bolus therapy or CSII when compared to those using NPH and rapid-acting bolus analogues (33,34). Insulin therapy should be individualized to reach A1C targets, minimize hypoglycemia and optimize quality of life.

Glucose Monitoring

Self-monitoring of blood glucose (SMBG) is an essential part of management of type 1 diabetes, and increased frequency has been associated with better clinical outcomes (35–37). Evidence of a strong association between frequency of SMBG and hemoglobin A1C levels has been found in T1D Exchange Clinic Registry participants (37). Subcutaneous continuous glucose sensors allow detection of asymptomatic hypoglycemia and hyperglycemia. In some studies, use of continuous glucose monitoring (CGM) has resulted in improved glycemic control with less hypoglycemia (38–40). In 1 larger randomized controlled trial of 322 adults and children, use of CGM was associated with improved glycemic control in adults but not in children and adolescents (41). Glycemic benefit correlated with duration of sensor use, which was much lower in children and adolescents (42). Recently, a built-in algorithm in an available CSII device with low glucose suspend feature has been shown to significantly lower overnight hypoglycemia (43,44).

Closed-Loop Pancreas System

The closed-loop pancreas system, also known as the artificial or bionic pancreas system, is one of the most rapidly evolving areas of clinical care for type 1 diabetes. It couples the use of an insulin pump with infusion of 1 or more hormones (insulin +/- glucagon), a glucose sensor and an algorithm for glucose control. The closed-loop system allows for decreasing excursions in blood glucose levels while reducing the overall burden of self-care. However, the system must ensure patient safety as well as prevent the occurrence of severe hypo- and hyperglycemia, as well as DKA. Results from several studies are promising for outcomes combining a lowering of the number of hypoglycemic events while optimizing per cent time in target range for glucose, fasting blood glucose and mean sensor glucose (45). However, most studies are short term and assessed the closed-loop system in different clinical settings. Larger randomized clinical trials in adults and youth are currently underway.

Nutrition

All children with type 1 diabetes should receive counselling from a registered dietitian experienced in pediatric diabetes. Children with

Table 2
Examples of carbohydrates for treatment of mild-to-moderate hypoglycemia

Patient age	<5 yrs	5 to 10 yrs	>10 yrs
Amount of carbohydrate	5 g	10 g	15 g
Carbohydrate Source			
Glucose tablet (4 g)	1	2 or 3	4
Dextrose tablet (3 g)	2	3	5
Apple or orange juice; regular soft drink; sweet beverage (cocktails)	40 mL	85 mL	125 mL

diabetes should follow a healthy diet as recommended for children without diabetes in *Eating Well with Canada's Food Guide* (46). This involves consuming a variety of foods from the 4 food groups (grain products, vegetables and fruits, milk and alternatives, and meat and alternatives). Children with diabetes have been found to consume a diet that is similar to children without diabetes, one that is higher in fat and lower in fibre than guidelines recommend for healthy eating (47). Carbohydrate counting is a commonly used method of matching insulin to carbohydrate intake that allows increased flexibility in diet, although fat and protein content also influence postprandial glucose levels. There is no strong evidence that one form of nutrition therapy is superior to another in attaining age-appropriate glycemic targets. Nutrition therapy should be individualized (based on the child's nutritional needs, eating habits, lifestyle, ability and interest) and must ensure normal growth and development without compromising glycemic control. This plan should be evaluated regularly and at least annually. Features suggestive of eating disorders and of celiac disease should be systematically sought out (48).

Treatment of Hypoglycemia

Hypoglycemia is a major obstacle for children with type 1 diabetes and can affect their ability to achieve glycemic targets. Children with early-onset diabetes are at greatest risk for disruption of cognitive function and neuropsychological skills, but the respective roles of hypoglycemia and hyperglycemia in their development are still questioned (16,49). Significant risk of hypoglycemia often necessitates less stringent glycemic goals, particularly for younger children. There is no evidence in children that one insulin regimen or mode of administration is superior to another for resolving nonsevere hypoglycemia. As such, treatment must be individualized (50). Frequent use of CGM in a clinical care setting may reduce episodes of hypoglycemia (51).

Severe hypoglycemia should be treated with pediatric doses of intravenous dextrose in the hospital setting or glucagon in the home setting. In children, the use of mini-doses of glucagon has been shown to be useful in the home management of mild or impending hypoglycemia associated with inability or refusal to take oral carbohydrate. A dose of 10 micrograms (mcg) per year of age (the equivalent of 1 unit on the syringe per year of age) (minimum dose 20 mcg (2 units), maximum dose 150 mcg (15 units)) is effective at treating and preventing hypoglycemia, with an additional doubled dose given if the BG has not increased in 20 minutes (52,53). Treatment of mild hypoglycemia is described in Table 2.

Chronic Poor Metabolic Control

A careful multidisciplinary assessment should be undertaken for every child with chronically poor metabolic control (e.g. A1C >10%) to identify potential causative and associated factors, such as depression (54), eating disorders (55), lower socioeconomic status, lower family support and higher family conflict (56,57), and to identify and address barriers to improved glycemic control. Use of a standardized measure of risk factors has been shown to identify those at high risk for poor control, emergency room visits and DKA (58). Glycemic control may be particularly challenging during adolescence due to physiologic insulin resistance, depression and other psychological issues, and reduced adherence during a time of growing independence. Multipronged interventions that target emotional, family and coping issues have shown a modest reduction in A1C with reduced rates of hospital admission (59–61).

Physical Activity

Inadequate levels of physical activity are common in all children, including those with diabetes. Increased physical activity is associated with better metabolic control. Two recent systematic reviews with meta-analyses have shown A1C reductions of ~0.5% with interventions aimed at increasing physical activity (62,63).

DKA

DKA occurs in approximately 40% of children with new-onset diabetes (range of 28% to 40% across United States centres and 11% to 67% across European centres), and at a frequency of one to 10 episodes per 100 patient-years in those with established diabetes (64,65). DKA continues to be the leading cause of morbidity and mortality in children with diabetes; subtle, persistent changes in brain structure and function ensuing from DKA are being increasingly appreciated (66–68). Children younger than 3 years of age and from areas with low prevalence of diabetes are especially at risk for moderate-to-severe DKA at the time of diagnosis (65). DKA can be prevented through earlier recognition and initiation of insulin therapy. Public awareness campaigns about the early signs of diabetes have significantly reduced the frequency of DKA in new-onset diabetes (69,70). In children with established diabetes, DKA results from failing to take insulin or poor sick-day management. Sick-day management includes more frequent SMBG, ketone measurement during hyperglycemia and adjustment of insulin dose in response to monitoring (71). Risk is increased in children with poor metabolic control or previous episodes of DKA, peripubertal and adolescent girls, children on CSII or long-acting basal insulin analogues, ethnic minorities, and children with psychiatric disorders and those with difficult family circumstances (72–75). The frequency of DKA in established diabetes can be decreased with education, behavioural intervention and family support (76,77), as well as access to 24-hour telephone services or telemedicine for parents of children with diabetes (78–80).

Management of DKA

While most cases of DKA are corrected without event, 0.5% to 1% of pediatric cases are complicated by cerebral edema (81), which is associated with significant morbidity (21% to 35%) and mortality (21% to 24%) (82). In contrast, cerebral edema has rarely been reported in adults (82). Although the cause of cerebral edema is still unknown, several factors are associated with increased risk (Table 3) (83–87). A bolus of insulin prior to infusion is not recommended since it does not offer faster resolution of acidosis (88,89) and may contribute to cerebral edema (90). Early insulin administration (within the first hour of fluid replacement) may increase the risk for cerebral edema (87). Special caution should be exercised in young children with DKA and new-onset diabetes or a greater degree of acidosis and extracellular fluid volume depletion because of the increased risk of cerebral edema.

Table 3
Risk factors for cerebral edema during treatment of diabetic ketoacidosis in children

- Younger age (<5 years)
- New-onset diabetes
- Greater severity of acidosis (lower pH and bicarbonate)
- High initial serum urea
- Low initial partial pressure of arterial carbon dioxide (pCO2)
- Rapid administration of hypotonic fluids
- IV bolus of insulin
- Early IV insulin infusion (within first hour of administration of fluids)
- Failure of serum sodium to rise during treatment
- Use of bicarbonate

IV, intravenous.

In some centres, it is common practice to initiate an intravenous insulin infusion at a rate of 0.05 units/kg/hour. One recent, prospective randomized controlled study suggests that an initial insulin infusion rate of 0.05 units/kg/hour is safe and effective, but this lower starting rate was not studied among those presenting in more severe or complicated DKA (91). Either mannitol or hypertonic saline can be used in the treatment of cerebral edema, but there is still insufficient evidence to favor one over the other; hypertonic saline use has been associated with increased mortality in a single, retrospective study (92). DKA should be managed according to published protocols for management of pediatric DKA (Figure 1) (93).

Vaccination

Historically, national guidelines have recommended influenza vaccination for children with type 1 diabetes (94,95). Currently, there is no evidence supporting increased morbidity or mortality from influenza in children with type 1 diabetes (96,97). However, the management of type 1 diabetes can be complicated by illness, requiring parental knowledge of sick-day management and increased attention during periods of illness. For this reason, parents may choose to have their children vaccinated.

Smoking Prevention and Cessation

Smoking is a significant risk factor for both cardiovascular (CV) and microvascular complications of diabetes (98) and, in adolescents, is associated with worse metabolic control (99). Smoking prevention should be emphasized throughout childhood and adolescence. The Canadian Paediatric Society website contains useful resources to promote smoking cessation among adolescents (http://www.cps.ca/en/documents/position/smoking-cessation) (100).

Alcohol and Substance Use

Adolescents with diabetes have similar rates of alcohol use and similar or higher rates of illicit drug use compared to adolescents without diabetes (101). Regular counselling should be provided around alcohol and substance use.

Contraception and Sexual Health Counselling

Adolescents with diabetes should receive regular counselling about sexual health and contraception. Unplanned pregnancies should be avoided, as pregnancy in adolescent females with type 1 diabetes with suboptimal metabolic control may result in higher risks of maternal and fetal complications than in older women with type 1 diabetes who are already at increased risk compared to the general population (102). Oral contraceptives, intrauterine devices and barrier methods can be used safely in the vast majority of adolescents (103).

Psychological Issues

For children, and particularly adolescents, there is a need to identify psychological disorders associated with diabetes and to intervene early to minimize the impact over the course of development. Children and adolescents with diabetes have significant risks for psychological problems, including diabetes distress (104), depression (105), anxiety (105), eating disorders and externalizing disorders (106–110). The risks increase during adolescence and emerging adulthood (111–113). Studies have shown that psychological disorders predict poor diabetes management and control (54,105,114–117) and, consequently, negative medical outcomes (118–121). Conversely, as glycemic control worsens, the probability of psychological problems increases (122).

The presence of psychological symptoms and diabetes problems in children and adolescents is often strongly affected by caregiver/family distress. Research has demonstrated that while parental psychological issues may distort perceptions of the child's diabetes control (123), they are often related to poor psychological adjustment and diabetes control (124–127). Maternal anxiety and depression are associated with poor diabetes control in younger adolescents and with reduced positive affect and motivation in older teens (128).

Eating disorders

Ten per cent of adolescent females with type 1 diabetes meet the *Diagnostic and Statistical Manual of Mental Disorders* (4th Edition) criteria for eating disorders compared to 4% of their age-matched peers without diabetes (129). Disordered eating with insulin restriction is also seen in youth with diabetes (130). Furthermore, eating disorders are associated with poor metabolic control (55) and earlier onset and more rapid progression of microvascular complications (131). Eating disorders should be suspected in those adolescent and young adult females who are unable to achieve and maintain metabolic targets, especially when insulin omission is suspected. It is important to identify individuals with eating disorders because different management strategies are required to optimize metabolic control and prevent microvascular complications (129,131,132).

Prevention and intervention

Children and adolescents with diabetes, along with their families, should be screened throughout their development for psychological disorders (133). Given the prevalence of psychological issues, screening in this area can be seen as equally important as screening for microvascular complications in children and adolescents with diabetes (134).

Psychological interventions with children and adolescents, as well as families, have been shown to improve mental health (106,135), including overall well-being and perceived quality of life (136), along with depressive symptoms (137,138). In addition, there is some evidence that psychosocial interventions can positively affect glycemic control (59,135,139). Most importantly, some studies have demonstrated that psychological interventions can increase diabetes treatment adherence, improve glycemic control and improve psychosocial functioning (140,141).

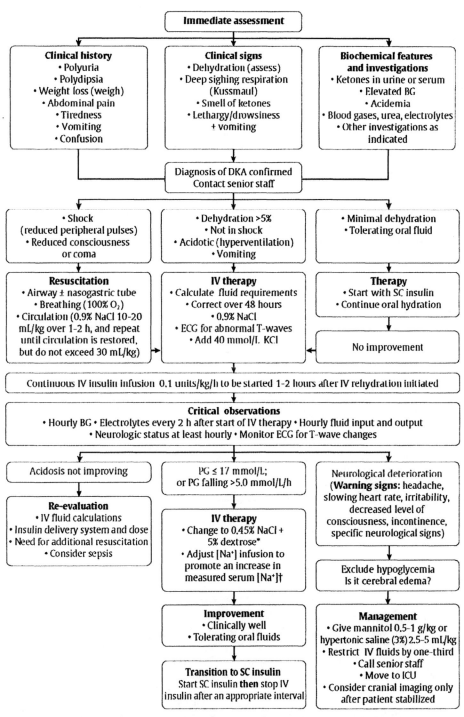

Figure 1. Immediate assessment and management of diabetic ketoacidosis in children.
BG, blood glucose; *D5W*; 5% dextrose in water; *D10W*; 10% dextrose in water; *D12.5W*; 12.5% dextrose in water; *DKA*; diabetic ketoacidosis; *ECG*, electrocardiogram; *ICU*, intensive care unit; *IV*, intravenous; *NaCl*; sodium chloride; *PG*, plasma glucose; *SC*, subcutaneous. Adapted with permission from reference 93.

Comorbid Conditions

Autoimmune thyroid disease

Clinical autoimmune thyroid disease (AITD) occurs in 15% to 30% of individuals with type 1 diabetes (142). The risk for AITD during the first decade of diabetes is directly related to the presence or absence of anti-thyroid antibodies (i.e. thyroid peroxidase antibodies) at diabetes diagnosis (143). Hypothyroidism is most likely to develop in girls at puberty (144). Early detection and treatment of hypothyroidism will prevent growth failure and symptoms of hypothyroidism (Table 4). Hyperthyroidism also occurs more

335

Table 4
Recommendations for screening for comorbid conditions in children with type 1 diabetes

Condition	Indications for screening	Screening test	Frequency
Autoimmune thyroid disease	All children with type 1 diabetes	Serum TSH level + thyroid peroxidase antibodies	At diagnosis and every 2 years thereafter; thyroperoxidase antibodies do not need to be repeated if previously positive
	Positive thyroid antibodies, symptoms of thyroid disease or goiter	Serum TSH level (+thyroid peroxidase antibodies if previously negative)	Every 6–12 months
Primary adrenal insufficiency	Unexplained recurrent hypoglycemia and decreasing insulin requirements	8 AM serum cortisol and serum sodium and potassium	As clinically indicated
Celiac disease	Recurrent gastrointestinal symptoms, poor linear growth, poor weight gain, fatigue, anemia, unexplained frequent hypoglycemia or poor metabolic control	Tissue transglutaminase + immunoglobulin A levels	As clinically indicated

TSH, thyroid-stimulating hormone.

Table 5
Screening for diabetes complications, dyslipidemia and hypertension in children with type 1 diabetes

Complication/ Comorbidity	Indications and intervals for screening	Screening method
Nephropathy	• Yearly screening commencing at 12 years of age in those with duration of type 1 diabetes >5 years	• First morning (preferred) or random urine ACR • Abnormal ACR requires confirmation at least 1 month later with a first morning ACR and, if abnormal, followed by timed, overnight or 24-hour split urine collections for albumin excretion rate • Repeated sampling should be done every 3–4 months over a 6- to 12-month period to demonstrate persistence
Retinopathy	• Yearly screening commencing at 15 years of age with duration of type 1 diabetes >5 years • Screening interval can increase to 2 years if good glycemic control, duration of diabetes <10 years and no retinopathy at initial assessment	• 7-standard field, stereoscopic-colour fundus photography with interpretation by a trained reader (gold standard); or • Direct ophthalmoscopy or indirect slit-lamp fundoscopy through dilated pupil; or • Digital fundus photography
Neuropathy	• Children ≥15 years with poor metabolic control should be screened yearly after 5 years of type 1 diabetes	• Question and examine for symptoms of numbness, pain, cramps and paresthesia, as well as skin sensation, vibration sense, light touch and ankle reflexes
Dyslipidemia	• Delay screening post-diabetes diagnosis until metabolic control has stabilized • Screen at 12 and 17 years of age • <12 years of age: screen only those with BMI >97th percentile, family history of hyperlipidemia or premature CVD	• Fasting or non-fasting TC, HDL-C, TG, calculated LDL-C. Measurement of non-fasting lipids may be considered if TG are not elevated.
Hypertension	• Screen all children with type 1 diabetes at least twice a year	• Use appropriate cuff size

ACR, albumin to creatinine ratio; BMI, body mass index; CVD, cardiovascular disease; HDL-C, high-density lipoprotein cholesterol; LDL-C, low-density lipoprotein cholesterol; TC, total cholesterol; TG, triglycerides.

frequently in association with type 1 diabetes than in the general population.

Primary adrenal insufficiency (Addison's disease)

Primary adrenal insufficiency is rare, even in those with type 1 diabetes (145). Targeted screening is required in those with unexplained recurrent hypoglycemia and decreasing insulin requirements (Table 4).

Celiac disease

Celiac disease can be identified in 4% to 9% of children with type 1 diabetes (142), but in 60% to 70% of these children, the disease is asymptomatic (silent celiac disease). Children with type 1 diabetes are at increased risk for classic or atypical celiac disease during the first 10 years of diabetes (146). There is good evidence that treatment of classic or atypical celiac disease with a gluten-free diet improves intestinal and extraintestinal symptoms (147), and prevents the long-term sequelae of untreated classic celiac disease (148). However, there is no evidence that untreated asymptomatic celiac disease is associated with short- or long-term health risks (149,150) or that a gluten-free diet improves health in these individuals (151). Thus, universal screening for and treatment of asymptomatic celiac disease remains controversial (Table 4).

Diabetes Complications

There are important age-related considerations regarding surveillance for diabetes complications and interpretation of investigations (Table 5). Risk for microvascular complications accelerates through puberty (152,153). In an observational study, children with type 1 diabetes with a mean duration of 7.9 years were found to have an age-adjusted prevalence of diabetic nephropathy of 5.8%, retinopathy 5.6%, peripheral neuropathy 8.5%, arterial stiffness 11.6%, hypertension 10.1% and cardiovascular (CV) autonomic neuropathy 14.4% (154).

Chronic kidney disease

Prepubertal children and those in the first 5 years of diabetes should be considered at very low risk for albuminuria (152,155). A first morning urine albumin to creatinine ratio (ACR) has high sensitivity and specificity for the detection of albuminuria (156,157). Although screening with a random ACR is associated with greater compliance than with a first morning sample, its specificity may be compromised in adolescents due to their higher frequency of exercise-induced proteinuria and benign postural proteinuria. Abnormal random ACRs (i.e. >2.5 mg/mmol) require confirmation with a first morning ACR or timed overnight urine collection (158).

The likelihood of transient or intermittent albuminuria is higher during the early peripubertal years (155). Individuals with intermittent albuminuria may progress to overt nephropathy (159). Abnormal screening results require confirmation and follow up to demonstrate persistent abnormalities, as albuminuria can and is more likely to regress in youth compared to older adults (160–162).

Treatment is indicated only for those adolescents with persistent albuminuria. One short-term randomized controlled trial in adolescents demonstrated that angiotensin-converting enzyme (ACE) inhibitors were effective in reducing albuminuria compared to placebo (163). However, there are no long-term intervention studies assessing the effectiveness of ACE inhibitors or angiotensin receptor blockers (ARBs) in delaying progression to overt nephropathy in adolescents with albuminuria. Therefore, treatment of adolescents with persistent albuminuria is based on the effectiveness of treatments in adults with type 1 diabetes (164).

Retinopathy

Retinopathy is rare in prepubertal children with type 1 diabetes and in postpubertal adolescents with good metabolic control (153,165–167). Earlier reductions in A1C during adolescence and attention to blood pressure (BP) control may stave off sight-threatening diabetic retinopathy in adulthood (153).

Neuropathy

When present, neuropathy is mostly subclinical in children (168). While prospective nerve conduction studies and autonomic neuropathy assessment studies have demonstrated increased prevalence of abnormalities over time (169), persistence of abnormalities is an inconsistent finding (170). There are very few studies assessing the diagnostic utility of noninvasive screening methods in children with diabetes; among them, vibration and monofilament testing have suboptimal sensitivity and specificity in adolescents. Normative thresholds vary with age and gender (171). With the exception of intensifying diabetes management to achieve and maintain glycemic targets, no other treatment modality has been studied in children and adolescents.

Dyslipidemia

Most children with type 1 diabetes should be considered at low risk for cardiovascular disease (CVD) associated with dyslipidemia (172–174). The exceptions are those with longer duration of disease, microvascular complications or other CV risk factors, including smoking, hypertension, obesity (175) and/or family history of premature CVD (176). Dyslipidemia screening should be targeted at those greater than 12 years of age and younger children with specific risk factors for dyslipidemia. Measurement of non-fasting lipids is now recommended for adults as long as triglycerides are not elevated. Evidence in children with diabetes is limited. Statin therapy has been studied specifically in children with diabetes, and while there is no evidence linking specific low-density lipoprotein cholesterol (LDL-C) cut-offs in children with diabetes with long-term outcomes, statin therapy has been shown to significantly lower LDL-C as well as lipoproteins (177). In pubertal children without diabetes but with familial hypercholesterolemia, statin therapy is known to be safe and effective at lowering LDL-C levels and attenuating progression of surrogate markers for future CVD (178). Different markers of future CVD are being explored to better predict when to intervene (179–182).

Hypertension

Up to 16% of adolescents with type 1 diabetes have hypertension (183). Twenty-four hour ambulatory BP monitoring has been used to exclude white coat hypertension and to identify loss of diurnal systolic rhythm (nondippers) with nocturnal hypertension in some normotensive adolescents with type 1 diabetes (184). These abnormalities may be predictive of future albuminuria (184). However, the role of ambulatory BP monitoring in routine care remains uncertain. Children with type 1 diabetes and confirmed hypertension should be treated according to the guidelines for children without diabetes (185).

Transition to Adult Care

Emerging adulthood, the developmental stage between ages 18 to 25 years, is a stage of life wherein the emerging adult is establishing his or her autonomy, personal identity, and making vocational and educational choices (186). For the emerging adult with diabetes, this stage is complicated by the transition from pediatric to adult care, a high-risk period characterized by inadequate medical follow up and self-management, deteriorating glycemic control, and an increased risk of adverse outcomes (187–190). Between 25% and 65% of young adults have no medical follow up during the transition from pediatric to adult diabetes care services (191–193). Those with no follow up are more likely to experience hospitalization for DKA during this period. Organized transition services may decrease the rate of loss of follow up and the risk of adverse outcomes (189,192,195–198). Further, initiating a transition plan in early adolescence (e.g. 12 years of age), that includes education in self-care behaviours, transition readiness assessments and identifying transition goals may be of benefit in preparing adolescents and their families for transition (199,200).

RECOMMENDATIONS

Delivery of Care

1. All children with diabetes should have access to an experienced pediatric DHC team that includes either a pediatric endocrinologist or pediatrician with diabetes expertise, dietician, diabetes nurse educator, social worker and mental health professional for specialized care starting at diagnosis [Grade D, Level 4 (1)].

2. Children with new-onset type 1 diabetes who are medically stable should receive their initial education and management in an outpatient setting, provided that appropriate personnel and daily communication with a DHC team are available [Grade B, Level 1A (6,7)].

3. To ensure ongoing and adequate diabetes care, adolescents should receive care from a specialized program aimed at creating a well-prepared and supported transition to adult care that is initiated early and includes a transition coordinator; patient reminders; and support and education promoting autonomy and self-care management skills [Grade C, Level 3 (189,191,192,194–197)].

Glycemic Targets

4. Children and adolescents <18 years of age should aim for an A1C target ≤7.5% [Grade D, Consensus]
   a. Attempts should be made to safely reach the recommended glycemic target, while minimizing the risk for severe or recurrent hypoglycemia. Treatment targets should be tailored to each child, taking into consideration individual risk factors for hypoglycemia [Grade D, Consensus]
   b. In children <6 years of age, particular care to minimize hypoglycemia is recommended because of the potential association in this age group between severe hypoglycemia and later cognitive impairment [Grade D, Level 4 (15)].

5. Children with persistently poor glycemic control (e.g. A1C >10%) should be assessed with a validated tool by a specialized pediatric DHC team for comprehensive interdisciplinary assessment and referred for

psychosocial support as indicated [Grade D, Consensus]. Intensive family and individualized psychological interventions aimed at improving glycemic control should be considered to improve chronically poor metabolic control [Grade A, Level 1A (59–61)].

Insulin Therapy

6. Children with new-onset diabetes should be started on boluses of rapid-acting insulin analogues combined with basal insulin (e.g. intermediate-acting insulin or long-acting basal insulin analogue) using an individualized regimen that best addresses the practical issues of daily life [Grade D, Consensus].

7. Insulin therapy should be assessed at each clinical encounter to ensure it still enables the child to meet A1C targets, minimizes the risk of hypoglycemia and allows flexibility in carbohydrate intake, daily schedule and activities [Grade D, Consensus]. If these goals are not being met, an intensified diabetes management approach (including increased education, monitoring and contact with diabetes team) should be used [Grade A, Level 1 (8) for adolescents; Grade D, Consensus for younger children], and treatment options may include the following:
   a. Increased frequency of injections [Grade D, Consensus]
   b. Change in the type of basal and/or bolus insulin [Grade B, Level 2 (29) for adolescents; Grade D, Consensus for younger children]
   c. Change to CSII therapy [Grade C, Level 3 (22)].

Treatment of Hypoglycemia

8. In children, the use of mini doses of glucagon (10 mcg per year of age with minimum dose 20 mcg and maximum dose 150 mcg) should be considered in the home management of mild or impending hypoglycemia associated with inability or refusal to take oral carbohydrate [Grade D, Level 4 (52)].

9. In the home situation, severe hypoglycemia in an unconscious child >5 years of age should be treated with 1 mg glucagon subcutaneously or intramuscularly. In children ≤5 years of age, a dose of 0.5 mg glucagon should be given. The episode should be discussed with the DHC team as soon as possible and consideration given to reducing insulin doses for the next 24 hours to prevent further severe hypoglycemia [Grade D, Consensus].

10. Dextrose 0.5 to 1 g/kg should be given intravenously over 1–3 minutes to treat severe hypoglycemia with unconsciousness when intravenous access is available [Grade D, Consensus].

Physical Activity

11. Regular physical activity ≥3 times per week for ≥60 minutes each time should be encouraged for all children with diabetes [Grade A, Level 1 (62,63)].

Diabetic Ketoacidosis

12. To prevent DKA in children with diabetes:
   a. Targeted public awareness campaigns should be considered to educate parents, other caregivers (e.g. teachers) and health-care providers about the early symptoms of diabetes [Grade C, Level 3 (70,76)]
   b. Immediate assessment of ketone and acid-base status should be done in any child presenting with new-onset diabetes [Grade D, Consensus]
   c. Comprehensive education and support services [Grade C, Level 3 (77)], as well as 24-hour telephone services [Grade C, Level 3 (78)], should be available for families of children with diabetes.

13. DKA in children should be treated according to pediatric-specific protocols [Grade D, Consensus]. If appropriate expertise/facilities are not available locally, there should be immediate consultation with a centre with expertise in pediatric diabetes [Grade D, Consensus].

14. In children in DKA, rapid administration of hypotonic fluids should be avoided [Grade D, Level 4 (84)]. Circulatory compromise should be treated with only enough isotonic fluids to correct circulatory inadequacy [Grade D, Consensus]. Replacement of fluid deficit should be extended over a 48-hour period with regular reassessments of fluid status [Grade D, Level 4 (84)].

15. In children in DKA, an intravenous insulin bolus should not be given [Grade D, Consensus]. The insulin infusion should not be started for at least 1 hour after starting fluid replacement therapy [Grade D, Level 4 (87)]. An intravenous infusion of short-acting insulin should be used at an initial dose of 0.05 to 0.1 units/kg/h, depending on the clinical situation [Grade A, Level 1A (91)].

16. In children in DKA, once blood glucose reaches ≤17.0 mmol/L, intravenous dextrose should be started to prevent hypoglycemia. The dextrose infusion should be increased, rather than reducing insulin, to prevent rapid decreases in glucose. The insulin infusion should be maintained until pH normalizes and ketones have mostly cleared [Grade D, Consensus].

17. In children in DKA, administration of sodium bicarbonate should be avoided except in extreme circulatory compromise, as this has been associated with cerebral edema [Grade D, Level 4 (83)].

18. In children in DKA, either mannitol or hypertonic saline may be used in the treatment of cerebral edema [Grade D, Level 4 (92)].

Microvascular Complications

19. Children ≥12 years with diabetes duration >5 years should be screened annually for CKD with a first morning urine ACR (preferred) [Grade B, Level 2 (157)] or a random ACR [Grade D, Consensus]. Abnormal results should be confirmed [Grade B, Level 2 (161,162)] at least 1 month later with a first morning ACR and, if abnormal, followed by timed, overnight or 24-hour split urine collections for albumin excretion rate [Grade D, Consensus]. Albuminuria (ACR >2.5 mg/mmol; AER >20 mcg/min) should not be diagnosed unless it is persistent, as demonstrated by 2 consecutive first morning ACR or timed collections obtained at 3- to 4-month intervals over a 6- to 12-month period [Grade D, Consensus].

20. Children ≥12 years with persistent albuminuria should be treated per adult guidelines (see Chronic Kidney Disease in Diabetes chapter, p. S201) [Grade D, Consensus].

21. Children ≥15 years with 5 years' diabetes duration should be annually screened and evaluated for retinopathy by an expert professional [Grade C, Level 3 (167)]. The screening interval can be increased to every 2 years in children with type 1 diabetes who have good glycemic control, duration of diabetes <10 years and no significant retinopathy (as determined by an expert professional) [Grade D, Consensus].

22. Children ≥15 years with 5 years' diabetes duration and poor metabolic control should be questioned about symptoms of numbness, pain, cramps and paresthesia, and examined for skin sensation, vibration sense, light touch and ankle reflexes [Grade D, Consensus].

Comorbid Conditions and Other Complications

23. Children and adolescents with diabetes, along with their families, should be screened regularly for psychosocial or psychological disorders [Grade D, Consensus] and should be referred to an expert in mental health and/or psychosocial issues for intervention when required [Grade D, Consensus].

24. Adolescents with type 1 diabetes should be regularly screened using nonjudgmental questions about weight and body image concerns, dieting, binge eating and insulin omission for weight loss [Grade D, Consensus].

25. Children with type 1 diabetes who are <12 years of age should be screened for dyslipidemia if they have other risk factors, such as obesity (body mass index >97th percentile for age and gender) and/or a family history of dyslipidemia or premature CVD. Routine screening for dyslipidemia should begin at 12 years of age, with repeat screening after 5 years [Grade D, Consensus].

26. Once dyslipidemia is diagnosed in children with type 1 diabetes, the dyslipidemia should be monitored regularly and efforts should be made to improve metabolic control and promote healthy behaviours. While it can be treated effectively with statins, a specific LDL cut-off to initiate treatment is yet to be determined in this age category [Grade D, Consensus].

27. All children with type 1 diabetes should be screened for hypertension at least twice annually [Grade D, Consensus].

28. Children with type 1 diabetes and BP readings persistently above the 95th percentile for age should receive healthy behaviour counselling, including weight loss if overweight [Grade D, Level 4 (201)]. If BP remains elevated, treatment should be initiated based on recommendations for children without diabetes [Grade D, Consensus].

29. Influenza vaccination should be offered to children with diabetes as a way to prevent an intercurrent illness that could complicate diabetes management [Grade D, Consensus].

30. Formal smoking prevention and cessation counselling should be part of diabetes management for children with diabetes [Grade D, Consensus].

31. Adolescents should be regularly counselled around alcohol and substance use [Grade D, Consensus].

32. Adolescent females with type 1 diabetes should receive counselling on contraception and sexual health in order to prevent unplanned pregnancy [Grade D, Level 4 (202)].

33. Children with type 1 diabetes who have anti-thyroid antibodies should be considered at high risk for autoimmune thyroid disease [Grade C, Level 3 (143)]. Children with type 1 diabetes should be screened at diabetes diagnosis with repeat screening every 2 years using a serum thyroid-stimulating hormone and thyroid peroxidase antibodies [Grade D, Consensus]. More frequent screening is indicated in the presence of positive anti-thyroid antibodies, thyroid symptoms or goiter [Grade D, Consensus].

34. Children with type 1 diabetes and symptoms of classic or atypical celiac disease (see Table 4) should undergo celiac screening [Grade D, Consensus] and, if confirmed, be treated with a gluten-free diet to improve symptoms [Grade D, Level 4 (147)] and prevent the long-term sequelae of untreated classic celiac disease [Grade D, Level 4 (148)]. Discussion of the pros and cons of screening and treatment of asymptomatic celiac disease should take place with children and adolescents with type 1 diabetes and their families [Grade D, Consensus].

Abbreviations

A1C, glycated hemoglobin; *ACR*, albumin to creatinine ratio; *ACE*, angiotensin-converting enzyme; *AER*, albumin excretion rate; *AITD*, autoimmune thyroid disease; *ARB*, angiotensin receptor blocker; *BP*, blood pressure; *CGM*, continuous glucose monitoring; *CKD*, chronic kidney disease; *CV*, cardiovascular; *CVD*, cardiovascular disease; *CSII*, continuous subcutaneous insulin infusion; *DHC*, diabetes health care; *DKA*, diabetic ketoacidosis; *LDL-C*, low-density lipoprotein cholesterol; *MDI*, multiple daily injections; *mcg*, micrograms; *SMBG*, self-monitoring of blood glucose.

Author Disclosures

Dr. Ho reports grants from Lilly, outside the submitted work. Dr. Huot reports support from Sanofi Aventis, Boehringer Ingelheim, and Merck, outside the submitted work. Dr. Legault reports personal fees from Medtronic and Insulet; other support from Novo Nordisk; and grants from Merck, Sanofi, and AstraZeneca, outside the submitted work; in addition, Dr. Legault has a patent IP issued in the field of artificial pancreas. Dr. Rosolowsky reports grants from the National Institutes of Health, outside the submitted work. No other author has anything to disclose.

References

1. Glasgow AM, Weissberg-Benchell J, Tynan WD, et al. Readmissions of children with diabetes mellitus to a children's hospital. Pediatrics 1991;88:98–104.
2. von Sengbusch S, Muller-Godeffroy E, Hager S, et al. Mobile diabetes education and care: Intervention for children and young people with type 1 diabetes in rural areas of northern Germany. Diabet Med 2006;23:122–7.
3. Pillay J, Armstrong MJ, Butalia S, et al. Behavioral programs for type 1 diabetes mellitus: A systematic review and meta-analysis. Ann Intern Med 2015;163:836–47.
4. Price KJ, Knowles JA, Fox M, et al. Effectiveness of the Kids in Control of Food (KICk-OFF) structured education course for 11–16 year olds with Type 1 diabetes. Diabet Med 2016;33:192–203.
5. Basarir H, Brennan A, Jacques R, et al. Cost-effectiveness of structured education in children with type-1 diabetes mellitus. Int J Technol Assess Health Care 2016;32:203–11.
6. Clar C, Waugh N, Thomas S. Routine hospital admission versus out-patient or home care in children at diagnosis of type 1 diabetes mellitus. Cochrane Database Syst Rev 2006;(2):CD004099.
7. Tonyushkina KN, Visintainer PF, Jasinski CF, et al. Site of initial diabetes education does not affect metabolic outcomes in children with T1DM. Pediatr Diabetes 2014;15:135–41.
8. The Diabetes Control and Complications Trial Research Group. The effect of intensive treatment of diabetes on the development and progression of long-term complications in insulin-dependent diabetes mellitus. N Eng J Med 1993;329:977–86.
9. Diabetes Control and Complications Trial Research Group. Effect of intensive diabetes treatment on the development and progression of long-term complications in adolescents with insulin-dependent diabetes mellitus: Diabetes control and complications trial. J Pediatr 1994;125:177–88.
10. Swift PG, Skinner TC, de Beaufort CE, et al. Target setting in intensive insulin management is associated with metabolic control: The Hvidoere childhood diabetes study group centre differences study 2005. Pediatr Diabetes 2010;11:271–8.
11. Maahs DM, Hermann JM, DuBose SN, et al. Contrasting the clinical care and outcomes of 2,622 children with type 1 diabetes less than 6 years of age in the United States T1D Exchange and German/Austrian DPV registries. Diabetologia 2014;57:1578–85.
12. Aye T, Barnea-Goraly N, Ambler C, et al. White matter structural differences in young children with type 1 diabetes: A diffusion tensor imaging study. Diabetes Care 2012;35:2167–73.
13. Barnea-Goraly N, Raman M, Mazaika P, et al. Alterations in white matter structure in young children with type 1 diabetes. Diabetes Care 2014;37:332–40.
14. Blasetti A, Chiuri RM, Tocco AM, et al. The effect of recurrent severe hypoglycemia on cognitive performance in children with type 1 diabetes: A meta-analysis. J Child Neurol 2011;26:1383–91.
15. Hershey T, Perantie DC, Warren SL, et al. Frequency and timing of severe hypoglycemia affects spatial memory in children with type 1 diabetes. Diabetes Care 2005;28:2372–7.
16. Gaudieri PA, Chen R, Greer TF, et al. Cognitive function in children with type 1 diabetes: A meta-analysis. Diabetes Care 2008;31:1892–7.
17. Robertson KJ, Schoenle E, Gucev Z, et al. Insulin detemir compared with NPH insulin in children and adolescents with Type 1 diabetes. Diabet Med 2007;24:27–34.
18. Chase HP, Arslanian S, White NH, et al. Insulin glargine versus intermediate-acting insulin as the basal component of multiple daily injection regimens for adolescents with type 1 diabetes mellitus. J Pediatr 2008;153:547–53.
19. Pihoker C, Badaru A, Anderson A, et al. Insulin regimens and clinical outcomes in a type 1 diabetes cohort: The SEARCH for Diabetes in Youth study. Diabetes Care 2013;36:27–33.
20. Phillip M, Battelino T, Rodriguez H, et al. Use of insulin pump therapy in the pediatric age-group: Consensus statement from the European Society for Paediatric Endocrinology, the Lawson Wilkins Pediatric Endocrine Society, and the International Society for Pediatric and Adolescent Diabetes, endorsed by the American Diabetes Association and the European Association for the Study of Diabetes. Diabetes Care 2007;30:1653–62.
21. Levy-Shraga Y, Lerner-Geva L, Modan-Moses D, et al. Benefits of Continuous Subcutaneous Insulin Infusion (CSII) therapy in preschool children. Exp Clin Endocrinol Diabetes 2013;121:225–9.
22. McMahon SK, Airey FL, Marangou DA, et al. Insulin pump therapy in children and adolescents: Improvements in key parameters of diabetes management including quality of life. Diabet Med 2005;22:92–6.
23. Misso ML, Egberts KJ, Page M, et al. Continuous Subcutaneous Insulin Infusion (CSII) versus multiple insulin injections for type 1 diabetes mellitus. Cochrane Database Syst Rev 2010;(1):CD005103.
24. Weinzimer SA, Sikes KA, Steffen AT, et al. Insulin pump treatment of childhood type 1 diabetes. Pediatr Clin North Am 2005;52:1677–88.
25. Johnson SR, Cooper MN, Jones TW, et al. Long-term outcome of insulin pump therapy in children with type 1 diabetes assessed in a large population-based case-control study. Diabetologia 2013;56:2392–400.
26. Overgaard Ingeholm I, Svensson J, Olsen B, et al. Characterization of metabolic responders on CSII treatment amongst children and adolescents in Denmark from 2007 to 2013. Diabetes Res Clin Pract 2015;109:279–86.
27. Bergenstal RM, Tamborlane WV, Ahmann A, et al. Effectiveness of sensor-augmented insulin-pump therapy in type 1 diabetes. N Engl J Med 2010;363:311–20.
28. Alemzadeh R, Berhe T, Wyatt DT. Flexible insulin therapy with glargine insulin improved glycemic control and reduced severe hypoglycemia among preschool-aged children with type 1 diabetes mellitus. Pediatrics 2005;115:1320–4.
29. Murphy NP, Keane SM, Ong KK, et al. Randomized cross-over trial of insulin glargine plus lispro or NPH insulin plus regular human insulin in adolescents with type 1 diabetes on intensive insulin regimens. Diabetes Care 2003;26:799–804.
30. Hassan K, Rodriguez LM, Johnson SE, et al. A randomized, controlled trial comparing twice-a-day insulin glargine mixed with rapid-acting insulin analogs versus standard neutral protamine Hagedorn (NPH) therapy in newly diagnosed type 1 diabetes. Pediatrics 2008;121:e466–72.
31. Thalange N, Bereket A, Larsen J, et al. Insulin analogues in children with type 1 diabetes: A 52-week randomized clinical trial. Diabet Med 2013;30:216–25.
32. Thalange N, Deeb L, Iotova V, et al. Insulin degludec in combination with bolus insulin aspart is safe and effective in children and adolescents with type 1 diabetes. Pediatr Diabetes 2015;16:164–76.
33. de Beaufort CE, Swift PG, Skinner CT, et al. Continuing stability of center differences in pediatric diabetes care: Do advances in diabetes treatment improve

outcome? The Hvidoere Study Group on Childhood Diabetes. Diabetes Care 2007;30:2245–50.

34. Rosenbauer J, Dost A, Karges B, et al. Improved metabolic control in children and adolescents with type 1 diabetes: A trend analysis using prospective multicenter data from Germany and Austria. Diabetes Care 2011;35:80–6.

35. Formosa N. Blood glucose monitoring in children and adolescents with type 1 diabetes mellitus. MMJ 2013;25:31–5.

36. Nordly S, Mortensen HB, Andreasen AH, et al. Factors associated with glycaemic outcome of childhood diabetes care in Denmark. Diabet Med 2005;22:1566–73.

37. Miller KM, Beck RW, Bergenstal RM, et al. Evidence of a strong association between frequency of self-monitoring of blood glucose and hemoglobin A1c levels in T1D exchange clinic registry participants. Diabetes Care 2013;36:2009–14.

38. Mauras N, Fox L, Englert K, et al. Continuous glucose monitoring in type 1 diabetes. Endocrine 2013;43:41–50.

39. Rachmiel M, Landau Z, Boaz M, et al. The use of continuous glucose monitoring systems in a pediatric population with type 1 diabetes mellitus in real-life settings: The AWeSoMe Study Group experience. Acta Diabetol 2015;52:323–9.

40. Hommel E, Olsen B, Battelino T, et al. Impact of continuous glucose monitoring on quality of life, treatment satisfaction, and use of medical care resources: analyses from the SWITCH study. Acta Diabetol 2014;51:845–51.

41. The Juvenile Diabetes Research Foundation Continuous Glucose Monitoring Study Group; Tamborlane WV, Beck RW, Bode BW, et al. Continuous glucose monitoring and intensive treatment of type 1 diabetes. N Engl J Med 2008;359:1464–76.

42. Matsuda E, Brennan P. The effectiveness of continuous glucose monitoring for type 1 diabetic adolescents using continuous subcutaneous insulin infusion pumps: A systematic review. JBI Database System Rev Implement Rep 2014;12:88–120.

43. Buckingham BA, Raghinaru D, Cameron F, et al. Predictive low-glucose insulin suspension reduces duration of nocturnal hypoglycemia in children without increasing ketosis. Diabetes Care 2015;38:1197–204.

44. Maahs DM, Calhoun P, Buckingham BA, et al. A randomized trial of a home system to reduce nocturnal hypoglycemia in type 1 diabetes. Diabetes Care 2014;37:1885–91.

45. Thabit H, Tauschmann M, Allen JM, et al. Home use of an artificial beta cell in type 1 diabetes. New Engl J Med 2015;373:2129–40.

46. Health Canada. Eating well with Canada's food guide. Ottawa, ON, Health Products and Food Branch, Office of Nutrition Policy and Promotion: Health Canada; 2011. Report No.: H164-38/1-2011E-PDF. Available from: http://www.hc-sc.gc.ca/fn-an/food-guide-aliment/order-commander/eating_well_bien_manger-eng.php.

47. Mehta SN, Volkening LK, Quinn N, et al. Intensively managed young children with type 1 diabetes consume high-fat, low-fiber diets similar to age-matched controls. Nutr Res 2014;34:428–35.

48. Markowitz JT, Butler DA, Volkening LK, et al. Brief screening tool for disordered eating in diabetes: Internal consistency and external validity in a contemporary sample of pediatric patients with type 1 diabetes. Diabetes Care 2010;33:495–500.

49. Naguib JM, Kulinskaya E, Lomax CL, et al. Neuro-cognitive performance in children with type 1 diabetes–a meta-analysis. J Pediatr Psychol 2009;34:271–82.

50. Garg S, Moser E, Dain MP, et al. Clinical experience with insulin glargine in type 1 diabetes. Diabetes Technol Ther 2010;12:835–46.

51. Juvenile Diabetes Research Foundation Continuous Glucose Monitoring Study Group. Effectiveness of continuous glucose monitoring in a clinical care environment: Evidence from the Juvenile Diabetes Research Foundation Continuous Glucose Monitoring (JDRF-CGM) trial. Diabetes Care 2010;33:17–22.

52. Hartley M, Thomsett MJ, Cotterill AM. Mini-dose glucagon rescue for mild hypoglycaemia in children with type 1 diabetes: The Brisbane experience. J Paediatr Child Health 2006;42:108–11.

53. Haymond MW, Schreiner B. Mini-dose glucagon rescue for hypoglycemia in children with type 1 diabetes. Diabetes Care 2001;24:643–5.

54. Kongkaew C, Jampachaisri K, Chaturongkul CA, et al. Depression and adherence to treatment in diabetic children and adolescents: A systematic review and meta-analysis of observational studies. Eur J Pediatr 2014;173:203–12.

55. Young V, Eiser C, Johnson B, et al. Eating problems in adolescents with type 1 diabetes: A systematic review with meta-analysis. Diabet Med 2013;30:189–98.

56. Neylon OM, O'Connell MA, Skinner TC, et al. Demographic and personal factors associated with metabolic control and self-care in youth with type 1 diabetes: A systematic review. Diabetes Metab Res Rev 2013;29:257–72.

57. Drotar D, Ittenbach R, Rohan JM, et al. Diabetes management and glycemic control in youth with type 1 diabetes: Test of a predictive model. J Behav Med 2013;36:234–45.

58. Schwartz DD, Axelrad ME, Anderson BJ. A psychosocial risk index for poor glycemic control in children and adolescents with type 1 diabetes. Pediatr Diabetes 2014;15:190–7.

59. Winkley K, Ismail K, Landau S, et al. Psychological interventions to improve glycaemic control in patients with type 1 diabetes: Systematic review and meta-analysis of randomised controlled trials. BMJ 2006;333:65.

60. Hood KK, Rohan JM, Peterson CM, et al. Interventions with adherence-promoting components in pediatric type 1 diabetes: Meta-analysis of their impact on glycemic control. Diabetes Care 2010;33:1658–64.

61. Armour TA, Norris SL, Jack L Jr, et al. The effectiveness of family interventions in people with diabetes mellitus: A systematic review. Diabet Med 2005;22:1295–305.

62. Quirk H, Blake H, Tennyson R, et al. Physical activity interventions in children and young people with Type 1 diabetes mellitus: A systematic review with meta-analysis. Diabet Med 2014;31:1163–73.

63. MacMillan F, Kirk A, Mutrie N, et al. A systematic review of physical activity and sedentary behavior intervention studies in youth with type 1 diabetes: Study characteristics, intervention design, and efficacy. Pediatr Diabetes 2014;15:175–89.

64. Lévy-Marchal C, Patterson CC, Green A, et al. Geographical variation of presentation at diagnosis of type I diabetes in children: The EURODIAB study. Diabetologia 2001;44:B75–80.

65. Klingensmith GJ, Tamborlane WV, Wood J, et al. Diabetic ketoacidosis at diabetes onset: Still an all too common threat in youth. J Pediatr 2013;162:330–4, e1.

66. Patterson CC, Dahlquist G, Harjutsalo V, et al. Early mortality in EURODIAB population-based cohorts of type 1 diabetes diagnosed in childhood since 1989. Diabetologia 2007;50:2439–42.

67. Cameron FJ, Scratch SE, Nadebaum C, et al. Neurological consequences of diabetic ketoacidosis at initial presentation of type 1 diabetes in a prospective cohort study of children. Diabetes Care 2014;37:1554–62.

68. Glaser NS, Wootton-Gorges SL, Buonocore MH, et al. Subclinical cerebral edema in children with diabetic ketoacidosis randomized to 2 different rehydration protocols. Pediatrics 2013;131:e73–80.

69. Vanelli M, Chiari G, Ghizzoni L, et al. Effectiveness of a prevention program for diabetic ketoacidosis in children. An 8-year study in schools and private practices. Diabetes Care 1999;22:7–9.

70. King BR, Howard NJ, Verge CF, et al. A diabetes awareness campaign prevents diabetic ketoacidosis in children at their initial presentation with type 1 diabetes. Pediatr Diabetes 2012;13:647–51.

71. Brink S, Joel D, Laffel L, et al. ISPAD clinical practice consensus guidelines 2014. Sick day management in children and adolescents with diabetes. Pediatr Diabetes 2014;15:193–202.

72. Keenan HT, Foster CM, Bratton SL. Social factors associated with prolonged hospitalization among diabetic children. Pediatrics 2002;109:40–4.

73. Hanas R, Lindgren F, Lindblad B. A 2-yr national population study of pediatric ketoacidosis in Sweden: Predisposing conditions and insulin pump use. Pediatr Diabetes 2009;10:33–7.

74. Karges B, Kapellen T, Neu A, et al. Long-acting insulin analogs and the risk of diabetic ketoacidosis in children and adolescents with type 1 diabetes: A prospective study of 10,682 patients from 271 institutions. Diabetes Care 2010;33:1031–3.

75. Maahs DM, Hermann JM, Holman N, et al. Rates of diabetic ketoacidosis: International comparison with 49,859 pediatric patients with type 1 diabetes rrom England, wales, the U.S., Austria, and Germany. Diabetes Care 2015;38:1876–82.

76. Drozda DJ, Dawson VA, Long DJ, et al. Assessment of the effect of a comprehensive diabetes management program on hospital admission rates of children with diabetes mellitus. Diabetes Educ 1990;16:389–93.

77. Ellis D, Naar-King S, Templin T, et al. Multisystemic therapy for adolescents with poorly controlled type 1 diabetes: Reduced diabetic ketoacidosis admissions and related costs over 24 months. Diabetes Care 2008;31:1746–7.

78. Hoffman WH, O'Neill P, Khoury C, et al. Service and education for the insulin-dependent child. Diabetes Care 1978;1:285–8.

79. Chiari G, Ghidini B, Vanelli M. Effectiveness of a toll-free telephone hotline for children and adolescents with type 1 diabetes. a 5-year study. Acta Biomed 2003;74:45–8.

80. Wagner DV, Stoeckel M, E Tudor M, et al. Treating the most vulnerable and costly in diabetes. Curr Diab Rep 2015;15:606.

81. Edge JA, Hawkins MM, Winter DL, et al. The risk and outcome of cerebral oedema developing during diabetic ketoacidosis. Arch Dis Child 2001;85:16–22.

82. Rosenbloom AL. Intracerebral crises during treatment of diabetic ketoacidosis. Diabetes Care 1990;13:22–33.

83. Glaser N, Barnett P, McCaslin I, et al. Risk factors for cerebral edema in children with diabetic ketoacidosis. The pediatric emergency medicine collaborative research committee of the American Academy of Pediatrics. N Engl J Med 2001;344:264–9.

84. Harris GD, Fiordalisi I, Harris WL, et al. Minimizing the risk of brain herniation during treatment of diabetic ketoacidemia: A retrospective and prospective study. J Pediatr 1990;117:22–31.

85. Harris GD, Fiordalisi I. Physiologic management of diabetic ketoacidemia. A 5-year prospective pediatric experience in 231 episodes. Arch Pediatr Adolesc Med 1994;148:1046–52.

86. Hale PM, Rezvani I, Braunstein AW, et al. Factors predicting cerebral edema in young children with diabetic ketoacidosis and new onset type I diabetes. Acta Paediatr 1997;86:626–31.

87. Edge JA, Jakes RW, Roy Y, et al. The UK case-control study of cerebral oedema complicating diabetic ketoacidosis in children. Diabetologia 2006;49:2002–9.

88. Fort P, Waters SM, Lifshitz F. Low-dose insulin infusion in the treatment of diabetic ketoacidosis: Bolus versus no bolus. J Pediatr 1980;96:36–40.

89. Lindsay R, Bolte RG. The use of an insulin bolus in low-dose insulin infusion for pediatric diabetic ketoacidosis. Pediatr Emerg Care 1989;5:77–9.

90. Hoorn EJ, Carlotti AP, Costa LA, et al. Preventing a drop in effective plasma osmolality to minimize the likelihood of cerebral edema during treatment of children with diabetic ketoacidosis. J Pediatr 2007;150:467–73.

91. Nallasamy K, Jayashree M, Singhi S, et al. Low-dose vs standard-dose insulin in pediatric diabetic ketoacidosis: A randomized clinical trial. JAMA Pediatr 2014;168:999–1005.

92. Decourcey DD, Steil GM, Wypij D, et al. Increasing use of hypertonic saline over mannitol in the treatment of symptomatic cerebral edema in pediatric diabetic ketoacidosis: An 11-year retrospective analysis of mortality. Pediatr Crit Care Med 2013;14:694–700.

93. Wolfsdorf JI, Allgrove J, Craig ME, et al. ISPAD clinical practice consensus guidelines 2014. Diabetic ketoacidosis and hyperglycemic hyperosmolar state. Pediatr Diabetes 2014;15:154–79.

94. National Advisory Committee on Immunization (NACI). NACI recommendations, statements and updates. Ottawa: Public Health Agency of Canada. 2016. http://www.phac-aspc.gc.ca/naci-ccni/. [Accessed June 10, 2016].

95. Moore DL; Canadian Paediatric Society, Infectious Diseases and Immunization Committee. Vaccine recommendations for children and youth for the 2015/2016 influenza season. Paediatr Child Health 2015;20:389–94.

96. Davies P, Nwokoro C, Leigh M. Vaccinations against influenza and pneumococcus in children with diabetes: Telephone questionnaire survey. BMJ 2004;328:203.

97. Irwin DE, Weatherby LB, Huang W-Y, et al. Impact of patient characteristics on the risk of influenza/ILI-related complications. BMC Health Serv Res 2001;1:8.

98. Scott LJ, Warram JH, Hanna LS, et al. A nonlinear effect of hyperglycemia and current cigarette smoking are major determinants of the onset of microalbuminuria in type 1 diabetes. Diabetes 2001;50:2842–9.

99. Hofer SE, Rosenbauer J, Grulich-Henn J, et al. Smoking and metabolic control in adolescents with type 1 diabetes. J Pediatr 2009;154:20–3, e1.

100. Harvey J, Chadi N, Canadian Paediatric Society Adolescent Health Committee. Strategies to promote smoking cessation among adolescents. Paediatr Child Health 2016;21:201–4.

101. Scaramuzza A, De Palma A, Mameli C, et al. Adolescents with type 1 diabetes and risky behaviour. Acta Paediatr 2010;99:1237–41.

102. Carmody D, Doyle A, Firth RG, et al. Teenage pregnancy in type 1 diabetes mellitus. Pediatr Diabetes 2010;11:111–15.

103. Codner E, Soto N, Merino PM. Contraception, and pregnancy in adolescents with type 1 diabetes: A review. Pediatr Diabetes 2012;13:108–23.

104. Hagger V, Hendrieckx C, Sturt J, et al. Diabetes distress among adolescents with type 1 diabetes: A systematic review. Curr Diab Rep 2016;16:1–14.

105. Buchberger B, Huppertz H, Krabbe L, et al. Symptoms of depression and anxiety in youth with type 1 diabetes: A systematic review and meta-analysis. Psychoneuroendocrinology 2016;70:70–84.

106. Fogel NR, Weissberg-Benchell J. Preventing poor psychological and health outcomes in pediatric type 1 diabetes. Curr Diab Rep 2010;10:436–43.

107. Lawrence JM, Standiford DA, Loots B, et al. Prevalence and correlates of depressed mood among youth with diabetes: The SEARCH for Diabetes in Youth study. Pediatrics 2006;117:1348–58.

108. Hood KK, Huestis S, Maher A, et al. Depressive symptoms in children and adolescents with type 1 diabetes: Association with diabetes-specific characteristics. Diabetes Care 2006;29:1389–91.

109. Adal E, Onal Z, Ersen A, et al. Recognizing the psychosocial aspects of type 1 diabetes in adolescents. J Clin Res Pediatr Endocrinol 2015;7:57–62.

110. Morgan E, Patterson CC, Cardwell CR. General practice-recorded depression and antidepressant use in young people with newly diagnosed type 1 diabetes: A cohort study using the Clinical Practice Research Datalink. Diabet Med 2014;31:241–5.

111. Northam EA, Matthews LK, Anderson PJ, et al. Psychiatric morbidity and health outcome on Type 1 diabetes–perspectives from a prospective longitudinal study. Diabet Med 2005;22:152–7. Available from:

112. Kakleas K, Kandyla B, Karayianni C, et al. Psychosocial problems in adolescents with type 1 diabetes mellitus. Diabetes Metab 2009;35:339–50.

113. Lasaite L, Dobrovolskiene R, Danyte E, et al. Diabetes distress in males and females with type 1 diabetes in adolescence and emerging adulthood. J Diabetes Complications 2016;30:1500–5.

114. McDonnell CM, Northam EA, Donath SM, et al. Hyperglycemia and externalizing behavior in children with type 1 diabetes. Diabetes Care 2007;30:2211–15.

115. Korbel CD, Wiebe DJ, Berg CA, et al. Gender differences in adherence to type 1 diabetes management across adolescence: The mediating role of depression. Child Health Care 2007;36:83–98. http://dx.doi.org/10.1080/02739610701316936.

116. Bryden KS, Neil A, Mayou RA, et al. Eating habits, body weight, and insulin misuse. A longitudinal study of teenagers and young adults with type 1 diabetes. Diabetes Care 1999;22:1956–60.

117. Herzer M, Hood KK. Anxiety symptoms in adolescents with type 1 diabetes: Association with blood glucose monitoring and glycemic control. J Pediatr Psychol 2010;35:415–25.

118. Chida Y, Hamer M. An association of adverse psychosocial factors with diabetes mellitus: A meta-analytic review of longitudinal cohort studies. Diabetologia 2008;51:2168–78.

119. Gonzalez JS, Peyrot M, McCarl LA, et al. Depression and diabetes treatment nonadherence: A meta-analysis. Diabetes Care 2008;31:2398–403.

120. Stewart SM, Rao U, Emslie GJ, et al. Depressive symptoms predict hospitalization for adolescents with type 1 diabetes mellitus. Pediatrics 2005;115:1315–19.

121. Garrison MM, Katon WJ, Richardson LP. The impact of psychiatric comorbidities on readmissions for diabetes in youth. Diabetes Care 2005;28:2150–4.

122. Hassan K, Loar R, Anderson BJ, et al. The role of socioeconomic status, depression, quality of life, and glycemic control in type 1 diabetes mellitus. J Pediatr 2006;149:526–31.

123. Hood KK. The influence of caregiver depressive symptoms on proxy report of youth depressive symptoms: A test of the depression-distortion hypothesis in pediatric type 1 diabetes. J Pediatr Psychol 2009;34:294–303.

124. Cunningham NR, Vesco AT, Dolan LM, et al. From caregiver psychological distress to adolescent glycemic control: The mediating role of perceived burden around diabetes management. J Pediatr Psychol 2011;36:196–205.

125. Butler JM, Skinner M, Gelfand D, et al. Maternal parenting style and adjustment in adolescents with type 1 diabetes. J Pediatr Psychol 2007;32:1227–37.

126. Jaser SS, Whittemore R, Ambrosino JM, et al. Mediators of depressive symptoms in children with type 1 diabetes and their mothers. J Pediatr Psychol 2008;33:509–19.

127. Eckshtain D, Ellis DA, Kolmodin K, et al. The effects of parental depression and parenting practices on depressive symptoms and metabolic control in urban youth with insulin dependent diabetes. J Pediatr Psychol 2010;35:426–35.

128. Cameron LD, Young MJ, Wiebe DJ. Maternal trait anxiety and diabetes control in adolescents with type 1 diabetes. J Pediatr Psychol 2007;32:733–44.

129. Jones JM, Lawson ML, Daneman D, et al. Eating disorders in adolescent females with and without type 1 diabetes: Cross sectional study. BMJ 2000;320:1563–6.

130. Bachle C, Stahl-Pehe A, Rosenbauer J. Disordered eating and insulin restriction in youths receiving intensified insulin treatment: Results from a nationwide population-based study. Int J Eat Disord 2016;49:191–6.

131. Rydall AC, Rodin GM, Olmsted MP, et al. Disordered eating behavior and microvascular complications in young women with insulin-dependent diabetes mellitus. N Engl J Med 1997;336:1849–54.

132. Young-Hyman DL, Davis CL. Disordered eating behavior in individuals with diabetes: Importance of context, evaluation, and classification. Diabetes Care 2010;33:683–9.

133. Schwartz DD, Cline VD, Hansen JA, et al. Early risk factors for nonadherence in pediatric type 1 diabetes: A review of the recent literature. Curr Diabetes Rev 2010;6:167–83.

134. Cameron FJ, Northam EA, Ambler GR, et al. Routine psychological screening in youth with type 1 diabetes and their parents: A notion whose time has come? Diabetes Care 2007;30:2716–24.

135. Harkness E, Macdonald W, Valderas J, et al. Identifying psychosocial interventions that improve both physical and mental health in patients with diabetes: A systematic review and meta-analysis. Diabetes Care 2010;33:926–30.

136. de Wit M, Delemarre-van de Waal HA, Bokma JA, et al. Monitoring and discussing health-related quality of life in adolescents with type 1 diabetes improve psychosocial well-being: A randomized controlled trial. Diabetes Care 2008;31:1521–6.

137. van der Feltz-Cornelis CM, Nuyen J, Stoop C, et al. Effect of interventions for major depressive disorder and significant depressive symptoms in patients with diabetes mellitus: A systematic review and meta-analysis. Gen Hosp Psychiatry 2010;32:380–95.

138. Rosello JM. Cognitive-behavioral group therapy for depression in adolescents with diabetes: A pilot study. Interam J Psychol 2006;40:219–26.

139. Alam R, Sturt J, Lall R, et al. An updated meta-analysis to assess the effectiveness of psychological interventions delivered by psychological specialists and generalist clinicians on glycaemic control and on psychological status. Patient Educ Couns 2009;75:25–36.

140. Delamater AM, Jacobson AM, Anderson B, et al. Psychosocial therapies in diabetes: Report of the Psychosocial Therapies Working Group. Diabetes Care 2001;24:1286–92.

141. Mendez FJ, Belendez M. Effects of a behavioral intervention on treatment adherence and stress management in adolescents with IDDM. Diabetes Care 1997;20:1370–5.

142. Barker JM. Clinical review: Type 1 diabetes-associated autoimmunity: Natural history, genetic associations, and screening. J Clin Endocrinol Metab 2006;91:1210–17.

143. Glastras SJ, Craig ME, Verge CF, et al. The role of autoimmunity at diagnosis of type 1 diabetes in the development of thyroid and celiac disease and microvascular complications. Diabetes Care 2005;28:2170–5.

144. Kordonouri O, Hartmann R, Deiss D, et al. Natural course of autoimmune thyroiditis in type 1 diabetes: Association with gender, age, diabetes duration, and puberty. Arch Dis Child 2005;90:411–14.

145. Marks SD, Girgis R, Couch RM. Screening for adrenal antibodies in children with type 1 diabetes and autoimmune thyroid disease. Diabetes Care 2003;26:3187–8.

146. Cerutti F, Bruno G, Chiarelli F, et al. Younger age at onset and sex predict celiac disease in children and adolescents with type 1 diabetes: An Italian multicenter study. Diabetes Care 2004;27:1294–8.

147. Mayer M, Greco L, Troncone R, et al. Compliance of adolescents with coeliac disease with a gluten free diet. Gut 1991;32:881–5.

148. Holmes GK, Prior P, Lane MR, et al. Malignancy in coeliac disease–effect of a gluten free diet. Gut 1989;30:333–8.

149. Mackinder M, Allison G, Svolos V, et al. Nutritional status, growth and disease management in children with single and dual diagnosis of type 1 diabetes mellitus and coeliac disease. BMC Gastroenterol 2014;14:99.

150. Lang-Muritano M, Molinari L, Dommann-Scherrer C, et al. Incidence of enteropathy-associated T-cell lymphoma in celiac disease: implications for children and adolescents with type 1 diabetes. Pediatr Diabetes 2002;38:42–5.

151. Rami B, Sumnik Z, Schober E, et al. Screening detected celiac disease in children with type 1 diabetes mellitus: effect on the clinical course (a case control study). J Pediatr Gastroenterol Nutr 2005;41:317–21.

152. Donaghue KC, Craig ME, Chan AK, et al. Prevalence of diabetes complications 6 years after diagnosis in an incident cohort of childhood diabetes. Diabet Med 2005;22:711–18.

153. Broe R, Rasmussen ML, Frydkjaer-Olsen U, et al. The 16-year incidence, progression and regression of diabetic retinopathy in a young population-based Danish cohort with type 1 diabetes mellitus: The Danish cohort of pediatric diabetes 1987 (DCPD1987). Acta Diabetol 2014;51:413–20.

154. Dabelea D, Stafford JM, Mayer-Davis EJ, et al. Association of type 1 diabetes vs type 2 diabetes diagnosed during childhood and adolescence with complications during teenage years and young adulthood. JAMA 2017;317:825–35.

155. Schultz CJ, Konopelska-Bahu T, Dalton RN, et al. Microalbuminuria prevalence varies with age, sex, and puberty in children with type 1 diabetes followed from diagnosis in a longitudinal study. Oxford Regional Prospective Study Group. Diabetes Care 1999;22:495–502.

156. Gatling W, Knight C, Hill RD. Screening for early diabetic nephropathy: Which sample to detect microalbuminuria? Diabet Med 1985;2:451–5.

157. Shield JP, Hunt LP, Baum JD, et al. Screening for diabetic microalbuminuria in routine clinical care: Which method? Arch Dis Child 1995;72:524–5.

158. Hogg RJ, Furth S, Lemley KV, et al. National Kidney Foundation's Kidney Disease Outcomes Quality Initiative clinical practice guidelines for chronic kidney disease in children and adolescents: Evaluation, classification, and stratification. Pediatrics 2003;111:1416–21.

159. Stone ML, Craig ME, Chan AK, et al. Natural history and risk factors for microalbuminuria in adolescents with type 1 diabetes: A longitudinal study. Diabetes Care 2006;29:2072–7.

160. Perkins BA, Ficociello LH, Silva KH, et al. Regression of microalbuminuria in type 1 diabetes. N Engl J Med 2003;348:2285–93.

161. Nazim J, Fendler W, Starzyk J. Metabolic control and its variability are major risk factors for microalbuminuria in children with type 1 diabetes. Endokrynol Pol 2014;65:83–9.

162. Houlihan CA, Tsalamandris C, Akdeniz A, et al. Albumin to creatinine ratio: A screening test with limitations. Am J Kidney Dis 2002;39:1183–9.

163. Cook J, Daneman D, Spino M, et al. Angiotensin converting enzyme inhibitor therapy to decrease microalbuminuria in normotensive children with insulin-dependent diabetes mellitus. J Pediatr 1990;117:39–45.

164. ACE Inhibitors in Diabetic Nephropathy Trialist Group. Should all patients with type 1 diabetes mellitus and microalbuminuria receive angiotensin-converting enzyme inhibitors? A meta-analysis of individual patient data. Ann Intern Med 2001;134:370–9.

165. Maguire A, Chan A, Cusumano J, et al. The case for biennial retinopathy screening in children and adolescents. Diabetes Care 2005;28:509–13.

166. Huo B, Steffen AT, Swan K, et al. Clinical outcomes and cost-effectiveness of retinopathy screening in youth with type 1 diabetes. Diabetes Care 2007;30:362–3.

167. Geloneck MM, Forbes BJ, Shaffer J, et al. Ocular complications in children with diabetes mellitus. Ophthalmology 2015;122:2457–64.

168. Karavanaki K, Baum JD. Coexistence of impaired indices of autonomic neuropathy and diabetic nephropathy in a cohort of children with type 1 diabetes mellitus. J Pediatr Endocrinol Metab 2003;16:79–90.

169. Olsen BS, Sjølie A, Hougaard P, et al. A 6-year nationwide cohort study of glycaemic control in young people with type 1 diabetes. Risk markers for the development of retinopathy, nephropathy and neuropathy. Danish Study Group of Diabetes in Childhood. J Diabetes Complications 2000;14:295–300.

170. Donaghue KC, Fung AT, Fairchild JM, et al. Prospective assessment of autonomic and peripheral nerve function in adolescents with diabetes. Diabet Med 1996;13:65–71.

171. Hirschfeld G, von Glischinski M, Blankenburg M, et al. Screening for peripheral neuropathies in children with diabetes: A systematic review. Pediatrics 2014;133:e1324–30.

172. Schwab KO, Doerfer J, Marg W, et al. Characterization of 33 488 children and adolescents with type 1 diabetes based on the gender-specific increase of cardiovascular risk factors. Pediatr Diabetes 2010;11:357–63.

173. Margeirsdottir HD, Larsen JR, Brunborg C, et al. High prevalence of cardiovascular risk factors in children and adolescents with type 1 diabetes: A population-based study. Diabetologia 2008;51:554–61.

174. Giurgea GA, Nagl K, Gschwandtner M, et al. Gender, metabolic control and carotid intima-media-thickness in children and adolescents with type 1 diabetes mellitus. Wien Klin Wochenschr 2015;127:116–23.

175. Redondo MJ, Rodriguez LM, Haymond MW, et al. Serum adiposity-induced biomarkers in obese and lean children with recently diagnosed autoimmune type 1 diabetes. Pediatr Diabetes 2014;15:543–9.

176. Celermajer DS, Ayer JGJ. Childhood risk factors for adult cardiovascular disease and primary prevention in childhood. Heart 2006;92:1701–6.

177. Canas JA, Ross JL, Taboada MV, et al. A randomized, double blind, placebo-controlled pilot trial of the safety and efficacy of atorvastatin in children with elevated low-density lipoprotein cholesterol (LDL-C) and type 1 diabetes. Pediatr Diabetes 2015;16:79–89.

178. Vuorio A, Kuoppala J, Kovanen PT, et al. Statins for children with familial hypercholesterolemia. Cochrane Database Syst Rev 2010;(7): CD006401.

179. McCulloch MA, Mauras N, Canas JA, et al. Magnetic resonance imaging measures of decreased aortic strain and distensibility are proportionate to insulin resistance in adolescents with type 1 diabetes mellitus. Pediatr Diabetes 2015;16:90–7.

180. Scaramuzza AE, Redaelli F, Giani E, et al. Adolescents and young adults with type 1 diabetes display a high prevalence of endothelial dysfunction. Acta Paediatr 2015;104:192–7.

181. Alman AC, Talton JW, Wadwa RP, et al. Cardiovascular health in adolescents with type 1 diabetes: The SEARCH CVD study. Pediatr Diabetes 2014;15:502–10.

182. Dabelea D, Talton JW, D'Agostino R Jr, et al. Cardiovascular risk factors are associated with increased arterial stiffness in youth with type 1 diabetes: The SEARCH CVD study. Diabetes Care 2013;36:3938–43.

183. Eppens MC, Craig ME, Cusumano J, et al. Prevalence of diabetes complications in adolescents with type 2 compared with type 1 diabetes. Diabetes Care 2006;29:1300–6.

184. Lurbe E, Redon J, Kesani A, et al. Increase in nocturnal blood pressure and progression to microalbuminuria in type 1 diabetes. N Engl J Med 2002;347:797–805.

185. Flynn JT, Kaelber DC, Baker-Smith CM, Blowey D, Carroll AE, Daniels SR, et al. Clinical practice guideline for screening and management of high blood pressure in children and adolescents. Pediatrics 2017;140.

186. Arnett JJ. Emerging adulthood. A theory of development from the late teens through the twenties. Am Psychol 2000;55:469–80.

187. Nakhla M, Daneman D, To T, et al. Transition to adult care for youths with diabetes mellitus: Findings from a Universal Health Care System. Pediatrics 2009;124:e1134–41.

188. Lotstein DS, Seid M, Klingensmith G, et al. Transition from pediatric to adult care for youth diagnosed with type 1 diabetes in adolescence. Pediatrics 2013;131:e1062–70.

189. Sheehan AM, While AE, Coyne I. The experiences and impact of transition from child to adult healthcare services for young people with type 1 diabetes: A systematic review. Diabet Med 2015;32:440–58.

190. Findley MK, Cha E, Wong E, et al. A systematic review of transitional care for emerging adults with diabetes. J Pediatr Nurs 2015;30:e47–62.

191. Frank M. Factors associated with non-compliance with a medical follow-up regimen after discharge from a pediatric diabetes clinic. Can J Diabetes Care 1996;20:13–20.

192. Van Walleghem N, MacDonald CA, Dean HJ. Evaluation of a systems navigator model for transition from pediatric to adult care for young adults with type 1 diabetes. Diabetes Care 2008;31:1529–30.

193. Mistry B, Van Blyderveen S, Punthakee Z, et al. Condition-related predictors of successful transition from paediatric to adult care among adolescents with type 1 diabetes. Diabet Med 2015;32:881–5.

194. Cadario F, Prodam F, Bellone S, et al. Transition process of patients with type 1 diabetes (T1DM) from paediatric to the adult health care service: A hospital-based approach. Clin Endocrinol (Oxf) 2009;71:346–50.

195. Holmes-Walker DJ, Llewellyn AC, Farrell K. A transition care programme which improves diabetes control and reduces hospital admission rates in young adults with type 1 diabetes aged 15–25 years. Diabet Med 2007;24:764–9.

196. Sequeira PA, Pyatak EA, Weigensberg MJ, et al. Let's Empower and Prepare (LEAP): Evaluation of a structured transition program for young adults with type 1 diabetes. Diabetes Care 2015;38:1412–19.

197. Schultz AT, Smaldone A. Components of interventions that improve transitions to adult care for adolescents with Type 1 diabetes. J Adolesc Health 2017;60:133–46.

198. O'Hara MC, Hynes L, O'Donnell M, et al. A systematic review of interventions to improve outcomes for young adults with type 1 diabetes. Diabet Med 2016;34:753–69.

199. Garvey KC, Foster NC, Agarwal S, et al. Health care transition preparation and experiences in a U.S. National Sample of young adults with type 1 diabetes. Diabetes Care 2017;40:317–24.

200. Garvey KC, Wolpert HA, Rhodes ET, et al. Health care transition in patients with type 1 diabetes: Young adult experiences and relationship to glycemic control. Diabetes Care 2012;35:1716–22.

201. Rocchini AP, Katch V, Anderson J, et al. Blood pressure in obese adolescents: Effect of weight loss. Pediatrics 1988;82:16–23.

202. Fischl AF, Herman WH, Sereika SM, et al. Impact of a preconception counseling program for teens with type 1 diabetes (READY-Girls) on patient-provider interaction, resource utilization, and cost. Diabetes Care 2010;33:701–5.

203. Moher D, Liberati A, Tetzlaff J, et al. Preferred reporting items for systematic reviews and meta-analyses: The PRISMA statement. PLoS Med 2009;6:e1000097.

Literature Review Flow Diagram for Chapter 34: Type 1 Diabetes in Children and Adolescents

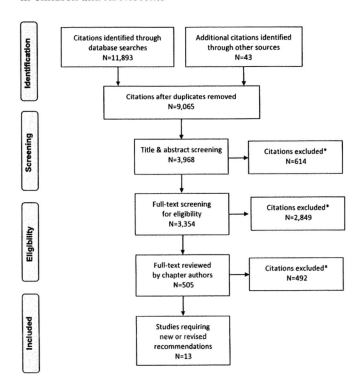

*Excluded based on: population, intervention/exposure, comparator/ control or study design.

From: Moher D, Liberati A, Tetzlaff J, Altman DG, The PRISMA Group (2009). *Preferred Reporting Items for Systematic Reviews and Meta-Analyses:* The PRISMA Statement. PLoS Med 6(6): e1000097. doi:10.1371/journal.pmed1000097 (203).

For more information, visit www.prisma-statement.org.

Journal of Pediatric Nursing (2016) 31, 123–131

ELSEVIER

Helping Adolescents with Type 1 Diabetes "Figure It Out"

Elizabeth Babler PhD, ARNP, CDE[a],*, Carolyn June Strickland PhD, RN[b]

[a]*Franklin, WI*
[b]*University of Washington School of Nursing, Psychosocial & Community Health, Seattle, WA*

Received 2 February 2015; revised 11 September 2015; accepted 12 October 2015

Key words:
Type 1 diabetes;
Adolescents;
Normalizing;
Self-management

Purpose: The aim of this study was to gain an understanding of adolescent's experiences living with diabetes and build a theoretical paradigm for future interventions in adolescents with type 1 diabetes mellitus (T1DM). The adolescent's quest for independence, balancing blood sugars, and integrating diabetes led to increased conflict with parents which contributed to difficulty coping. One code in this study, **"figuring it out"**, is the focus of this manuscript.
Methods: Grounded theory with 15 in depth interviews were conducted with adolescents ages 11 to 15 with T1DM.
Results: A theoretical model about the concept of **"normalizing"** was identified. Normalizing was defined as the ability to integrate diabetes into the background of one's daily life to make diabetes 'part of me'. The fifth phase of normalizing was **"Figuring it out"** which had 4 sub codes: (1) learning to accept diabetes, (2) believing it's possible to manage their diabetes, (3) showing responsibility, and (4) staying on track, and the normalizing task was **"accepting the new normal"**.
Conclusions: Adolescents with T1DM develop the understanding that diabetes is their 'new normal'. The use of motivational interviewing, goal setting, and promotion of self-management may be important interventions in supporting adolescents with T1DM to normalize their life.
© 2016 Elsevier Inc. All rights reserved.

CHILDREN WITH TYPE 1 diabetes mellitus (T1DM) who reach adolescence struggle with maintaining their hemoglobin A1C (A1C) in a safe range (Hoey, 2009) recommended for their age and dramatically decrease testing blood glucose (BG) and administering insulin (Anderson, Ho, Brackett, Finkelstein, & Laffel, 1997). There are approximately 208,000 children under the age of 20 with T1DM (ADA, 2014), and diabetes is the 7th leading cause of death in the United States. The total cost for people diagnosed with diabetes in 2012 was $245 billion, and it is estimated that $69 billion was due to decreased productivity (CDC, 2014). Multiple interventions and utilizing a psychological and/or behavioral approach have been

employed to improve outcomes in this age group with no long term improvements in A1Cs (Grey, Boland, Davidson, Li, & Tamborlane, 2000; Hood, Peterson, Rohan, & Drotar, 2009; Hood, Rohan, Peterson, & Drotar, 2010; Nansel et al., 2009). The purpose of this study was to gain an understanding of adolescents' experiences in living with diabetes and build a theoretical paradigm to create future interventions for adolescents with T1DM. Findings are of value to health care providers and educators aiming to support adolescents with T1DM in successfully normalizing their life with diabetes.

During adolescence only 10% of adolescents are still testing their BG the recommended four times daily (Anderson et al., 1997). Studies have shown that a decrease in BG monitoring leads to higher A1C levels (Anderson et al., 1997; Evans et al., 1999; Iannotti et al., 2006; Ingerski, Anderson, Dolan, & Hood, 2010; Ziegler et al., 2010) and an increased risk for hospitalization due to diabetic ketoacidosis

---

* Corresponding author: Elizabeth K. Babler, PhD, ARNP, CDE.
E-mail address: bethbabler@gmail.com.

http://dx.doi.org/10.1016/j.pedn.2015.10.007
0882-5963/© 2016 Elsevier Inc. All rights reserved.

(DKA) (Levine et al., 2001; Ziegler et al., 2010). Hospital admissions are approximately 40% of the total overall cost of diabetes care (Holmes-Walker, Llewellyn, & Farrell, 2007). Higher rates of anxiety, depression, problems coping, and poor self-esteem (Grey, Cameron, & Thurber, 1991; Grey, Whittemore, & Tamborlane, 2002; Hood et al., 2006; Kovacs, Goldston, Obrosky, & Bonar, 1997; Kovacs, Obrosky, Goldston, & Drash, 1997) are seen in adolescents with T1DM. Adolescents with T1DM also struggle with relationships with their peers (Buchbinder et al., 2005; Grey et al., 1991) and parents (Anderson et al., 2002; Dashiff, Vance, Abdullatif, & Wallander, 2009; Davidson, Penney, Muller, & Grey, 2004; Ingerski et al., 2010) which leads to increased levels of conflict (Anderson et al., 2002; Dashiff et al., 2009).

Less than one third of adolescents are able to maintain their A1C in target range for their age (Hoey, 2009). Ongoing high BG levels, poor adherence to diet and exercise, and missing insulin doses persist into adulthood with only one third of adults able to maintain their A1C <7.5% and over 12% having very high A1C levels over 10% (Toljamo & Hentinen, 2001). As adolescents take on more self-care, they perceive diabetes to be a burden (Davidson et al., 2004) but often believe their parents are too controlling and do not want supervision for their care (Grey et al., 2009; Hoey, 2009). Parental support (Hanna & Guthrie, 2001; Kyngas & Rissanen, 2001; Leonard, Garwick, & Adwan, 2005) and peer (Kyngas, Hentinen, & Barlow, 1998; Kyngas & Rissanen, 2001) support have been shown to be helpful for adolescents in increasing BG monitoring and lowering A1Cs.

A recent meta-analysis of 15 studies with interventions to improve adherence (Hood et al., 2010) found a mean effect size of 0.11 for pre to post treatment group changes when comparing the control and intervention group, but did show that adding interventions around emotional, social, and family issues was better than behavior change alone. Two studies utilizing coping skills training showed minimal change in A1Cs (Grey et al., 2000, 2009). Additionally, a study on enhancing problem solving skills showed an increase in A1Cs during the study period (Nansel et al., 2009) and another with no change (Mulvaney, Rothman, Wallston, Lybarger, & Dietrich, 2010).

In summary, interventions aimed at improving diabetes self-management (DSM) for adolescents with T1DM have not had a major influence on A1Cs. Limited research has provided insights into the perspectives of adolescents experiencing T1DM. A theoretical model has also not been developed in this area to guide intervention design and practice as was the aim of this study. The theoretical paradigm of the concept of normalizing provides important information about strategies adolescents use as they **'figure it out'** (Babler & Strickland, 2013). This research builds on adolescent perceptions and strengths; it fosters understanding of the conditions present that allow adolescents success in DSM and helps move nursing science forward. These findings focus on positive reinforcement and the development of strategies to assist adolescents as they **'accept their new normal'**. Hypotheses were generated for future interventional research to improve health outcomes for adolescents with T1DM.

Methods

The purpose of this study was to gain an understanding of adolescents' experiences in living with diabetes and build a theoretical paradigm to create future interventions for adolescents with T1DM. This paper provides more detail on phase 5 of the paradigm; the methods, data analysis, and full model were previously described in detail in previous work (Babler & Strickland, 2013, 2015) and will not be fully repeated here.

Study Design

This was a qualitative study that utilized grounded theory (Glaser & Strauss, 1967). Grounded theory was selected because it best supported the aims of this study which were to understand the adolescents' experiences in T1DM management, to build a theory model, and to generate hypotheses to support interventional design. Gaining insight into the conditions under which behaviors occur strengthens the theory and provides a deeper understanding of interventions that may be plausible (Bowers, 1988; Glaser & Strauss, 1967). The theoretical framework for grounded theory is symbolic interactionism (Blumer, 1969).

Recruitment

All eligible participants were mailed a recruitment letter, in clinic recruitment posters were displayed, and postcard handouts were provided. Parents interested in having their adolescents participate contacted the researcher directly and completed a verbal questionnaire to determine study eligibility. A $25 gift card was given to study participants at the end of their interview.

Study Sample

The study sample was comprised of adolescents ages 11 to 15 (mean, 13.9) with T1DM. Average hemoglobin A1C of participants was 8.2% (range, 7.2%–9.2%; median, 8.4) per parent report. Sampling, coding, and data analysis were done simultaneously. A total of 15 in home private interviews with 11 participants (3 boys, 27.3% and 8 girls, 72.7%) were conducted each lasting approximately 1 hour. Interviews were digitally recorded and transcribed verbatim. Interviews were continued until data saturation had been reached. Data analysis followed the methods described by Babler and Strickland (2015) and Glaser and Strauss (1967) to create an integrated paradigm. First line coding was done on the interviews looking for gerund codes (-ing words) indicating behaviors that were occurring. This was followed by second line coding in which codes were grouped into clusters. Constant comparative analysis was used to understand the relationship of the various clusters or categories and to identify the core phenomenon that was occurring. The paradigm created describes the codes and their relationships, the behaviors and conditions when they occur, along with the major tasks of each phase and hypotheses. Credibility, fittingness, and auditability were assured by reviewing findings with some adolescents and through the use of a focus group (Guba & Lincoln, 2005; Lincoln & Guba, 1985).

Study Questions

The following open ended questions were used initially with all participants and included: (1) *Let's discuss your experiences of living with diabetes.* (2) *Let's talk about taking care of or managing your diabetes. Can you tell me about that?* Further probe questions used were provided in detail in another manuscript (Babler & Strickland, 2013, 2015) and included: *(1) What is it like for you to take care of your diabetes?* and *(2) Tell me about taking your insulin and testing your BG.* Additional questions about emerging codes were added to later interviews to fully saturate the codes and included: *(1) Some people talk about coming to a place that says "I can take care of my diabetes," tell me about that.*

Human Subjects

IRB approval was obtained from the study site and the University of Washington. Consents were signed by parents and assents by adolescents prior to participation.

Results

A theoretical model of normalizing was developed (Babler & Strickland, 2013). This model has six phases: (1) Remembering the beginning of the journey with the normalizing task of "recognizing my life is changing", (2) Balancing the blood sugars/preventing a crisis with the normalizing task of "taking action to prevent crisis", (3) Integrating diabetes into the world outside the home with the normalizing task of "disclosing to engage support", (4) Moving the journey towards independence with the normalizing task of "taking on the burden of care", (5) Figuring it out with the normalizing task of "accepting the new normal", and (6) Helping others with the normalizing task of "hoping for a normal future". Each phase contains in-depth information about the major task the adolescent is trying to accomplish, a definition, related sub-codes, and conditions when adolescents are or are not able to meet the tasks (Babler & Strickland, 2013, 2015). This paper is focused on phase 5 'Figuring it out' (Figure 1). Phase 5 is a critical phase in DSM; in earlier phases of the journey, adolescents often have trouble learning to cope and manage their diabetes. Adolescents have difficulty transitioning into phase 5 which leads to feelings of being different and viewing diabetes as a burden which then contribute to ongoing conflict with others and poor DSM. Once adolescents are successful in figuring out how to manage diabetes in phase 5, they then gain confidence in their DSM which allows them to move to phase 6 of the model which is being able to help others with diabetes.

In phase 5 adolescents realize that things need to change and they learn how to self-manage (SM) their diabetes indepen-

dently from their parents. The definition of 'figuring it out' is the ability to realize that you can manage your diabetes and maintain your glucose control, when you are able to accept diabetes and stay on track. This also includes having developed the skills to simplify and integrate diabetes into the activities of normal daily living. The adolescents have a shift in their mental framework that helps them understand that diabetes is part of their life. When they complete this phase, they finally accept diabetes and realize their life with diabetes is their 'new normal'. The adolescents realize that diabetes is not so hard, and they begin to believe they can SM diabetes. This changing awareness allows them to make positive changes, and thus they take on more responsibility for diabetes care. Adolescents gain an understanding of how to care for themselves and develop confidence to stay on track and keep their BG balanced. The major task in Phase 5, "Figuring it out" is **learning to cope with diabetes**. The normalizing task is **'accepting the new normal'**. Codes include: **accepting diabetes, believing it's possible to manage diabetes, showing responsibility, and staying on track.** *"you don't think about it as being extremely hard... you start to figure out it's not as hard as people think, once you... get used to the motion of it, it becomes just a really simple thing." Interview #4 p. 13.*

Accepting Diabetes is defined as understanding that diabetes is part of you and that having diabetes is normal. As adolescents move past the grief, anger, sadness, denial, and rebellion of having diabetes, they realize that diabetes is not going away and must be accepted. They understand the consequences of not taking care of diabetes and believe that they are capable of dealing with diabetes and feeling normal. Adolescents shared the process of coping and accepting that diabetes "is" their new normal. Sub-codes include: (1) realizing diabetes is forever, (2) believing you are trapped, (3) understanding things need to change, (4) learning to cope, and (5) accepting the new normal. *"It (diabetes) is there, it will never go, but it is just how much you let it get to you is just the key to it, it never goes away it is always a part of you, until you just accept it, it is always just there." Interview #6 p. 16–17.*

Realizing diabetes is forever is defined as knowing that you will not be able to get rid of the diabetes and must learn to live with it. *"you are sitting alone at night and you are like shit, I'm going to have this forever — like FOREVER and then ... how am I going to do that, and you get that panic moment of oh my God, what am I going to do." Interview #11 p. 12.*

In examination of conditions related to recognizing that diabetes is not going away, it was found that adolescents have to first move out of denial of diabetes. Therefore, a hypothesis is helping adolescents understand the permanence of diabetes may be important in moving them forward with acceptance.

Believing you are trapped is defined as believing that there is no way out and you are stuck forever, therefore, you may as well adjust to having diabetes and accept it. *"(it's) ridiculously hard sometimes because you feel like trapped,*

Figuring it Out

1.0 Accepting diabetes
    1.1 Realizing diabetes is forever
    1.2 Believing you are trapped
    1.3 Understanding things need to change
    1.4 Learning to cope
        1.4.1 Gaining a positive outlook
            1.4.1.1 Understanding you are important
        1.4.2 Seeing diabetes as not scary
        1.4.3 Talking to a friend with diabetes
        1.4.4 Finding solutions
        1.4.5 Realizing it's not a big deal
    1.5 Accepting the new normal
        1.5.1 Getting used to having diabetes
        1.5.2 Realizing diabetes is part of my life
2.0 Believing it's possible to manage diabetes
    2.1 Changing the attitude
        2.1.1 Realizing it's not hard
    2.2 Knowing how to do everything
    2.3 Realizing diabetes is manageable
    2.4 Making diabetes a priority
    2.5 Gaining confidence that you can do what you want
3.0 Showing responsibility
    3.1 Putting in an effort
4.0 Staying on track
    4.1 Maintaining health
        4.1.1 Understanding how to control blood sugars
            4.1.1.1 Testing blood sugars
            4.1.1.2 Giving insulin
            4.1.1.3 Managing diet
            4.1.1.4 Managing exercise
            4.1.1.5 Making diabetes part of your routine
        4.1.2 Overcoming fear
    4.2 Setting goals
        4.2.1 Recognizing blood sugars are high or low
        4.2.2 Demonstrating to others you can meet recommendations
        4.2.3 Encouraging myself
        4.2.4 Setting goals for A1C and blood sugars
        4.2.5 Measuring success by attaining goals
        4.2.6 Seeing effects of your actions
    4.3 Maintaining motivation
        4.3.1 Encouraging myself
        4.3.2 Urging yourself
        4.3.3 Receiving offerings of help from others
        4.3.4 Pushing myself
        4.3.5 Receiving urging from others

Figure 1   Figuring it out — phase 5 of normalizing my life with diabetes during adolescence.

then you're just like, well people deal with a lot worse" *Interview #11 p. 12.*

Understanding things need to change is defined as developing an awareness that it is the high blood sugars that cause illness, and they need to do something different to control their diabetes to prevent themselves from getting sick, yet realizing that this task is not easy to accomplish. *"It was just really horrible because my BS were just constantly running high and it didn't even seem like insulin would really get it down and it was like they were up in the 500's and my A1C's were way up there and I was throwing up almost every day ... this is one of those times ... you need to start thinking about what you are doing ... if you don't do it something could go wrong ... I saw that it wasn't going to be easy." Interview #4 p. 8–9.*

Conditions that related to understanding that things need to change included having multiple episodes of feeling sick leading to DKA and realizing that by taking insulin they were less likely to get sick. Thus it was hypothesized that helping adolescents understand that crisis can be prevented through regular blood glucose monitoring (BGM) and insulin dosing will decrease DKA admissions and increase understanding that things need to change, and they have control over this change.

Learning to cope is defined as the steps needed to emotionally handle having a chronic illness. Sub-codes include: (*a*) *gaining a positive outlook, (b) seeing diabetes as not scary, (c) talking to a friend with diabetes, (d) finding solutions, and (e) realizing it's not a big deal. "The longer I live with it the more I can kind of find ways to kind of cope with it easier." Interview #10 p. 1.* The sub-code *seeing diabetes as not scary* is important as parents' reactions to blood sugars sometimes make it hard for adolescents to not be scared. *Talking to a friend with diabetes* is defined as being able to receive support and understanding from friends who have diabetes to help with coping. *"One thing I found really helpful...to talk about it with someone who really knows exactly what you are going thru...I've found one way to cope ... I'll talk to a friend that has diabetes." Interview #10 p. 7–8.*

Conditions when adolescents cope include when they have support from family, friends, and others with diabetes. Conditions when adolescents are not able to cope are when others are not supportive and when parents are afraid of high or low blood sugars. Thus it was hypothesized that working with families, schools, and peers to increase supportive behaviors will enhance coping. It was also hypothesized that providing counseling and education for parents to raise awareness that their fears contribute to fear for the adolescent, and assisting with parental coping, may be expected to be of value in fostering coping for the adolescent.

Accepting the new normal is defined as realizing that my life includes diabetes which is now a 'part of my being' and 'who I am'. Sub-codes include: (*a*) *getting used to having diabetes and (b) realizing that diabetes is part of my life. "After a few years I started to get used to the thought that diabetes was a part of me, ... sometimes things just happen and you've got to work with it." Interview #4 p. 2.*

Conditions when adolescents are able to accept diabetes as the new normal include when they have a positive attitude and realize that this is their life. A condition when adolescents do not accept diabetes is when they are in denial. A hypothesis is that by having role models who successfully manage their own diabetes mentor adolescents, the adolescents will be more likely to accept diabetes and move forward.

The major goal in this phase of the journey, "Figuring it out" is accepting diabetes and understanding that diabetes is not going to go away, learning to deal with it, and making it

part of your life. Acceptance is an important aspect of normalizing life for adolescents with diabetes.

Believing it's possible to manage diabetes is when the adolescent has the confidence to know how to manage diabetes in terms of decision making skills and in the desire to control diabetes successfully. Part of this process is when adolescents begin to make diabetes a priority in their life instead of trying to ignore it to 'fit in' with their friends. Sub-codes include: (1) changing the attitude, (2) knowing how to do everything, (3) realizing that diabetes is manageable, (4) making diabetes a priority, and (5) gaining confidence that you can do what you want.

Changing the attitude is defined as a willing emotional state that allows you to believe in your ability to manage diabetes. There is an attitude change when they realize that diabetes is not hard which coincides with glucose control. During phase 4 adolescents described taking care of diabetes as overwhelming, and juggling responsibilities made them feel that diabetes was hard. *"I was kind of all over it (my diabetes), my BS leveled out so I felt better...that kind of changed my attitude and everything turned around." Interview #11 p. 9.* Included is *realizing it's not hard. "I guess now it's not really a hard thing it's just kind of an everyday thing, it's something that you can't just forget about one day." Interview #4 p. 18.*

Knowing how to do everything is defined as when you feel you have adequate knowledge and are capable of managing your diabetes. Adolescents shared that it takes a while to not only understand how to do the tasks needed to do their care, but also learn how their choices are going to affect their BG value. Once they have mastered these skills, they share this is when they believe they can be truly independent in their care. *"When you first start doing it yourself it is a harder thing because you're not sure what you are doing...you have always had someone else...doing it for you ...ok, what am I supposed to do." Interview #4 p. 17.*

A condition when adolescents know how to do everything is when they understand the process of how to take care of themselves and all the steps needed. Thus it was hypothesized that providing careful, positive support and feedback for adolescents in learning the process of self-management may be expected to move the adolescent forward in knowing how to do everything.

Realizing diabetes is manageable is defined as developing and understanding of the steps necessary to take care of diabetes in order to keep blood sugars controlled. The adolescents shared that they do not feel that diabetes was as hard as other things people have to do, and as long as they take their insulin every day, it no longer felt like such a burden to them. *"I always think there are a lot of people that have a lot harder stuff to deal with than diabetes, mine is manageable, I take insulin every day — I am good to go." Interview #11 p. 12.*

Making diabetes a priority is defined as an attitude change that includes stopping a current activity to manage diabetes instead of ignoring it. *"Taking care of myself is my top priority...I don't have a problem like stopping what I'm doing now to make sure my blood sugar is ok and it is just a priority, so I just make sure that my health comes first."* Interview #10 p.17.

Gaining confidence that you can do what you want is defined as believing you have the ability to successfully manage your diabetes to be able to meet whatever goal or aspiration you have in life. *"You can be anyone...you want to be."* Interview #4 p. 15.

A condition when adolescents make diabetes a priority is when they have the ability to understand that taking care of their diabetes will affect both their short and long term health.

Showing responsibility is defined as the mental ability to see the consequences of their actions and understand why being responsible is important. A sub-code is putting in an effort which is defined as taking the time to care for oneself. The adolescents shared that they begin to put in an effort to take care of their diabetes as they take on additional responsibility for care, and that is seen in their ability to keep their blood sugar more level. They share that they need to stop being lazy and take care of their diabetes. *"I was putting an effort in and it was showing, I was putting an effort in keeping my blood sugar level."* Interview #11 p. 9.

A condition when the adolescents are more likely to be able to show responsibility is when they understand there are consequences to their actions. Conditions when the adolescents are not likely to show responsibility include when they are experiencing rebellion and are not putting forth effort. It was hypothesized that enhancement of adolescent readiness to take responsibility might be improved through positive supportive actions by parents during transition to DSM through active listening (Babler & Strickland, 2013, 2015).

Staying on track is defined as learning to manage diabetes in a way that is physically and emotionally healthy. Steps that help adolescents stay on track: (1) maintaining health, (2) setting goals, and (3) maintaining motivation.

Maintaining health is defined as the ability to control diabetes by taking the necessary steps to address blood sugars to meet goals. Sub-codes include: *(a) understanding how to control blood sugars and (b) overcoming fear.* *"Now if I take care of myself later on I'll be a lot healthier and so... one of my biggest goals is just to maintain my health while I am young."* Interview #10 p. 16. Understanding how to control blood sugars through testing blood sugars, giving insulin, managing diet, managing exercise, and making diabetes part of your routine provide information on steps adolescents believe are part of gaining control by creating routines to perform the tasks needed for DSM. *Overcoming fear* of giving shots is defined as mentally preparing oneself to give a shot. With the needle fear that the adolescents have described throughout this process of their journey of diabetes, the adolescents shared that it is an important step for them when they are finally able to overcome their fear of needles. *"Something came over me and I just wasn't scared anymore, I just overcame my fear and that was the best day of my life actually because I took control."* Interview #2 p. 9.

Setting Goals is defined as making a decision about what outcomes are attainable in diabetes care to maintain health. Sub-codes include: *(a) recognizing blood sugars are high or low, (b) demonstrating you can meet recommendations, (c) encouraging myself, (d) setting goals for A1C and blood sugars, (e) measuring success by attaining goal, and (f) seeing effects of your actions.*

A condition for setting goals was when adolescents became disappointed in results of A1C or blood sugars. A condition for not setting goals was not seeing the value in goal setting. A hypothesis is that by helping adolescents to test their blood sugar regularly, take the correct dose of insulin, count carbohydrates carefully, and stay active, they will be better able to maintain blood sugar control. Helping adolescents understand the "value" of goal setting through counseling was hypothesized as a strategy to address the importance of setting goals.

Maintaining motivation is defined as the ability to maintain the energy and focus and gather resources needed to consistently maintain a positive attitude. In phase 4 adolescents described not being motivated which is partly what led to their difficulties in their diabetes management. Steps in the process of maintaining motivation include: *(a) encouraging myself, (b) urging yourself, (c) receiving offerings of help from others, (d) pushing myself, and (e) receiving urging from others.* Adolescents shared that praise from doctors, parents, and others was helpful, and nagging and criticism were not. They also noted that being constantly told that they are doing things wrong did not help their motivation. *"To stay motivated I just keep pushing myself ...just keep doing it and you will accomplish everything you want...I'm very, very proud of myself, I feel very accomplished for all the things I have done."* Interview #14 p. 3.

A condition that allows the adolescent to stay motivated is not wanting to hear nagging from others. A condition that does not allow the adolescents to stay motivated is being told they are doing everything wrong. Thus it was hypothesized that motivating adolescents to care for themselves with a positive attitude and encouraging words and refraining from criticizing may be expected to enhance motivation.

Discussion

Adolescents in this study provided rich details about how they were able to **'figure it out'** in their effort to integrate managing diabetes while maintaining a normal life. The findings in this study provide greater understanding of the tasks adolescents are addressing in trying to "figure it out" as they integrate diabetes with normal life and conditions that are supportive. Identifying strengths that the adolescents utilize in figuring out how to self-manage their diabetes is critical, and developing this theoretical framework provides a model to guide future research in understanding DSM in adolescents.

Previous research has described the relationship of some developmental tasks during adolescence including autonomy and self-image on adolescent adherence and self-efficacy

(Chih, Jan, Shu, & Lue, 2010; Fritz & McQuaid, 2000; Greene, Mandleco, Roper, Marshall, & Dyches, 2010). Blood glucose control is improved if parents are able to continue with supervision (Ellis et al., 2007) and provide ongoing support (Kyngas & Rissanen, 2001). The type of interaction from the parent is extremely important in this interaction with helpful reminders viewed as positive, but disagreements, humiliation, blame, shame and nagging seen as negative (Viklund & Wikblad, 2009). An exploratory study described the importance of feeling good about self-care and gaining approval from others (Hanna & Guthrie, 2000) during the transition from parents' management. In a secondary analysis, researchers reviewed qualitative transcripts of communication between parents and adolescents, and one of the themes identified was making diabetes normal (Ivey, Wright, & Dashiff, 2009). These studies are critical to understanding this important transition time of moving to DSM, but this study focuses on the perspective of adolescents, and the theory of normalizing adds important information to this knowledge of not only the steps adolescents take to self-managing their diabetes but also how they 'figure it out'. These findings, which provide details of how adolescents "figure out" the management of diabetes and the related conditions, contribute to the design of more effective management interventions.

In previous research, adults of children with chronic illness describe 'altering their regimen to normalize their life' (Bossert, Holaday, Harkins, & Turner-Henson, 1990); in another study adults with cystic fibrosis describe the importance of 'maintaining routines' (Widerman, 2004). These findings are both similar to this phase of normalizing 'accepting the new normal' in this study. The findings of our study provides a novel model of normalizing that describes the process adolescents go through, their behaviors, and conditions when they are or are not able to complete these tasks.

It is critical to move adolescents into this stage of figuring their diabetes out as they transition to DSM. Practitioners and diabetes educators can now help adolescents reframe diabetes and increase acceptance of their diabetes as their 'new normal'. Helping the adolescent find strategies to believe that they can manage their diabetes on their own through goal setting, and maintaining their motivation through positive feedback, is expected to be very beneficial for intervention design. In this study we found that providing support and encouragement, reducing fears, and addressing the interactions with parents, may be expected to be helpful in the adolescents' ability to complete the tasks of integration of their diabetes into normal life. Practitioners and parents often become upset and focus on what the adolescent is not doing rather than framing office visits and education with a positive focus using strategies to improve motivation and success. This study provides new and important information from the adolescents' perspective that advances both nursing science as well as nursing practice.

Recommendations

Recommendations for diabetes educators and practitioners include: (a) Discuss current coping strategies with the adolescent to foster diabetes acceptance and provide positive feedback. Focus on positive habits that increase feelings of accomplishment. (b) Discuss with parents ways to support the adolescent with their self-management, focusing on providing positive feedback and fostering independent decision making while decreasing nagging, and address parental fears about diabetes. (c) Strategize with parents if a 'reward system' for completing tasks that improve diabetes care such as BGM and keeping a BG log while providing positive feedback on their successes would be helpful in keeping their adolescent on track. (d) Engage school nurses and counselors in supporting adolescent self-management with positive comments that contribute to building self-esteem and examining their policies to determine if change is needed to better support adolescents with T1DM.

Future intervention studies might focus on enhancing acceptance of diabetes, motivation and goal setting in the adolescent, and engaging parents in reducing fear and utilizing supportive behaviors. Building skills in DSM, coping, and acceptance while fostering positive reinforcement were found to be important elements in supporting adolescents in "figuring it out" and integrating diabetes with normal life.

Conclusion

The major task in this phase of **"figuring it out"** was to figure out how to take control of balancing blood sugar and strive for a normal life. The key process in normalizing was **'accepting the new normal'**. As adolescents proceeded through this phase, they learned to cope and maintain their motivation to accept that diabetes is their new life. An important condition for this acceptance was achieving success in their BGM and believing in themselves.

The four major codes in **"figuring it out"** included the following: (1) accepting diabetes, (2) believing it's possible to manage diabetes, (3) showing responsibility, and (4) staying on track. Key hypotheses include the following: (a) helping adolescents understand that crisis can be prevented through regular BGM and insulin dosing will decrease DKA admissions and understanding that things need to change and they have control over this change. (b) working with families, schools and peers to increase supportive behaviors, will enhance coping, (c) by helping adolescents to set and achieve goals they will be better able to maintain blood sugar control, (d) enhancement of adolescent readiness to take responsibility might be improved through positive supportive actions by parents during transition to DSM through active listening, and (e) motivating adolescents to care for themselves with a positive attitude and encouraging words and refraining from criticizing may be expected to enhance motivation. The major task for adolescents in managing their diabetes is **learning to cope with diabetes**, and the normalizing task during this phase is **'accepting the new normal'**.

In this discussion we focused on the phase of normalizing, "figuring it out", which was part of a larger grounded theory research effort about adolescents with T1DM perspectives on diabetes management. In so doing the major tasks the adolescents were attempting to accomplish were identified, as well as recognizing the conditions that were and were not supportive to their achievement of these tasks. This understanding contributed to the creation of a theoretical model, generation of hypotheses, and provisions of recommendations for interventions. Quantitative research is now needed to move this work into intervention design to further advance both nursing science and practice in diabetes management.

Acknowledgments

This work was supported through the Warren G. Magnuson, the Hester McLaws, the Gladys N. Stevenson, the Joyce Carr, and the Hahn Scholarships and by NNCRR Grant TL1 RR 025016. Blinded interview data and journals are available from lead author upon request.

References

ADA (2014). American Diabetes Association. http://www.diabetes.org/diabetes-basics/statistics/

Anderson, B., Ho, J., Brackett, J., Finkelstein, D., & Laffel, L. (1997). Parental involvement in diabetes management tasks: Relationships to blood glucose monitoring adherence and metabolic control in young adolescents with insulin-dependent diabetes mellitus. *Journal of Pediatrics, 130*, 257–265 (doi: S0022-3476(97)70352-4 [pii]).

Anderson, B. J., Vangsness, L., Connell, A., Butler, D., Goebel-Fabbri, A., & Laffel, L. M. (2002). Family conflict, adherence, and glycaemic control in youth with short duration type 1 diabetes. *Diabetic Medicine, 19*, 635–642 (doi: 752 [pii]).

Babler, E. K., & Strickland, C. J. (2013). Normalizing: Adolescent experiences in living with type 1 diabetes. from http://hdl.handle.net/1773/23599

Babler, E., & Strickland, C. J. (2015). Normalizing: Adolescent experiences living with type 1 diabetes. *The Diabetes Educator. 41*, 351–360.

Blumer, H. (1969). *Symbolic interactionism; perspective and method.* Englewood Cliffs, N.J.: Prentice-Hall.

Bossert, E., Holaday, B., Harkins, A., & Turner-Henson, A. (1990). Strategies of normalization used by parents of chronically ill school age children. *Journal of Child and Adolescent Psychiatric and Mental Health Nursing, 3*, 57–61.

Bowers, B. J. (1988). Grounded theory. In B. Sarter (Ed.). *Paths to knowledge: Innovative research methods for nursing* (pp. 33–59). New York, NY: National League for Nursing.

Buchbinder, M. H., Detzer, M. J., Welsch, R. L., Christiano, A. S., Patashnick, J. L., & Rich, M. (2005). Assessing adolescents with insulin-dependent diabetes mellitus: A multiple perspective pilot study using visual illness narratives and interviews. *Journal of Adolescent Health, 36*, 71 e79-13. http://dx.doi.org/10.1016/j.jadohealth.2004.02.019.

CDC (2014). Center for Disease Control. http://www.cdc.gov/diabetes/pubs/statsreport14/national-diabetes-report-web.pdf (accessed 9.17.14)

Chih, A. H., Jan, C. F., Shu, S. G., & Lue, B. H. (2010). Self-efficacy affects blood sugar control among adolescents with type I diabetes mellitus. *Journal of the Formosan Medical Association, 109*, 503–510. http://dx.doi.org/10.1016/S0929-6646(10)60084-8 (S0929-6646(10)60084-8 [pii]).

Dashiff, C., Vance, D., Abdullatif, H., & Wallander, J. (2009). Parenting, autonomy and self-care of adolescents with type 1 diabetes. *Child: Care, Health and Development, 35*, 79–88. http://dx.doi.org/10.1111/j.1365-2214.2008.00892.x (CCH892 [pii]).

Davidson, M., Penney, E. D., Muller, B., & Grey, M. (2004). Stressors and self-care challenges faced by adolescents living with type 1 diabetes. *Applied Nursing Research, 17*, 72–80 (doi: S0897189704000266 [pii]).

Ellis, D. A., Podolski, C. L., Frey, M., Naar-King, S., Wang, B., & Moltz, K. (2007). The role of parental monitoring in adolescent health outcomes: Impact on regimen adherence in youth with type 1 diabetes. *Journal of Pediatric Psychology, 32*, 907–917. http://dx.doi.org/10.1093/jpepsy/jsm009 (jsm009 [pii]).

Evans, J. M., Newton, R. W., Ruta, D. A., MacDonald, T. M., Stevenson, R. J., & Morris, A. D. (1999). Frequency of blood glucose monitoring in relation to glycaemic control: Observational study with diabetes database. *British Medical Journal, 319*, 83–86.

Fritz, G. K., & McQuaid, E. L. (2000). Chronic medical conditions: Impact on development. In A. J. L. Sameroff, Michael Miller, & M. Suzanne (Eds.), *Handbook of developmental psychopathology* (pp. 277–289) (2nd ed.). New York: Kluwer Academic.

Glaser, B. G., & Strauss, A. L. (1967). *The discovery of grounded theory; strategies for qualitative research.* Chicago: Aldine Pub. Co.

Greene, M. S., Mandleco, B., Roper, S. O., Marshall, E. S., & Dyches, T. (2010). Metabolic control, self-care behaviors, and parenting in adolescents with type 1 diabetes: A correlational study. *Diabetes Educator, 36*, 326–336. http://dx.doi.org/10.1177/0145721710361270 (0145721710361270 [pii]).

Grey, M., Boland, E. A., Davidson, M., Li, J., & Tamborlane, W. V. (2000). Coping skills training for youth with diabetes mellitus has long-lasting effects on metabolic control and quality of life. *Journal of Pediatrics, 137*, 107–113. http://dx.doi.org/10.1067/mpd.2000.106568 (S0022-3476(00)61563-9 [pii]).

Grey, M., Cameron, M. E., & Thurber, F. W. (1991). Coping and adaptation in children with diabetes. *Nursing Research, 40*, 144–149.

Grey, M., Whittemore, R., Jaser, S., Ambrosino, J., Lindemann, E., Liberti, L., ... Dziura, J. (2009). Effects of coping skills training in school-age children with type 1 diabetes. *Research in Nursing & Health, 32*, 405–418. http://dx.doi.org/10.1002/nur.20336.

Grey, M., Whittemore, R., & Tamborlane, W. (2002). Depression in type 1 diabetes in children: Natural history and correlates. *Journal of Psychosomatic Research, 53*, 907–911 (doi: S0022399902003124 [pii]).

Guba, E. G., & Lincoln, Yvonna S. (2005). Paradigmatic controversies, contradictions, and emerging confluences. In N. K. Denzin, & Yvonna S. Lincoln (Eds.), *The Sage handbook of qualitative research* (pp. 191–215). Thousand Oaks: Sage Publications.

Hanna, K. M., & Guthrie, D. (2000). Adolescents' perceived benefits and barriers related to diabetes self-management—Part 1. *Issues in Comprehensive Pediatric Nursing, 23*, 165–174.

Hanna, K. M., & Guthrie, D. (2001). Parents' and adolescents' perceptions of helpful and nonhelpful support for adolescents' assumption of diabetes management responsibility. *Issues in Comprehensive Pediatric Nursing, 24*, 209–223.

Hoey, H. (2009). Psychosocial factors are associated with metabolic control in adolescents: Research from the Hvidoere Study Group on Childhood Diabetes. *Pediatric Diabetes, 10*, 9–14. http://dx.doi.org/10.1111/j.1399-5448.2009.00609.x (PDI609 [pii]).

Holmes-Walker, D. J., Llewellyn, A. C., & Farrell, K. (2007). A transition care programme which improves diabetes control and reduces hospital admission rates in young adults with type 1 diabetes aged 15–25 years. *Diabetic Medicine, 24*, 764–769. http://dx.doi.org/10.1111/j.1464-5491.2007.02152.x (DME2152 [pii]).

Hood, K. K., Huestis, S., Maher, A., Butler, D., Volkening, L., & Laffel, L. M. (2006). Depressive symptoms in children and adolescents with type 1 diabetes: Association with diabetes-specific characteristics. *Diabetes Care, 29*, 1389–1391. http://dx.doi.org/10.2337/dc06-0087 (29/6/1389 [pii]).

Hood, K. K., Peterson, C. M., Rohan, J. M., & Drotar, D. (2009). Association between adherence and glycemic control in pediatric type 1 diabetes: A meta-analysis. *Pediatrics, 124*, e1171–e1179. http://dx.doi.org/10.1542/peds.2009-0207 (peds.2009-0207 [pii]).

Hood, K. K., Rohan, J. M., Peterson, C. M., & Drotar, D. (2010). Interventions with adherence-promoting components in pediatric type 1 diabetes: Meta-analysis of their impact on glycemic control. *Diabetes Care, 33,* 1658–1664. http://dx.doi.org/10.2337/dc09-2268 (dc09-2268 [pii]).

Iannotti, R. J., Nansel, T. R., Schneider, S., Haynie, D. L., Simons-Morton, B., Sobel, D. O., ... Clark, L. (2006). Assessing regimen adherence of adolescents with type 1 diabetes. *Diabetes Care, 29,* 2263–2267. http://dx.doi.org/10.2337/dc06-0685 (29/10/2263 [pii]).

Ingerski, L. M., Anderson, B. J., Dolan, L. M., & Hood, K. K. (2010). Blood glucose monitoring and glycemic control in adolescence: Contribution of diabetes-specific responsibility and family conflict. *Journal of Adolescent Health, 47,* 191–197. http://dx.doi.org/10.1016/j.jadohealth.2010.01.012 (S1054-139X(10)00035-2 [pii]).

Ivey, J. B., Wright, A., & Dashiff, C. J. (2009). Finding the balance: Adolescents with type 1 diabetes and their parents. *Journal of Pediatric Health Care, 23,* 10–18.

Kovacs, M., Goldston, D., Obrosky, D. S., & Bonar, L. K. (1997). Psychiatric disorders in youths with IDDM: Rates and risk factors. *Diabetes Care, 20,* 36–44.

Kovacs, M., Obrosky, D. S., Goldston, D., & Drash, A. (1997). Major depressive disorder in youths with IDDM. A controlled prospective study of course and outcome. *Diabetes Care, 20,* 45–51.

Kyngas, H., Hentinen, M., & Barlow, J. H. (1998). Adolescents' perceptions of physicians, nurses, parents and friends: Help or hindrance in compliance with diabetes self-care? *Journal of Advanced Nursing, 27,* 760–769.

Kyngas, H., & Rissanen, M. (2001). Support as a crucial predictor of good compliance of adolescents with a chronic disease. *Journal of Clinical Nursing, 10,* 767–774.

Leonard, B. J., Garwick, A., & Adwan, J. Z. (2005). Adolescents' perceptions of parental roles and involvement in diabetes management. *Journal of Pediatric Nursing, 20,* 405–414. http://dx.doi.org/10.1016/j.pedn.2005.03.010 (S0882-5963(05)00066-7 [pii]).

Levine, B. S., Anderson, B. J., Butler, D. A., Antisdel, J. E., Brackett, J., & Laffel, L. M. (2001). Predictors of glycemic control and short-term adverse outcomes in youth with type 1 diabetes. *Journal of Pediatrics, 139,* 197–203. http://dx.doi.org/10.1067/mpd.2001.116283 (S0022-3476(01)75473-X [pii]).

Lincoln, Y. S., & Guba, E. G. (1985). *Naturalistic inquiry.* Beverly Hills, Calif.: Sage Publications.

Mulvaney, S. A., Rothman, R. L., Wallston, K. A., Lybarger, C., & Dietrich, M. S. (2010). An internet-based program to improve self-management in adolescents with type 1 diabetes. *Diabetes Care, 33,* 602–604. http://dx.doi.org/10.2337/dc09-1881 (dc09-1881 [pii]).

Nansel, T. R., Anderson, B. J., Laffel, L. M., Simons-Morton, B. G., Weissberg-Benchell, J., Wysocki, T., ... Lochrie, A. S. (2009). A multisite trial of a clinic-integrated intervention for promoting family management of pediatric type 1 diabetes: Feasibility and design. *Pediatric Diabetes, 10,* 105–115. http://dx.doi.org/10.1111/j.1399-5448.2008.00448.x (PDI448 [pii]).

Toljamo, M., & Hentinen, M. (2001). Adherence to self-care and glycaemic control among people with insulin-dependent diabetes mellitus. *Journal of Advanced Nursing, 34,* 780–786 (doi: jan1808 [pii]).

Viklund, G., & Wikblad, K. (2009). Teenagers' perceptions of factors affecting decision-making competence in the management of type 1 diabetes. *Journal of Clinical Nursing, 18,* 3262–3270. http://dx.doi.org/10.1111/j.1365-2702.2009.02963.x (JCN2963 [pii]).

Widerman, E. (2004). The experience of receiving a diagnosis of cystic fibrosis after age 20: Implications for social work. *Social Work in Health Care, 39,* 415–433.

Ziegler, R., Heidtmann, B., Hilgard, D., Hofer, S., Rosenbauer, J., & Holl, R. (2010). Frequency of SMBG correlates with HbA1c and acute complications in children and adolescents with type 1 diabetes. *Pediatric Diabetes.* http://dx.doi.org/10.1111/j.1399-5448.2010.00650.x (PDI650 [pii]).